COMPLETE HOMOEOPATHIC MATERIA MEDICA

AT A
GLANCE
WITH VIVA NOTES

By
DR RAVI N. BHOSALE, MD

Prinicipal – Sawkar Homoeopathic Medical College, Satara
Member – Central Council of Homoeopathy, Delhi

DR ANURADHA .V. CHAVAN, MD
Assistant-Professor in Materia Medica,
at Sawkar Homoeopathic Medical College, Satara

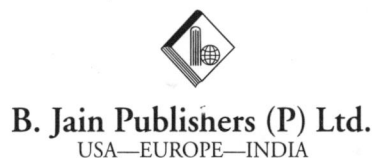

B. Jain Publishers (P) Ltd.
USA—EUROPE—INDIA

COMPLETE HOMOEOPATHIC MATERIA MEDICA AT A GLANCE

First Edition: 2014

3rd Impression: 2019

All rights reserved. No part of this book may be reproduced, stored in a retrieval system or transmitted, in any form or by any means, mechanical, photocopying, recording or otherwise, without any prior written permission of the publisher.

© with the author

Published by Kuldeep Jain for

B. JAIN PUBLISHERS (P) LTD.
B. Jain House, D-157, Sector-63,
NOIDA-201307, U.P. (INDIA)
Tel.: +91-120-4933333 • *Email:* info@bjain.com
Website: **www.bjain.com**

Printed in India by

ISBN: 978-81-319-3201-8

HIPPOCRATIC OATH

I swear by Apollo the physician, Asclepius, Hygieia, Panacea, and by all the Gods and Goddesses, making them my witnesses, that I will carry out, according to my ability and judgment, this oath and this indenture:

To regard my teacher in this art as equal to my parents; to make him partner in my livelihood, and when he is in need of money to share mine with him; to consider his offspring equal to my brothers; to teach them this art, if they require to learn it, without fee or indenture; and to impart, oral instruction, and all the other learning, to my sons, to the sons of my teacher, and to pupils who have signed this indenture and sworn obedience to the Physicians Law, but to none other.

I will use treatment to help the sick according to my ability and judgement, but I will never use it to injure or wrong them. I will not give poison to anyone even if I am asked to do so, nor will I suggest such a plan. Similarly, I will not give a pessary to a woman to cause abortion. But in purity and in holiness, I will guard my life and my art.

I will not use the knife either on sufferers from stone, but I will give place to such as are craftsmen therein. Into whosoever house I enter, I will do so to help the sick, keeping myself free from all intentional wrong-doing and harm, especially from fornication with woman or man, bond or free. Whatsoever in the course of practice I see or hear (or even outside my practice in social intercourse) that ought never be published abroad, I will not divulge, but consider such things to be holy secrets.

Now if I keep this oath and break it not, may I enjoy honour, in my life and art, among all men for all time; but if I transgress and forswear myself, may the opposite befall me.

Source: W.H.S. Jones, The Doctor's Oath. (Cambridge: Cambridge UP, 1924), 11, 12.

"NO INDIVIDUAL HAS DONE MORE GOOD TO THE MEDICAL PROFESSION THAN SAMUEL HAHNEMANN"

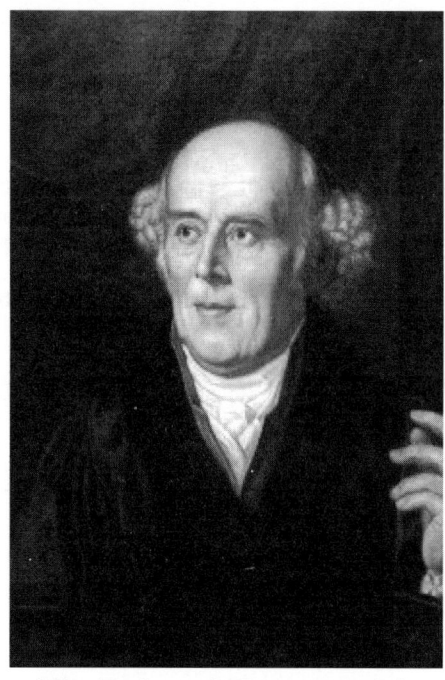

(The Father of Homoeopathy).

**Christian Friedrich Samuel Hahnemann
(1755-1843)**

DEDICATION

Dedicated

to my loving parents

Adv T.R. Bhosale & Mrs Satyavati Bhosale

who have inspired me

to pursue my passion for Homoeopathy

Homoeopathy cures a greater percentage of cases than any other method of treatment. Homoeopathy is the latest and refined method of treating patients economically and non-violently

"Homoeopathy …. cures a larger percentage of cases than any other method of treatment and is beyond doubt safer and more economical and most complete medical science.

— **Mahatma Gandhi**

PREFACE

"WE TREAT HE CURES"

The curative power of Homoeopathy is immense and known to us all with wide ranging options available to us. For homoeopaths to treat any ailment, choosing the right drug is a difficult task which depends on the totality of symptoms. The effectiveness and the curative power of Homoeopathy is known to us all. This required results and relief for the patients. Homoeopathy is incomplete without a thorough knowledge of Materia Medica, Organon of Medicine, Pharmacy, and Repertory which are used in various combinations as per the requirement and merits of each case. But the most important subject within Homoeopathy is no doubt Materia Medica.

"THE ARMOURY OF HOMOEOPATHY". Though a large number of books have been written about Materia Medica and abundant literature is available on this subject, there is a major lacuna that was noticed by me during the study of this subject i.e there are few literature which tell us as to how to use this subject effectively and in a practical way, when the student of Materia Medica start their clinical practice.

In this book, we have tried to overcome the above mentioned hurdles. This book is an attempt to provide a concise yet complete information of each remedy with its sphere of action, source, ailments from, mind, constitution, temperament, thermal, miasm, keynote symptoms, clinical diagnosis, remedy relationship, modality of the remedy at a glance. The main principle of Homoeopathy is that each human being is different and unique, even twins are not alike as far as our intrinsic core is concerned. Individualisation is the basis of Homoeopathic practice. Similarly, each remedy is different and unique as different individuals.

"Materia medica is the study of collection of symptoms obtained by drugs which are proved on healthy human beings of different sex, ages and constitutions in an anatomical way according to Hahnemannian schema".

Source of Materia medica: Proving on healthy human beings, Proving on healthy animals, Clinical observation, Accidental source, Toxicological source, Chemical source, Empirical source, Doctrine of signature.

Source of Drugs: Vegetable kingdom, Animal kingdom, Mineral kingdom, Nosodes, Sarcodes, Imponderabilia.

Drug action: Action of a drug depends upon the dose and general receptive capacity of the body. The arithmetical data of homoeopathic drug action is not fully known. The latent dynamic spiritual power with its pharmacological message is liberated from material bonds and acts upon the dynamicity of the living cell of the human organism.

When a medicine is given it produces a mechanical or chemical action on the person according to the nature of the drug, when the primary action is over, the vital force produces a reaction to the primary action and this is called the secondary action. Potentised drugs act through the oral receptors, the specific message goes to the brain through afferent nerves in the form of an electric impulse in the cortex of the brain. Then, an appropriate response goes through the efferent nerves particularly, autonomic efferent to correct abnormal condition.

Constitution: Constitution is defined as a person's physical and mental make up which is revealed through his physical built, his characteristic desires and aversions and reactions as well as emotional and intellectual attributes.

The three constitutions of Grauvogl:

1. The hydrogenoid constitution.

2. The oxygenoid constitution.

3. The carbo-nitrogenoid constitution.

Thermals: Relation with heat and cold: Hot patient, Chilly patient, Ambithermal.

Temperament: Temperament is our inborn, God given nature, it is given to us at conception and remains constant throughout our life; Sanguine, Choleric, Melancholic, Phlegmatic, Nervous

Miasm: The true simillimum is always based on the existing miasm. Fundamental miasm and Dominant miasm. Psora, Sycosis, Tubercular, Syphilitic.

- **Psoric miasm:** The reaction of the body on exposure to environmental stimuli, to ones surroundings, like noise, light, and odours, producing functional disturbances.
- **Sycotic miasm:** Hypersensitive (hypertrophic) response to something specific, arising from the deficiency of normal response like tumors, allergies.
- **Syphilitic miasm**: Tissue destruction like gangrene, ulceration. Body and mind destroy itself.
- **Tubercular miasm:** Recurrence of complaints, changing symptoms, vague complaints, weakness, pain shifting in location, depletion, dissatisfaction, lack of tolerance.

Mind: State of mind (including fears, anxieties, attitudes, dreams, will, emotion, intellect, understanding etc.) The mental symptoms are of special importance in homoeopathic prescribing. They reflect the deepest aspects of the patients who experience them and the remedies which evoke them; in many cases they take precedence over general and local symptoms, even when these have constituted the original complaint; and when correctly selected and matched, they can lead to a lasting cure.

Social and psychological stress can trigger or aggravate a wide variety of diseases. Stress therefore, can cause physical symptoms even though no physical disease may be present. The body responds physiologically to emotional stress. A skilled homoeopath should know the relationship between the mind and the body. Many a times, chronic cases like that of migraine and peptic ulcer, which had their origin after a mental trauma or prolonged stress, disappear with a few doses of correctly prescribed homoeopathic medicine. Psychological symptoms often play a primary role in the selection of correct medicine.

Keynote symptoms: The keynote in music is defined as "the fundamental note or tone on which the whole piece is accommodated". In pathology, the term "pathognomonic symptom" expresses what might be called the keynote of the disease, or that which differentiates it from other diseases of a similar character. "The most striking, singular, uncommon and peculiar (characteristic) signs and symptoms of the case are chiefly and almost solely to be kept in view; for it is more particularly, these similar list of symptoms that must correspond with the selected medicine, in order to constitute it the most suitable for effecting the cure.

Clinical diagnosis: Disease is correctly defined as the loss of harmony in function and sensation. Today, with the advancement in medical field and awareness amongst the people about the implications and complications of a disease or ailment, it is rather essential that we not only have to diagnose the ailment of the patient but also have to satisfy the patient's knowledgeable queries and also have to confirm our own diagnosis.

For a homoeopath, many times a diagnostic report will help in minimizing the sphere of selection of a drug, achieved by elimination of common symptoms of that particular disease and concentrating more on peculiar guiding symptoms. By this process, we are able to provide rapid relief. The importance of diagnosis are as follows:

- The management of the case will be easy if the diagnosis is known.
- It helps us to know the common symptoms of the diseases. These common symptoms will, thus help us to know the uncommon symptoms.
- The uncommon symptoms help us to find the similimum.

- The seat of the disease tells us which potency to choose.
- That will also help in repetition of medicines.
- The prognosis will tell us whether there is disease aggravation or medicinal aggravation and thus, help in differentiation from homoeopathic aggravations.
- The probable diagnosis helps us to know what lab investigations or special investigations are to be adviced to confirm the diagnosis.
- To know about a diagnosis, helps us to refer the case to an emergency or refer for surgery which will save the life of the patient.
- The most important thing a patient wants from a doctor is A DIAGNOSIS.

Modality refers to the circumstances and conditions that affect or modify a symptom, or a condition. "The modalities of a drug are the pathognomonic symptoms of the Materia Medica". "Aggravation" means an increase or intensification of an already existing symptom by some appreciable circumstance or condition. "Amelioration" is technically used to express the modification of relief, or diminution of intensity in any of the symptoms, or in the state of the patient as a whole, by medication, or by the influence of any agency, circumstance or condition. The symbol "<" means "worse from" and the symbol ">" means "better from".

Remedy relationship:

- **Antidotes** – To the effects of massive and molecular doses; chemical antidotes in poisoning
- **Collateral** – Side relations (congeners) belonging to the same or allied botanical family or chemical group.
- **Compatible** – Drugs following well.
- **Complementary** – Completes the action of the previous remedy.
- **Inimical** – Drugs disagreeing, incompatible, do not follow well.
- **Similar** – Drugs suggested for comparison by reason of their similarity.

In this book, we have tried our best to cover all the topics considering the systemic affections of living beings like: skin, gastrointestinal system, circulatory system, respiratory system, endocrine, head and the most important is the mind section. Specific disease affections with most liking and suitable homoeopathic remedies and with differential diagnosis and therapeutic indications, all these aspects combined together make this book an easy reference guide and we hope our sincere efforts of writing this book will prove to be helpful to all students and homoeopathic practitioners.

We have also recommended clinical suggestions of many drugs so far proved, thus making available an avenue to experiment and in future by proving, add to our existing armoury.

The purpose of writing this book is sharing the vast experience gathered during the years of practice and making Homoeopathy an interesting subject.

I hope after reading this book any student interested in practicing classical homoeopathy will never in his dreams think of practicing any other alternative pathy except pure, classical and constitutional prescribing according to Hahnemannian homoeopathy.

HAHNEMANNIAN OATH:

"On my honour I swear that I shall practice the teaching of Homoeopathy, perform my duty, render justice to my patients and help the sick, whosoever come to me for treatment.

May the teachings of Master Hahnemann inspire me and may I have the strength for fulfillment of my mission".

Dr Anuradha .V. Chavan M.D
Homoeopath

ACKNOWLEDGEMENTS

I acknowledge with Joy and Pleasure.

After writing my earlier books on Materia Medica and on subjects of use to students of Homoeopathy, writing this sixth book has been a totally different journey. The subject itself is so vast that doing justice to all its aspects was really very difficult. However, as this subject is very close to my heart (and my favorite subject since my college days) I was ready to put in any amount of efforts required to write this book. Of course, this would not have been possible without the unstinted support of all my family members, assistants, professional associates, friends, students and my patients.

The purpose of writing this book was to share the vast experience gathered during 19 years of my practice and teaching of Homoeopathy at Sawkar H C Satara.

I am grateful to God and my parents who gave me this opportunity to learn and practice this art and science of Homoeopathy.

I wish to express my gratitude to my family members who have been the nurturing force behind me while writing this book. I wish to express my gratitude to Mr Dhairyasheel Bhosale for his kind co-operation

I am also thankful to Adv T R Bhosale and Mrs Satyavati Bhosale who encouraged me throughout the writing of this book.

My heartfelt thanks to my husband Lt Col Vikram Chavan who has stood by me like a rock and ensured that I had my space for this creative venture.

My thanks to Dr Hemalata Karkar, Adv. Aarti Jadhav, Dr Aishwarya Patil, Mrs Kusum Chavan who have inspired me to complete this book.

I am also thankful to Mr. Arvind Gavali, Chairman, Sawkar H C, Satara and all my colleagues there, where I got the opportunity to teach and learn Homoeopathy further. I would also like to thank the Principal and teachers of D.S.H. College, Pune from where I completed my BHMS and the Principal and teachers of YMTH College, Navi Mumbai from where I completed my MD.

A very special thanks to all my well wishers and distinguished personalities and senior physicians.

Dr Ramjee Singh, Dr Arun Bhasme, Dr Arya, Dr S.K.Phansalkar, Dr K.C.Shah, Dr Ajit Kulkarni, Dr Solanki, Dr P.Page, Dr D.Bagal, Dr Anita Jadhav, Dr Vishpale Parthsarthy, Dr Tiwari, Dr Rajan Sankaran, Dr Mahendra Singh, Dr Dhawale, Dr Vijaykar, Dr N.L Tiwari, Dr Jawahar Shah, Dr Kavishwar, Dr Kothe, Dr Sahani, Dr Shekar Bhosale, Dr Dinesh Bakshi, Dr Kavita, Dr Jathkar, Dr Girish Patel, Dr Chimthanawala, Dr Vibha Bakshi

My thanks to Kshitija Karkar, Asmita, Ajinka, Shalaka, Tejasvini, Riya

The team of my publishers – B Jain has been extremely cooperative and helpful.

My thanks to Mr Kuldeep Jain (Publisher), Mr Nishant Jain, Dr Geeta Arora, Dr Isha Gupta and Mr Abhijit Morgaonkar for their kind support.

I would also like to thank all the patients whom I have treated and those who had faith in Homoeopathy. Finally, I hope that this book will be a helpful guide to the BHMS and MD level students and also to all practitioners of Homoeopathy.

I am open to any suggestions from the readers.

Thank you all.

Dr Anuradha Chavan, MD
Consulting Homoeopath
Satara , Maharashtra,
INDIA
09960135936
anuradhac2014@rediffmail.com

PUBLISHER'S NOTE

Homeopathic Materia Medica is one subject which can never be memorized or learnt completely. At the same time reading Materia Medica is something which cannot be avoided or stopped by any homeopathic practitioner. People devise ways to learn and write Materia Medica. Dr Anuradha Chavan book is also one such concept where immense information about each drug has been compiled and arranged in a very systematic fashion so as to make it easy, accessible and comprehensible at the same time. This is an example of a work where the whole Materia Medica has been simplified but has gone through a lot of work before it was done so. It's a work which has had efforts of the authors for more than 5 years and a similar level of efforts has been done by the editorial team, so that the author's efforts take a good shape and form, which it deserves. There are more than 340 drugs covered in this book. Each remedy has been covered under the headings like sphere of action, mind, modalities, constitution, clinical and remedy relationship. Thus, it subtly covers all aspects of a drug and this looks simple and readable as it is all covered on one page.

This work would not have been completed without Dr Taru Bhagat hard editorial work and accurate information. It was a hard and laborious task to compile and collect all the information given in this book from various sources.

This book has been designed keeping in mind that all aspects of a drug can be seen through at one glance and one doesn't have to refer to different Materia Medica books. Hope this books serves the purpose it has been written for.

Kuldeep Jain
C.E.O., B. Jain Publishers (P) Ltd.

CONTENTS

Hippocratic Oath .... *iii*

Dedication .... *v*

Preface .... *vii*

Acknowledgements .... *xi*

Publisher's Note .... *xiii*

1. Abies canadensis 1
2. Abies nigra 2
3. Abrotanum 3
4. Acalypha indica 4
5. Aceticum acidum 5
6. Aconitum napellus 6
7. Actaea racemosa (Cimicifuga racemosa) 7
8. Actaea spicata 8
9. Adonis vernalis 9
10. Adrenalinum 10
11. Aesculus hippocastanum 11
12. Aethusa cynapium 12
13. Agaricus muscarius 13
14. Agnus castus 14
15. Agraphis nutans 15
16. Ailanthus glandulosa 16
17. Aletris farinosa 17
18. Alfalfa 18
19. Allium cepa 19
20. Allium sativum 20
21. Aloe socotrina 21
22. Alumina 22
23. Ambra grisea 23
24. Ammonium carbonicum 24
25. Ammonium causticum 25
26. Ammonium muriaticum 26
27. Anacardium orientale 27
28. Anthracinum 28
29. Antimonium arsenicosum 29
30. Antimonium crudum 30
31. Antimonium tartaricum 31
32. Apis mellifica 32
33. Apocynum cannabinum 33
34. Aralia racemosa 34
35. Aranea diadema 35
36. Argentum metallicum 36
37. Argentum nitricum 37
38. Arnica montana 38
39. Arsenicum album 39
40. Arsenicum bromatum 40
41. Arsenicum iodatum 41
42. Arsenicum sulfuratum flavum 42
43. Artemesia vulgaris 43

44.	Arum triphyllum	44	70.	Caladium seguinum	70
45.	Asafoetida	45	71.	Calcarea arsenicosa	71
46.	Asparagus officinalis	46	72.	Calcarea carbonica ostrearum	72
47.	Aspidosperma quebracho	47	73.	Calcarea fluorica	73
48.	Asterias rubens	48	74.	Calcarea phosphorica	74
49.	Aurum metallicum	49	75.	Calcarea silicata	75
50.	Aurum muriaticum natronatum	50	76.	Calcarea sulphurica	76
51.	Avena sativa	51	77.	Calendula officinalis	77
52.	Bacillinum burnett	52	78.	Camphora officinalis	78
53.	Badiaga	53	79.	Cannabis sativa	79
54.	Baptisia tinctoria	54	80.	Cantharis vesicatoria	80
55.	Baryta carbonica	55	81.	Capsicum annuum	81
56.	Baryta muriatica	56	82.	Carbo animalis	82
57.	Belladonna	57	83.	Carbo vegetabilis	83
58.	Bellis perennis	58	84.	Carbolicum acidum	84
59.	Benzoicum acidum	59	85.	Carcinosinum	85
60.	Berberis vulgaris	60	86.	Carduus marianus	86
61.	Bismuthum subnitricum	61	87.	Caulophyllum thalictroides	87
62.	Blatta orientalis	62	88.	Causticum hahnemanni	88
63.	Borax veneta	63	89.	Ceanothus americanus	89
64.	Bothrops lanceolatus	64	90.	Cedron	90
65.	Bovista lycoperdon	65	91.	Chamomilla	91
66.	Bromium	66	92.	Chelidonium majus	92
67.	Bryonia alba	67	93.	Chimaphila umbellata	93
68.	Bufo rana	68	94.	Chininum arsenicosum	94
69.	Cactus grandiflorus	69	95.	Chininum sulphuricum	95

96.	Cholesterinum	96
97.	Cicuta virosa	97
98.	Cina maritima	98
99.	Cinchona officinalis	99
100.	Cinnabaris	100
101.	Cinnamomum zeylanicum	101
102.	Cistus canadensis	102
103.	Clematis erecta	103
104.	Cobaltum metallicum	104
105.	Coca	105
106.	Coccinella septempunctata	106
107.	Cocculus indicus	107
108.	Coccus cacti	108
109.	Coffea cruda	109
110.	Colchicum autumnale	110
111.	Collinsonia canadensis	111
112.	Colocynthis	112
113.	Conium maculatum	113
114.	Corallium rubrum	114
115.	Crataegus oxyacantha	115
116.	Crocus sativus	116
117.	Crotalus horridus	117
118.	Croton tiglium	118
119.	Cuprum metallicum	119
120.	Cyclamen europaeum	120
121.	Digitalis purpurea	121
122.	Dioscorea villosa	122
123.	Diphtherinum	123
124.	Dolichos pruriens	124
125.	Drosera rotundifolia	125
126.	Duboisinum	126
127.	Dulcamara	127
128.	Echinacea angustifolia	128
129.	Elaterium	129
130.	Electricitas	130
131.	Equisetum hymale	131
132.	Erigeron canadense	132
133.	Eucalyptus globulus	133
134.	Eugenia jambos	134
135.	Eupatorium perfoliatum	135
136.	Euphrasia officinalis	136
137.	Fagopyrum esculentum	137
138.	Ferrum iodatum	138
139.	Ferrum metallicum	139
140.	Ferrum phosphoricum	140
141.	Ferrum picricum	141
142.	Ficus religiosa	142
143.	Fluoricum acidum	143
144.	Formica rufa	144
145.	Gambogia	145
146.	Gelsemium sempervirens	146
147.	Ginseng quinquefolia	147

148.	Glonoinum	148
149.	Glycerinum	149
150.	Gnaphalium polycephalum	150
151.	Graphites	151
152.	Gratiola officinalis	152
153.	Grindelia robusta	153
154.	Guaiacum officinale	154
155.	Hamamelis virginiana	155
156.	Hecla lava	156
157.	Helleborus niger	157
158.	Heloderma	158
159.	Helonias dioica	159
160.	Hepar sulphuris calcareum	160
161.	Hydrastis canadensis	161
162.	Hydrocotyle asiatica	162
163.	Hydrocyanicum acidum	163
164.	Hyoscyamus niger	164
165.	Hypericum perforatum	165
166.	Iberis amara	166
167.	Ignatia amara	167
168.	Insulinum	168
169.	Iodium	169
170.	Ipecacuanha	170
171.	Iris versicolor	171
172.	Jalapa	172
173.	Kalium bichromicum	173
174.	Kalium bromatum	174
175.	Kalium carbonicum	175
176.	Kalium muriaticum	176
177.	Kalium phosphoricum	177
178.	Kalium sulphuricum	178
179.	Kalmia latifolia	179
180.	Kreosotum	180
181.	Lac caninum	181
182.	Lac defloratum	182
183.	Lachesis mutus	183
184.	Laurocerasus	184
185.	Ledum palustre	185
186.	Leptandra virginica	186
187.	Lilium tigrinum	187
188.	Lithium carbonicum	188
189.	Lobelia inflata	189
190.	Lycopodium clavatum	190
191.	Lycopus virginicus	191
192.	Lyssinum	192
193.	Magnesia carbonica	193
194.	Magnesia muriatica	194
195.	Magnesia phosphorica	195
196.	Malaria officinalis	196
197.	Manganum aceticum	197
198.	Medorrhinum	198
199.	Melilotus officinalis	199

200.	Menyanthes trifoliata	200	226. Oleander	226
201.	Mephitis putorius	201	227. Oleum animale	227
202.	Mercurius corrosivus	202	228. Oleum jecoris aselli	228
203.	Mercurius cyanatus	203	229. Onosmodium virginianum	229
204.	Mercurius dulcis	204	230. Opium	230
205.	Mercurius solubilis	205	231. Oxalicum acidum	231
206.	Mezereum	206	232. Oxytropis lamberti	232
207.	Millefolium	207	233. Paeonia officinalis	233
208.	Morgan gaertner	208	234. Palladium metallicum	234
209.	Morphinum	209	235. Pareira brava	235
210.	Moschus moschiferus	210	236. Paris quadrifolia	236
211.	Murex purpurea	211	237. Passiflora incarnata	237
212.	Muriaticum acidum	212	238. Petroleum	238
213.	Myrica cerifera	213	239. Phellandrium aquaticum	239
214.	Myristica sebifera	214	240. Phosphoricum acidum	240
215.	Naja tripudians	215	241. Phosphorus	241
216.	Naphthalinum	216	242. Physostigma venenosum	242
217.	Natrium carbonicum	217	243. Phytolacca decandra	243
218.	Natrium muriaticum	218	244. Picricum acidum	244
219.	Natrium phosphoricum	219	245. Pinus sylvestris	245
220.	Natrium sulphuricum	220	246. Piper methysticum	246
221.	Nitricum acidum	221	247. Pix liquida	247
222.	Nuphar luteum	222	248. Platinum metallicum	248
223.	Nux moschata	223	249. Plumbum metallicum	249
224.	Nux vomica	224	250. Podophyllum peltatum	250
225.	Oenanthe crocata	225	251. Polygonum hydropiperoides	251

#	Entry	Page
252.	Primula obconica	252
253.	Prunus spinosa	253
254.	Psorinum	254
255.	Ptelea trifoliata	255
256.	Pulex irritans	256
257.	Pulsatilla nigricans	257
258.	Pyrogenium	258
259.	Radium bromatum	259
260.	Ranunculus bulbosus	260
261.	Raphanus sativus	261
262.	Ratanhia peruviana	262
263.	Rhamnus californica	263
264.	Rheum palmatum	264
265.	Rhododendron chrysanthum	265
266.	Rhus glabra	266
267.	Rhus toxicodendron	267
268.	Rhus venenata	268
269.	Robinia pseudocacia	269
270.	Rumex crispus	270
271.	Ruta graveolens	271
272.	Sabadilla	272
273.	Sabal serrulata	273
274.	Sabina	274
275.	Salix nigra	275
276.	Sambucus nigra	276
277.	Sanguinaria canadensis	277
278.	Sanicula aqua	278
279.	Sarcolacticum acidum	279
280.	Sarsaparilla officinalis	280
281.	Scrophularia nodosa	281
282.	Secale cornutum	282
283.	Selenium metallicum	283
284.	Senecio aureus	284
285.	Sepia officinalis	285
286.	Serum anguillae	286
287.	Silicea terra	287
288.	Sinapis nigra	288
289.	Solidago virgaurea	289
290.	Spigelia anthelmia	290
291.	Spongia tosta	291
292.	Squilla maritima	292
293.	Stannum metallicum	293
294.	Staphysagria	294
295.	Stellaria media	295
296.	Sticta pulmonaria	296
297.	Stigmata maydis	297
298.	Stramonium	298
299.	Strontium carbonicum	299
300.	Strophanthus hispidus	300
301.	Sulphur	301
302.	Symphoricarpus racemosus	302
303.	Symphytum officinale	303

304. Syphilinum	304
305. Syzygium jambolanum	305
306. Tabacum	306
307. Taraxacum officinale	307
308. Tarentula cubensis	308
309. Tarentula hispanica	309
310. Terebinthiniae oleum	310
311. Teucrium marum verum	311
312. Thallium metallicum	312
313. Thea chinensis	313
314. Theridion curassavicum	314
315. Thlaspi bursa pastoris	315
316. Thuja occidentalis	316
317. Thyroidinum	317
318. Trifolium pratense	318
319. Trillium pendulum	319
320. Triticum repens	320
321. Trombidium muscae domesticae	321
322. Tuberculinum bovinum kent	322
323. Uranium nitricum	323
324. Urtica urens	324
325. Ustilago maydis	325
326. Uva ursi	326
327. Vaccininum	327
328. Valeriana officinalis	328
329. Vanadium metallicum	329
330. Variolinum	330
331. Veratrum album	331
332. Veratrum viride	332
333. Verbascum thapsus	333
334. Vespa crabro	334
335. Viburnum opulus	335
336. Vinca minor	336
337. Viola odorata	337
338. Viola tricolor	338
339. Vipera berus	339
340. Viscum album	340
341. X-ray	341
342. Xanthoxylum fraxineum	342
343. Xerophyllum tenax	343
344. Yohimbinum	344
345. Zincum metallicum	345
346. Zingiber officinale	346
347. Origin of Homoeopathy	347
348. Preparation of Homoeopathic Remedies	349
349. Clinical Case History	351
350. Potency Selection	353
351. Homoeopathic Remedy	355
352. Homoeopathic Pulse	363
353. Homoeopathic Tongue	367
354. Homoeopathic Dreams	371
355. Miasmatic Evolution	373
356. Trios of Remedies	375
Bibliography	*393*

SPHERE OF ACTION

- Mind
- Gastrointestinal system
- Heart
- Female genital system

INTRODUCTION

- **Common name:** Hemlock spruce
- **Family:** *Pinaceae*
- **Source:** Vegetable kingdom
- **Part used:** Bark
- **Prover:** Gatchell

CONSTITUTION

- For cases with peculiar and chilly sensations, especially in women with uterine displacements – a result of defective nutrition
- For old people with gastric derangements, having a tendency to over eat
- **Temperament:** Nervous, bilious
- **Thermal:** Chilly
- **Miasm:** Psora, Sycosis, Syphilis

MIND

- Vanishing of thoughts, confusion and stupefaction of mind, as if intoxicated
- Greedy while eating
- Mental exhaustion
- Irritability, moody
- Feels light headed
- Sadness

ABIES CANADENSIS

CLINICAL

- Debility
- Prostration
- Vertigo
- Pyrosis
- Bulimia
- Flatulence
- Dyspepsia
- Indigestion
- Gastritis
- Duodenal ulcer
- Diarrhoea
- Dysentery
- Uterine displacement
- Gleet
- Night sweat
- Fever

KEYNOTE SYMPTOMS

- Cold shiverings
- Prostration, debility
- Gnawing, hungry, faint feeling at the epigastrium
- **Tendency to eat far beyond the capacity for digestion – bulimia**
- **Peculiar cravings for meat, pickles, radishes, turnips, artichokes, coarse food**
- Over eating and indigestion
- Burning and distention in abdomen with palpitations; rumbling
- Canine hunger with a torpid liver
- Respiration and action of heart laboured
- Suited to women with uterine displacements, probably due to defective nutrition and debility; prolapsus uteri with little or no local congestion
- Uterine displacements. **Sensation as if womb is soft and feeble; sensation as if she will abort**

MODALITIES

- **Aggravation:** Flatulence increases heart's action, after eating
- **Amelioration:** Rest, lying down

REMEDY RELATIONSHIP

- **Compare:** Abies-n., Sabin., Thuj., and other conifers; also Nux-v., Chin., Am-m.

SPHERE OF ACTION

- Mind
- Gastrointestinal system
- Respiratory system
- Heart

INTRODUCTION

- **Common name:** Amber resin, Black spruce
- **Family:** *Pinaceae*
- **Source:** Vegetable kingdom
- **Part used:** Distilling the volatile oil obtained from the oleo-resin of the plant
- **Prover:** Leyman

CONSTITUTION

- For dyspeptic troubles of the aged with heart complaints
- **Temperament:** Nervous, bilious
- **Thermal:** Chilly
- **Miasm:** Sycosis, Syphilis

ABIES NIGRA

MIND

- Abusive or insulting
- Sad, despondent, dejected, mentally depressed, gloomy
- Anxiety about health; hypochondriacal
- Functions mentally like an old man
- Dullness, sluggishness with difficulty in thinking, comprehending
- Vanishing of thoughts
- Low spirited and dull during the day; wakeful and restless at night; with hunger, unable to think

KEYNOTE SYMPTOMS

- Hiatus hernia. Sensation of a boiled egg at the cardiac end of stomach (location of hiatus hernia)
- Those cases of dyspepsia which do not seem to have recovered despite abstinence from any particular food or by a strict diet
- Gastric disorders, lump in abdomen; waterbrash and indigestion in abusers of tea and tobacco
- Dyspepsia with **sensation of a hard boiled egg lodged at the cardiac end of stomach**
- **Pain in stomach comes on immediately after eating. Total loss of appetite in the morning but great craving for food at noon and at night.**
- Compressed choking sensation in the throat
- Painful sensation as if something was loaded in the chest, has to cough it up
- Sharp, cutting pain in the region of the heart; tachycardia marked, also bradycardia can be seen
- Wakeful and restless at night due to hunger

CLINICAL

- Prostration
- Vertigo
- Halitosis
- Eructations
- Indigestion
- Dyspepsia
- Hiatus hernia
- Dysentery
- Constipation
- Dyspnoea
- Tachycardia
- Bradycardia
- Night sweat
- Chronic fever

MODALITIES

- **Aggravation:** After eating, after abuse of tea and tobacco
- **Amelioration:** Rest

REMEDY RELATIONSHIP

- **Compare:** Chin., Bry., Puls., Thuj., Sabin., Cupre-l., Nux-v., Kali-c.

ABROTANUM

INTRODUCTION
- **Common name:** Southernwood, Lady's love
- **Family:** *Compositae*
- **Source:** Vegetable kingdom
- **Part used:** Leaf and young shoot

SPHERE OF ACTION
- Mind
- Gastrointestinal system
- Nerves
- Fibrous tissues
- Serous membranes
- Skin

MIND
- Great anxiety
- Depression
- Cruel, peevish and ill-natured
- Irritable and violent
- Dullness and feebleness of mind
- Incapability to think, gets easily fatigued by conversation or on making a mental effort
- No humanity; inhuman
- Cross, irritable, anxious
- Taciturnity

MODALITIES
- **Aggravation:** Cold air, at night, wet weather, checked secretions
- **Amelioration:** From loose stools, motion

KEYNOTE SYMPTOMS
- Ill-effects of suppressed conditions
- **Marasmus in lower extremities with ravenous hunger. Progressive wasting disease. Appetite good with emaciation.**
- Metastasis of states and symptoms – like metastasis of rheumatism from joints to heart to spine
- **Extreme weakness; stomach feels as if swimming or hanging in water, feels cold**
- Oozing of blood and moisture from umbilicus
- Alternate diarrhoea and constipation. Piles. Food passes undigested; frequent urging, bloody stool.
- Raw feeling. Impeded respiration; dry cough following diarrhoea. Pain across the chest.
- Rheumatic condition with cardiac irritation
- Painful contraction of limbs, arms and wrists
- Skin flabby, loose. Falling out of hair
- Angioma of the face. Skin becomes purplish after suppression of eruptions
- **Face is wrinkled, pale, old looking, cold with blue rings around the eyes**
- Exudative processes like exudative pleurisy, tuberculous peritonitis

CONSTITUTION
- For marasmus, especially in children, of the legs; marked emaciation, skin is flabby and hangs in folds
- For tendency to rheumatism and gout
- **Temperament:** Anaemic
- **Thermal:** Chilly
- **Miasm:** Sycosis

CLINICAL
- Marasmus
- Metastasis
- Alopecia areata
- Angioma of face
- Epistaxis
- Comedones
- Tuberculous peritonitis
- Anal fissure
- Haemorrhoids
- Respiration difficult
- Pleurisy
- Hydrothorax
- Empyema
- Hydrocoele
- Rheumatic arthritis
- Rheumatism
- Gout
- Chilblains

REMEDY RELATIONSHIP
- **Compare:** Cham., Cina, Graph; Nux-v. and Agar. in chilblains; Iod. and Nat-m. in marasmus; benz-ac. in gout
- **Follows well:** Hep. in furuncle; after Acon. and Bry. in pleurisy

ACALYPHA INDICA

SPHERE OF ACTION
- Gastrointestinal system
- Respiratory system
- Female genital system

INTRODUCTION
- **Common name:** Indian nettle
- **Family:** *Euphorbiaceae*
- **Source:** Vegetable kingdom
- **Part used:** Whole plant
- **Prover:** Dr Tonnere

CONSTITUTION
- Adapted to old people suffering from morning cough; tubercular constitution and tendency for haemorrhages
- **Temperament:** Nervous, bilious, haemorrhagic
- **Thermal:** Chilly
- **Miasm:** Psora, Sycosis, Syphilis

MIND
- **Gloomy but unwilling to die**

CLINICAL
- Arterial haemorrhage
- Diarrhoea
- Jaundice
- Rectal haemorrhage
- Cough
- Incipient phthisis
- Lung cancer
- Menorrhagia

KEYNOTE SYMPTOMS
- Arterial haemorrhage but no febrile disturbances
- **Very weak in the morning, gains strength during the day**
- Progressive emaciation
- Rumbling distention in abdomen; spluttering diarrhoea with noisy and forcible expulsion of flatus
- Burning in pharynx, stomach, intestines
- Incipient phthisis; **hard racking cough, bloody expectoration**
- Respiratory system – cough dry and hard followed by haemoptysis, worse morning and night
- Haemoptysis – blood bright red and profuse in the morning. All pathological haemorrhages have an aggravation in the morning
- Dullness of chest on percussion
- Constant, severe pain in chest

MODALITIES
- **Aggravation:** In the morning, cough is worse at night
- **Amelioration:** Rest

REMEDY RELATIONSHIP
- **Compare:** Mill., Phos., Acet-ac., Kali-n., Ham., Ip.
- **Antidoted by:** Calc.

ACETICUM ACIDUM

INTRODUCTION
- **Common name:** Glacial acetic acid
- **Group:** Organic acid
- **Source:** Mineral kingdom
- **Formula:** CH_3COOH
- **Prover:** Berridge

SPHERE OF ACTION
- Gastrointestinal system
- Nervous system
- Heart
- Urinary system
- Female genital system

MIND
- Anxiety and fear, driving him from place to place
- Debility; very dull and low spirited
- Grieves about sickness and children. Worried about business
- Forgetful about what recently happened, does not know her own children
- Irritability with headache, and abdominal and liver complaints
- Lamenting, wailing with delirium; with swelling of abdomen
- Hysteria; crawling and rolling on the floor
- Borrows troubles
- Stupor and delirium alternate

MODALITIES
- **Aggravation:** Cough worse on inhaling
- **Amelioration:** Back pains relieved by lying on the abdomen

KEYNOTE SYMPTOMS
- **Great prostration after surgical injuries, after anaesthesia**
- Severe anaemia with dropsy; with great debility and dyspnoea, especially in nursing women
- **Anasarca; dropsy of legs and abdomen, with marked thirst, and pale, washy skin**
- Excessive wasting and debility. Chronic weakness and other wasting diseases of children; weakness, diabetes, tuberculosis
- Has ability to dissolve albuminous and fibrous deposits
- Tendency to haemorrhage from any part; especially after labour; from bowels
- Nervous headache, especially after abuse of narcotics
- **Burning thirst, insatiable, even for large quantities but no thirst during fever**
- Sensation of sinking in the abdomen
- Burning pain, as of an ulcer in the stomach; Cancer of stomach
- Sour belching and vomiting, especially of pregnancy; waterbrash; violent burning pain in stomach and chest followed by coldness of skin and cold sweat on the forehead
- Irritation of trachea and bronchorrhoea; hoarseness
- Putrid, hectic fevers with drenching night sweat; ebullitions
- **In fever, red spot on left cheek, drenching cold night sweat. Thirstless during fever**
- **Cannot sleep on back, rests better lying on belly**

CONSTITUTION
- Suits pale, lean persons with lax flabby muscles; face pale and waxy, suffer from chronic weakness
- For wasting diseases of children and old people with emaciation
- **Temperament:** Tubercular
- **Thermal:** Hot
- **Miasm:** Sycosis, Syphilis

CLINICAL
- Injuries
- Bruises
- Emaciation
- Marasmus
- Haemorrhages
- Anaemia
- Terminal stages of heart disease
- Anasarca
- Oedema
- Varicose veins
- Scurvy
- Epithelioma of lip
- Gastralgia
- Ascitis
- Membranous croup
- Diphtheria
- Kidney diseases
- Mastitis
- Catamenia
- Diabetes

REMEDY RELATIONSHIP
- **Compare:** Am-act., Benzo. (night sweats); Ars., Chin., Dig., Liat. (general anasarca in heart and kidney disease, dropsy, and chronic diarrhoea)
- **Antidotes:** Anesthetic vapours, fumes of charcoal and gas; Op. and Stram.
- **Follows well:** After Chin., in haemorrhage; after Dig. in dropsy

ACONITUM NAPELLUS

INTRODUCTION

- **Common name:** Monkshood, Wolf's bane
- **Family:** *Ranunculaceae*
- **Source:** Vegetable kingdom
- **Part used:** Whole plant
- **Prover:** Hahnemann

SPHERE OF ACTION

- Mind
- Eyes
- Nervous system
- Respiratory system
- Female genital system
- Serous membranes
- Joints

CONSTITUTION

- For acute and recent cases, especially in plethoric individuals who lead a sedentary life; easily affected by atmospheric changes
- Suits persons with rigid fibres, dark hair and eyes leading a sedentary life; one cheek red, the other pale. Warm blooded.
- **Temperament:** Plethoric, sanguine
- **Thermal:** Chilly
- **Miasm:** Psora, Sycosis

MIND

- Fright followed by panic and shock; ailments from fright
- Phobias, nightmares
- Fear, anxiety and restlessness accompany all symptoms
- For ailments from mental and emotional shocks; never well since
- Tension, anguish, nervous excitability. Panic attacks. Despair from pains.
- **Fear of death, predicts date and hour of death.** Clairvoyance.
- **Restless, tosses about in agony; one of the trios of restless remedies**
- Music is unbearable, makes patient sad
- Fear and frights; terror stricken; anticipation
- Delirium with unhappiness, worry, anxiety and fear; fear of crossing the road, crowds, to get out of the house

KEYNOTE SYMPTOMS

- **Marked physical and mental restlessness**
- Acute, sudden and violent onset of symptoms; remains for a short while; periodicity of symptoms seen
- Sudden and rapid onset with high fever, and great smaking of strength
- Pains sticking and tearing. Parts remain sore or numb after pains. Tingling, coldness and numbness.
- *Aconitum napellus* **causes no pathological changes. Indicated in only functional disturbances**
- Tension in arteries or emotional and physical tension
- Complaints caused due to exposure to dry cold weather, checked perspiration or very hot weather
- Dryness, heat, especially of skin with **thirst for large quantities of cold water – unquenchable thirst**
- Red, inflamed eyes. Lids dry, hot. Photophobia.
- Smell acutely sensitive
- Haemorrhage of bright red blood
- Vomiting bilious, mucoid, bloody, greenish, of bitter taste; haematemesis
- Colic in abdomen – no position relieves. Abdomen sensitive to touch
- Pressure in the stomach with dyspnoea
- Oppressed breathing on least motion; shortness of breath
- Urine scanty, red, hot, painful with tenesmus; burning at neck of bladder. Retention of urine, especially after child birth with screaming
- Suppressed menses or impending miscarriage from fright or variation or cold. Severe after – pains with fear and restlessness
- In inflammations and associated fevers, this remedy should be thought of first. Sudden chills or fever. Fever with thirst and restlessness.

CLINICAL

- Shock
- Anxiety
- Dropsy
- Epilepsy
- Conjunctivitis
- Blepharitis
- Photophobia
- Trigeminal Neuralgia
- Gingivitis
- Mumps
- Haematemesis
- Dysentry
- Cholera
- Diarrhoea
- Haemorrhoids
- Otalgia
- Otitis media
- Influenza
- Coryza
- Epistaxis
- Tonsillitis-first stage
- Whooping cough
- Bronchitis
- Chest affections
- Asthma
- Pneumonia
- Nephritis
- Tenesmus
- Haematuria
- Retention of urine
- Orchitis
- Fever
- Pruritus
- Measles
- Purpurea miliaris

MODALITIES

- **Aggravation:** Evening and night, in a warm room, when rising from bed, lying on affected side, dry cold winds, fright, shock, sleeping in the sun
- **Amelioration:** In the open air, rest, sitting still

REMEDY RELATIONSHIP

- **Complementary:** Coff. and Cham. in pain and sleeplessness; to Arn. in traumatism; to Bapt. and Pyrog. in high fever with sudden onset; to Bry. in effects of cold, dry winds
- **Aconite is the acute of Sulph.**; it often completes the action that Acon. starts

ACTAEA RACEMOSA (CIMICIFUGA RACEMOSA)

INTRODUCTION

- **Common name:** Cimicifuga, Macrotys, Black snakeroot, Black cohosh
- **Family:** *Ranunculaceae*
- **Source:** Vegetable kingdom
- **Part used:** Rhizome
- **Prover:** Jeanes

SPHERE OF ACTION

- Mind
- Central nervous system
- Gastrointestinal system
- Heart
- Muscular system
- Female genital system

MIND

- **Sensation as if a heavy, black cloud has settled all over her; all is darkness and confusion**
- **Great depression, with dreams of impending evil**
- Fears riding in a closed carriage, of being obliged to jump out
- Incessant talking
- Puerperal mania or melancholia; tries to injure herself; hysterical, thinks she is going crazy
- Delirium tremens
- Mania following disappearance of neuralgia
- **Illusions of rats and mice running from under the chair**
- Thinks she is going crazy

MODALITIES

- **Aggravation:** During menstruation: the more profuse the flow the greater the suffering, heat and cold, change of weather, morning, damp cold air, puberty, emotions
- **Amelioration:** Warmth, pressure, eating, open air, continuous motion

KEYNOTE SYMPTOMS

- **For agitation and pains like electric shocks**
- **Tongue pointed and trembling.** Gnawing pain in stomach
- Sinking sensation in epigastrium; gnawing pains
- Tenderness in uterine region; pain across pelvis, from hip to hip
- Has ensured safe delivery in women who have previously born dead children without any discovered cause
- **Given before term, it renders labour easier, cures sickness of pregnancy, after-pains**
- False labour-like pains
- Labour pains displaced, felt more in hips, back or thighs
- Pain just before menses; menses profuse, dark, coagulated and offensive with backache
- Heart's action ceases suddenly; impending suffocation. Numbness in left arm
- **Infra-mammary pains, worse on left side**
- Irregular, slow, trembling pulse. Action of the heart ceases suddenly, threatening suffocation
- Stitching, cramping, muscular pains of neurotic origin in every part of the body
- Rheumatic pain in muscles of neck, back; spine sensitive. Excessive muscular soreness

CONSTITUTION

- For rheumatic, plump, delicate, nervous people, particularly women with ovarian irritation, cramps in the uterus and heavy limbs; during menopausal period
- For facial blemishes in young women
- **Temperament:** Nervous
- **Thermal:** Chilly
- **Miasm:** Psora

CLINICAL

- Hysteria
- Chorea
- Cramps
- Paralysis
- Hyperaemia
- Migraine
- Meningitis
- Asthenopia
- Ciliary neuralgia
- Nausea
- Vomiting
- Angina pectoris
- Intercostal rheumatism
- Amenorrhoea
- Ovarian neuralgia
- Uterine disorders
- False labour pains
- Rheumatic dysmenorrhoea
- Puerperal fever
- Puerperal mania
- Menopause
- Stiff neck
- Febrile irritation

REMEDY RELATIONSHIP

- **Similar to:** Caul. Lil-t., Agar., Sep. and Puls. in uterine and rheumatic affections, to Rham-cal. in rheumatism; to Arist-m, in pain in tendo-Achilles; to Der. in neuralgic headache of rheumatic origin

ACTAEA SPICATA

SPHERE OF ACTION
- Mind
- Gastrointestinal system
- Respiratory system
- Musculoskeletal system
- Joints

INTRODUCTION
- **Common name:** Baneberry
- **Family:** *Ranunculaceae*
- **Source:** Vegetable kingdom
- **Part used:** Roots
- **Prover:** Petroz

CONSTITUTION
- For rheumatic complaints of small joints. It is especially suited to men
- **Temperament:** Nervous, bilious
- **Thermal:** Chilly
- **Miasm:** Psora, Sycosis, Syphilis

MIND
- For bad effects of fatigue and fright; over exertion of mind or mental anxiety
- Absentmindedness; alternating with confusion of mind
- Raving, raging delirium in fever
- Fearful, starts easily
- Fear of being alone, fear of death at night in bed

KEYNOTE SYMPTOMS
- Sudden lassitude after eating or talking
- Pulsations all over the body, especially in the hepatic and renal regions
- **Right sided affections**
- Vertigo with tearing pains in the head
- Rush of blood to head excited by drinking coffee
- Cramp-like pain in stomach and epigastrium with difficulty in breathing
- Pain and tenderness in liver region
- **Red tip of nose with fluent coryza**
- Great oppression; shortness of breath on exposure to cold air. Difficult inspiration
- Cardiovascular spasm, pulsations
- Rheumatic remedy. Small joints, especially wrist affected
- **Wrist rheumatism, worse any motion. Rheumatism of fingers**
- **Slight fatigue causes swelling of joints. Violent tearing, drawing and tingling pains, worse by touch, movement. Wrist is swollen and red.**
- Paralytic weakness and lame feeling in hands and arms

CLINICAL
- Lassitude
- Pulsations
- Cramps
- Vertigo
- Dandruff
- Dyspepsia
- Diarrhoea
- Dysentery
- Hepatitis
- Coryza
- Cardiovascular spasm
- Arthritis
- Rheumatism
- Wrist pain

MODALITIES
- **Aggravation:** Touch, motion, cold air, night, mental or physical exertion
- **Amelioration:** Rest, open air

REMEDY RELATIONSHIP
- **Compare:** Cimic., Caul., Led.
- **Complementary:** Caul., Coloc., Sabin., Stict., Viol-o.

ADONIS VERNALIS

SPHERE OF ACTION
- Heart
- Respiratory system
- Urinary system

INTRODUCTION
- **Common name:** Pheasant's eye
- **Family:** *Ranunculaceae*
- **Source:** Vegetable kingdom
- **Part used:** Whole plant

CONSTITUTION
- Suits people with low vitality, weak heart and a slow, weak pulse
- For rapid, feeble action of heart, dropsy and scanty urine with casts and albumin
- **Temperament:** Nervous, bilious
- **Thermal:** Chilly
- **Miasm:** Psora, Sycosis, Syphilis

MIND
- Anxiety, arising from the stomach causing restlessness and nervousness
- Anxious, frightful dreams.
- Morose, cross, irritable, peevish
- Apprehensiveness

KEYNOTE SYMPTOMS
- **Tongue dirty, yellow, sore, feels scalded or burnt**
- Heart affected after rheumatism, influenza or nephritis; where the muscles of the heart are in the stage of fatty degeneration; Rheumatic endocarditis
- **Frequent desire to take a long breath; sensation of weight on chest**
- Pulse rapid, irregular
- A good cardiac remedy for precordial pain, palpitation and dyspnoea present
- Mitral and aortic regurgitation with marked venous engorgement
- Valvular heart disease, cardiac dropsy, cardiac asthma
- Compensatory hypertrophy of heart in cardiac stenosis and mitral regurgitation
- **Irregular cardiac action with sensation of constriction**
- Kidney diseases – nephritis. Oily pellicle on urine. Urine scanty, with albumin. Urging to urinate.

CLINICAL
- Anasarca
- Oedema
- Vertigo
- Tinnitus
- Ascitis
- Hydrothorax
- Cardiac dropsy
- Cardiac asthma
- Myocarditis
- Chronic aortitis
- Valvular heart disease
- Kidney disease
- Urinary tract infection
- Nephritis
- Cystitis
- Albuminuria
- Bright's disease

MODALITIES
- **Aggravation:** Cold, on lying down
- **Amelioration:** Walking in open air, exertion

REMEDY RELATIONSHIP
- **Compare:** Adonin. it is a cardiac tonic and diuretic; Dig., Crat., Conv., Stroph-h.

ADRENALINUM

INTRODUCTION
- **Common name:** Adrenaline
- **Group:** Sarcode
- **Source:** Internal secretion or extract of adrenal gland
- **Prover:** Gatman

SPHERE OF ACTION
- Mind
- Gastrointestinal system
- Respiratory system
- Musculoskeletal system
- Arteries
- Adrenal gland
- Vasomotor system

MIND
- Nervous, despondent
- Anxious and restless
- Aversion to mental activity, cannot concentrate, lack of interest. Apathy, no ambition, no mental stamina or will power
- Ailments from stress and over work

MODALITIES
- **Aggravation:** Stress, overwork, in the evening
- **Amelioration:** Pressure, rubbing, rest

KEYNOTE SYMPTOMS
- Adrenaline is the active principle of medulla of the suprarenal gland. It is employed as a chemical messenger for the regulation of the activities of the body, especially for the stimulation of sympathetic nerves
- Acts on sympathetic nerve endings by stimulating them
- Causes constiction of peripheral arterioles resulting in an increase in blood pressure
- Act on arteries, heart, suprarenal bodies and vasomotor system – they are prominently affected
- **Exceedingly rapid pulse; heart beat irregular and intermitting**
- It is a haemostatic because of its vasoconstriction action
- Acute congestion of lungs, sphenoidal and ethmoidal sinuses
- Prolonged contraction of the general muscular system. Great loss of strength, rapid emaciation

CONSTITUTION
- **It is a powerful astringent and haemostatic as it has a predominant vasoconstriction action**
- Medulla and suprarenal gland affected, sympathetic nerve stimulated
- **Temperament:** Nervous, anxious, haemorrhagic
- **Thermal:** Chilly
- **Miasm:** Psora, Sycosis, Syphilis

CLINICAL
- Chlorosis
- Anaemia
- Shock
- Addison's disease
- Grave's disease
- Allergies
- Neuralgia
- Neuritis
- Haemorrhages
- Haemophilia
- Headache
- Hyperaemia of conjunctiva
- Asthma
- Hay fever
- Acute bronchospasm
- Arteriosclerosis
- Tachycardia
- High blood pressure
- Angina pectoris
- Acute urticaria
- Bronzed skin

REMEDY RELATIONSHIP
- **Compare:** Thyr., Iod.

AESCULUS HIPPOCASTANUM

INTRODUCTION
- **Common name:** Horse chestnut
- **Family:** *Sapindaceae*
- **Source:** Vegetable kingdom
- **Part used:** The ripe nut excluding the outer shell
- **Prover:** Helbig

SPHERE OF ACTION
- Veins
- Gastrointestinal system
- Respiratory system
- Musculoskeletal system
- Female genital system

CONSTITUTION
- Suits old people with haemorrhoidal tendency, during pregnancy, lactation, leucorrhoea
- For persons suffering from gastric, bilious and catarrhal troubles
- **Temperament:** Nervous, bilious
- **Thermal:** Chilly
- **Miasm:** Psora, Sycosis, Syphilis

MIND
- Looses temper easily, gains control slowly, miserably cross
- Confused, dullness or sluggishness
- Depressed and extremely irritable
- Attempts to escape from the window
- Gloomy, despondent
- Dullness and sluggishness on waking in the morning, or on waking at night; wakes with mental confusion

KEYNOTE SYMPTOMS
- It is a great venous remedy; engorged veins; venous stasis; feeling of fullness in internal parts
- Glandular swellings present
- Mucous membranes are dry, swollen, raw and burning
- **Flying pains all over**
- Vertigo when sitting and walking
- **Frequent inclination to swallow**
- Marked action on lower bowel producing engorged haemorrhoidal veins with characteristic backache, with absence of actual constipation
- **Aching in rectum with feeling as if full of small sticks;** during pregnancy, prolapse
- Burning in anus with chills up and down the back
- **Haemorrhoids blind, painful, purplish, with severe lumbosacral backache, must sit or lie**
- Dryness and heat in rectum; constipation, intense pain in anus for hours
- Jaundice, portal circulation stasis and torpor
- Follicular pharyngitis, dry throat with stitching pain. Pharyngeal veins distended
- Constrant throbbing behind symphysis pubis
- **Dark, yellow, sticky, corroding leucorrhoea with lameness of the back**
- Weakness of sacro-iliac joint. Backache of sacrum and hips, worse walking, stooping. Spine feels weak. Degenerative hip disease.

CLINICAL
- Congestion
- Venous stasis
- Ascarides
- Jaundice
- Haemorrhoids
- Laryngitis
- Atrophic pharyngitis
- Varicose veins
- Leucorrhoea
- Arthritis
- Rheumatism
- Cervical spondylosis
- Lumbago

MODALITIES
- **Aggravation:** Motion, walking, stooping, winter, cold weather, on waking, after eating, after stool
- **Amelioration:** Summer, cool open air, bathing

REMEDY RELATIONSHIP
- **Similar to:** Aloe, Coll., Ign., Mur-ac., Nux-v., Sulph., in haemorrhoids
- Useful after Coll., Nux-v. and Sulph. have improved, but failed to cure piles

AETHUSA CYNAPIUM

INTRODUCTION
- **Common name:** Fool's parsley
- **Family:** *Umbelliferae*
- **Source:** Vegetable kingdom
- **Part used:** Whole plant
- **Prover:** Nenning

SPHERE OF ACTION
- Mind
- Gastrointestinal system
- Nervous system
- Glandular system
- Skin

CONSTITUTION
- In puffiness of the face with marked linea nasalis and an experession of great anxiety. Physically, the child is so weak that he is unable to stand or hold the head up
- Suits teething children and summer complaints of elderly and children
- **Temperament:** Anxious
- **Thermal:** Hot
- **Miasm:** Psora

MIND
- Mentally idiotic, confused and unable to think. Brain fag
- Great weakness, mentally and physically
- Inability to fix attention
- Expression of great anxiety and pain
- Irritability, especially in open air
- Restlessness and anxiety
- Unconscious
- Delirious sees rats, cats, dogs
- **Animal lovers; talks to them and look after them well**

KEYNOTE SYMPTOMS
- Great physical weakness, child cannot hold the head up. Sleepiness is well marked
- Glandular swelling of lymphatic glands
- Epileptic spasms with clenched thumb, red face, eyes turned downwards, pupils fixed, dilated and sharp; pulse is small, hard, quick. Weakness, prostration
- Fingers and thumb clenched or bent inwards numbness of hands and feet; violent spasms
- Weakness of lower limbs
- Dryness and aphthae in mouth. **Burning thirst with no appetite**
- Indigestion of teething children
- **Vomiting is violent, sudden, projectile; of frothy, milky white substance followed by curdled milk and cheesy matter. Vomiting with retching, sweat, marked prostration and sleepiness. Hungry after vomiting. Vomiting during pregnancy.**
- **Intolerance of milk in any form; milk is vomited as soon as it is swallowed and as large curds**
- Regurgitation of food an hour or so after eating. Nausea at the sight of food
- Cholera in children and elderly; discharge of indigested, thin, green stools preceeded by colic and tenesmus
- Herpetic eruptions at the tip of the nose. Body surface covered with clammy perspiration
- **Complete absence of thirst with great heat during fever; must cover during sweat stage**

CLINICAL
- Mental retardation
- Brain fag
- Idiocy
- Delirium
- Epilepsy
- Convulsions
- Paralysis
- Marasmus
- Malnutrition
- Anasarca
- Vertigo
- Headache
- Photophobia
- Intolerance of milk
- Stomach disorders
- Hiccough
- Vomiting
- Dyspepsia
- Pyloric stenosis
- Infantile diarrhoea
- Cholera infantum
- Cough

MODALITIES
- **Aggravation:** From milk, after eating or drinking, after vomiting, after stool, after spasm, 3 to 4 am, and in the evenings, warmth, summers
- **Amelioration:** In open air, in company

REMEDY RELATIONSHIP
- **Compare:** Ant-c., Ars., Calc., Sanic.
- **Complementary to:** Calc., Sil.
- **Antidotes:** Op.

AGARICUS MUSCARIUS

INTRODUCTION

- **Common name:** Toad stool, Bug agaric
- **Family:** *Agaricaceae*
- **Source:** Vegetable kingdom
- **Part used:** The whole fruit body except the outer skin
- **Prover:** Stapf

SPHERE OF ACTION

- Mind
- Eye
- Spinal cord
- Nervous system
- Medulla
- Gastrointestinal system
- Respiratory system
- Skin

CONSTITUTION

- For people with light hair and lax skin and muscles
- For old people with weak, indolent circulation
- **Temperament:** Nervous
- **Thermal:** Chilly
- **Miasm:** Sycosis, Tubercular

MIND

- Depression and languor; awkward and clumsy
- Dull and dizzy, as if drunk; alcoholism
- Aversion to work, indifference; indisposed to perform any kind of work, especially mental; cannot do anything new
- **Fearlessness, or fear of cancer, fear after going to bed**
- Great mental excitement alternates with melancholy
- Increased cheerfulness, full of ecstasy; embraces and kisses hands
- **Furious and raging delirium; wants to injure self**
- Anxiety about health
- Loquacity, talks of one subject and then another, but does not answer any question; disinclined to answer questions
- Dependent, fearful
- Delirium accompanied by singing, shouting, muttering; and loquacity; makes verses and prophesies; tries to get out of bed; especially in typhoid or typhus

KEYNOTE SYMPTOMS

- **Symptoms appear diagonally – right arm and left leg**
- Symptoms appear slowly. Pains are accompanied by coldness, numbness and tingling
- **Cold sensation, as if pierced by cold or hot needles**
- Yawning before complaints, before pain or spasm. Paroxysms of yawning
- Nervous prostration after sexual excesses
- Involuntary movements when awake, cease on sleeping
- Bad effects of a debauch
- More vertigo and delirium when intoxicated. Vertigo from sunlight
- Epilepsy from suppressed eruptions, with great exertion of strength
- Twitching, jerking fasciculations, spasms, convulsions, chorea, grimaces, trembling and itching
- Twitching of eyelids. Difficult to read as letters seem to swim before eyes. Diplopia; short sighted.
- **Tongue white; aphthae at roof of mouth. Tremulous tongue**
- Stitching pain in abdomen, especially liver and spleen region; stitch in the side of runners
- Spasmodic cough at night on falling asleep with easy expectoration like little balls of mucous; cough ends in a sneeze
- Awkwardness in arms and legs
- Low back pain along cerebrospinal axis; spine sensitive to touch
- **Frostbites and chilblains that are red, and itch and burn intolerably**

CLINICAL

- Anxiety
- Depression
- Delirium
- Neuromyopathy
- Multiple sclerosis
- Tremors
- Twitching
- Paraesthesia
- Seizure disorder
- Chorea
- Neuralgia
- Alcoholism
- Delirium tremens
- Vertigo
- Bell's palsy
- Myopia
- Diplopia
- Blepharitis
- Epistaxis
- Diarrhoea
- Prolapse
- Sciatica
- Spinal irritation
- Chilblains
- Frostbite
- Herpes
- Gangrene

MODALITIES

- **Aggravation:** After eating, after coitus, cold air, mental application, before a thunderstorm, after a debauch, alcohol, in the morning
- **Amelioration:** Moving about slowly

REMEDY RELATIONSHIP

- **Compare:** Cimic., Calc., Cann-i., Hyos., Kali-p., Lach., Nux-v., Op., Stram., in delirium of alcoholism and chorea; to Mygal., Tarent., Zinc., in chorea; Ars. in hot needles like sensation

AGNUS CASTUS

INTRODUCTION

- **Common name:** The Chaste tree
- **Family:** *Verbenaceae*
- **Source:** Vegetable kingdom
- **Part used:** Fruit
- **Prover:** Hahnemann

SPHERE OF ACTION

- Mind
- Gastrointestinal system
- Male genital system
- Female genital system
- Urinary system

MIND

- Ailments from masturbation and sexual excesses
- Sexual vitality is lowered, with corresponding mental depression and loss of nervous energy
- Lack of courage; fear of death
- **Has to read a sentence twice before he can comprehend; forgetful. Poor memory, cannot fix attention**
- Absentmindedness
- Illusions of smell – herring, musk
- Nervous debility in unmarried people
- Great sadness, depression, with a fixed idea of approaching death
- Prematurely old with apathy and melancholy

MODALITIES

- **Aggravation:** From sexual excess, sexual loss, sprains, masturbation, over lifting
- **Amelioration:** Scratching, pressure

KEYNOTE SYMPTOMS

- Spleen swollen, indurated and sore, especially after intermittent fever
- **Distention of abdomen after meals; sensation as if intestines were pressed downwards**
- History of repeated gonorrhoea or masturbation
- Premature old age from abuse of sexual power
- Self-contempt from sexual abuse. Sexual melancholy
- Weakness from masturbation
- Infertility in both sexes, especially men
- Women with excessive sexual desire and lasciviousness or sterility and loss of sexual desire
- Male genitals cold and relaxed with impotence; lack of sexual power and lack of self-confidence, with depression and mental apathy. No erection
- **Yellow discharge from urethra; drawing pain along spermatic cord**
- Loss of prostatic fluid on straining. Weakness of sexual organs or impotency
- Sprains and strains, especially from over lifting

CONSTITUTION

- Suits lymphatic and sycotic constitution
- Adapted sexual melancholy; premature old age from abuse of sexual power with apathy and melancholy
- **Temperament:** Anaemic
- **Thermal:** Ambithermal
- **Miasm:** Sycosis

CLINICAL

- Hysteria
- Weak memory
- Depression
- Weakness
- Sprains
- Strains
- Nausea
- Spleen swollen
- Splenomegaly
- Ascitis
- Fissures
- Epistaxis
- Tachycardia
- Sexual weakness
- Sterility
- Agalactia
- Leucorrhoea
- Gonorrhoea
- Orchitis
- Impotence

REMEDY RELATIONSHIP

- Calad. and Sel. follow well after Agn. in weakness of sexual organs or impotence
- **Compare:** Sel., Con., Nat-m., Sep., Sabal., Ph-ac., Camph., Lyc., Olnd.

AGRAPHIS NUTANS

SPHERE OF ACTION
- Gastrointestinal system
- Ears
- Throat
- Respiratory system
- Mucous membranes

INTRODUCTION
- **Common name:** Bluebell
- **Family:** *Liliaceae*
- **Source:** Vegetable kingdom
- **Part used:** Whole plant
- **Prover:** Cooper

CONSTITUTION
- Suited to those who have a tendency to take cold on exposure to cold winds
- **Temperament:** Anxious
- **Thermal:** Chilly
- **Miasm:** Psora

MIND
- Irritability, worse contradiction
- Fear of being alone
- Obstinate
- Desires company

KEYNOTE SYMPTOMS
- **Generally relaxed condition of the system**
- Tendency to take cold on exposure to cold winds
- **Mutism of childhood unconnected with deafness**
- Mucous diarrhoea from cold; or mucous diarrhoea after suppressed cold
- Throat and ear troubles with a tendency to free discharges from mucous membranes
- Catarrhal conditions of ears, nose and throat
- **One of the leading remedies in cases of adenoids**
- Deafness from adenoids
- Obstruction of the nostrils, especially from adenoids
- Enlarged tonsils

CLINICAL
- Mutism
- Mucoid diarrhoea
- Deafness
- Otitis media
- Tympanitis
- Obstruction of nostrils
- Coryza
- Cough
- Pharyngitis
- Laryngitis
- Adenoids
- Tonsillitis

MODALITIES
- **Aggravation:** Exposure to cold air, mucous diarrhoea after suppressed cold
- **Amelioration:** From shelter

REMEDY RELATIONSHIP
- **Compare:** Hydr., All-c., Calc-p., Sul-i., Calc-i., Squil.

AILANTHUS GLANDULOSA

SPHERE OF ACTION

- Eyes
- Mouth
- Gastrointestinal system
- Blood
- Mucous membranes
- Skin

INTRODUCTION

- **Common name:** Chinese sumach
- **Family:** *Simarubacea*
- **Source:** Vegetable kingdom
- **Part used:** Stem, bark of young shoots and well developed flowers
- **Prover:** Hering and Lippe

CONSTITUTION

- Patient is stupid, dull, delirious and weak
- Nervous, sensitive, stout and robust persons with a haemorrhagic diathesis
- **Temperament:** Bilious
- **Thermal:** Ambithermal
- **Miasm:** Sycosis

MIND

- Stupor; or stoic indifference, with sighing
- Dullness, must read a subject several times or figures over and over again
- **Sensation of animals creeping on him, crawling up his leg**
- All the antecedents are forgotten
- Constant, muttering delirium; with sleeplessness and restlessness
- Raging delirium, with brilliant eyes
- Confused mind
- Mental depression

KEYNOTE SYMPTOMS

- Low forms of the disease as it disorganizes blood
- Unconsciousness and coma in scarlatina, after suppressed eruptions. Semiconscious; delirious; weak pulse.
- **Feels snakes in, and around her**
- Extreme prostration at the very onset of a disease; general stupor with sighing
- Lividity, stupor, torpor and malignancy are marked
- Mucous membranes – haemorrhagic and ulcerative. Discharges are thin, acrid, especially from the nose
- Headache – frontal, with drowsiness and suffused, dilated eyes
- **Teeth – covered with sordes; foetor**
- **Tongue – dry, brown, parched, cracked**
- Vomiting, sudden and violent on sitting up
- Diarrhoea and dysentery with great weakness; stools are thin, watery and offensive
- Neck – tender, swollen
- Throat – diphtheria, follicular tonsillitis, streptococcal infection
- Throat inflamed, oedematous, dusky red. **Pains on swallowing, extending to the ears**
- Skin has livid or purplish eruptions; patchy, irregular
- Rash, coming out in patches; returning annually

CLINICAL

- Adynamia
- Stupor
- Lividity
- Malignancy
- Streptococcus infection
- Haemorrhage, ulceration
- Meningitis
- Dysphagia
- Diarrhoea
- Dysentery
- Ulcerative colitis
- Diphtheria
- Follicular tonsillitis
- Raynaud's disease
- Low fevers
- Eruptions
- Measles

MODALITIES

- **Aggravation:** From suppressions, raising up, sitting up, motion
- **Amelioration:** By hot drinks, lying on the right side

REMEDY RELATIONSHIP

- **Antidotes:** Rhus-t., Nux-v.
- **Compare:** Am-c., Bapt., Arn., Mur-ac., Lach., Phyt., Rhus-t.

ALETRIS FARINOSA

INTRODUCTION

- **Common name:** Star grass, Colic root
- **Family:** *Liliaceae*
- **Source:** Vegetable kingdom
- **Part used:** Rhizome and root
- **Prover:** Hale

SPHERE OF ACTION

- Mind
- Head
- Gastrointestinal system
- Female genital system
- Male genital system
- Blood

CONSTITUTION

- For chlorotic girls and pregnant women. Weak, emaciated people who are anaemic, debilitated and relaxed
- **Temperament:** Anaemic
- **Thermal:** Chilly
- **Miasm:** Sycosis

MIND

- Prostration of mind
- Mental exhaustion
- Brain fag
- Indolence
- Aversion to work
- Confused feeling
- Cannot concentrate
- Weakness of mind
- Power and energy weakened

KEYNOTE SYMPTOMS

- Patient is fatigued and tired all the time; mental and physical weariness
- Fainting attacks with vertigo
- Sensation of weight in occiput, as if it would draw the head back
- Much frothy saliva, frothy eructations, frothy expectoration
- **Want of appetite; disgust for food.** Least food causes distress. Vomiting of pregnancy.
- **Nausea returns with gagging at sight, smell or thought of fatty food**
- Rectum loaded with faeces
- Stools – large, hard, difficult, pass with great pain. Constipation
- Suits females who always feel tired and suffer from prolapses, leucorrhoea and rectal distress
- Heaviness of parts. Uterus seems heavy, sensation of weight in uterine region
- Premature and profuse menses with labour pains
- Muscular pains during pregnancy
- Habitual tendency to abortion leading to weakness of mind and body
- **Leucorrhoea – white, stringy; from anaemia and weakness**

CLINICAL

- Anaemia
- Chlorosis
- Debility
- Fatigue
- Fainting
- Haemorrhage
- Vertigo
- Vomiting
- Colic
- Sterility
- Leucorrhoea
- Metrorrhagia
- Uterine prolapse
- Abortions

MODALITIES

- **Aggravation:** Loss of fluids
- **Amelioration:** Passing flatus, bending backwards

REMEDY RELATIONSHIP

- **Compare:** Chin., Hydr., Sabin., Senec., Sep., Helon., Dios., in colic worse bending forward; Alum.

SPHERE OF ACTION

- Mind
- Sympathetic nerves
- Gastrointestinal system
- Nervous system
- Muscular system

INTRODUCTION

- **Common name:** Medicago sativa, California clover, Lucerne
- **Family:** *Leguminosae*
- **Source:** Vegetable kingdom
- **Part used:** Whole plant excluding roots
- **Prover:** Blackwood

CONSTITUTION

- Suits weak, emaciated and broken down constitutions due to malnutrition
- **Temperament:** Rheumatic, nervous
- **Thermal:** Chilly
- **Miasm:** Psora

MIND

- Bain fag, mental prostration
- Lack of confidence
- Fearfulness
- Dull, drowsy, stupid, sluggish
- Nervousness, heavy, dull feeling
- Gloomy and irritable, worse in the evening
- Mental exhilaration, cheerful, vivacious. General feeling of well being
- State of exhilaration, clearness of thoughts
- Aversion to mental work

ALFALFA

CLINICAL

- Nervousness
- Neurasthenia
- Anaemia
- Hypoglycaemia
- Marasmus
- Anorexia
- Weakness
- Exhaustion
- Malnutrition
- Alopecia areata
- Flatulence
- Distension
- Chronic appendicitis
- Bronchitis
- Asthma
- Polyuria
- Cystitis
- Diabetes insipidus
- Deficient lactation
- Impotency
- Rheumatoid arthritis
- Sleeplessness

KEYNOTE SYMPTOMS

- Influences nutrition and regulates metabolism
- Helps children who fail to thrive
- Dull heavy feeling in occiput. **Pain in left side of head. Violent headache.**
- **Helps toning up the appetite and digestion; hungry in the forenoon**
- Reduced appetite with weight loss or hungry all the time, must eat frequently. **Increased thirst, desires sweet. Nibbles food.**
- Frequent loose, yellow, painful stools with excoriating flatulence
- Flatulance with distension
- Chronic appendicitis; also useful in other inflammatory conditions like – colitis, peritonitis, enteritis, etc.
- **Stuffed feeling in eustachian tubes**
- Kidneys inactive and weak with frequent urging to micturition, polyuria
- **Increases quality and quantity of milk in nursing mothers**
- Sleeps better early in the morning. Insomnia or sleeplessness during convalescence

MODALITIES

- **Aggravation:** Towards evening (head and mental symptoms)
- **Amelioration:** Eating frequently

REMEDY RELATIONSHIP

- **Compare:** Aven., Dip., Gels., Hydr., Kali-p., Ph-ac., Zinc.

ALLIUM CEPA

SPHERE OF ACTION

- Mind
- Eyes
- Ears
- Gastrointestinal system
- Respiratory system
- Skin

INTRODUCTION

- **Common name:** Red onion
- **Family:** *Liliaceae*
- **Source:** Vegetable kingdom
- **Part used:** Red, mature bulbs
- **Prover:** Hering

CONSTITUTION

- Suits young people with catarrhal tendency
- Suits psoric and allergic constitutions
- **Temperament:** Nervous, phlegmatic
- **Thermal:** Chilly
- **Miasm:** Psora, Tubercular

MIND

- **Absentmindedness and confusion of mind after wine or coffee in the afternoon; with irritation of the brain**
- Dreams of battles, fights, being let down into wells or precipices
- **Dreams of being near water, of high waves; vexation, during convalescence**
- Anxiety with catarrh; about health; dullness of intellect
- Fear that pain will become intolerable

KEYNOTE SYMPTOMS

- Left sided medicine, symptoms go from left to right
- **For neuralgic pain like a fine thread after operation, amputation, injury to nerves**
- **Desire for raw onions**
- Diarrhoea with flatulence
- **Profuse, watery and acrid nasal discharge with profuse bland lachrymation (opposite of Euphr. – bland nasal discharge and acrid lachrymation)**
- Most commonly indicated in ear aches of children, coryza, sneezing and laryngitis
- Coryza with a lot of sneezing and profuse, acrid discharge, corroding the upper lip and nose
- Catarrhal laryngitis; grasps the larynx; hacking cough, feels as if cough would tear it; cough on inhaling cold air
- Itching at the back of the throat with hoarseness and change of voice
- Phlebitis after forceps delivery
- Ulcers on feet, heels
- A raw onion eaten just before going to bed is a popular remedy for sleeplessness
- Yawning, with headache and drowsiness

CLINICAL

- Allergies
- Traumatic neuritis
- Blepharitis
- Conjunctivitis
- Photophobia
- Toothache
- Colic
- Abdominal pain
- Diarrhoea
- Haemorrhoids
- Fissure in anus
- Sneezing
- Coryza
- Rhinitis
- Hay fever
- Sinusitis
- Nasal polyp
- Catarrhal laryngitis
- Whooping cough
- Phlebitis
- Panaritia

MODALITIES

- **Aggravation:** Predominantly in the evening and in a warm room, rest, damp weather
- **Amelioration:** In a cold room, open air (Puls.), bathing

REMEDY RELATIONSHIP

- **Complementary:** Phos., Puls., Sars., Thuj.
- **Followed by:** Calc. and Sil. in polypus
- **Compare:** Euphr., All-s., Acon., Puls., Gels.

SPHERE OF ACTION

- Head
- Gastrointestinal system
- Respiratory system
- Female genital system
- Mucous membranes
- Musculoskeletal system

INTRODUCTION

- **Common name:** Garlic
- **Family:** *Liliaceae*
- **Source:** Vegetable kingdom
- **Part used:** The mature bulb
- **Prover:** Petroz

CONSTITUTION

- Adapted to extremely pale and fleshy subjects, suffering from dyspepsia, used to high living and suffer from catarrhal affections
- **Temperament:** Bilious
- **Thermal:** Chilly
- **Miasm:** Psora, Sycosis

MIND

- Impatient and restless; must move, impulse to run away, worse when alone
- Fear that he will never get well; fear cannot bear any medicine; of being poisoned
- Wants many things, pleased with nothing
- Child is drowsy, lifeless
- Sensitive
- Sad; when alone, weeps during sleep
- Anxious and impatient
- Poor memory

ALLIUM SATIVUM

CLINICAL

- Catarrhal affections
- Arterial hypertension
- Sweetish saliva
- Appetite, voracious
- Peristalsis increased
- Dyspepsia
- Colitis
- Deafness
- Koch's disease
- Haemoptysis
- Bronchitis
- Vasodilation
- Breast affections
- Hip joint disease
- Rheumatism of hips
- Pimples

KEYNOTE SYMPTOMS

- Stinging, burning pains; increase gradually till they reach their climax, then decline gradually
- Patients who eat a great deal, especially meat, than they drink. **Desire for butter**
- **Tongue pale, with red papillae. Sensation of a hair on the tongue**
- **Much sweetish saliva, after meals, at night**
- Incarcerated flatus; pressing pain in epigastrium
- Acts on intestinal mucous membranes, increasing peristalsis
- Pain in transverse colon, darting pain
- Cough and expectoration when smoking
- Cough with foetid breath; bronchial catarrh with profuse, gelatinous, difficult expectoration
- Pulmonary tuberculosis and haemoptysis – it reduces the cough and expectoration and brings temperature down to normal
- Pain in hip, psoas and iliac muscles, cannot walk
- Swelling and pain in breasts

MODALITIES

- **Aggravation:** Change in temperature, drinking bad water, in morning on waking, in evening and at night
- **Amelioration:** Sitting bent

REMEDY RELATIONSHIP

- **Compare:** Caps., Ars., Seneg., Kali-n.
- **Complementary:** Ars.
- **Antidote:** Lyc.

ALOE SOCOTRINA

SPHERE OF ACTION
- Mind
- Gastrointestinal system
- Urinary system
- Female genital system
- Skin

INTRODUCTION
- **Common name:** Socotrine aloes
- **Family:** *Liliaceae*
- **Source:** Vegetable kingdom
- **Part used:** The inspissated juice of the leaves
- **Prover:** Helbig

CONSTITUTION
- For old weary people, especially women of relaxed phlegmatic habit; averse to mental or physical labour
- Adapted to old beer drinkers
- **Temperament:** Nervous, bilious, lymphatic, hypochondriacal
- **Thermal:** Hot
- **Miasm:** Psora, Sycosis, Syphilis

MIND
- Extremely irritable and excited
- Patient hates people and repels everyone
- Lives a sedentary life
- Indolent, weary person
- Aversion to mental or physical labour
- Dissatisfied, angry about himself, worse when constipated
- Bad humour, especially in cloudy weather
- Hypochondriacal

KEYNOTE SYMPTOMS
- Profuse, jelly-like mucous from all mucous membranes, especially, throat and rectum
- Taste bitter, sour
- Epistaxis in the morning on getting up
- **Has to rush to the toilet after eating or drinking**
- Lumpy, watery stool, colic before stool. **Stool passes effortlessly. Jelly-like stools with soreness of rectum after stool.**
- Abdomen feels heavy, hot, bloated. Marked flatus, pressing downwards.
- Passage of burning, copious flatus
- Sensation of plug between symphysis pubis and coccygial os
- Sensation of heaviness in the rectum with much flatus; sensation of insecurity of rectum when passing flatus
- Diarrhoea alternates with constipation and piles; diarrhoea, early in the morning, driving patient out of bed; hungry after diarrhoea
- **Piles, like a bunch of grapes; bleeding, sore, tender and hot; relieved by cold water application. Portal congestion**
- Incontinence of urine, especially in aged, with bearing down sensation and an enlarged prostate
- Climacteric haemorrhage; uterus feels heavy. Bearing down pains in rectum, worse during menses and when standing
- Lumbago alternating with haemorrhoids or headache
- Itch starts every year in winters, preventing sleep

CLINICAL
- Prostration
- Conjunctivitis
- Flatulence
- Colic
- Colitis
- Diarrhoea
- Dysentery
- Obstinate constipation
- Haemorrhoids
- Fissure
- Proctalgia
- Asthma
- Incontinence
- Dysmenorrhoea
- Menorrhagia
- Enlarged prostate
- Lumbago
- Insomnia
- Itch

MODALITIES
- **Aggravation:** Early morning, sedentary life, hot dry weather, summer, after eating or drinking, standing or walking
- **Amelioration:** Cold water, cold weather, discharge of flatus and stool

REMEDY RELATIONSHIP
- **Compare:** Am-m., Gamb., Nux-v., Podo., Merc, Aesc.; Sulph. in many chronic diseases with abdominal plethora and congestion of portal circulation; develops suppressed eruptions.
- **Complementary:** Sulph.

ALUMINA

INTRODUCTION

- **Common name:** Oxide of aluminium, Argilla, Aluminium hydroxide
- **Group:** Metal hydroxide
- **Source:** Mineral kingdom
- **Formula:** $Al(OH)_3$
- **Prover:** Hahnemann

SPHERE OF ACTION

- Mind
- Spinal cord
- Gastrointestinal system
- Female genital system
- Musculoskeletal system
- Mucous membranes
- Skin

MIND

- Weak memory
- **Suicidal tendency on seeing a knife or blood**
- **Fears loss of reason. Consciousness of reality and judgement is disturbed as if guilty of crime**
- Impressions reach consciousness slowly
- Great mental confusion as to his personal identity itself. Alternating moods
- An hour seems half a day; time passes too slowly
- Everything is viewed in sad light, depressed on awakening, on the other hand, fears his own impulses
- Illusion of being large, numb, smooth, heavy
- Makes mistakes in speaking, writing
- Dullness, slowness, disorientation, senile dementia
- Hurried and hasty

MODALITIES

- **Aggravation:** In cold except headache, during winter, while sitting, from eating potatoes, periodically, on alternate days, at new and full moon, warmth of room or bed
- **Amelioration:** Evening, as the day advances, open air, damp weather

KEYNOTE SYMPTOMS

- Dryness of the skin, and all the mucous membranes of the body, inability to perspire
- It affects the cerebrospinal axis causing disturbance in co-ordination and paretic effects, paraesthesia, spinal degeneration
- Deficient in animal heat and relieved by warmth; tendency to take colds
- Discharges are profuse, thin, acrid, irritating
- Pulsations are felt in various parts
- **Desires starchy food, especially indigestible things such as starch, chalk, charcoal, coffee, but potatoes disagree; potato causes bitter eructations**
- Aversion to meat, potatoes and beer
- **Can swallow only small mortels of food at a time**
- Diarrhoea when urinating or worse on alternate days
- **Obsinate constipation** with hard, dry knotty stools – **has to strain even for soft stool, stool sticks to the rectum like clay; has to strain at stool to urinate; no desire for stool**
- Menses short, scanty, pale; followed by severe prostration
- **Leucorrhoea is acrid, profuse, transparent, ropy; running down the heels**
- Legs fall asleep, especially when sitting with legs crossed. Staggers on walking. Numbness of heels
- Inability to walk with eyes closed in darkness
- Severe itching when getting warm in bed; scratches till it bleeds. Dry, tettery, itchy eruptions, worse in winters
- Sore throat of clergymen who are thin
- Throat dry and sore, inducing frequent clearing of throat in the evening

CONSTITUTION

- For people leading a sedentary life and suffering from chronic diseases or for elderly people with lack of vital heat
- Suits bottle fed, constipated babies or big bellied children
- Dry, thin subjects of dark complexion, wants to lie down but this increases the fatigue.
- **Temperament**: Bilious
- **Thermal**: Chilly
- **Miasm**: Psora

CLINICAL

- Depression
- Dementia
- Fatigue
- Paralysis
- Ataxia
- Myopathy
- Paraesthesia
- Multiple sclerosis
- Parkinson's disease
- Alzheimer's disease
- Vertigo
- Halitosis
- Gingivitis
- Heartburn
- Painter's colic
- Colic
- Constipation
- Ozaena
- Hoarseness
- Clergyman's sore throat
- Urinary retention
- Leucorrhoea
- Eczema
- Brittle nails

REMEDY RELATIONSHIP

- **Antidotes:** Lead poisoning
- **Complementary:** Bry., Plb.
- **Follows well:** Bry., Lach., Sulph.
- **Alumina is the chronic of Bryonia**
- **Compare:** Bar-c., Con., in ailments of old people; Alumn., Arg-n., for clergymen's sore throat

AMBRA GRISEA

INTRODUCTION

- **Common name:** Ambergis
- **Group:** Nosode
- **Source:** Morbid secretion of the whale
- **Prover:** Hahnemann

SPHERE OF ACTION

- Mind
- Nervous system
- Gastrointestinal system
- Respiratory system
- Male genital system

MIND

- Claustrophobia
- Forgetful, dull, mentally slow; indifference
- Sad, sits weeping; dwells upon unpleasant things, melancholic
- Shy, timid, introvert
- Hysterical, has fantastic illusions
- Time passes slowly
- **Music aggravates symptoms;** causes weeping and trembling
- Impossible to express himself and communicate
- Bashful, embarrassed in company – blushes, loses confidence, becomes bashful, avoids people
- Memory impaired – slow comprehension
- Mental and emotional disorders marked by intense shyness and introversion in early stage followed later by silliness and marked loquacity

MODALITIES

- **Aggravation:** Warm drinks, warm room, music, in the presence of others, from any unusual things
- **Amelioration:** Slow motion, open air, cold drinks, lying on painful side

KEYNOTE SYMPTOMS

- Suits patients who are weakened by age or over work
- **Weakness, coldness and numbness of single parts like fingers, hands, etc. especially in the morning**
- Affinity for nerves causing twitching, jerking, nervousness
- Strong sexual desire; patients masturbate and feel guilty
- Erratic symptoms; symptoms change place suddenly
- One sided complaints like – tearing in muscles and joints of one side only
- Sensation of coldness and numbness, generally of single parts
- Eructations with violent cough; acid eructations like heartburn
- Sensation of coldness in the abdomen; distention of stomach and abdomen after midnight
- Cannot have others presence when passing urine or stool
- Asthmatic breathing; nervous spasmodic cough, worse in the presence of other people
- Conscious of pulse; pulsations and ebullitions all over the body, especially after taking a walk in open air
- Palpitation with pressure on chest, as if from a lump
- Menses too early, profuse. Discharge of blood between periods. **Profuse, bluish leucorrhoea. Itching of pudenda with swelling and soreness**
- Cramps in hands, fingers; numbness of arms
- Cannot sleep from worry, especially after business embarrassments

CONSTITUTION

- For hysterical, nervous 'dried up', people, especially women who are prematurely old
- Suits thin, lean, emaciated people who take cold easily
- For old people with numbness, weakness and impairment of all functions; nerves worn out
- **Temperament:** Nervous, bilious
- **Thermal:** Chilly
- **Miasm:** Sycosis

CLINICAL

- Weakness
- Emaciation
- Vertigo
- Headache
- Ranula
- Halitosis
- Colitis
- Epistaxis
- Hearing impaired
- Asthma
- Spasmodic cough
- Hypertension
- Nymphomania
- Voluptuous itching of scrotum
- Cramps in hands
- Anxious dreams
- Insomnia

REMEDY RELATIONSHIP

- **Compare:** Asaf., Cimic., Coca, Ign., Mosch., Phos., Valer., Ars., Coff., Sec., Bov., Psor.
- **Antidotes:** Staph.
- Mosch. generally follows it well

AMMONIUM CARBONICUM

SPHERE OF ACTION
- Mind
- Heart
- Respiratory system
- Gastrointestinal system
- Female genital system

INTRODUCTION
- **Common name:** Carbonate of ammonia, Ammonium carbonate
- **Group:** Salt
- **Source:** Mineral kingdom
- **Formula:** $NH_4HCO_3NH_4CO_2NH_2$

CONSTITUTION
- Suits children who dislike washing or scrofulous, stout, nervous, fleshy women leading a sedentary life, with a tendency to use a smelling bottle and catch cold readily
- For fat people with weak hearts and a feeling of suffocation
- **Temperament:** Bilious, scrofulous
- **Thermal:** Chilly
- **Miasm:** Sycosis

MIND
- Sad, weepy, timid
- Vacant mind; absentminded; makes mistakes in reading and writing
- Loss or weakness of memory, vexation
- Hearing others talk or talking himself affects him
- Aversion to work
- Peevish, fretting, as if a crime has been committed
- Active, but soon exhausted
- Forgetful, ill-humoured, gloomy, during stormy weather
- Headless and unruly, disobedience
- Depressed, with weakness of intellect
- Aversion to opposite sex
- Disposed to uncleanliness

KEYNOTE SYMPTOMS
- Haemorrhagic tendency; from nose, gums, haemorrhoids, during menses
- Uncleanliness of body – leads to erythema, vesication and finally gangrene
- **Pressing teeth together sends shocks through the head, eyes and ears**
- Scorbutic condition of bleeding gums
- Bleeding piles, aggravated during menses
- **Epistaxis when washing the face and hands in the morning, from left nostril, after eating**
- Stopping of nose mostly at night; must breathe through the mouth; snuffles of infants
- Enlarged tonsils and glands of neck
- Marked anxiety in cardiac region with faintness and palpitations
- Menses frequent, profuse, clotted and premature
- Leucorrhoea watery, burning, itching; swelling, burning in pudenda
- **Cholera-like symptoms at the commencement of menses**
- Muscles are soft and flabby. Numbness and stiffness of arms and hands

CLINICAL
- Anxiety
- Fainting
- Uncleanliness
- Haemorrhages
- Obesity
- Constipation
- Haemorrhoids
- Epistaxis
- Allergy
- Sinusitis
- Rhinitis
- Pharyngitis
- Cough
- Bronchitis
- Pulmonary oedema
- Pneumonia
- Emphysema
- Thyroiditis
- Congestive cardiac failure
- Dysmenorrhoea
- Menorrhagia
- Erysipelas
- Gangrene

MODALITIES
- **Aggravation:** Cold wet weather, wet poultices, from washing, during menses, motion, falling asleep
- **Amelioration:** Lying on abdomen, on painful side, in dry weather

REMEDY RELATIONSHIP
- **Antidotes:** Poisoning with Rhus-t. and stings of insects
- **Inimical:** Lach.
- **Compare:** Ant-t., Carb-v., Glon., Lach., Mur-ac., Rhus-t.

AMMONIUM CAUSTICUM

INTRODUCTION

- **Common name:** Hydrate of ammonia, Ammonia water, Ammonium hydroxide
- **Group:** Base
- **Source:** Mineral kingdom
- **Formula:** NH_4OH
- **Prover:** Wibmer

SPHERE OF ACTION

- Nose
- Throat
- Gastrointestinal system
- Respiratory system
- Muscular system

CONSTITUTION

- Used as a powerful cardiac stimulant in syncope, haemorrhages, snake bites, etc. by inhalation
- **Temperament:** Nervous
- **Thermal:** Chilly
- **Miasm:** Psora

MIND

- Timidity, great tendency to get frightened
- Great anguish
- Makes mistakes in talking
- Great excitement in the evening
- Restlessness
- Nervousness at night

CLINICAL

- Exhaustion
- Oedema
- Syncope
- Ulceration
- Snake bites
- Muscular debility
- Excoriating discharges
- Haemorrhage
- Aphonia
- Croup
- Nasal diphtheria
- Respiration difficult
- Spasm of glottis
- Thrombosis
- Cardiac failure
- Arthritis
- Rheumatism of shoulder

KEYNOTE SYMPTOMS

- Severe exhaustion and muscular debility
- Powerful cardiac stimulant; can be used by inhalation in syncope
- Burning sensation experienced especially in throat, gullet and rectum
- **White patches on tongue and inside of cheeks**
- **Intense thirst; contents of the stomach are ejected violently**
- Useful in membranous croup with burning in oesophagus
- **Uvula covered with white mucous**
- Aphonia, loss of voice. Voice low and weak. Speech broken. A good all round remedy in aphonia.
- Burning rawness in throat. Scraping and burning in throat and oesophagus. Pain in oesophagus on breathing deeply.
- Difficult respiration. Accumulation of mucous with incessant coughing; patient gasps for breath

MODALITIES

- **Aggravation:** After eating or drinking, in the evening

REMEDY RELATIONSHIP

- **Compare:** Am-c., Caust.

AMMONIUM MURIATICUM

SPHERE OF ACTION
- Mind
- Eyes
- Gastrointestinal system
- Respiratory system
- Musculoskeletal system
- Female genital system
- Skin

INTRODUCTION
- **Common name:** Sal ammoniac, Ammonium chloride
- **Group:** Salt
- **Source:** Mineral kingdom
- **Formula:** NH_4Cl
- **Prover:** Nenning

CONSTITUTION
- Adapted to fat, puffy, sluggish people with thin legs and a tendency to respiratory problems
- **Temperament:** Nervous, bilious
- **Thermal:** Chilly
- **Miasm:** Psora, Sycosis, Syphilis

MIND
- Involuntary aversion to certain people
- Melancholic and apprehensive; as from internal grief
- Desire to cry, but cannot
- Great anguish, as from vexation or cares with inclination to shed tears
- Fear of darkness
- Irritability, worse contradiction

KEYNOTE SYMPTOMS
- **Body is fat and large with large buttocks but thin legs**
- Profuse glairy mucous discharges with many complaints
- Boiling sensation; blood seems to be in constant turmoil, sensation of pulsations
- Chronic congestion of liver
- Scanty, hard, crumbly stool, covered with glairy mucous
- Blood from anus, or diarrhoea during menses
- Feeling of tension and tightness, as if muscles and tendons are too short
- Haemorrhoids after suppressed leucorrhoea
- Watery, acrid coryza. Scanty expectoration. Nose feels stuffy and obstructed.
- Noisy, rattling tenacious mucous in chest
- Hoarseness in larynx with burning
- **Leucorrhoea like the white of an egg; pain around naval before discharge; however, after urination, it becomes brown, slimy and painless**
- Menorrhagia, flow more at night
- **Sensation of coldness in back between shoulders in catarrhal conditions and chest affections such as cough**

CLINICAL
- Cataract
- Haemorrhoids
- Catarrh
- Sneezing
- Coryza
- Anosmia
- Tonsillitis
- Hoarseness
- Bronchitis
- Polyuria
- Menorrhagia
- Prolapse
- Lumbago
- Sciatica
- Fatty tumours

MODALITIES
- **Aggravation:** Head and chest symptoms are worse in the morning, abdominal symptoms in the afternoon, walking erect
- **Amelioration:** Open air, motion, warm bath

REMEDY RELATIONSHIP
- **Antidotes:** Coff., Nux-v., Caust.
- **Compare:** Calc., Seneg., Caust., Nat-m., Valer., Mur-ac., Rhus-t.

ANACARDIUM ORIENTALE

INTRODUCTION

- **Common name:** Marking nut
- **Family:** *Ancardiaceae*
- **Source:** Vegetable kingdom
- **Part used:** The resinous juice of the seed

SPHERE OF ACTION

- Mind
- Gastrointestinal system
- Respiratory system
- Nerves
- Musculoskeletal system
- Urinary system

MIND

- Great weakness of memory; sudden loss of memory
- Lack of confidence
- **Illusion of duality–as if possessed by two persons or wills; as if an angel or demon is sitting on his shoulder telling him to do good or bad**
- Physical and mental lack of power. Weakness, fatigue, brain fag
- Absentminded
- Religious mania, as if possessed
- Fear of examination
- Nervous exhaustion from over study
- Fear of failure, of someone behind him
- Fear or delusion, or dreams of being pursued; suspicious
- Suicidal – maniacal depressed; suspicious
- Tendency to curse and swear
- Malicious; tends towards wickedness
- Ailments from humiliation; victims of abuse – verbal, sexual or physical

MODALITIES

- **Aggravation:** On application of hot water, mental exertion, abuse and mortification, draft of air, open air, fasting
- **Amelioration:** From eating, lying on side, rubbing, heat

KEYNOTE SYMPTOMS

- Lack of physical and mental powers. Weakness of all senses; objects appear far away (eyes); sense of smell perverted (nose)
- **Eating temporarily relieves all symptoms; worse fasting**
- Ailments from anger, fright, care, sedentary habits, examination, mental exertion, over study; consequences of mortification, suppressed eruptions in different parts
- **Sensation of a plug, or a band, or a hoop in various parts like head, rectum, bladder, etc.**
- Eructation, nausea, vomiting
- Empty sensation in stomach with weakness and irritability
- Pressing headache, as if from a plug, worse mental exertion, better eating
- Inactive bowels. **Rectum feels powerless; soft stools passed with difficulty, ineffectual desire for stool.** Sensation as if rectum is plugged up
- Dull pressure in shoulder as if from weight with palpitation
- Cramp-like pains in muscles; contraction of joints; injured or strained tendons

CONSTITUTION

- Adapted to neurasthenic, hypochondriacal, hysterical women with diminished sense of smell, sight and hearing
- Suits maniac depressives
- **Temperament:** Nervous
- **Thermal:** Ambithermal
- **Miasm:** Syphilis

CLINICAL

- Neurasthenia
- Behavioural problems
- Phobia
- Maniacal depression
- Paranoia
- Inferiority complex
- Suicidal tendencies
- Schizophrenia
- Weak memory
- Dementia
- Hallucinations
- Vertigo
- Halitosis
- Nausea
- Vomiting
- Dyspepsia
- Gastritis
- Peptic ulcer
- Haemorrhoids
- Deafness
- Pericarditis
- Rheumatism
- Rhus poisoning
- Eczema
- Urticaria
- Insomnia
- Lichen planus

REMEDY RELATIONSHIP

- **Antidotes:** Grin., Coff., Jug-c., Rhus-t., Eucal.
- **Compare:** Anac-oc. erysipelas, vesicular facial eruptions, anaesthetic variety of leprosy; warts, corns, ulcers, cracking of skin on soles of feet; Rhus-t., Cypr., Chel., Xero.
- **Follows well:** Plat.

SPHERE OF ACTION

- Gastrointestinal system
- Mucous membranes
- Nervous system
- Muscular system
- Skin

INTRODUCTION

- **Common name:** Bacillus anthracis
- **Group:** Nosode
- **Part used:** Sterile lysate of the anthrax poison
- **Prover:** Lux

CONSTITUTION

- For boils, acne, carbuncles, malignant ulcers and a dirty look
- **Temperament:** Cancerous
- **Thermal:** Ambithermal
- **Miasm:** Syphilis

ANTHRACINUM

MIND

- Depressed and irritable; melancholic
- Confused
- Restless and nervous at night
- Feels death is approaching

KEYNOTE SYMPTOMS

- Very vulnerable to malignant and septic inflammation of connective or cellular tissue
- Terrible burning with great prostration, weakness and enervations
- **Haemorrhages – thick, black, tar-like from any orifice; rapidly decomposing**
- Glands are swollen; cellular tissue is oedematous and indurated
- Enlarged lymphatic glands; **hard, stony swelling of right lower jaw and submaxillary glands**
- Septic fevers with great prostration. Sinking pulse, delirium and fainting
- Dissecting wounds turn gangrenous. Septic inflammations; carbuncles and malignant ulcers with induration of cellular tissue
- Septicaemia, tendency to boils, acne; ulceration with terrible, burning pains and sloughing
- Malignant ulcers, carbuncles, succession of boils and carbuncles

CLINICAL

- Prostration
- Haemorrhages
- Enlarged lymphatic glands
- Parotitis, gangrenous
- Septicaemia
- Fever
- Malignant ulcers
- Boils
- Abscesses
- Carbuncles
- Gangrene
- Dissecting wounds
- Insect stings
- Acne
- Erysipelas
- Cellulitis

MODALITIES

- **Aggravation:** Cold application
- **Amelioration:** Warm application

REMEDY RELATIONSHIP

- **When Ars. or the best selected remedy fails to relieve the burning pain of carbuncle or malignant ulceration.**
- **Compare to:** Ars., Carb-ac., Lach., Sec., Pyrog., Tarent-c., Echi. in malignant and septic conditions.
- **Follows well:** Ars.

ANTIMONIUM ARSENICOSUM

SPHERE OF ACTION
- Gastrointestinal system
- Respiratory system
- Blood
- Circulatory system

INTRODUCTION
- **Common name:** Arsenite of antimony, Antimony arsenate
- **Group:** Salt
- **Source:** Mineral kingdom
- **Formula:** $SbAsO_4$

CONSTITUTION
- Suits people with a tendency to lung affections – emphysema and excessive dyspnoea
- **Temperament:** Bilious, anxious
- **Thermal:** Chilly
- **Miasm:** Psora, Syphilis

MIND
- Sadness
- Irritability, worse contradiction
- Fearful
- Desires company
- Restlessness

KEYNOTE SYMPTOMS
- Prostration, sense of weakness
- Increased thirst
- **Affects preferably the upper left lung**
- Emphysema with excessive dyspnoea and cough, with much mucous secretion. Rattling of mucous in the chest
- Equally effective in old, right sided cases of pneumonia and catarrhal pneumonia in children
- Catarrhal pneumonia associated with influenza
- Pleurisy, especially of left side with exudation, pericarditis and effusion
- Cardiac with weakness and myocarditis

CLINICAL
- Diarrhoea
- Dysentery
- Haemorrhoids
- Influenza
- Dyspnoea
- Asthma
- Catarrhal pneumonia
- Emphysema
- Pleurisy
- Broncho-pneumonia
- Bronchitis
- Pericarditis

MODALITIES
- **Aggravation:** Eating, lying down, left side

REMEDY RELATIONSHIP
- **Compare:** Other Antimony salts; Ars., Aur., Lach., Puls., Sulph.

ANTIMONIUM CRUDUM

INTRODUCTION
- **Common name:** Black sulphide of antimony trisulphide
- **Group:** Salt
- **Source:** Mineral kingdom
- **Formula:** Sb_2S_3

SPHERE OF ACTION
- Mind
- Gastrointestinal system
- Respiratory system
- Musculoskeletal system
- Female genital system

MIND
- Bad effects of disappointed love
- Great anxiety about his fate
- Inclination to shoot himself
- Fretful, cross and peevish; extremely irritable
- Cries, if looked at, or touched, or washed, especially in children
- Adults are sulky, do not wish to speak with anyone
- Loathing of life, of food, of bathing
- Ecstasy and exalted love
- Excitability
- **Dreamy, sentimental mood in moonlight and twilight, during diarrhoea, before menses**
- Soft, sensitive and emotional
- **Disposed to talk in rhymes and verses**

MODALITIES
- **Aggravation:** After eating, cold baths, acids or sour wine, after heat of sun or fire, extremes of cold, or heat, cold water, moonlight; getting drunk
- **Amelioration:** In open air, during rest, after a warm bath

KEYNOTE SYMPTOMS
- Irritable, peevish children who cannot bear to be touched or looked at
- Moroseness and loathing of life after long illness or disappointment in love
- **All symptoms are aggravated by heat or cold bathing**
- **Thick, white coating of tongue like a fur with gastric complaints**
- **Loss of appetite; desire for acids and pickles**
- Eructations taste of ingesta; constant belching, chronic indigestion
- Gastric complaints from bread, pastry, acids, hot weather, cold things. Bloating after eating. Distended abdomen with much rumbling.
- **Thirst in the evening**
- Vomiting after eating and drinking
- Alternate diarrhoea and constipation; stool in hard lumps mixed with a watery discharge. Constipation from abuse of laxative
- Loss of voice from becoming overheated
- Feet covered with large horny corns. Warts
- Eczema accompanies gastric derangements; thick, hard, honey coloured scabs
- Callosities from slight pressure

CONSTITUTION
- For old people with a tendency to morning diarrhoea continuous drowsiness
- Adapted to children and young with a tendency to grow fat
- **Temperament:** Nervous, scrofulous
- **Thermal:** Chilly
- **Miasm:** Sycosis, Syphilis

CLINICAL
- Depression
- Chronic fatigue syndrome
- Obesity
- Headache
- Blepharitis
- Glossitis
- Heartburn
- Vomiting
- Peptic ulcer
- Gastritis
- Diarrhoea
- Constipation
- Haemorrhoids
- Proctitis
- Laryngitis
- Menopausal complaints
- Arthritis
- Callosities
- Chickenpox
- Urticarea
- Impetigo
- Warts

REMEDY RELATIONSHIP
- **Complementary:** Squil., Sulph.
- **Compare:** Bry., Ip., Lyc., Puls.,
- **Follows well:** Puls., Ip.

SPHERE OF ACTION

- Head
- Gastrointestinal system
- Respiratory system
- Skin

INTRODUCTION

- **Common name:** Tartar emetic, Tartarate of antimony and potash
- **Group:** Acid
- **Source:** Mineral kingdom
- **Formula:** $K(SbO)C_4H_4O_6 \cdot \frac{1}{2} H_2O$
- **Prover:** Hottereb and Trinks

CONSTITUTION

- It is the hydrogenoid constitution of Grauvogl; torpid, phlegmatic persons
- Suits old people and children; gouty, worn out subjects
- **Temperament:** Nervous
- **Thermal:** Chilly
- **Miasm:** Sycosis

ANTIMONIUM TARTARICUM

MIND

- Fear of being alone
- Bad humour. Despondent
- Frightened at every trifle
- Muttering delirium
- Stupid on awakening
- Apathy or easily annoyed; wants to be left alone
- Despair of recovery
- Child continuously wishes to be carried erect, unwilling to be looked at, or touched
- Child clings to attendants; irritable, peevish, whining and moaning
- Overwhelming sleepiness

KEYNOTE SYMPTOMS

- Lack of vital reaction; patient is physically and mentally prostrated
- Ill-effects of vaccination
- Debility, drowsiness (an irresistible desire to sleep) and sweat accompany all symptoms
- Vertigo alternates with drowsiness, dullness and confusion, band-like feeling over forehead
- Face is cold, blue, pale, covered with cold sweat
- **Absence of thirst**
- Nausea, retching, vomiting; nausea is in waves. Bitter, sour substance vomited
- **Craving for apples, fruits and acids**
- Congestion and catarrh of respiratory system; **rattling of mucous with scanty expectoration, death rattle**
- Lungs seem full of mucous, yet very less is raised
- Cough, cold, coryza with rattling of mucous but scanty, difficult expectoration, unable to get it out; suffocation, shortness of breath

CLINICAL

- Sepsis
- Vertigo
- Spasmodic colic
- Cholera morbus
- Asphyxia
- Respiratory infections
- Hoarseness
- Bronchitis
- Chronic obstructive pulmonary disease
- Pneumonia
- Pertussis
- Congestive heart failure
- Cyanosis
- Cystitis
- Urethritis
- Orchitis
- Intermittent fever
- Impetigo
- Chickenpox
- Warts
- Pustular eruptions

MODALITIES

- **Aggravation:** In the evening, from lying down at night, from warmth, in damp cold weather, from all sour things and milk
- **Amelioration:** Sitting erect, eructation, expectoration, vomiting

REMEDY RELATIONSHIP

- **Antidotes:** Puls., Bar-c., Bry., Caust., Sep.
- **Compare:** Kali-s., Ip., Acon., Ars., Bry., Verat., Op., Thuj.
- **Follows well:** Sil. in dyspnoea; Puls in nausea, in chest and gonorrheal suppression

APIS MELLIFICA

INTRODUCTION
- **Common name:** Honey bee
- **Family:** *Apidae*
- **Source:** Animal kingdom
- **Part used:** The live bee

SPHERE OF ACTION
- Mind
- Eyes
- Gastrointestinal system
- Respiratory system
- Urinary system
- Genital system
- Mucous membranes
- Serous membranes

CONSTITUTION
- For a strumous constitution with indurated and enlarged glands
- Adapted to women, especially widows who are awkward and drop things easily
- **Temperament:** Nervous
- **Thermal:** Hot
- **Miasm:** Psora

MIND
- Absentminded, cannot concent-rate
- Indifferent or apathetic
- Awkward, lets things fall from her hands and laughs
- Unconsciousness, impaired memory and slow march of ideas
- Weepiness, cannot help crying
- Cannot bear to be left alone, busy and restless
- Depression, as if she would die
- Mania from sexual irritation. Increased sexual desire in widows with much jealousy
- Fear of being poisoned
- Low muttering delirium following suppressed eruptions

KEYNOTE SYMPTOMS
- **Right side is affected.** Symptoms proceed from right to left
- Bad effects or ailments from fright, grief, jealousy, vexation and rage
- **Sensitiveness to touch with a general soreness; even the touch of hair is painful**
- Burning, stinging, pains with redness and swelling accompany most symptoms
- Puffiness and oedema of various parts. Oedematous swellings, local or general, with skin whitish, waxen, almost transparent. In general dropsy, skin is alternately dry and perspiring.
- Prostration upto fainting
- Sudden shrill, piercing cries or shrieks, especially in children. Sensitive. Rolls the head.
- Adipsia with oedema; but thirsty during chill. Burning heat
- Urine scanty, high coloured; Incontinence of urine; burning when micturating last few drops burn and smart
- Tension, swelling and stiffness of limbs. Tired and bruised all over
- **Intermittent fever; afternoon chill, at 3 pm with thirst;** worse warmth and external heat
- Swelling after bites, urticaria; erysipelas; carbuncles; cellulitis
- Allergic oedema of face, eyelids, lips, mouth and throat. Also, redness and swelling with pain, burning and stinging in eyes, eyelids, ears, face, lips, tongue, anus, throat, testicles
- **Large urticaria like bee stings with intolerable itching at night**
- Puffy, allergic eyelids like water bags. Intense chemosis of conjunctiva. Suppurative inflammation of eyes

CLINICAL
- Malignancy
- Allergy
- Neuralgia
- Angioneurotic oedema
- Meningitis
- Conjunctivitis
- Corneal ulcer
- Keratitis
- Fistula lachrymalis
- Diarrhoea
- Constipation
- Pharyngitis
- Throat swollen
- Pleurisy
- Pneumonia
- Cystitis
- Nephritis
- Pyelonephritis
- Premenstrual syndrome
- Abortions
- Arthritis
- Scoliosis
- Psoriasis
- Urticaria
- Herpes zoster
- Insect bites
- Bee stings
- Erysipelas
- Rashes
- Dermatitis

MODALITIES
- **Aggravation:** Heat, touch, pressure, late in the afternoon, after sleeping, is closed and heated rooms, suppressed eruptions
- **Amelioration:** In open cool air, uncovering, cold bathing, motion

REMEDY RELATIONSHIP
- **Complementary: Nat-m. is the chronic of Apis;** also Bar-c., if lymphatics are involved
- **Inimical:** Rhus-t. in eruptive diseases
- **Compare:** Zinc., Canth., Vesp., Lach., Puls., Bell., Ars., Bry., Rhus-t.

APOCYNUM CANNABINUM

INTRODUCTION

- **Common name:** Hemp
- **Family:** *Apocynaceae*
- **Source:** Vegetable kingdom
- **Part used:** Rhizome and roots
- **Prover:** Freitag

SPHERE OF ACTION

- Gastrointestinal system
- Cardiovascular system
- Respiratory system
- Urinary system
- Serous membranes

MIND

- Alcoholism, dipsomania
- Loss of ambition
- **Anxiety, especially felt in the abdomen after stool**
- Mentally confused, especially during paroxysm of pain; cannot think
- Bewildered, low-spirited at night
- Nervous
- Desires company
- Restlessness, especially at night

MODALITIES

- **Aggravation:** Cold weather, cold drinks, uncovering, lying down, after sleep
- **Amelioration:** Warmth

KEYNOTE SYMPTOMS

- Dropsy – acute, inflammatory – with or without organic diseases
- **Oedema or dropsy everywhere with scanty discharges of sweat or urine. Patient feels that if only he could sweat, he would feel better.**
- Increases mucous and serous secretions causing dropsy and oedema
- **Faints when raised from pillow**
- Loss of power; loss of muscular power, relaxed sphincters
- Severe vomiting, food and water are immediately thrown off, sinking sensation in the stomach
- Abdomen – bloated sensation; ascites
- Anxiety before stool; watery stool with soreness of anus
- Short, dry cough; takes cold easily
- **Must take frequent deep inspirations; short, unsatisfactory breaths; suffocation**
- Pulse is slow, irregular or weak, dropsical
- Pulse intermittent, fluttering, at times feeble. Darting and oppressed feeling in the cardiac region
- Tricuspid and mitral regurgitation
- Congestive cardiac failure, weak heart leading to oedema, especially of the heart, pericardium and limbs

CONSTITUTION

- Adapted to sanguine constitutions, especially of; young girls with dropsy of abdomen and extremities
- **Temperament:** Nervous
- **Thermal:** Chilly
- **Miasm:** Sycosis

CLINICAL

- Dropsy
- Anasarca
- Hydrocephalus
- Vomiting
- Gastritis
- Diarrhoea
- Ascites
- Pleural effusion
- Hypotension
- Fatty degeneration of the heart
- Mitral regurgitation
- Tricuspid regurgitation
- Cardiac dropsy
- Fluttering of heart
- Renal disease
- Nephritis
- Nephrotic syndrome
- Bright's disease

REMEDY RELATIONSHIP

- **Compare:** Acet-ac., Apis., Ars., Chin., Dig., in dropsical affections; Stroph-h., in extreme cardiac depression with gastric disturbance
- Blatta-o. has cured bad cases of general dropsy, after Apis, Apoc., and Dig. failed

ARALIA RACEMOSA

INTRODUCTION

- **Common name:** American spikenard
- **Family:** *Araliaceae*
- **Source:** Vegetable kingdom
- **Part used:** Roots
- **Prover:** Dr S.A. Jones

SPHERE OF ACTION

- Nose
- Throat
- Gastrointestinal system
- Respiratory system
- Nervous system

CONSTITUTION

- Adapted to weak, relaxed, exhausted and nauseated patients
- **Temperament:** Nervous, bilious
- **Thermal:** Chilly
- **Miasm:** Psora, Sycosis

MIND

- Fear of lung diseases that cannot be overcome
- Sensitiveness
- Dullness
- Restlessness
- Anxiety

KEYNOTE SYMPTOMS

- Patient is weak, relaxed, exhausted and nauseated. **Drenching night sweats**
- Biliousness and acrid mucous secretions
- Extreme sensitiveness to draughts of cold air
- **The least current of cold air causes frequent sneezing, hay fever, rawness and burning**
- Tendency to **acrid mucous secretions**
- Dry cough coming on after first sleep, on lying down, worse 11 pm. Sensation of a foreign body in the throat
- Copious, watery, excoriating nasal discharge of salty, acrid taste in hay fever
- Asthmatic conditions, with wheezing respiration immediately aggravated on lying down at night, after first sleep

CLINICAL

- Flatulence
- Diarrhoea
- Constipation
- Haemorrhoids
- Fissure-in-ano
- Rhinitis
- Sinusitis
- Sneezing
- Hay fever
- Coryza
- Cough
- Asthma
- Pneumonia
- Bronchitis
- Amenorrhoea
- Leucorrhoea

MODALITIES

- **Aggravation:** Around 11 pm (cough), draft of air, short nap
- **Amelioration:** Lying with head high, sitting up

REMEDY RELATIONSHIP

- **Compare:** Pect. in humid asthma; Ars-i., Naphtin., All-c., Rosa, Sabad., Sin-n., Gins., Hed., Calc.
- **Complementary:** Lob.

ARANEA DIADEMA

SPHERE OF ACTION
- Mind
- Gastrointestinal system
- Respiratory system
- Nervous system
- Musculoskeletal system
- Female genital system

INTRODUCTION
- **Common name:** Papal-cross spider
- **Family:** *Arachnidae*
- **Source:** Animal kingdom
- **Part used:** Whole spider

CONSTITUTION
- Suits hydrogenoid constitution; patient feels cold to the very bones, not relieved by anything
- **Temperament:** Nervous, phlegmatic
- **Thermal:** Chilly
- **Miasm:** Psora, Sycosis

MIND
- Nervous temperament
- Despondent
- Longs for death
- Delusion that he is swollen
- Confusion; better by smoking in open air
- **Frightful dreams, waking him up screaming**
- Morose, peevish, sad during intermittent fever
- Inner unrest, irritability
- Objects and people seem unreal
- Alternately depressed and happy

KEYNOTE SYMPTOMS
- **Marked periodicity of symptoms**
- Abnormal susceptibility to damp and cold. **Inability to live near fresh water, river, lakes, etc. or in damp, chilly places. Chilly day and night**
- **Patient feels cold to the very bones, cannot get warm enough**
- Patient is subject to neuralgias due to humid cold. Periodic neuralgias; facial neuralgia, trigeminal neuralgia, of occipital nerves and limbs
- Tendency to haemorrhages from any part, especially from wounds and lungs – violent haemoptysis
- Restless, wakes up frequently, sensation of swelling
- Feeling as if parts are enlarged and heavier, feeling twice their natural size; splenomegaly
- **Head feels numb and pains; better by smoking or in open air**
- Gastric, intestinal and urinary complaints are accompanied by cramping pains
- Quietness and sleep in cardiac affections
- Pain in os calcis. **Coldness, with pain in long bones; sensation as if bones were made of ice**
- Very early and very copious menses with pain in lumbar and sacral regions
- **Menstrual discharge smells of ammonia**

CLINICAL
- Neuralgia
- Haemorrhage
- Malarial poisoning
- Headache
- Toothache
- Diarrhoea
- Splenomegaly
- Haemoptysis
- Phthisis
- Asthma
- Menorrhagia
- Arthritis
- Cramps
- Periostitis
- Calcanean spur
- Plantar fasciitis
- Punctured wounds
- Insomnia

MODALITIES
- **Aggravation:** Damp weather, cold weather, late in the afternoon, at midnight
- **Amelioration:** Smoking tobacco, open air, summer, movement

REMEDY RELATIONSHIP
- **Compare:** Cedr., Mygal., Tarent., Ip., Nux-v., Apis., Ther., Tela
- **Antidotes:** Chin., Merc.

ARGENTUM METALLICUM

SPHERE OF ACTION
- Mind
- Larynx
- Respiratory system
- Female genital system
- Mucous membranes
- Ligaments
- Cartilages
- Bones

INTRODUCTION
- **Common name:** Silver
- **Group:** Metal
- **Source:** Mineral kingdom
- **Formula:** Ag
- **Prover:** Hahnemann

CONSTITUTION
- For broken down constitutions; suffer from loss of muscular power and trembling; emaciation
- **Temperament:** Nervous
- **Thermal:** Chilly
- **Miasm:** Sycosis

MIND
- Mental exertion aggravates complaints
- Apprehensive about their health
- Disinclination to talk
- Imbecility from disorders of intellect and memory
- Forgetful
- Loss of control over mind or body
- Hurried feeling
- Time passes slowly
- Melancholic, depressed
- Neurosis from worry; restless anxiety
- Epileptic attacks followed by delirious rage, jumping about, striking those near

KEYNOTE SYMPTOMS
- **Left sided complaints**
- Ill-effects of onanism, sunstroke, anger, fear, fright, overuse of voice
- Emaciation, a gradual drying up
- Symptoms appear gradually but are progressive and deep penetrating
- **Desires for fresh air, dyspnoea**
- **Secretions of mucous membranes are thick, grey, tenacious or like boiled starch; for example, jelly-like mucous from the throat; expectoration like boiled starch; turbid urine**
- Chief action causes – thickening of the tissues, especially cartilages
- Hoarseness or aphonia in professional singers
- **Raw feeling, weakness of chest; worse use of voice**
- Leucorrhoea – foul, corroding, of bloody water; cervix is spongy and eroded
- Haemorrhage during menopause; abdomen feels sore
- Rheumatic affection of joints, swelling of ankles, involuntary contraction of fingers, paralysis of forearm
- Cartilage affections; thickening of cartilage in articulations
- Cramps in muscles, limps feel powerless

CLINICAL
- Infiltrations
- Induration
- Cysts
- Tumours
- Ulcerations
- Epithelioma
- Paralysis
- Vertigo
- Laryngitis
- Aphonia
- Coryza
- Polyuria
- Ovarian cyst
- Chronic gonorrhoea
- Rheumatism
- Arthritis
- Writer's cramps

MODALITIES
- **Aggravation:** Touch, towards noon, using voice, sun, entering a warm room
- **Amelioration:** Open air, cough at night when lying down (opposite Hyos.), motion, wrapping up

REMEDY RELATIONSHIP
- **Antidotes:** Merc., Puls., Zinc., Pall., Stann.
- **Compare:** Sel., Alum., Plat., Stann., Ampe-qu., Arg-n., Sep., Calc., Med., Psor.
- **Follows well:** Alum., Plat.

ARGENTUM NITRICUM

SPHERE OF ACTION
- Mind
- Eyes
- Gastrointestinal system
- Respiratory system
- Musculoskeletal system
- Urinary system

INTRODUCTION
- **Common name:** Nitrate of silver, Silver nitrate
- **Group:** Salt
- **Source:** Mineral kingdom
- **Formula:** $AgNO_3$
- **Prover:** Hahnemann

CONSTITUTION
- Suits dried up, old looking persons with anticipatory anxiety; they are hurried and worried
- **Temperament**: Nervous, bilious
- **Thermal**: Hot
- **Miasm**: Sycosis

MIND
- Time passes slowly
- **Great apprehension, especially when getting ready for church, opera, examination, or any other engagement, diarrhoea sets in**
- Full of fears and phobias – of impending doom, of being poisoned
- Full of anticipation; dreads ordeals; performance anxiety
- **Great fear of projecting buildings on street corners, which creates a sensation as if it would fall over him**
- Heights make the patient dizzy
- Suicidal tendency prevails on crossing a bridge, at high places or looking out through a window; melancholic
- Impulsive, wants to do things in a hurry
- Unexplainable, foolish, peculiar impulses
- Obstinate, against whatever was proposed he had the queerest objection
- Nervous. Brain fag. Lack of ambition.

KEYNOTE SYMPTOMS
- **Splinter – like sensation in throat, difficult swallowing; strangulated feeling**
- Acute or chronic diseases from unusual or long continued mental exertion
- Trembling of affected parts
- Pains increase and decrease gradually; splinter-like pains are characteristic
- Loss of control, inco-ordination mentally and physically
- Epilepsy from fright
- Intolerance of heat
- Mucous membranes are inflamed and ulcerated, causing muco-purulent discharges and splinter-like pains. Violent pains as if sticking deep inside, like a splinter or sharp shooting pains
- Dull chronic headache of students
- Acute conjuctivitis; eyes appear scarlet red, like raw beef
- Ophthalmia neonatorum
- **Craves sugar, which aggravates**
- Flatulent distention of abdomen with bursting sensation and colic
- Loud explosive belching upwards and downwards
- Gastric ulcers-gnawing, ulcerating pains which radiate
- Stools expelled with much fluttering
- **Diarrhoea–green like chopped spinach; especially after eating**
- High notes cause cough. Chronic laryngitis of singers.
- Paraplegia from exhaustion; emaciation, especially of lower extremities

MODALITIES
- **Aggravation:** Cold food, cold drinks, eating sugar, ice cream, sweets, unusual mental exertion, anxiety, apprehension
- **Amelioration:** Open air, craves the wind blowing on his face, bathing with cold water, cool air, hard pressure, belching

CLINICAL
- Anxiety
- Panic attacks
- Examination funk
- Agoraphobia
- Abusive
- Epilepsy
- Brain fag
- Acute conjuctivitis
- Blepharitis
- Iritis
- Ophthalmia neonatorum
- Gastric ulcer
- Flatulence
- Emotional diarrhoea
- Rectal abscess
- Otitis media
- Tonsillitis
- Laryngitis
- Pharyngitis
- Sinusitis
- Dyspnoea
- Asthma
- Croup
- Bronchitis
- Pleurisy
- Dysuria
- Urethral stricture
- Urethritis
- Diabetes
- Gonorrhoea
- Mastitis
- Balanitis
- Multiple sclerosis
- Addisons disease
- Locomotor ataxia
- Eczema
- Paronychia
- Acne
- Ulcers
- Herpes

REMEDY RELATIONSHIP
- **Compare to:** Nat-m., Nit-ac., Lach., Aur., Cupr., Kali-bi., Thuj., Ars., Merc., Phos.
- Nat-m. for the bad effects of cauterizing with nitrate of silver.
- Coffea increases nervous headache.
- After Verat.; Lyc. follows well in flatulent dyspepsia

ARNICA MONTANA

INTRODUCTION

- **Common name:** Leopard's bane
- **Family:** *Compositae*
- **Source:** Vegetable kingdom
- **Part used:** Whole plant
- **Prover:** Hahnemann

SPHERE OF ACTION

- Mind
- Gastrointestinal system
- Respiratory system
- Heart
- Musculoskeletal system
- Female genital system
- Skin

CONSTITUTION

- Acts best in sanguine, plethoric persons disposed to cerebral congestion
- Used in debilitated persons with impoverished blood
- **Temperament:** Nervous, bilious
- **Thermal:** Chilly
- **Miasm:** Psora, Sycosis

MIND

- Useful in severe mental stress or mental, emotional shocks
- Stupor, can be aroused, answers correctly and then slips into coma
- **Says nothing is the matter with him and sends the doctor away**
- Fear of being struck, or touched, or approached. Agrophobia.
- Fear of wind, sudden death
- Wants to be left alone. Indifference.
- Delirious
- Nervous. Oversensitive. Restlessness.
- Depression following head injury
- Any injury or stroke causes mental dysfunctions

KEYNOTE SYMPTOMS

- Ailments from injuries, falls, blows, excessive hard work, concussion, excessive use of any organ, contusion, for trauma in any form
- Trauma, mental or physical, and their effects, recent or remote
- **Sore, lame, bruised feeling all over the body as if beaten. Everything lain on, even bed seems too hard. Body is oversensitive to touch**
- Stupor with involuntary discharge of urine and stool
- Cerebral congestion
- Nose feels cold
- Foetid breath, vomiting, stool; putridity; septic conditions
- Whooping cough or violent, spasmodic cough, causing bloodshot eyes or epistaxis
- Palpitation or angina after shock or injury. Heart strained after violent running.
- Bladder affections after mechanical injuries
- Soreness from overexertion; limbs feel as if beaten; muscles sore and aching during influenza
- Back achy and sore from over lifting, overuse and strain
- **During fever, heat of upper part of body and coldness of lower**
- **Crops of small boils; acne characterised by bilateral symmetry. Tendency to blue black spots**

CLINICAL

- Injury
- Trauma
- Concussion
- Contusion
- Neuralgia
- Shock
- Septic condition
- Extravasation of blood
- Stroke
- Ecchymosis
- Thrombosis
- Concussion of brain
- Apoplexy
- Vertigo
- Asthenopia
- Tinnitus
- Diplopia
- Black eye
- Epistaxis
- Dysentery
- Pneumonia
- Pleurisy
- Cystitis
- Emphysema
- Haematocoele
- Rheumatism
- Sprains
- Pimples
- Petechiae
- Boils
- Acne
- Bedsores
- Traumatic fever
- Typhoid

MODALITIES

- **Aggravation:** Least touch, motion, rest, wine, damp, cold, over exertion, sprains, after sleep
- **Amelioration:** Lying down, or lying with head low

REMEDY RELATIONSHIP

- **Antidotes:** Camph.
- **Complementary:** Acon., Ip.
- **Compare:** Acon., Bapt., Bell-p., Ham., Rhus-t., Hyper., Symph.
- **Follows well:** Acon., Ip., Apis, Verat.

ARSENICUM ALBUM

INTRODUCTION

- **Common name:** Arsenious acid, Arsenic trioxide
- **Group:** Acid
- **Source:** Mineral kingdom
- **Formula:** As_2O_3
- **Prover:** Hahnemann

SPHERE OF ACTION

- Mind
- Gastrointestinal system
- Respiratory system
- Cardiovascular system
- Blood
- Urinary system
- Mucous membranes

MIND

- Mentally very anxious, highly sensitive
- Anguish, lack of courage, begs for help
- Anxiety about health
- Insecurity, feels vulnerable in an unsafe world
- **Fastidious, obsessed with order and tidiness. Fault-finding**
- Violence, self-torture, pulls her hair, bites her own nails and tears at own body
- **Restless mentally but physically too weak to move**
- Fears being alone, of cancer, robbers, poverty. Fear of death, comes at the later stage of disease, thinks it is useless to take medicine, as disease is incurable
- Moans and groans
- Despair drives the patient from one place to another
- Mania, insanity, suicidal impulses, wants to be held
- Patient is very domineering and demanding

MODALITIES

- **Aggravation:** Wet weather, after midnight, from cold (except headache), cold drinks or food, seashore, right side, around midnight, exertion
- **Amelioration:** Heat, from head elevated, warm drinks, hot dry applications, company

KEYNOTE SYMPTOMS

- A deep acting remedy for all nervous, mental and physical ailments
- **Burning pains, affected parts burn like fire;** better by heat
- Periodicity; alternation of symptoms like asthma alternates with skin symptoms
- Hugs the fire all the time with evidence of destruction of tissues causing ulceration, putridity, acridity, irritability
- **Suffering is directly proportional to anxiety, restlessness and fear of death**
- Excessive exhaustion and weakness with extreme restlessness and anxiety
- Prostration, out of proportion to the rest of the illness
- Tendency to septic infections; low vitality
- Discharges are thin, acrid and scanty, with putrid, cadaveric odour
- Oedematous inflammation of serous membranes with copious effusion
- Burning in eyes with hot, acrid discharge or lachrymation; severe photophobia
- **Cannot bear smell or sight of food**
- **Marked thirst, drinks little and often**
- Food poisoning, especially from fruits; watery fruits, melons; bad meat etc.
- **Vomits as soon as cold drinks reach the stomach**
- Haemorrhoids, burn like fire, better heat; excoriation of anus
- Peptic ulcer at the pyloric end; burning in stomach, stomach cancer
- Stool dark, offensive, painful, accompanied by prostration
- Diuretic in all forms of dropsy, albuminuria
- Sneezing; hay fever; thin, watery, excoriating discharge from the nose
- Asthma, worse around midnight, suffocative attack during sleep, must sit up. Frothy scanty expectoration. Fear of suffocation, therefore does not lie down
- Itching, burning eruptions – dry, rough, scaly; urticaria, psoriasis, carbuncles, gangrene

CONSTITUTION

- For broken down constitutions, who suffer from loss of muscular power and tremble
- Suits emaciated and exhausted people of full plethoric habits
- **Temperament:** Nervous, anxious
- **Thermal:** Chilly
- **Miasm:** Psora

CLINICAL

- Anxiety
- OCD
- Nervousness
- Anaemia
- Chlorosis
- Alcoholism
- Haemorrhage
- Allergies
- Cancer
- Leukaemia
- Epithelioma
- Destructive inflammation
- Motor paralysis
- Ascites
- Nausea
- Vomitting
- Food poisoning
- Gastroenteritis
- Diarrhoea
- Dysentery
- Constipation
- Haemorrhoids
- Hay fever
- Coryza
- Asthma
- Pneumonia
- Angina pectoris
- Fatty degeneration of heart
- Valvular disease
- Cystitis
- Bright's disease
- Albuminuria
- Urethritis
- Ovaritis
- Menorrhagia
- Endometritis
- Arthritis
- Fevers
- Malaria
- Eczema
- Psoriasis
- Urticaria
- Gangrene

REMEDY RELATIONSHIP

- **Complementary:** Rhus-t., Carb-v., Phos., Thuj., Sec.
- Antidotal to lead poisoning.
- **Antidotes:** Op., Carb-v., Chin., Hep., Nux-v.
- **Chemical antidotes:** Charcoal; Hydrated peroxide of iron; Lime water.
- **Compare:** Arsenicum stibiatum 3x. Cench., Iod., Phos., Chin., Verat., Carb-v., Kali-p. Epil., Strych-g., Bry., Sarcol-ac.

SPHERE OF ACTION

- Endocrine system
- Gastrointestinal system
- Pancreas
- Musculoskeletal system
- Skin

MIND

- Sensitiveness
- Dullness
- Great restlessness, wants to be carried all the time
- Anxiety
- Depression
- Sadness
- Irritability
- Fear of disease

MODALITIES

- **Aggravation:** Spring (for acne)
- **Amelioration:** From being carried (restlessness)

INTRODUCTION

- **Common name:** Bromide of arsenic, Arsenious bromide
- **Group:** Acid
- **Source:** Mineral kingdom
- **Formula:** $AsBr_3$

ARSENICUM BROMATUM

KEYNOTE SYMPTOMS

- Great antipsoric and antisyphilitic remedy
- Weakness, itching, burning, swelling and oedema
- Tendency to herpetic eruptions, syphilitic excrescences, glandular tumours and indurations
- Diabetes mellitus and insipidus. In diabetes, three drops, three times a day in a glass of water is prescribed
- **Acne rosacea,** with violet papules on the nose, worse in spring. Acne in young people
- Eruptions; dry, rough skin with restlessness and scrubs
- Inactivity of bowels, weak and slow digestion, constipation
- **Presence of an irregular, brown stripe in center of tongue**
- Obstinate cases of intermittent fever with unbearable neuralgia
- **Marked thirst for large quantities of water**

CONSTITUTION

- Adapted to a cancerous diathesis with weakness
- **Temperament:** Nervous, bilious
- **Thermal:** Chilly
- **Miasm:** Psora, Syphilis

CLINICAL

- Glandular tumours
- Carcinoma
- Dandruff
- Asthma
- Diabetes mellitus
- Diabetes insipidus
- Rheumatism
- Arthritis
- Locomotor ataxia
- Intermittent fever
- Eruptions
- Eczema
- Herpes
- Acne rosacea

REMEDY RELATIONSHIP

- **Compare:** Ant-c., Berb-aq., Eug., Kreos., Carb-an., Psor., Sulph., in acne

ARSENICUM IODATUM

INTRODUCTION

- **Common name:** Iodide of arsenic, Arsenous iodatum
- **Group:** Acid
- **Source:** Vegetable kingdom
- **Formula:** AsI_3

SPHERE OF ACTION

- Ears
- Glands
- Gastrointestinal system
- Respiratory system
- Heart
- Nerves
- Muscles

CONSTITUTION

- Suits those who have a tendency to allergies and enlarged, scrofulous glands
- **Temperament:** Tubercular, Hyperactive
- **Thermal:** Chilly
- **Miasm:** Syphilis, Tubercular

MIND

- **Tremendous restlessness, especially at night, driving the patient out of bed**
- Hyperactive children
- Hurried, impatient, excitable
- Unable to study; study causes headache; worse mental exertion
- Highly sensitive to sensual impressions
- Anguish, anxiety
- Anxiety about health
- Angry, sudden impulse to kill

KEYNOTE SYMPTOMS

- Marked prostration, debility, emaciation with a rapid; irritable pulse, recurring fever and sweats, especially night sweats
- Bad effects of malaria or quinine; enlarged spleen
- Discharges of mucous membranes are persistently acrid, irritating, profuse; thin in acute conditions; thick, gluey, yellow like honey in chronic affections; cause burning and excoriation of parts over which they flow
- Affinity for glands – enlarged, scrofulous glands, fever or sore throat with enlarged glands, goitre, etc.
- Epithelioma of lip; cancer of lips
- Aching in malar bones
- **Intense thirst with uncontrollable desire for cold water, but water is immediately ejected**
- Tendency to watery diarrhoea during tuberculosis
- Otitis with foetid, corrosive discharge; hypertrophy of eustachian canal with deafness
- Hay fever; thin, acrid, corroding, watery nasal discharge with intense sneezing
- Chronic catarrh of nose and middle ear
- **Bronchial tree irritation with yellow-green, foul expectoration**
- Indicated in chronic pneumonia when an abscess is about to be formed with mucopurulent expectoration; dyspnoea and night sweats
- Wheezing in chest on lying down
- Tuberculosis; especially early stage with severe prostration, repeated fevers and drenching night sweats
- Tuberculosis with hoarse, racking cough, profuse expectoration of purulent nature, cardiac weakness, emaciation, general debility and scrofulous glands
- Cardiac weakness, senile heart, fatty degeneration of heart

CLINICAL

- Haemorrhage
- Haemolysis
- Malignant tissue
- Goitre
- Epithelioma of lip
- Vomiting
- Rhinitis
- Hay fever
- Influenza
- Sinusitis
- Diphtheria
- Pleuritis
- Dyspnoea
- Pneumonia
- Asthma
- Chronic lung disease
- Tuberculosis
- Breast cancer
- Artriosclerosis
- Myocarditis
- Chronic aortitis
- Arthritis
- Acne
- Psoriasis
- Eczema
- Ichthyosis
- Night sweats

MODALITIES

- **Aggravation:** Dry, cold weather, foggy weather, tobacco smoke, exertion
- **Amelioration:** Open air, after eating

REMEDY RELATIONSHIP

- **Compare:** Tub.; Ant-i. in hay fever; Aral., Naphtin., Rosa, Sangin-n., All-c, Ars., Kali-br., Tub., Bac., Arum-t.
- **Complementary:** Phos.
- **Antidote:** Ars., Bry., which relieves pain and heartburn

ARSENICUM SULFURATUM FLAVUM

SPHERE OF ACTION

- Gastrointestinal system
- Respiratory system
- Mucous membranes
- Skin

INTRODUCTION

- **Common name:** Yellow sulphuret of arsenic, Orpiment, Arsenic tri-sulphide
- **Group:** Salt
- **Source:** Mineral kingdom
- **Formula:** As_2S_3
- **Prover:** Hahnemann

CONSTITUTION

- For skin and mucous membrane affections, especially regular and malignant ulcerations with intense anxiety, apprehension and restlessness
- **Temperament:** Nervous
- **Thermal:** Chilly
- **Miasm:** Sycosis

MIND

- Intense torturing anxiety and apprehension
- Hasty, restless
- Obstinate
- Vanishing of thoughts
- Does not like to be spoken

KEYNOTE SYMPTOMS

- Marked periodicity in complaints
- General debility with lameness, staggering and trembling
- **Stitching, tearing, rheumatic pains, moving from place to place**
- **Sensation of needle pricks from within outwards**
- Ulceration, especially of the stomach with severe burning pains, vomiting and diarrhoea
- Difficult respiration, great prostration, high temperature, purulent discharge
- Sciatica and pain around the knee
- Skin itching, dry, cracked with rhagades
- Leucoderma and squamous syphilides
- Chafing of skin about genitals and behind ears of children
- **Starting in sleep; also in falling asleep; as if he would fall out of bed**

CLINICAL

- Apprehension
- Anxiety
- Debility
- Trembling
- Vomiting
- Gastric ulcer
- Diarrhoea
- Dysentery
- Influenza
- Arthritis
- Rheumatism
- Sciatica
- Pellagra
- Acne
- Psoriasis
- Eczema
- Chapped skin
- Leucoderma

MODALITIES

- **Aggravation:** Every afternoon and evening
- **Amelioration:** Steam, hot water, lying down

REMEDY RELATIONSHIP

- **Compare:** Ars-s-r., Calc.

ARTEMESIA VULGARIS

INTRODUCTION
- **Common name:** Mugwort
- **Family:** *Compositae*
- **Source:** Vegetable kingdom
- **Part used:** Roots (collected in dry season) taking care not to wash them
- **Prover:** Gatchell

SPHERE OF ACTION
- Mind
- Central nervous system
- Gastrointestinal system
- Female genital system

CONSTITUTION
- For epileptic convulsions during childhood and in girls at puberty
- **Temperament:** Nervous, bilious
- **Thermal:** Chilly
- **Miasm:** Sycosis, Tubercular

MIND
- Ailments from fright, grief or bad news
- Violent emotions, anger
- Patient is excitable and irritable before an attack of epilepsy
- Stupor after convulsions
- Inclination to steal
- Peevish
- Inclined to weep
- Irritable
- Depressed

KEYNOTE SYMPTOMS
- Ailments caused by a blow on the head or from fright, grief, or bad news
- Convulsions in children, or in girls at puberty, without an aura; from physical exertion, photic stimulation, on becoming cool, after masturbation or sexual excitement
- **Convulsive attacks accompanied by profuse offensive sweat, having a garlic-like odour and seminal emission**
- Convulsive diseases with congestion of the brain
- **Right side of the body is convulsed, left side is paralysed**
- Produces petit mal type of convulsion – frequent attacks followed by a period of long rest
- Irritability and excitability before an attack of epilepsy or convulsion
- Chorea during daytime, better at night, with inability to swallow
- Coloured light produces dizziness
- Irregular or deficient menses with epileptic seizures; violent contractions of uterus, especially a pregnant uterus; spasms during menses

CLINICAL
- Somnabulism
- Convulsions
- Seizure disorder
- Chorea
- Petit mal epilepsy
- Grand mal epilepsy
- Hydrocephalus
- Mastoiditis
- Dyspepsia
- Flatulence
- Dysentery
- Worm infestation
- Coryza
- Pharyngitis
- Dysmenorrhoea
- Gonorrhoea
- Checked lochia
- Eclampsia
- Phimosis

MODALITIES
- **Aggravation:** After fright, bad news, daytime (chorea)
- **Amelioration:** Chorea better at night

REMEDY RELATIONSHIP
- **Compare:** Absin., Cina, Cic., Abrot., Cham., Arn.

ARUM TRIPHYLLUM

INTRODUCTION
- **Common name:** Jack-in-the-pulpit
- **Family:** *Araceae*
- **Source:** Vegetable kingdom
- **Part used:** Roots / corn

SPHERE OF ACTION
- Mind
- Head
- Mouth
- Salivary glands
- Respiratory system
- Skin

MIND
- Delirium with picking at nose or lips
- Indifference, irritability, restlessness
- Anxiety
- Very cross and stubborn
- Forgetful and absentminded
- Bites nails till they bleed when nervous

MODALITIES
- **Aggravation:** Northwest wind, lying down, talking, singing

KEYNOTE SYMPTOMS
- **Left sidedness of most complaints**
- **Great redness and irritation around the mouth and lower half of the face**
- Chapped lips; **persistent picking at the nose and lips at one spot until they bleed; raw bleeding surface, very painful – screams with pain, but keeps up the boring**
- Children, particularly pick at the ends of fingers or keep boring into the nose
- Bores head into the pillow, indicating brain affections. Headache, worse hot coffee, worse very warm clothing
- Twitching or quivering of the left eyelid
- Raw, acrid, ichorous discharge from the nose, excoriating the inside of the nose, alae and upper lip
- Coryza – acrid; fluent acidity causing soreness of nostril, scab formation, pain over root of nose
- Raw, burning sensation on roof and palate of mouth, and in throat
- Hoarseness, especially in public speakers, are unable to finish their speech

CONSTITUTION
- Suits children who lose their appetite, lax flesh, don't want to play and complaints of headaches; constantly pick their lips or bore finger in their nose
- For those who have or tendency to pick at one spot or at dry lips
- **Temperament:** Irritable, excitable, nervous
- **Thermal:** Chilly
- **Miasm:** Syphilis

CLINICAL
- Allergy
- Meningitis
- Headache
- Gingivitis
- Enlarged submaxillary gland
- Stomatitis
- Hoarseness
- Nasal obstruction
- Coryza
- Hay fever
- Laryngitis
- Diphtheria
- Scarlet fever
- Eczema
- Fissures
- Impetigo contagiosa
- Pemphigus

REMEDY RELATIONSHIP
- **Compare:** Am-c., Ail., All-c., Cina., Am-c., Ars., Canth., Caps., Hep., Nit-ac.
- **Antidoted by:** Buttermilk; Acet-ac., Puls.
- **Incompatible:** Calad.
- **Complementary:** Nit-ac.

ASAFOETIDA

INTRODUCTION
- **Common name:** Gum of the Stinkasand
- **Family:** *Umbelliferae*
- **Source:** Vegetable kingdom
- **Part used:** Gum resin

SPHERE OF ACTION
- Mind
- Eyes
- Gastrointestinal system
- Respiratory system
- Heart
- Bones
- Female genital system
- Skin

MIND
- Presents a perfect picture of hysteria – with hysterical restlessness and anxiety
- Intolerably nervous and over-sensitive
- Irritable, constantly complaining of her troubles; fickleness, cannot preserve in anything, wants a new thing and then another
- Magnifies her symptoms, craves sympathy. Hypochondriacal.
- Fainting during pain
- Hysteria from sudden suppression of symptoms
- Mental and physical oversensitivity; like, faints from emotional excitement, noise, crowds, etc.
- Very irritable during menses; alternates with indifference
- Dissatisfied with self

MODALITIES
- **Aggravation:** At night, from touch, left side, during rest, warm applications, after eating or drinking after, suppressions
- **Amelioration:** Open air, from motion, pressure

KEYNOTE SYMPTOMS
- Great offensiveness of all discharges and secretions
- Pains from within outwards; pressing pains with numbness; nocturnal pains
- Orbits bruised, sore and sensitive
- **Ball rises in throat, difficult eructation; globus hystericus**
- Hiccough – like contractions of diaphragm
- **Stone rancid taste in mouth after belching**
- Flatulence and regurgitation of liquids; and food. Great distention, hysterical flatulency, pressing upwards in the abdomen
- Sensation as if everything in the abdomen would burst through the mouth
- **Diarrhoea, extremely offensive, with meteorism. Also, obstinate constipation**
- Spasmodic tightness of chest, as if lungs cannot be fully expanded
- Mammae turgid with milk in non-pregnant women. Deficient milk with oversensitivity after confinement
- Caries of bones. Ulcerations. Extreme sensitiveness. Decay of bones.
- Periosteum painful, swollen
- Itching better by scratching

CONSTITUTION
- Indicated commonly in women, who are hysterical, with a plethoric appearance, puffed face, bloated even dropsical; venous, purple, a very troublesome face suggesting cardiac disturbance and venous stasis
- **Temperament:** Nervous, bilious, oversensitive
- **Thermal:** Chilly
- **Miasm:** Psora, Sycosis, Syphilis

CLINICAL
- Oversensitivity
- Hysteria
- Corneal ulcers
- Syphilitic iritis
- Globus hystericus
- Flatulence
- Regurgitation
- Reverse peristalsis
- Reflux oesophagitis
- Diarrhoea
- Otorrhoea
- Mastoiditis
- Deficient milk
- Bone affections
- Bone caries
- Periosteal pains
- Bone decay
- Ulcers

REMEDY RELATIONSHIP
- **Antidotes:** Chin., Merc.
- **Compare:** Mosch., Chin., Merc., Aur., Lach.
- **Complementary:** Caust., Puls.

SPHERE OF ACTION

- Cardiovascular system
- Gastrointestinal system
- Respiratory system
- Urinary system
- Muscular system

INTRODUCTION

- **Common name:** Common garden asparagus
- **Family:** *Liliaceae*
- **Source:** Vegetable kingdom
- **Part used:** Young shoots
- **Prover:** Buchner

CONSTITUTION

- Suits weakness, cardiac depression urinary complaints and dropsy
- For predisposition to kidney stones
- **Temperament:** Nervous, bilious
- **Thermal:** Chilly
- **Miasm:** Psora, Sycosis, Syphilis

ASPARAGUS OFFICINALIS

MIND

- Excitement, excitable
- Constant anxiety; anxious expression on face; apprehension
- Morose, peevish, ill-humoured, fretful
- **Constant desire to be carried around in arms**
- Disturbed by trifles

KEYNOTE SYMPTOMS

- Complaints from suppression of perspiration
- Severe coryza with profuse secretion of thin, whitish fluid; frequent, violent sneezing
- **Profuse discharge of tenacious mucous in the throat which cannot be loosened easily; brought up by hawking or paroxysms of cough**
- Marked oppression in chest when breathing and when walking; hydrothorax
- Palpitations with oppression of chest; palpitations are visible and audible and accompanied by anxious restlessness
- Pulse intermittent, feeble, weak and accelerated
- Cardiac depression and dropsy, with urinary disturbances
- Rheumatic constricting pain in the cardiac region when voiding last drops, forcing him to cry out, face may turn blue
- **Urine has peculiar odour like that of cat's urine. Greasy sediments; brown, like beer; loaded with phosphates and urates of ammonia**
- Frequent micturation with fine stitches in urethral orifice
- **Pain about left shoulder and heart, associated with bladder disturbances**
- Rheumatic pain in the back

CLINICAL

- Hydrophobia
- Migraine
- Coryza
- Bronchitis
- Asthma
- Hydrothorax
- Palpitation
- Angina pectoris
- Cardiac dropsy
- Cystitis
- Polyurea
- Urinary calculi
- Kidney disorders
- Rheumatism

MODALITIES

- **Aggravation:** Left side; palpitations worse on motion, ascending stairs, when seated and after a meal; pain in limbs worse on being seated, in the morning, on waking and on extending limb

REMEDY RELATIONSHIP

- **Antidotes:** Acon., Apis.
- **Compare:** Alth. in irritable bladder, throat and bronchi, Physal-al., Dig., Sars., Spig., Arn., Aur-m., Cann-i., Conv.

ASPIDOSPERMA QUEBRACHO

SPHERE OF ACTION

- Heart
- Gastrointestinal system
- Respiratory system
- Urinary system
- Skin

INTRODUCTION

- **Common name:** White quebracho
- **Family:** *Apocynaceae*
- **Source:** Vegetable kingdom
- **Part used:** Bark
- **Prover:** Hale

CONSTITUTION

- Suits pulmonary hypertension with respiratory and cardiac dyspnoea
- Stimulates the respiratory center
- **Temperament:** Nervous, bilious
- **Thermal:** Chilly, ambithermal
- **Miasm:** Psora, Sycosis, Syphilis

MIND

- Restlessness
- Sadness
- Melancholy
- Anxiety

KEYNOTE SYMPTOMS

- It stimulates the respiratory centres and increases the oxygen in blood. **Good lung tonic, also called 'Digitalis of the lungs'**
- Removes temporary obstruction to oxidation of blood by stimulating respiratory centres, increasing oxidation and excretion of carbonic acid
- Want of breath during exertion; dyspnoea, difficult respiration. Uraemic dyspnoea
- Asthma, cardiac asthma with respiratory paralysis and a slow heart rate
- Thrombosis of pulmonary artery; pulmonary hypertension

CLINICAL

- Diarrhoea
- Dysentery
- Breathlessness
- Dyspnoea
- Bronchiectasis
- Asthma
- Emphysema
- Cardiac asthma
- Pulmonary artery stenosis
- Thrombosis
- Cyanosis
- Uraemia
- Eczema
- Urticaria

MODALITIES

- **Aggravation:** Exertion, motion
- **Amelioration:** Rest

REMEDY RELATIONSHIP

- **Compare:** Ars., Coca, Coff.

ASTERIAS RUBENS

SPHERE OF ACTION
- Head
- Central nervous system
- Gastrointestinal system
- Respiratory system
- Breasts

INTRODUCTION
- **Common name:** Red starfish
- **Family:** *Asteriadae*
- **Source:** Vegetable kingdom
- **Part used:** Entire animal
- **Prover:** Petroz

CONSTITUTION
- Suits sycotic diathesis; lymphatic constitution in flabby people with a red face
- For the climacteric period
- **Temperament:** Nervous, bilious
- **Thermal:** Chilly
- **Miasm:** Psora, Sycosis, Syphilis

MIND
- **Delusion that he is away from home, in the amidst of strangers, hears voices and replies**
- Fear of apoplexy with sensation as if head would burst; of misfortune, better weeping
- Easily excited from any emotion, especially contradictions
- Weeps from least emotion
- Nervous disturbance
- Excitement in both sexes
- Very irritable, patient wants to quarrel with someone

KEYNOTE SYMPTOMS
- Left sided complaints
- Pulsations and congestions, especially of head, chest and uterus
- Drawn back feeling in the eyes and nipples
- Nervous disturbances like neuralgias, epilepsy, hysteria and chorea; pains lancinating at night
- Apoplexy with a red face and hard, throbbing carotids; sensation as if head is surrounded by hot air, rush of blood to head. Shocks in the brain
- Sensation as if head would burst, especially before a stroke
- Epilepsy preceeded by twitching all over the body
- **Severe, obstinate constipation; stools hard, in round balls like olives**
- Stools, are brown, watery, gushing like a jet. Involuntary diarrhoea
- Indicated in cancer, especially cancer of the breast, even in the ulcerative stage
- **Breast, particularly the left one feels as if pulled inwards; acute lancinating pains in tumour**
- Axillary glands swollen, hard, knotted
- Increased sexual desire, sexual excitement
- Numbness of hands and fingers, especially of the left side
- Unsteady gait. Muscles do not obey will
- Chorea, particularly when hands are in the pocket. Tendency to pimples during adolescence. Acne with a black tipped puncta

CLINICAL
- Hysteria
- Cancer
- Neuralgia
- Chorea
- Epilepsy
- Ulceration
- Diarrhoea
- Constipation
- Sexual disorders
- Breast cancer
- Mastitis
- Herpes
- Psoriasis
- Pimples

MODALITIES
- **Aggravation:** Coffee, night, cold damp weather, left side, motion
- **Amelioration:** Discharge of menses

REMEDY RELATIONSHIP
- **Antidotes:** Plb., Zinc.
- **Compare:** Con., Carb-v., Ars., Cund., Murx., Sep., Carc., Thuj., Bell., Grat., Jatr.
- **Incompatible:** Nux-v., Coff.

AURUM METALLICUM

INTRODUCTION
- **Common name:** Metallic gold
- **Group:** Metal
- **Source:** Mineral kingdom
- **Formula:** Au

SPHERE OF ACTION
- Mind
- Eyes
- Nerves
- Bones
- Glands
- Cardiovascular system
- Respiratory system
- Genitourinary system

CONSTITUTION
- For scrofulous constitutions broken down by bad effects of syphilis and mercury
- Suits sanguine people with black hair and eyes, blue about nose and lips; low spirited, lifeless
- Pining boys, old people
- **Temperament:** Nervous, hysterical, depressed
- **Thermal:** Chilly
- **Miasm:** Syphilis

MIND
- Profound melancholia. Person is intelligent, having good position, but has negative thinking, does not take part in emotional problems of others, instead wants mental support.
- Grief and depression. Workaholic, duty bound. Religious mania.
- **Self-condemnation**
- The future looks dark, worried over trifles
- Depressive insanity, low spirited, peevish, abusive. Hopelessness
- **Constantly dwelling on suicide; suicidal tendency**
- Hurried, worried
- Boredom
- Confusion
- Frightful dreams
- Oversensitivity, especially to contradiction

KEYNOTE SYMPTOMS
- **Sunset to sunrise aggravation**
- Oversensitive to touch, smell
- Syphilitic and mercurial bone affections; exostosis and bone decay with nocturnal bone pains; especially affects cranial, nasal and palatine bones
- Caries of nasal, palatine and mastoid bones
- **Only sees the lower part of any object – hemiopia**
- **Appetite and thirst increased with swelling in the epigastrium. Taste putrid, bitter**
- Right hypochondrium hot, painful
- Constipation; stools hard and knotty. Nocturnal diarrhoea with burning in rectum
- Obstinate, foetid otorrhoea
- Adenopathy; nose ulcerated, painful, swollen; foetid discharge, sensitive to smell; putrid smell from nose
- High blood pressure; sensation as if the heart stopped beating for 2-3 seconds; palpitations with rush of blood to chest
- Painful retention of urine; urine turbid with thick sediment
- Sterility; vaginismus, uterus enlarged, prolapsed – for uterine disorders with depressions
- Chronic induration of testicles. Underdeveloped testicles in puny boys, Hydrocoele. Atrophy of testicles in boys
- Chronic insomnia, with depressions. Moans and cries out in sleep. Sleep disturbed by bone pains

CLINICAL
- Depressions
- Agoraphobia
- Sepsis
- Caries
- Photophobia
- Hemiopia
- Diplopia
- Iritis
- Blepharitis
- Rectal abscess
- Ozaena
- Otitis media
- Laryngitis
- Pharyngitis
- Sinusitis
- Tonsillitis
- Croup
- Bronchitis
- Pneumonia
- Asthma
- Pleurisy
- Arteriosclerosis
- Hypertension
- Palpitations
- Hypertrophy of heart
- Endocarditis
- Urethral stricture
- Urethritis
- Sterility
- Vaginitis
- Mastitis
- Prostatitis
- Balanitis
- Bone decay
- Exostosis
- Eczema
- Abcess
- Paronychia

MODALITIES
- **Aggravation:** In cold air, when getting cold, in winters, while lying down, mental exertion, cloudy weather; from sunset to sunrise
- **Amelioration:** In warm air, when growing warm, in the morning, during summer, from music

REMEDY RELATIONSHIP
- Aurum follows, and is followed well by Syph.
- **Compare:** Asaf. in caries of bones of ear and nose; Bell., Caps., in caries of mastoid; Calc., in night terrors; Kali-i, Hep., Merc., Mez., Nit-ac., Phos., Syph. in Syphilis; also Tarent., Lach., Lyc., Merc., Nit-ac., Dig.
- **Antidotes:** Bell., Chin., Merc., Cupr.

AURUM MURIATICUM NATRONATUM

INTRODUCTION

- **Common name:** Sodium chloroaurate
- **Group:** Salt
- **Source:** Mineral kingdom
- **Formula:** $NaAuCl_4 \cdot 2H_2O$
- **Prover:** Lembke

SPHERE OF ACTION

- Head
- Cardiovascular system
- Gastrointestinal system
- Female genital system
- Skeletal system
- Skin

MIND

- Ailments from vexation, chagrin, fright, grief
- Impatient and restless
- Fear of failure or rejection
- Hysteria; puerperal mania
- Anxiety of consciousness, remorse
- Fear to undertake anything new
- Sarcastic
- Full of self pity

MODALITIES

- **Aggravation:** Cold wet weather, rest

CONSTITUTION

- **It is a female remedy, for uterine tumours and palpitation in young girls**
- **Temperament:** Nervous, bilious
- **Thermal:** Chilly, ambithermal
- **Miasm:** Sycosis, Syphilis

KEYNOTE SYMPTOMS

- Old cases of rheumatism and gout
- **Boring pains** are very marked; **drawing, pressing over left eye, skull, chest, tibia, bones**
- Tendency for high blood pressure, with beating of carotids and temporal arteries in sturdy built individuals, with a gloomy nature due to disturbed function of nervous mechanism
- Suppuration of glands
- **Burning and stiching on tip of tongue; induration of tongue; warts on tongue**
- **Periosteal swellings on lower jaw**
- Coldness in abdomen
- Leucorrhoea with spasmodic contraction of vagina; corrosive leucorrhoea, corroding parts
- Sterility from ovarian dropsy. Ovarian induration, ossified uterus, subinvolution, prolapse
- Deficient sexual desire
- Induration of one part of uterus, softening of another part; cysts, tumours of the uterus; miscarriage from uterine induration

CLINICAL

- Gastroenteritis
- Cirrhosis
- Arteriosclerosis
- Hypertension
- Amenorrhoea
- Ovary indurated
- Prolapse of uterus
- Ovarian dropsy
- Metritis
- Leucorrhoea
- Uterine tumours
- Fibroids
- Ulceration of cervix
- Subinvolution of uterus
- Testicular swelling
- Rheumatism
- Arthritis
- Gout
- Periosteal swelling
- Psoriasis syphilitica

REMEDY RELATIONSHIP

- **Compare:** Arg-n., Ars., Bry., Con., Graph., Hep., Iod., Kali-bi., Lyc., Merc., Nit-ac., Phos., Sulph., Thuj.

AVENA SATIVA

INTRODUCTION
- **Common name:** Common oat
- **Family:** *Gramineae*
- **Source:** Vegetable kingdom
- **Part used:** Seeds

SPHERE OF ACTION
- Mind
- Gastrointestinal system
- Respiratory system
- Heart
- Musculoskeletal system
- Female genital system

CONSTITUTION
- For weakness, prostration – nervous and muscular
- **Temperament:** Nervous, bilious
- **Thermal:** Chilly
- **Miasm:** Psora, Sycosis, Syphilis

MIND
- Mental prostration, mental exhaustion, brain fag
- Nervous exhaustion, sexual debility, morphine habit
- Debility after exhausting diseases or mental exertion
- Inability to keep mind on one subject
- Dullness; sluggishness with difficulty in thinking, comprehending
- Nervousness

CLINICAL
- Alcoholism
- Morphinism
- Neurasthenia
- Nerve tremors
- Epilepsy
- Chorea
- Paralysis
- Diarrhoea
- Dysentery
- Acute coryza
- Diphtheria
- Carditis
- Endocarditis
- Rheumatic heart
- Amenorrhoea
- Dysmenorrhoea
- Spermatorrhoea
- Impotency
- Rheumatism
- Insomnia

KEYNOTE SYMPTOMS
- Alcoholism, dipsomania, drug addictions, nervous exhaustions; bad effects of ingesting morphine
- **It improves the nutrition of the brain and nervous system**
- Helps to stimulate the brain
- Nervous tremors of the aged, with paralysis agitans, chorea, epilepsy, nervous palpitations
- General debility, strength of hands reduced or diminished. Numbness of limbs, as if paralysed
- Nervous state of women, amenorrhoea or dysmenorrhoea with weak circulation
- Nervous headaches at menstrual period
- Nervous exhaustion or affections in females or aged after exhausting diseases
- Unable to keep the mind on any subject due to masturbation; tendency to masturbate
- Spermatorrhoea or impotency from over indulgence; sexual emission aggravates
- Insomnia, sleeplessness, especially in alcoholics and drug addicts

MODALITIES
- **Aggravation:** Exertion – mental or physical, after exhausting diseases, alcohol, morphine, masturbation, over indulgence in sex
- **Amelioration:** Rest

REMEDY RELATIONSHIP
- **Compare:** Alf. as a general tonic similar to Aven.—also in scanty and suppressed urine; Pani., Valer.

BACILLINUM BURNETT

SPHERE OF ACTION
- Eyes
- Teeth
- Respiratory system
- Gastrointestinal system
- Skin

INTRODUCTION
- **Common name:** Bacillinum
- **Group:** Nosode
- **Source:** Maceration of a tuberculous lung
- **Part used:** From human tuberculous sputum
- **Prover:** Burnett

CONSTITUTION
- Adapted to a tubercular diathesis – people who are lean, thin, emaciated and suffer from lung diseases
- For tubercular constitution with syphilitic taints
- **Temperament:** Nervous
- **Thermal:** Chilly
- **Miasm:** Tubercular

MIND
- Taciturn, sulky, snappy, fretful
- Irritable, morose
- Tendency to whine and complain
- **Tendency to be frightened; fear of dogs**
- Does not want to be disturbed
- Depressed, melancholic, to the point of insanity

KEYNOTE SYMPTOMS
- Defective growth. Retarded mental development
- Susceptibility to cold, wet weather
- **Perspiration on forehead, axilla; palms of hands**
- Tendency to enlarged and tender glands, and great weakness
- Eczema of eyelids
- Imperfectly developed teeth; grinds teeth in sleep
- **Sudden diarrhoea before breakfast**
- Tendency to catch cold and sore throat; chronic, recurring disposition for cough
- Lungs weak in children and old people suffering from chronic catarrh and nocturnal suffocation
- Lung congestion, humid asthma with much bubbling rales and muco-purulent expectoration
- Oppression of chest; catarrhal dyspnoea. This remedy often relieves congestion of the lungs
- **For tuberculosis which is better in sunny weather; after taking this remedy, the sputum becomes less purulent**
- Enlarged glands in groins. Tabes mesenterica
- Emaciated women with profuse menses
- Chronic recurrent fever

CLINICAL
- Lymphadenopathy
- Headache
- Tubercular meningitis
- Eczema of eyelids
- Pyorrhoea
- Tartar of teeth
- Diarrhoea
- Obstinate constipation
- Coryza
- Cough
- Bubbling rales
- Tonsillitis
- Asthma
- Bronchorrhoea
- Bronchitis
- Dyspnoea
- Tuberculosis
- Ringworm
- Eczema

REMEDY RELATIONSHIP
- **Complementary:** Calc-p., Kali-c., Lach.
- **Compare:** Its effects seem to be identical to that of Koch's Tuberculinum. In the early stages of tubercular diseases of glands, joints, skin and bones. Psor. seems to be its chronic equivalent; Phos., Dros., Merc., Bac-t., Ant-t., Iod., Ars-i.

MODALITIES
- **Aggravation:** Night and early morning, cold air

BADIAGA

SPHERE OF ACTION
- Eyes
- Gastrointestinal system
- Respiratory system
- Cardiovascular system
- Female genital system
- Skin

INTRODUCTION
- **Common name:** Fresh water sponge
- **Family:** *Spongillidae*
- **Source:** Animal kingdom
- **Part used:** Whole sponge
- **Prover:** Bedford

CONSTITUTION
- For swollen, enlarged; cancerous glands; tendency for skin eruptions
- **Temperament:** Nervous, bilious
- **Thermal:** Chilly
- **Miasm:** Psora, Sycosis, Syphilis

MIND
- After pleasurable emotions, palpitations
- Mind clear and active despite headache
- Delusions, imagination that body parts are enlarged
- Irritability from noise
- Desire for mental work
- Frightful dreams
- Oversensitive

KEYNOTE SYMPTOMS
- Induration or swelling of glands
- Marked general soreness, as if beaten
- **Dandruff – in excess or dry, tetter-like appearance of scalp; scalp sore to touch. Dry hair**
- Sensation of enlargement and fullness of head; headache better after sleep
- Mucous flies out of mouth and nostrils. Mouth hot and thirsty
- Pain in stomach extends to vertebra and scapula
- Metrorrhagia, worse at night
- Cancer of breasts
- Muscles stiff, sore, as if beaten worse motion, worse friction of clothes
- Soreness of integuments and muscles, as if beaten, very sensitive. General paresis
- Chronic rheumatism, worse cold air, stormy weather, ascending; better in a warm room
- **Awakens at 3-4 am with frightful dreams and severe cramps in metatarsals of both feet**

CLINICAL
- Cancer
- Dandruff
- Gingivitis
- Diarrhoea
- Dysentery
- Influenza
- Asthma
- Cough
- Breast cancer
- Metrorrhagia
- Syphilis
- Bubo
- Chancre
- Rheumatism
- Freckles
- Rhagades

MODALITIES
- **Aggravation:** Cold weather, cold air, pressure, touch, motion
- **Amelioration:** Heat, warm room

REMEDY RELATIONSHIP
- **Compare:** Merc. similar but opposite modalities; Spong., Phydr., Kali-i., Phyt., Con., Calc-s., Carb-an. in indurations, buboes; Grind., in respiration ceasing on sleeping; Cist. in scrofula
- **Complementary:** Sulph., Merc., Iod.

SPHERE OF ACTION

- Mind
- Blood
- Gastrointestinal system
- Respiratory system
- Mucous membranes

INTRODUCTION

- **Common name:** Wild indigo
- **Family:** *Leguminoseae*
- **Source:** Vegetable kingdom
- **Part used:** Root
- **Prover:** Thompson

CONSTITUTION

- Suits patients with a flushed, dusky and dark red face; expression is stupid and besotted, looks like a drunkard
- **Temperament:** Lymphatic
- **Thermal:** Chilly
- **Miasm:** Psora

BAPTISIA TINCTORIA

MIND

- Confused mind and perfect indifference; as if intoxicated
- Does not want to do any mental work; aversion to mental exertion
- **Patient feels that his head and body are scattered around the bed. He is in three pieces and is unable to keep them covered**
- Muttering delirium, feels too large and heavy
- Melancholy
- Falls off to sleep while being spoken to or while answering a question
- Restlessness

KEYNOTE SYMPTOMS

- Left side of the body is affected
- Septic conditions of blood; malarial poisoning, epidemic influenza with severe prostration
- **In whatever position the patient lies, the part rested upon feels sore and bruised**
- Rapid and profound prostration, muscles feel sore, heavy and achy
- Foetid discharges, like – stool, urine, sweat, breath, ulcers, body, etc.
- **Tongue coated yellowish-white, feels burnt or scalded; feels swollen and numb.**
- Contraction of cardiac orifice, oesophagus
- Pain in the epigastric region. Sensation of a hard substance; dreadful sinking sensation in the stomach
- Stool offensive, thin, dark, bloody
- Dysentery in old people. Diarrhoea, offensive, day and night
- Soreness of abdomen, in region of liver. Distention and rumbling
- Epidemic influenza with a besotted look; bleary eyes, headache, sore throat and soreness all over
- Dark red tonsils, soft palate; painless sore throat. Can swallow liquids only; difficulty in swallowing solid foods
- Septic sore throat with offensive discharges
- Threatened miscarriage from mental depression, puerperal fever. Menses too early, too profuse
- Dynamic fever, septic fever; high fever with sudden onset

CLINICAL

- Delirium
- Prostration
- Toxaemia
- Ulceration
- Headache
- Halitosis
- Stomatitis
- Diarrhoea
- Dysentery
- Intestinal toxemia
- Influenza
- Spasm of glottis
- Loss of voice
- Tonsillitis
- Nasal diphtheria
- Asthma
- Cardiac failure
- Thrombosis
- Menorrhagia
- Threatened miscarriage
- Rheumatism of shoulder
- Typhoid fever
- Hectic fever
- Enteric fever

MODALITIES

- **Aggravation:** Humid heat, fog, indoors, pressure, swallowing solids, mental exertion
- **Amelioration:** Drinking liquids, motion, open air

REMEDY RELATIONSHIP

- **Compare:** Bry. and Ars. may be needed to complete the favorable reaction; Ail. differs, being more painful. Bapt. is more painless; Rhus-t., Mur-ac., Arn., Echi., Pyrog.
- **Follow well:** Ars.

BARYTA CARBONICA

INTRODUCTION

- **Common name:** Carbonate of baryta, Barium carbonate
- **Group:** Salt
- **Source:** Mineral kingdom
- **Formula:** $BaCO_3$
- **Prover:** Hahnemann

SPHERE OF ACTION

- Mind
- Nutrition
- Glands
- Throat
- Circulatory system
- Male genital system
- Nerves
- Lymphatic system

CONSTITUTION

- **For dwarfish babies with stunted growth, are fatty with a swollen abdomen and puffed face**
- For dwarfish, hysterical women and old maids who are always chilly and have scanty menses
- Suits fat, old cachectic people with gouty complaints and degenerative changes; for childish old people or children
- **Temperament:** Nervous, anxious
- **Thermal:** Chilly
- **Miasm:** Sycosis, Psora, Tubercular

MIND

- Emotionally, tends to lack self-confidence; childish, timid, insecure and unable to make decisions; deficient mentally, idiotic. Mentally retarded
- Senile dementia
- Silly, bashful cowardly
- Mental and physical dwarfism, unable to learn anything. Can't learn the art of walking.
- Baby doesn't want to play, sits in a corner of the room or street doing foolish things
- Becomes serious on laughable matters and laughs at serious matters
- Loss of memory
- Mental weakness, inability to concentrate
- Loss of confidence
- Aversion to meeting strangers
- Homesickness

KEYNOTE SYMPTOMS

- Children, both physically and mentally weak, that is, physically and mentally dwarfish
- For early senility when degenerative changes begin early in men in the brain, heart and vascular system
- Chilly patient; tendency to catch cold easily; prone to suppuration
- **Aversion to fatty, rich foods; desires meat and sweets. Can only swallow liquids**
- Always have swollen tonsils. Quinsy. Swelling and induration or incipient suppuration of glands. Glands are enlarged.
- Softening of blood vessels causing their distention, aneurysm or rupture
- **Sensation of a cobweb on the face; as if the white of an egg hardened on the face**
- Cough on getting feet wet or on least exposure to cold air
- Constipation with hard, knotty stools. Haemorrhoids protrude on micturition
- Submaxillary gland swollen; tendency to tonsillitis; especially the suppurative variety
- Sensation as if they are inhaling smoke
- Burning in urethra, burning micturition
- Problems of old men like – hypertrophy of prostate and testes
- Feels as if legs are cut off and he is walking on his knees
- Offensive, foetid foot sweat; toes and soles get sore; tendency to bite nails

CLINICAL

- Down syndrome
- Dwarfism
- Senile dementia
- Mental retardation
- Glandular swelling
- Fatty tumours
- Apoplexy
- Brain affections
- Vertigo
- Hiccough
- Weak digestion
- Constipation
- Haemorrhoids
- Coryza
- Laryngitis
- Tonsillitis
- Quinsy
- Pleurisy
- Heart affections
- Hypertension
- Aneurysm
- Urethritis
- Enlarged prostate
- Wens
- Lipomas
- Foot sweat

MODALITIES

- **Aggravation:** While thinking of symptoms, from washing, lying on painful side, sitting, cold, suppressed foot sweat, mental exertion
- **Amelioration:** Walking in open air, warmth, when alone

REMEDY RELATIONSHIP

- **Compare:** Dig., Rad-br., Arag., Oxyt., Astrag., Alum, Ant-t., Bell., Calc., Con., Dulc., Merc., Sil.
- **Complementary:** Dulc., Sil., Psor.
- **Incompatible:** Calc.

BARYTA MURIATICA

INTRODUCTION

- **Common name:** Barium chloride, Barri chloridum
- **Group:** Salt
- **Source:** Mineral kingdom
- **Formula:** $BaCl_2 \cdot 2H_2O$

SPHERE OF ACTION

- Mind
- Gastrointestinal system
- Respiratory system
- Cardiovascular system
- Central nervous system
- Musculoskeletal system
- Urinary system
- Female genital system

MIND

- Mania, insanity from increased sexual drive
- Dullness of mind, sluggish; difficulty in thinking and comprehending
- Imbecility, idiocy
- Answers confusingly, as if thinking of something else
- Sadness in the morning
- Talking in sleep at night
- Biting at night
- Childish behaviour with increased sexual desire
- Suspiciousness, nymphomania and satyriasis

MODALITIES

- **Aggravation:** Tonsillitis is worse in spring and autumn
- **Amelioration:** Earache is better by sipping cold water

KEYNOTE SYMPTOMS

- With arteriosclerosis as the background there are cerebral, cardiac or vascular troubles of the aged or the retarded
- White blood corpuscles increased
- Glandular enlargements and indurations; of parotid, inguinal, pancreas, tonsils
- All kinds of mania with increased sexual desire
- Marked general lassitude, especially in the morning, with muscular stiffness and weakness of legs
- **Icy coldness of the body with paralysis**
- Epilepsy with loss of voluntary muscular power but complete sensibility. Multiple sclerosis of brain and cord
- **Convulsions with electric-like shocks; occur periodically**
- Hard in hearing
- Narrowing of the cardiac orifice with pain immediately after eating
- Bronchial affections, aids expectoration. Senile asthma
- Paresis after influenza and diphtheria
- Chronic hypertrophy of tonsils; suppurations of tonsils
- Arteriosclerosis causing high systolic pressure and relatively low diastolic pressure
- Hypertension and vascular degeneration; aneurysm
- Great increase in uric acid; urine very offensive

CONSTITUTION

- For dwarfism – mental and physical, especially in old people and scrofulous children
- Suits children who always have their mouths open and talk from their nose
- **Temperament:** Nervous, anxious
- **Thermal:** Chilly
- **Miasm:** Sycosis

CLINICAL

- Glandular induration
- Glandular enlargement
- Leukaemia
- Multiple sclerosis
- Convulsions
- Paralysis
- Vertigo
- Headache
- Cerebral anaemia
- Pancreatitis
- Diarrhoea
- Dysentery
- Tonsillitis
- Hypertension
- Cardiac dilation
- Arteriosclerosis
- Aneurysm
- Infertility
- Ovarian affections
- Nymphomania

REMEDY RELATIONSHIP

- **Compare:** Plb., Plb-i., in sclerotic degenerations, especially of spinal cord, liver and heart; also Aur-m., Iod., Kali-i., Sel.
- Useful after Ars. in extravasation of blood

BELLADONNA

INTRODUCTION

- **Common name:** Deadly nightshade
- **Family:** *Solanaceae*
- **Source:** Vegetable kingdom
- **Part used:** Whole plant
- **Prover:** Hering

SPHERE OF ACTION

- Mind
- Eyes
- Ears
- Glands
- Gastrointestinal system
- Respiratory system
- Nervous system
- Cardiovascular system
- Skin

CONSTITUTION

- Suits women and children with light hair, blue eyes, fair complexion, delicate skin; lymphatic, plethoric constitution
- For people who are lively when well but violent and delirious when unwell
- **Temperament:** Nervous, bilious, tubercular
- **Thermal:** Chilly
- **Miasm:** Psora

MIND

- **Nervous, imagines seeing a ghost, hideous face, black animal, dog, wolves, monster; visions of fire**
- Horrible visions in the dark
- Fear of imaginary things, especially animals wants to run away from them
- Violent, furious delirium. Disposition to bite, spit, strike and tear things. Breaks into fits of laughter, tries to escape.
- Visual hallucinations
- Very restless
- Stammering

KEYNOTE SYMPTOMS

- Marked violence of attack with sudden onset of symptoms
- **Severe burning, redness and dryness predominate all symptoms**
- Profound action on nervous system producing congestion, furious excitement, twitching, convulsions, pain and perverted special senses
- Pains or neuralgia come suddenly, go suddenly, last indefinitely. Pains usually in short attacks; worse light, noise, jar
- **Pain accompanied with throbbing of carotids, and redness of face and eyes**
- Great tendency to take cold
- Swollen, red, tender glands. Fullness and congestion, especially of head.
- Flushed face, dilated pupils, throbbing carotids and hot, red skin
- Convulsions during teething, with fever; come on suddenly, with hot head and cold feet
- Vertigo when stooping, when rising after stooping
- **Throbbing, hammering headache, with a red face and fullness of forehead; worse light, noise, jar, after haircut, washing hair or draft of cold air**
- Severe conjunctivitis with marked inflammation and photophobia. Conjunctiva red and dry; staring, brilliant eyes
- **Desires cold water or lemonade**
- Abdomen tender, distended, worse least jar, even of the bed
- Pain in right ileo-cecal region, worse slightest touch. Transverse colon protrudes like a pad.
- Right side of throat red, congested, dry and hot; throat feels constricted; difficult deglutition. Tonsillitis with fever
- Acute urinary infection; cystitis. Retention of urine which is scanty, dark and turbid
- Dryness and heat of vagina
- Menses profuse, bright red, too early
- Breasts feel heavy, hard, with tumour
- Diminished lochia; menses and lochia offensive and hot
- Prostatic hypertropy and orchitis
- Skin dry, smooth, hot, burning; alternate redness and paleness
- **High fever without thirst and burning,** pungent heat; delirium with fever

CLINICAL

- Delirium
- Hallucinations
- Mania
- Exophthalmic goitre
- Hydrophobia
- Neuralgia
- Convulsions
- Epilepsy
- Hydrocephalus
- Meningitis
- Photophobia
- Vertigo
- Headache
- Haematoma
- Conjunctivitis
- Diplopia
- Teething troubles
- Glossitis
- Gastritis
- Colic
- Diarrhoea
- Dysentery
- Epistaxis
- Coryza
- Sinusitis
- Rhinitis
- Tonsillitis
- Otitis media
- Ear infections
- Laryngitis
- Pneumonia
- Cough
- Retention of urine
- Haematuria
- Mastitis
- High fever
- Acne rosacea
- Erysipelas
- Boils
- Abscesses

MODALITIES

- **Aggravation:** Touch, motion, noise, draft of air especially on head, looking at bright shining objects, after 3 pm, night, summer sun, lying down, jar, checked sweat, pressure
- **Amelioration:** Rest, standing, warm room, leaning head against something

REMEDY RELATIONSHIP

- **Complementary:** Calc., **Bell. is the acute of Calc.,** which is often required to complete a cure; Borx., Hep., Merc., Nat-m.
- **Compare:** Acon., Bry., Cic., Gels., Glon., Hyos., Meli., Op., Stram.

BELLIS PERENNIS

INTRODUCTION
- **Common name:** Daisy
- **Family:** *Compositae*
- **Source:** Vegetable kingdom
- **Part used:** Whole plant
- **Prover:** Burnett

SPHERE OF ACTION
- Nerves
- Muscles
- Gastrointestinal system
- Female genital system
- Blood vessels

MIND
- Impulse to move
- Despair with pain
- Cheerfulness, gaity, happiness, when thunder and lightening occur
- Confusion of mind, regarding surroundings
- Irritable
- Anxious, nervous
- Sleeplessness, dreams of anger

MODALITIES
- **Aggravation:** Left side, injury, blow, sprain, exertion, lifting, touch, hot bath, warmth of bed, before storms, cold bathing, cold wind, cold drinks
- **Amelioration:** Continuos motion, pressure, cold application

KEYNOTE SYMPTOMS
- Left sided remedy
- **Effects of trauma, contusions, sprains, bruises, lacerations, incisions, falls or blows**
- Venous congestion from mechanical causes
- Post-operative pains and ecchymosis; soreness
- Sore, lame, bruised feeling all over the body
- Fagged and overworked individuals with an impulse to keep moving
- Injury to the deeper, internal organs or tissues
- Tumour or cyst from injury, especially breast tumour
- Pains aching, squeezing or throbbing
- Giddiness of elderly people
- Acute and chronic dyspepsia from eating ice
- Soreness of the abdominal wall, especially during pregnancy
- Yellow painless diarrhoea, with foul odour and bloated rumbling in the bowels
- Sore, bruised feeling in pelvic regions worse after delivering
- **During pregnancy, unable to walk**
- Wrist feels contracted, as if it is an elastic band
- Varicose veins in limbs with bruised, sore feeling
- Should not be given close to bedtime, may cause sleeplessness

CONSTITUTION
- Useful principally in women, during pregnancy or in old workmen, labourers, elderly people who are, overworked and fagged
- Stasis and fag; ill-effect of masturbation
- **Temperament:** Nervous, bilious
- **Thermal:** Ambithermal
- **Miasm:** Psora, Sycosis, Syphilis

CLINICAL
- Injury
- Sprains
- Bruises
- Splenomegaly
- Diarrhoea
- Breast tumours
- Railway spine
- Rheumatism
- Tendonitis
- Carpal tunnel syndrome
- Varicose veins
- Acne
- Boils
- Exudation

REMEDY RELATIONSHIP
- **Compare:** Arn., Ars., Staph., Ham., Bry.; Vanad. in degenerative states; Sep. in affects of child birth

BENZOICUM ACIDUM

INTRODUCTION
- **Common name:** Benzoic acid
- **Group:** Acid
- **Source:** Mineral kingdom
- **Formula:** $C_7H_6O_2$

SPHERE OF ACTION
- Mind
- Gastrointestinal system
- Respiratory system
- Heart
- Musculoskeletal system
- Urinary system

CONSTITUTION
- For gouty and asthmatic constitution; uric acid diathesis
- In circumscribed redness of cheeks and red spots on skin
- **Temperament:** Nervous, bilious
- **Thermal:** Chilly
- **Miasm:** Sycosis

MIND
- Prone to dwell upon unpleasant things in the past
- Omits words in writing
- Child cross, wants to be held in the arms, will not be laid down
- Shudders if he sees anyone deformed, fear following hurry
- Anxiety while sitting
- Delusion, hears confused voices, worse swallowing or walking in open air
- Anxiety when sitting
- Increased mental activity, when at work, followed by anxiety
- Dull
- Irritability
- Depression

KEYNOTE SYMPTOMS
- Pains suddenly change their location but are mostly felt in the region of heart or they alternate with urinary symptoms
- **Tongue spongy on surface with deep cracks and spreading ulcers in gouty persons**
- **Diarrhoea of children–white, very offensive, exhausting, liquid stools, running right through the diaper**
- Rectum feels constricted or puckered
- Cough with expectoration of green mucous
- Throat symptoms better after eating. Sensation of a lump in the throat
- Asthma with rheumatic complaints
- **Urine very offensive, hot and of a deep red or brown colour; offensive urine in old men**
- Joints crack on motion, pain in tendo-achillis
- Bunion of great toe; tearing pain of great toe
- Painful gouty nodes; gouty deposits; joints crack on motion
- Pain in achillis tendon at on calci with pain in heart
- Sweat, internal heat on awakening

CLINICAL
- Uric acid diathesis
- Vertigo
- Diarrhoea
- Constipation
- Asthma
- Pneumonia
- Rheumatic heart disease
- Renal insufficiency
- Urinary calculi
- Cystitis
- Enuresis
- Gonorrhoea
- Contractures
- Gout
- Wens
- Blisters
- Bunions
- Ganglion

MODALITIES
- **Aggravation:** In open air, by uncovering, cold, changing weather
- **Amelioration:** Heat, profuse urination

REMEDY RELATIONSHIP
- Useful after Colch. fails in gout; after Cop. in gonorrhoea
- **Compare:** Nit-ac., Am-be., Sabin.; Trop. in foetid urine
- **Antidote:** Cop.
- **Incompatible:** Wine

Benzoicum acidum

BERBERIS VULGARIS

INTRODUCTION
- **Common name:** Barberry
- **Family:** *Berberidaceae*
- **Source:** Vegetable kingdom
- **Part used:** Bark of root
- **Prover:** Hesse

SPHERE OF ACTION
- Mind
- Gastrointestinal system
- Respiratory system
- Genitourinary system
- Mucous membranes

CONSTITUTION
- Adapted to persons suffering from nerve affections; anaemic persons
- **Temperament:** Nervous
- **Thermal:** Chilly
- **Miasm:** Sycosis, Syphilis

MIND
- Apathy and indifference, disinclined to talk
- Sensitive to noise
- Aversion to work and talk
- Child repeats everything said to it
- Melancholy, grief; inclined to weep
- Lethargic
- Cerebral depression
- Nervous exhaustion and defective vitality
- Patients, especially children see terrifying apparitions in twilight
- **Vanishing of thoughts on interruption**

KEYNOTE SYMPTOMS
- Persons mentally and physically tired, does not want to do anything
- **Rapid change of symptoms, pains changing in regard to place and character, thirst alternating with thirstlessness, hunger with loss of appetite**
- Wandering, radiating pains; worse standing, acute exercise, pressure
- Venous engorgements as seen in pelvic engorgement and haemorrhoids
- Dryness of all mucous membranes – mouth, vagina, rectum, etc.
- **Sensation of a tight cap pressing upon the entire scalp**
- Nausea before breakfast
- Gall stone colic; radiating, shooting outwards; sticking, burning, smarting, sore, insensible; gall bladder catarrh
- Phthisis after fistula-in-ano
- Pains in thighs and loins on urinating. Soreness and sensitivity in kidney region; burning pains; bubbling sensation
- Inflammation of kidneys; haematuria has thick mucous and a bright red mealy sediment. Passes small calculi
- Neuralgic pains under finger nails with swelling of finger joints
- Gout with scanty urine

CLINICAL
- Emaciation
- Dropsy
- Styes
- Flatulence
- Liver degeneration
- Phthisis
- Fistula-in-ano
- Hypertension
- Diuresis
- Cystitis
- Renal stone
- Nephritis
- Enuresis
- Gout

MODALITIES
- **Aggravation:** Motion, standing, jar, stepping hard, fatigue, deep pressure
- **Amelioration:** Open air, urination

REMEDY RELATIONSHIP
- **Compare:** Convo-d., Aloe, Lyc., Nux-v., Sars., Xanrhoe.
- **Antidotes:** Camph., Bell.
- **Complementary:** Mag-m.
- **Follows well:** Bry., Kali-bi., Rhus-t., Sulph.

BISMUTHUM SUBNITRICUM

SPHERE OF ACTION

- Tongue
- Gastrointestinal system
- Respiratory system
- Musculoskeletal system

INTRODUCTION

- **Common name:** Precipitated sub-nitrate of bismuth, Bismuth subnitrate
- **Family:** Salt
- **Source:** Mineral kingdom
- **Formula:** $6Bi_2O_3 5N_2O_5 \cdot 9H_2O$ (approximately)
- **Prover:** Hahnemann

CONSTITUTION

- Suits irritation and catarrhal inflammation of alimentary canal
- **Temperament:** Nervous, bilious
- **Thermal:** Chilly
- **Miasm:** Psora, Sycosis, Syphilis

MIND

- Solitude is unbearable, wants company
- Anxious patient, therefore moves about frequently; never sits, walks, lies long in one place
- Irritability during daytime, better in the evening
- Anguish
- Discontented, dissatisfied
- Restless, apathetic
- Fear of death
- Fickle, does one thing only for a short time

KEYNOTE SYMPTOMS

- Restless on account of voluptuous dreams; sleepy in the morning, a few hours after eating
- Pains are tearing, which ameliorates gastric symptoms pinching, burning, screwing
- Headache extending to the root of the nose; alternates with stomach pain
- **Craves cold drinks; great thirst with frequent micturation**
- **Tongue swollen, black, gangrenous; profuse salivation; sweetish taste.** Gums swollen
- Vomiting of water in large quantities as soon as it reaches the stomach; burning in stomach, sensation of a load
- Catarrhal inflammation of alimentary tract with purging, vomiting and prostration
- Eructation, foetid belching with slow digestion
- **Food presses like a load on one spot; cancer of stomach**
- Abdomen distended; bloated in ridges
- Pain in abdomen in small spots
- Painless diarrhoea; cholera infantum in children, during summers, when vomiting predominates
- Dyspnoea from burning and constriction in chest
- Cramps in hands and feet, tearing in the wrist, pain in the tip of the fingers

CLINICAL

- Paralysis
- Convulsions
- Cramps
- Headache
- Gingivitis
- Toothache
- Gagging
- Vomiting
- Gastralgia
- Gastritis
- Gastroenteritis
- Colitis
- Diarrhoea
- Cholera
- Gastric cancer
- Pain after laparotomy
- Angina pectoris
- Insomnia

MODALITIES

- **Aggravation:** Motion, eating especially over-eating, when alone
- **Amelioration:** Cold drinks, cold application, bending backwards

REMEDY RELATIONSHIP

- **Antidotes:** Nux-v., Caps., Calc.
- **Compare:** Ant-c., Ars., Bell., Bry., Kreos., Phos., Lach., Lyc., Merc., Puls., Sep., Sil.

BLATTA ORIENTALIS

SPHERE OF ACTION
- Gastrointestinal system
- Respiratory system
- Heart
- Urinary system

INTRODUCTION
- **Common name:** Indian cockroach
- **Family:** *Orthoptera*
- **Source:** Animal kingdom
- **Part used:** Whole insect
- **Prover:** Ray

CONSTITUTION
- Suits young girls with yellow complexion; old people with asthma
- Acts best in obese, stout, corpulent people
- **Temperament:** Nervous, bilious, tubercular
- **Thermal:** Chilly
- **Miasm:** Psora, Sycosis, Syphilis

MIND
- Oversensitivity
- Nervousness
- Anxiety, especially regarding health
- Sadness
- Weariness

KEYNOTE SYMPTOMS
- Patient is obese and seems strong and robust. Despite this apparent vitality, the patient suffers from dyspnoea and shortness of breath from slightest exertion
- **Primarily, an asthma remedy; shortness of breath, dyspnoea from slightest exertion, with rattling of pus-like mucous**
- **Usually there is great allergy or sensitivity to mould, mildew or rotting leaves**
- Asthma associated with bronchitis or pain in urethra on micturating
- Cough with dyspnoea in bronchitis and phthisis, with much pus-like mucous; severe suffocation due to great accumulation of mucous
- Higher potencies are prescribed in more chronic cases; acts well when *Arsenicum album* fails

CLINICAL
- Obesity
- Spasms
- Jaundice
- Ascites
- Allergy
- Cold
- Dyspnoea
- Cough
- Bronchitis
- Bronchial asthma
- Pneumonia
- Tuberculosis
- Urethritis

REMEDY RELATIONSHIP
- **Compare:** Ars., Hydr., Puls., Sil., Kali-s.

MODALITIES
- **Aggravation:** From dust, during rain, in winters, exertion, moulds
- **Amelioration:** From expectoration

SPHERE OF ACTION

- Hair
- Gastrointestinal system
- Female genital system
- Mucous membranes
- Skin

INTRODUCTION

- **Common name:** Borate of sodium
- **Group:** Salt
- **Source:** Mineral kingdom
- **Formula:** $Na_2B_4O_7 \cdot 10H_2O$

CONSTITUTION

- Adapted to screaming children who are excessively nervous and have dread of downward motion
- Suits those with a pale, earthy face with an expression of suffering. Face swollen with pimples on face
- **Temperament:** Nervous
- **Thermal:** Chilly
- **Miasm:** Psora

BORAX VENETA

MIND

- Dread of downward motion. Fear of falling in children, when they are carried downstairs
- Fidgety; difficult to settle down to any definite work
- Fear of being infected by some contagious disease, of infection, of falling, of bridges, of thunder
- Mental symptoms better 11 pm
- Confusion, better after stool, cheerful
- Extreme anxiety; anxious expression on face
- Excessively nervous, easily frightened
- Sensitive to sudden noises
- Irritable, ill-humoured, fretful, indolent

KEYNOTE SYMPTOMS

- **Dread of downward motion** accompanies most complaints
- Excessively nervous; easily frightened or startled by the sound of sneezing or rustling of paper
- Extremely sensitive to slightest noise; not so much disturbed by louder ones
- **Hair become frowsy, tangled, splits, sticks together**
- **Sensation of a cobweb on the face**
- Eyelids and nose loaded with gummy exudation, stoppage of nostrils. Eyelashes turn inwards
- Aphthae in the mouth; mouth hot and tender. Painful gum boils. Oral thrush and oral herpes
- **Hot, smarting pain in orifice, pungent smell, child afraid to micturate**
- Shrieking from cystitis
- Pain in opposite breast when nursing
- **Galactorrhoea, increases; flow of milk; pain in opposite breast when nursing**
- **Leucorrhoea like white of an egg, as if warm water flowing down the legs**
- Menses too profuse, too soon; membranous dysmenorrhoea
- Helps in conception
- Unhealthy skin, least injury suppurates; psoriasis

CLINICAL

- Seasickness
- Epilepsy
- Plica polonica
- Entropion
- Stomatitis
- Aphthae
- Glossitis
- Candidiasis
- Thrush
- Nausea
- Diarrhoea
- Pleurisy
- Cystitis
- Vaginitis
- Leucorrhoea
- Dysmenorrhoea
- Premenstrual syndrome
- Infertility
- Galactorrhoea
- Nightmares
- Insomnia
- Herpes
- Psoriasis

REMEDY RELATIONSHIP

- **Follows well:** Calc., Psor., Sanic., Sulph.
- **Is followed by:** Ars., Bry., Lyc., Phos., Sil.
- **Incompatible:** Should not be used before or after Acet-ac., vinegar and wine
- **Compare:** Calc. Bry., Nux-v., Lyc., Merc., Puls., Rhus-t., Sil., Sulph.

MODALITIES

- **Aggravation:** Downward motion, from sudden slight noises, smoking which may bring on diarrhoea, damp cold weather, before urinating
- **Amelioration:** Pressure, holding painful side with hand, 11 pm

BOTHROPS LANCEOLATUS

SPHERE OF ACTION
- Mind
- Blood vessels
- Gastrointestinal system
- Respiratory system
- Skin

INTRODUCTION
- **Common name:** Yellow viper
- **Family:** *Crotalidae*
- **Source:** Animal kingdom
- **Part used:** Venom

CONSTITUTION
- Haemorrhagic constitution
- For the climacteric condition
- **Temperament:** Nervous, bilious
- **Thermal:** Chilly
- **Miasm:** Psora, Sycosis, Syphilis

MIND
- Forgetfulness of words
- While speaking, hunts for words
- Makes mistakes while talking, uses wrong words
- Desire to be silent, taciturn, indisposed to talk
- Slowness, lassitude, forgetfulness
- Inability to articulate
- Sluggishness
- Stupefaction, as if intoxicated

KEYNOTE SYMPTOMS
- Haemorrhages, blood becomes extremely fluid and dark, sometimes spouts out in jets from every orifice of the body
- **Diagonal course of symptoms prominent**
- Septic condition with slight shivering, followed by profuse sweat and nervous trembling
- Marked lassitude and sluggishness; sudden debility or emaciation. Nervous trembling and syncope
- Amaurosis due to retinal haemorrhage
- **Hemiplegia, right sided with aphasia, without affections of the tongue. Inability to articulate**
- Black vomiting – haematemesis, bloody stools with tympanitis
- Epigastric distress
- **Pain in right big toe**
- Leg severely infected after surgery for varicose veins. Muscular tissue filled with black blood
- Black spots on the skin as if from excessive contusions
- Skin swollen, livid, cold with haemorrhagic infiltrations; malignant erysipelas

CLINICAL
- Sluggishness
- Lassitude
- Haemorrhages
- Thrombosis
- Phlebitis
- Trembling
- Septic states
- Hemiplegia
- Amaurosis
- Conjunctival haemorrhage
- Haematemesis
- Aphasia
- Dysphagia
- Tympanitis
- Pulmonary congestion
- Erysipelas – malignant
- Gangrene
- Gangrenous ulcers
- Anthrax

MODALITIES
- **Aggravation:** Right side

REMEDY RELATIONSHIP
- **Compare:** Lach., Bell., in night blindness; Toxi., Trach.

BOVISA LYCOPERDON

INTRODUCTION

- **Common name:** Puff-ball
- **Family:** *Lycoperdaceae*
- **Source:** Vegetable kingdom
- **Part used:** Ripe bovista (fungus)

SPHERE OF ACTION

- Gastrointestinal system
- Respiratory system
- Blood
- Musculoskeletal system
- Urinary system
- Female genital system
- Skin

CONSTITUTION

- Suits those with acne; cheeks and lips are swollen, crusts about the nostrils
- Adapted to old maids with palpitations, who suffer from tettery type of eruptions or stammering children
- **Temperament:** Nervous, bilious, haemorrhagic
- **Thermal:** Ambithermal
- **Miasm:** Sycosis, Syphilis

MIND

- Awkward, everything falls from hands
- Absentminded, absorbed, buried in thoughts, dullness, sluggishness, difficulty of thinking
- Indifferent
- Sluggish
- Changeable moods – alternately laughing and crying
- Restless
- Mental depression; sad
- Sleep disturbed by anxious and frightful dreams
- Sensitive

KEYNOTE SYMPTOMS

- Discharges from all mucous membranes very tough, stringy and tenacious
- Causes relaxations of capillaries, producing of a haemorrhagic diathesis
- General puffiness and bloating of the body, causing easy indentations with blunt instruments
- **Sweat in axilla smells like onion**
- Sensation as if head was enlarged
- **Intolerance of tight clothing around the waist**
- **Sensation of a lump of ice in the stomach**
- Nose stopped up, can't breath. Stringy, tough discharge from nose
- **Colic with red urine**
- Diarrhoea before or during menses
- Menses profuse, starts or markedly increases at night; traces of menses between menstruation
- Leucorrhoea – thick, tough, greenish, acrid
- Impression on finger from using blunt instruments like scissors, knife, etc.
- Great weakness of the joints, they feel lax and loose
- Intolerable itching at the tip of the coccyx
- Pimples cover the entire body; scurvy; herpetic eruptions
- Acne worse in summers
- Dry and moist eruptions with urticaria; urticaria covers whole body; appears especially on excitement
- Eczematous eruptions on the back of the hands; eczema forms moist, thick crusts

CLINICAL

- Stammering
- Haemorrhages
- Oedema
- Pellagra
- Varicose veins
- Cerebral abscess
- Headache
- Stomatitis
- Hepatitis
- Ozaena
- Nasal catarrh
- Diarrhoea
- Colic
- Ulceration in frontal sinus
- Tubercles on alae nasi
- Laryngitis
- Tonsillitis
- Cough
- Asthma
- Tuberculosis
- Ovarian cyst
- Leucorrhoea
- Metrorrhagia
- Dysmenorrhoea
- Typhoid fever
- Septic fever
- Acne
- Urticaria
- Smallpox
- Eczema

MODALITIES

- **Aggravation:** Before and during menses, hot weather, after eating especially cold food, wine, coffee
- **Amelioration:** Bending double, eating hot food

REMEDY RELATIONSHIP

- **Compare:** Am-c., Bell., Calc., Mag-s.; Sep. in menstrual irregularities;
- **Antidotes,** effects of local applications of tar; suffocation from gas
- When Rhus-t. seems indicated but fails to cure, in chronic urticaria

BROMIUM

INTRODUCTION
- **Common name:** Bromine
- **Group:** Halogen
- **Source:** Mineral kingdom
- **Formula:** Br
- **Prover:** Hering

SPHERE OF ACTION
- Gastrointestinal system
- Respiratory system
- Heart
- Thyroid gland
- Musculoskeletal system
- Genital system

CONSTITUTION
- Suits scrofulous children with enlarged glands; tendency to infiltrate glands
- Adapted to people with light blue eyes, blond hair, fair, delicate skin
- **Temperament:** Nervous, tubercular
- **Thermal:** Chilly
- **Miasm:** Psora, Sycosis

MIND
- Anxious, apprehensive, with great depression of spirits
- **Expects to see things, jumps around the floor as if someone was behind him**
- **Sits in room doing nothing, looking in one direction only**
- Delusion that strange people are looking over his shoulder
- Quarrelsome, bad humour
- Loss of ideas
- Wants to be carried
- Aversion to any kind of work

KEYNOTE SYMPTOMS
- Left sided affections like left sided mumps
- Complaints from being over heated
- Swelling, induration and stony hardness of glands, especially of lower jaw and throat
- **Weak and easily heated, then very sweaty and extremely sensitive to cold drafts**
- Profuse sweat with great weakness. Tremulous all over
- Tendency to spasmodic attacks
- Sensation of a cobweb on the face
- Fan-like motion of alae nasi
- Nosebleed accompanies many complaints; especially those of the respiratory tract
- Laryngeal diphtheria with membrane formation in larynx spreading upwards. Throat feels raw. Laryngospasm.
- **Cough worse on entering a warm room**
- Spasmodic cough with rattling of mucous
- Cough – dry with hoarseness and burning pain behind the sternum
- Cold sensation in chest on inspiring
- Complaints from being overheated
- **Asthmatic complaints of sailors when they come ashore, but are relieved on going back to the sea**
- Discharge of flatus from the vagina
- Swelling of testicles with soreness induration

CLINICAL
- Emaciation
- Glandular indurations
- Adenopathy
- Goitre
- Cancer
- Tumours
- Mumps
- Haemorrhoids
- Malena
- Rhinitis
- Epistaxis
- Laryngitis
- Laryngospasm
- Pharyngitis
- Tonsillitis
- Hoarseness
- Diphtheria
- Croup
- Asthma
- Breast tumour
- Physometra
- Dysmenorrhoea
- Ovarian cysts
- Orchitis
- Indurated testicles
- Acne

MODALITIES
- **Aggravation:** From evening till midnight, when sitting in a warm room, warm damp weather, when at rest and lying on the left side, dust
- **Amelioration:** Any motion, exercise, at sea, nosebleed

REMEDY RELATIONSHIP
- **Antidotes:** Am-c., Camph.
- Salt inhibits the action of Brom
- **Compare:** Con., Spong., Iod., Aster., Arg-n., Spong., Ant-t., Hep.
- Avoid milk when taking Brom.

SPHERE OF ACTION

- Head
- Mucous membranes
- Serous membranes
- Gastrointestinal system
- Respiratory system
- Musculoskeletal system
- Sleep
- Skin

MIND

- Very irritable and ugly in behaviour; bad temper
- **Determined. Child doesn't like to be carried or raised**
- Taciturn, quarrelsome
- **Delirium – wants to go home, thinking he is not there, worse at night; constant motion of left leg and left hand**
- Talks of business
- Fear of poverty
- Wants to be left alone
- Averse to being disturbed
- Desire for things which are rejected when offered
- Homesickness
- Capricious, hard to please or satisfy

MODALITIES

- **Aggravation:** Warmth, any motion, morning, eating, hot weather, exertion, touch, anger, vexation, deep breathing
- **Amelioration:** Lying on the painful side, pressure, rest, cold things, being quiet, bandaging

INTRODUCTION

- **Common name:** Wild hop, Black berried bryony
- **Family:** *Cucurbitaceae*
- **Source:** Vegetable kingdom
- **Part used:** Roots (to be collected before flowering)

BRYONIA ALBA

KEYNOTE SYMPTOMS

- Right sided remedy
- Injury, trauma, sprains, fractures, especially of joints
- Physical weakness; complaints develop slowly
- All mucous membranes are dry; with scanty and adherent discharges
- Affects all serous membranes and subsequently the viscera they contain, causing inflammation and exudation
- Severe stitching, tearing, bursting pains; any spot in the body painful to pressure; worse touch or least motion; better absolute rest and lying on the painful side or pressure
- **Excessive dryness.** Lips dry, cracked; bitter taste; cough dry; urine dark and scanty; stool, as if burnt; tongue parched; etc.
- Vertigo, on rising up; worse on least motion; with nausea
- Bursting, splitting headache, especially in the occiput; worse motion
- **Extremely thirsty for large quantities of water, at infrequent intervals**
- **Tongue coated white, yellowish-brown at centre**
- Vomiting of water and bile, vomited immediately after eating, worse warm drinks; pressure in stomach after eating, as of a stone; stomach sensitive to touch
- **No desire for stools for a number of days. Stools large, dry, hard; constipation**
- **Dry, hacking cough with stitches in the chest; must sit up; worse after eating and drinking**
- **Vicarious menstruation, nosebleed when menses should appear**
- Stony hardness and heaviness of the breasts; must support them
- Rheumatic pains and swelling with dropsical effusion in synovial and serous membranes
- **Red, hot, swollen joints, worse least motion**
- Muscles become hard after neuralgia
- Fevers – all kinds of fever bilious, typhoid, remittent, etc.

CONSTITUTION

- Rheumatic or gouty diathesis
- Suits people with dark hair and complexion; dry, firm muscular fibre, robust people
- Adapted to business oriented people with a fear of poverty; marked irritability, want to be left alone
- **Temperament:** Nervous, bilious
- **Thermal:** Ambithermal
- **Miasm:** Psora, Sycosis, Syphilis

CLINICAL

- Injuries
- Lymphangitis
- Coma
- Meningitis
- Headache
- Migraine
- Toothache
- Dyspepsia
- Hiccoughs
- Appendicitis
- Gastroenteritis
- Jaundice
- Constipation
- Diarrhoea
- Influenza
- Epistaxis
- Meniere's disease
- Tinnitus
- Cough
- Whooping cough
- Tuberculosis
- Pleurisy
- Pleurodynia
- Bronchitis
- Asthma
- Pneumonia
- Nephritis
- Mastitis
- Ovaritis
- Arthritis
- Lumbago
- Sciatica
- Bursitis
- Tendonitis
- Relapsing fever
- Remittent fever
- Typhoid
- Rheumatic fever

REMEDY RELATIONSHIP

- **Complementary:** Upa when Bry. fails; Rhus-t., Alum.
- **Antidotes:** Acon., Cham., Nux-v.
- **Compare:** Asc-t., Tub., Kali-m., Ptel., Rhus-t., Kali-c., Acon., Ant-c., Arn., Ars., Bell., Nat-m.

BUFO RANA

INTRODUCTION
- **Common name:** Toad
- **Family:** *Bufonidae*
- **Source:** Animal kingdom
- **Part used:** Venom, poison of the toad
- **Prover:** Carl Hencke

SPHERE OF ACTION
- Gastrointestinal system
- Respiratory system
- Nervous system
- Cardiovascular system
- Female genital system
- Male genital system
- Skin

CONSTITUTION
- Suits mentally retarded or feeble-minded children; prematurely senile people
- **Temperament:** Nervous, bilious
- **Thermal:** Chilly
- **Miasm:** Psora, Sycosis, Syphilis

MIND
- Amorous disposition, shameless; moral depravity
- Disposition to handle genitals
- Desire for solitude to practice masturbation
- Cretinism; mentally slow and unrefined
- Talks nonsense, then angry if not understood
- Anger before convulsions
- Stupefaction between convulsions
- Unconsciousness after convulsions
- Music is unbearable
- Weeping easily in epilepsy
- Feeble minded
- Anxious about health
- **Fears animals, cancer, strangers, mirrors in a room**
- Idiotic, talks nonsense and then gets angry if not understood

KEYNOTE SYMPTOMS
- Low minded and develops low type of diseases; arouses lowest passions
- Convulsions, epilepsy; especially at night, connected to the sexual sphere
- Paralytic condition of eyelids
- Blisters form on the eyes; cornea ulcerated
- **Stammering, speech is difficult. Tongue is cracked and bluish-black**
- Constantly licks the lips
- Delirium, headache and insomnia during dysentery
- **Heart feels too large. Sensation as if heart swimming in water**
- Spasm or epileptic attack comes on during coition
- Burning and swelling in ovaries and uterus; ulceration of cervix
- Involuntary emissions, ejaculation too quick – impotence; spasms during coition; buboes. Tendency to masturbation
- Injury of fingers; pain runs in streaks up the arm
- Red streaks under the skin – lymphangitis
- Slightest injury suppurates; epidemic or infections, carbuncles

CLINICAL
- Mental retardation
- Epilepsy
- Convulsions
- Seizures
- Paralysis agitans
- Cancer
- Lymphangitis
- Epistaxis
- Metrorrhagia
- Milk leg
- Uterine polyp
- Cervix ulcerated
- Mammae indurated
- Breast cancer
- Bubo
- Masturbation
- Onanism
- Impotency
- Arthritis
- Rheumatism
- Panaritium
- Pemphigus
- Varicose veins
- Carbuncles

MODALITIES
- **Aggravation:** In a warm room, on awakening, from masturbation, sexual excitement
- **Amelioration:** Bathing, cold air, from putting feet in hot water

REMEDY RELATIONSHIP
- **Compare:** Bar-c., Aster., Salam. in epilepsy and softening of brain; Ars., Canth., Lach., Tarent. in epilepsy; Calc., Sil., Nux-v.
- **Antidoted by:** Lach., Seneg.
- **Complementary:** Salam., Helo., Amph.

SPHERE OF ACTION

- Mind
- Gastrointestinal system
- Cardiovascular system
- Musculoskeletal system
- Urinary system

INTRODUCTION

- **Common name:** Night-blooming cereus
- **Family:** *Cactaceae*
- **Source:** Vegetable kingdom
- **Part used:** Flowering stem

CONSTITUTION

- Adapted to old people with heart complaints; haemorrhagic tendency and sanguine constitution
- **Temperament:** Sanguine, plethoric
- **Thermal:** Chilly
- **Miasm:** Sycosis, Psora

CACTUS GRANDIFLORUS

MIND

- **Fear of death, believes the disease is incurable; fear of heart disease**
- Sadness; weeps without knowing why
- Apprehension
- Taciturn
- Tendency to be easily frightened on waking
- Irresistible desire to cry
- Melancholic
- Ill-humoured
- Screams with pain
- Anxiety, especially on walking
- Irritability, worse consolation
- Frightful dreams
- Loves solitude – wants to be alone and not speak to anyone
- Easily frightened

KEYNOTE SYMPTOMS

- Haemorrhage; it favours formation of clots speedily
- **Constriction sensation in various parts of the body; contraction as of an iron band. The whole body feels as if caged and each wire is being twisted tighter and tighter.**
- **Periodicity marked;** periodic neuralgia; periodic attacks of suffocation, **fever paroxysm returns at 11 am and/or 11 pm**
- Throbbing of carotids, right sided prosopalgia and pulsations in ears
- Constriction or heaviness in stomach; weight and distress in stomach after eating
- Sensation of weight in anus
- Constriction of chest, impeding respiration; oppressed breathing
- **Angina pectoris with suffocation, cold sweat, palpitation and vertigo; worse at the approach of menses and lying on the left side**
- **Heart feels clutched and released, alternately by an iron hand**
- Endocarditis with mitral insufficiency, together with violent and rapid action; endocardial murmur; cardiac hypertrophy
- Cardiac ailments with swelling of left hand and numbness of left arm
- Suits aneurysm of heart and large arteries
- Constriction of neck of bladder causing urine retention
- Haemorrhage from bladder; urine has red sand deposits
- Constriction of ovaries. Menstrual flow ceases on lying down
- Oedema of hands and feet; **rheumatism, beginning in upper limbs**

CLINICAL

- Hysteria
- Hypochondriasis
- Oedema
- Dropsy
- Haemorrhage
- Vertigo
- Haemoptysis
- Epistaxis
- Melena
- Heart trouble
- Aneurysm
- Arteriosclerosis
- Angina pectoris
- Tobacco heart
- Myocarditis
- Mitral insufficiency
- Haematuria
- Bladder paralysis
- Menorrhagia
- Dysmenorrhoea
- Vaginismus
- Rheumatism
- Insomnia

MODALITIES

- **Aggravation:** Around noon, lying on the left side, walking, going upstairs, 11 am and/or 11 pm
- **Amelioration:** Open air, pressure on vertex

REMEDY RELATIONSHIP

- **Antidoted by:** Acon., Camph., Chin.
- **Compare:** Dig., Spig., Conv., Kalm., Naja, Magn-gr., Dig., Lach., in mental symptoms; Bell., Glon., in congestion of head
- **Compatible:** Dig. in heart affections

SPHERE OF ACTION

- Mind
- Gastrointestinal system
- Respiratory system
- Musculoskeletal system
- Female genital system
- Male genital system
- Urinary system
- Skin

MIND

- Masturbation and its bad effects in men
- Lascivious men, though impotent, ogle at women on the street
- When nervous, craves tobacco
- Restless, cannot control himself after smoking, nervous excitation
- Sensitive to noise. Slightest noise startles from sleep
- Very forgetful
- Dreads motion
- Careful about health, fears catching a disease

MODALITIES

- **Aggravation:** Motion, sexual excess, tobacco smoking
- **Amelioration:** After sweat, after sleeping in the daytime, cold air

INTRODUCTION

- **Common name:** American arum
- **Family:** *Araceae*
- **Source:** Vegetable kingdom
- **Part used:** Whole plant
- **Prover:** Hering

CALADIUM SEGUINUM

KEYNOTE SYMPTOMS

- Nervous excitation
- **There is a great desire to lie down and aversion to motion; if he makes an effort, he is strong enough to move**
- Dryness of parts which are usually moist
- **Modifies craving for tobacco. Tobacco heart**
- Confused headache with pressure in the eyes, forehead and shoulders
- **Red, dry stripe down the centre of tongue, widening towards the tip**
- **Thirstless; thirst for only warm water**
- Acrid vomiting; gnawing and fluttering sensation in the stomach
- Stomach feels full of dry food
- Asthma alternates with an itching rash; catarrhal asthma with difficult expectoration which ameliorates on being expectorated
- Pruritus valvae in females which sometimes may be due to threadworms finding their way into the vagina inducing masturbation and even nymphomania
- Impotence with sexual desire and excitement; relaxed penis; no emission or orgasm during an embrace
- Pruritus of glans penis
- **Sweet sweat attracts flies**
- Intense burning and itching after insect or mosquito bites

CONSTITUTION

- For persons of lax, phlegmatic temperament
- Suits people with dread of motion, confused headache and sighing respiration
- **Temperament:** Nervous, phlegmatic
- **Thermal:** Chilly
- **Miasm:** Psora, Sycosis, Syphilis

CLINICAL

- Headache
- Eructations
- Gastritis
- Threadworms
- Catarrhal asthma
- Tobacco heart
- Nymphomania
- Pruritis vulvae
- Impotence
- Hydrocoele
- Masturbation
- Spermatorrhoea
- Balanitis
- Arthritis
- Rheumatism
- Insect bites
- Eczema
- Erysipelas
- Lichen planus
- Urticaria

REMEDY RELATIONSHIP

- **Incompatible:** Arum-t.
- **Complementary:** Nit-ac.
- **Compare:** Caps., Phos., Caust., Sel., Lyc.

CALCAREA ARSENICOSA

INTRODUCTION
- **Common name:** Arsenite of lime
- **Group:** Salt
- **Source:** Mineral kingdom
- **Formula:** $Ca_3(AsO_3)_2$
- **Prover:** Hering

SPHERE OF ACTION
- Mind
- Liver
- Spleen
- Kidneys
- Cardiovascular system

CONSTITUTION
- For people, especially women who are fair, fat and flabby, with a pale face, and are approaching menopause. Scrofulous constitution
- **Temperament:** Nervous, bilious
- **Thermal:** Chilly
- **Miasm:** Psora, Sycosis, Syphilis

MIND
- Anger, depression and anxiety
- Delirium in the evening, in the dark
- Restlessness after midnight, at 3 am
- Slightest emotion causes severe palpitation
- Fear of birds
- Desire for company
- Confusion, delusions, illusions, great mental depression
- Wonderful vision passing before the eyes. Often an indescribable feeling of health, 'as if in heaven'
- Anxiety about the future, about health
- Sensation as if flying or swimming – feet do not touch the ground

KEYNOTE SYMPTOMS
- Slightest emotions cause palpitation of heart, worse least exertion
- Complaints of drunkards after abstaining from alcohol; craving for alcohol
- Low haemoglobin and red blood cell count
- Rush of blood to the head or congestion of head before an attack of epilepsy. Aura is felt in the cardiac region
- Epilepsy from valvular heart disease
- Tasteless belching with salivation and palpitation. **Tongue dry**
- Enlarged spleen and liver of children and infants
- Loss of voice with dryness of larynx
- **Thirsty with no desire to eat.** Eructations and vomiting after eating
- Distention of abdomen
- Pancreatic disease, cancer of pancreas
- Cardiac disorders associated with kidney failure, nephritis
- Palpitations and oppression of chest causing insomnia; feeble heart
- Pain in cardiac region with fear of suffocation
- Kidney region sensitive to pressure in nephritis
- Urine is burning and scanty. **Albumin and casts are present in the urine.** Albuminuria and dropsy
- Burning pains in the uterus and vagina; carcinoma of uterus
- Menses early, scanty; dysmenorrhoea, metrorrhagia
- Weariness and lameness of lower limbs
- **Oedema of upper limbs, especially back of hands with albuminuria**

CLINICAL
- Delusions
- Anxiety
- Alcoholism
- Dropsy
- Obesity
- Lipoma
- Epilepsy
- Vertigo
- Gastric ulcer
- Peptic ulcer
- Hepato-splenomegaly
- Liver cirrhosis
- Colitis
- Pancreatic affections
- Cancer of pancreas
- Asthma
- Palpitation
- Valvular heart diseases
- Cardiac disorders
- Nephritis
- Albuminuria
- Malaria

MODALITIES
- **Aggravation:** From slight exertion, cold air, errors in diet
- **Amelioration:** Rest, open air

REMEDY RELATIONSHIP
- **Compare:** Con., Glon., Lith-c., Puls., Nux-v., Ars., Phos., Dig., Carb-v.
- **Follows well:** After Coni., in lymphatic, psoric or tuberculous persons
- Acts well in cases overdosed by quinine

CALCAREA CARBONICA OSTREARUM

INTRODUCTION

- **Common name:** Carbonate of lime, Calcarea ostrearum
- **Group:** Salt
- **Source:** Mineral kingdom
- **Formula:** $CaCO_3$
- **Prover:** Hahnemann

SPHERE OF ACTION

- Head
- Glands
- Eyes
- Ears
- Gastrointestinal system
- Respiratory system
- Female genital system
- Musculoskeletal system
- Skin

CONSTITUTION

- Suits fat, fair, flabby patients who become easily fatigued and tired on walking, much sweating, slow in movement
- Tendency to grow fat; impaired nutrition
- A scrofulous, anti-psoric remedy with tendency to take cold and increased mucous secretions
- **Temperament:** Nervous, leucophlegmatic, scrofulous
- **Thermal:** Chilly
- **Miasm:** Psora, Sycosis

MIND

- Ailments from getting over worked and exhausted
- Hard working, capable, conscientious, over responsible, people who take on too much responsibility; worse on getting over worked
- Life is all about completing your task-list. Cannot relax. Works to exhaustion then must give up job all together.
- Practical, down to earth
- Timid and restless as if an evil was impending over her, weakness of mind, lack of confidence and determination
- Aversion to others. Indifference, apathy to conversation
- Fears places at a height, mice, insects, rats, spiders, dogs and darkness
- Restlessness, depression. Apprehension, worse in the evening
- Obstinate, forgetful, confused
- Fears loss of reason, misfortune
- Desire to be magnetized
- Intelligent but slow comprehension
- Over crowding of ideas prevents sleep
- Horrid visions on opening eyes. Night mares; dreams of monsters

KEYNOTE SYMPTOMS

- Extremely sensitive to cold and damp; dreads open air
- **Profuse perspiration** – local and general; **especially on the back of the head and neck – wets pillow**
- **Craving for eggs, indigestible things like chalk, pencils, dirt**
- Diseases arising from defective assimilation and ossification; malnutrition, tendency to curvature of bones, especially back and long bones
- **Delayed milestones in children;** open fontanelles; defective nutrition of glands, bones and skin
- Glandular swellings – enlarged and hard, especially cervical and bronchial glands
- Pituitary and thyroid dysfunction. Hypothyroidism
- Exostosis; polypi, in nose, ear, uterus
- **Sourness of all discharges;** sour taste in mouth, sour eructations, sour vomiting, stools sour, urine sour, sour foot sweat
- Diarrhoea, in children from eating indigestible things
- Constipation – first part of stools hard
- Umbilical hernia; gall stone colic
- Inguinal and mesenteric glands are swollen and painful; distention of abdomen with hardness. Increase of fat in the abdomen
- Mucopurulent otorrhoea and enlarged glands
- Frequent colds, at every change of weather; nostrils sore, ulcerated
- Chest sensitive to touch, pressure or percussion. Suffocating spells
- Genitals relaxed; easy displacement of uterus
- Menses too early, too profuse, too long lasting with toothache and cold damp feet
- Tender and swollen breasts before menses
- Cold, damp feet/knees, as if damp stockings were worn
- Tendency to easily strain muscles and joints; weak ankles
- Warts on face and hands

CLINICAL

- Phobic disorders
- Malnutrition
- Adenopathy
- Obesity
- Connective tissue disease
- Polyps
- Multiple sclerosis
- Muscular dystrophy
- Systemic lupus erythmatosis
- Goitre
- Seizure disorder
- Hydrocephalus
- Lachrimal fistula
- Blepharitis
- Corneal ulcers
- Cataract
- Photophobia
- Toothache
- Dentitional disorders
- Dysphagia
- Umbilical hernia
- Peritonitis
- Diarrhoea
- Constipation
- Worms
- Otitis media
- Tonsillitis
- Asthma
- Incipient phthisis
- Premenstrual syndrome
- Uterine fibroid
- Arthritis
- Rheumatism
- Scoliosis
- Rickets
- Exostosis
- Osteomyelitis
- Osteoporosis
- Scleroderma
- Abscesses
- Warts

MODALITIES

- **Aggravation:** Cold air, wet weather, cold water, from washing (Ant-c.), morning, during full moon, milk, dentition, ascending
- **Amelioration:** Dry weather, lying on painful side (Bry., Puls.), after breakfast, magnetization

REMEDY RELATIONSHIP

- **Complementary to: Bell., which is the acute of Calc.**
- Calcarea acts best before, Lyc., Nux-v., Phos., Sil.
- **It follows:** Nit-ac., Puls., Sulph.
- According to Hahnemann, Calc. must not be used before Nit-ac. and Sulph.; may produce unnecessary complications
- In children it may be often repeated
- In aged people it should not be repeated; especially if the first dose benefited, it will usually do harm

CALCAREA FLUORICA

INTRODUCTION
- **Common name:** Fluoride of lime, Calcii flourica, Calcium fluoride, Fluorspar, Fluorite
- **Source:** Mineral kingdom
- **Formula:** CaF_2
- **Prover:** Schussler

SPHERE OF ACTION
- Eyes
- Ears
- Gastrointestinal system
- Respiratory system
- Heart
- Musculoskeletal system
- Female genital system
- Glands

CONSTITUTION
- Patient is fair and fat with varicosed veins
- **Temperament:** Nervous, bilious, sluggish
- **Thermal:** Chilly
- **Miasm:** Syphilis, Psora, Sycosis

MIND
- Depressed
- **Fear of poverty, groundless fear of financial loss, heights, mice**
- Grief from sudden, unexpected losses
- **Dreams of dead people, of cutting a woman up for salting**
- Anxiety about health
- Indecisive

KEYNOTE SYMPTOMS
- Indurations of stony hardness, threatening suppuration
- Glands enlarge and become stony hard
- Tendency to bony growths, osteosarcoma, exostosis, especially after injury
- Slow processes, sluggishness
- Tendency to suppurations–chronic middle ear suppuration, follicular sore throat, fistulous ulcers discharging pus, etc.
- **Discharges turn grass green**
- Congenital syphilis manifesting as caries and necrosis with burning pains and heat
- Reduces formation of adhesions post-surgery
- **Deficient enamel of teeth; teeth crumble and break easily**
- **Tongue cracked, fissured, indurated, hard**
- Diarrhoea with gout, stools gushing, watery, foetid; anal fissure
- Bleeding haemorrhoids, internal and blind piles with constipation
- Tonsils – rough, ragged, plugs of mucous forming in the crypts of tonsil; adenoids
- Tendency to varicoses and aneurysms. Veins dilate and become varicosed, inflamed.
- When tuberculous toxins affect the heart and blood vessels
- Tendons have nodules or growths post injury or after overuse
- **Fissures and cracks; on palms, anus, tongue**
- **Tendency to hard swelling on the cheek with toothache; hard swelling on jaw bone**

CLINICAL
- Enlarged glands of old
- Tumours
- Thyroid nodules
- Goitre
- Conjuctivitis
- Phlyctenular keratitis
- Palpebral cysts
- Cataract
- Cholelithiasis
- Constipation
- Chronic otitis media
- Ozaena
- Rheumatic heart
- Mitral stenosis
- Arteriosclerosis
- Aneurysm
- Uterine fibroids
- Cancer of breast
- Syphilis
- Bone deformities
- Bony spurs
- Ganglion
- Arthritis
- Scoliosis
- Varicosities
- Exostosis
- Backache

MODALITIES
- **Aggravation:** During rest, changes of weather, cold wet weather, beginning of motion
- **Amelioration:** Heat, warm applications, rubbing

REMEDY RELATIONSHIP
- **Compare:** Con., Lap-a., Bar-m., Hecla, Rhus-t., Nat-m., Calc-st-s. acts as a haemostatic and absorptive in uterine myoma; Mangi. in varicose veins

Calcarea fluorica

CALCAREA PHOSPHORICA

INTRODUCTION

- **Common name:** Phosphate of lime
- **Group:** Salt
- **Source:** Mineral kingdom
- **Formula:** $Ca_3(PO_4)_2$
- **Prover:** Hering

SPHERE OF ACTION

- Mind
- Bones
- Gastrointestinal system
- Respiratory system
- Genitourinary system

CONSTITUTION

- **For tall, scrawny, school going children, especially girls at puberty**
- Suits chlorotic; anaemic, spare subjects with dark hair, eyes and complexion, cold extremities and feeble digestion
- **Temperament:** Nervous, scrofulous
- **Thermal:** Chilly
- **Miasm:** Psora, Sycosis, Syphilis

MIND

- Mental dullness or weakness
- Sighing involuntarily
- Fear of dark, thunderstorms
- Ailments on hearing bad news, from grief, disappointment in love
- Discontented, dissatisfied, obstinate
- Constantly complaining, peevish, bored
- Friendly, open, sensitive
- **Strong desire to travel, wants to go somewhere**
- Child irritable, whiny, requires constant attention and needs to be carried
- Forgetful, especially after grief, vexation; weak memory
- Complaints are worse thinking about them
- Temper tantrums

KEYNOTE SYMPTOMS

- Anaemia after acute diseases and chronic wasting diseases
- **Change of weather aggravates all symptoms**
- Sensation of numbness and crawling accompany most symptoms
- Affinity for places where bones form sutures and symphyses
- Soft, thin bones. Malassimilation. Delayed closure of fontanelles; non-union of fractured bones
- **Pain along the suture lines, originating in the cervical region**
- Headaches in school going children
- Numbness; crawling sensation on top of head, as if ice was lying on the upper part of occiput
- Perspiration on head at night, while in bed
- Vertigo from constipation, worse drafts of air
- Delayed dentition and teething problems; problems incident to dentitional period
- Headache with abdominal flatulence
- Chronic abdominal colic in school going children
- Flabby, sunken abdomen, festering navel
- **Diarrhoea from juicy fruits during dentition; green, slimy, hot, undigested**
- Fistula-in-ano alternates with chest complaints
- Menorrhagia with intense backache
- Leucorrhoea like white of an egg

CLINICAL

- Depression
- Delayed development
- Obesity
- Anaemia
- Chronic fatigue syndrome
- Headache
- Opacity of cornea
- Dentitional complaints
- Caries of teeth
- Diarrhoea
- Haemorrhoids
- Otitis media
- Hoarseness
- Tubercular laryngitis
- Adenoids
- Prolapse of uterus
- Rickets
- Osteoporosis
- Osteomyelitis
- Arthritis
- Carpal tunnel syndrome
- Cervical spondylosis
- Lumbago
- Scoliosis
- Fractures

MODALITIES

- **Aggravation:** Exposure to damp, cold changeable weather, east winds, melting snow, mental exertion, during dentition, puberty, thinking of symptoms
- **Amelioration:** In summers, warm dry atmosphere, rest

REMEDY RELATIONSHIP

- **Complementary:** Ruta, Hep.
- **Compare:** Carb-an., Calc-f., Calc., Fl-ac., Kali-p.; to, Psor. in debility remaining after acute diseases; to, Sil. but sweat of head is wanting.
- Acts best before Iod., Psor., Sanic., Sulph.; after Ars., Tub.

CALCAREA SILICATA

INTRODUCTION
- **Common name:** Silicate of lime, Calcium silicate
- **Group:** Salt
- **Source:** Mineral kingdom
- **Prover:** Usher

SPHERE OF ACTION
- Eyes
- Face
- Respiratory system
- Gastrointestinal system
- Skin

CONSTITUTION
- Suits weak, emaciated, cold patient worse from being overheated
- Hydrogenoid constitution
- **Temperament:** Nervous
- **Thermal:** Chilly
- **Miasm:** Sycosis

MIND
- Want of self-confidence
- Confusion of mind from mental exertion; absentminded
- Lack of confidence; fearful
- **Talks with dead people, converses with or dreams of them; generally obsessed with dead friends or relatives. Dreams of dead bodies, dead people**
- Attempts to escape from the window
- Frightened easily, especially during an afternoon nap
- Irresolution, indecision
- Sadness, despondency, dejection, mental depression, gloom, melancholy, causeless sadness

KEYNOTE SYMPTOMS
- Deep, long acting remedy for complaints which come on slowly and reach their final development after long periods
- **Patient is weak, emaciated, cold, chilly, but is worse from being overheated; lack of vital heat**
- Sensitiveness all over due to pain. Dreads to be touched; sore internally, sensitive to jar
- Aversion to open air, sensitive to drafts, to bathing, especially if cold
- **Sensation of coldness in stomach, especially if empty**
- Flatulence and distention after eating. Vomiting and eructations
- Cough with coldness, weakness, emaciation and copious, yellowish-green mucous

CLINICAL
- Obesity
- Polyps
- Neuralgia
- Goitre
- Vertigo
- Corneal affections
- Rheumatic iritis
- Cataract
- Dyspepsia
- Enteritis
- Peritonitis
- Constipation
- Asthma
- Cystitis
- Metrorrhagia
- Uterine prolapse
- Rheumatism
- Sciatica
- Abscesses
- Warts
- Pimples
- Comedones
- Ulcers
- Acne
- Wens
- Insomnia

MODALITIES
- **Aggravation:** Change of weather, becoming cold, cold wet weather, exertion, from being overheated

REMEDY RELATIONSHIP
- **Compare:** Ars., Tub., Bar-c., Iod.

CALCAREA SULPHURICA

INTRODUCTION

- **Common name:** Sulphate of lime, Plaster of Paris
- **Group:** Salt
- **Source:** Mineral kingdom
- **Formula:** $CaSO_4 \cdot 2H_2O$
- **Prover:** Clarence Conant

SPHERE OF ACTION

- Mind
- Head
- Gastrointestinal system
- Respiratory system
- Musculoskeletal system
- Heart
- Female genital system
- Urinary system
- Skin

MIND

- Strong personality
- Argumentative, bossy
- Changeable moods
- Anxiety in the evening in bed, at night, better in open air
- Timidity
- Confusion from mental exertion
- Frightful hallucinations
- Forgetful
- Fear of death, insanity, misfortune
- Sluggish mind
- Great anxiety, irritability and depression in the morning
- Jealousy

MODALITIES

- **Aggravation:** From drafts, cold wet weather, touch, standing
- **Amelioration:** In open air, bathing, eating, uncovering

KEYNOTE SYMPTOMS

- **Tendency to suppuration; pus is thick, yellow, lumpy, bloody**
- Unhealthy skin; does not heal rapidly
- Tendency to form abscesses; when ruptured, are slow to heal and have a continuous discharge of yellow pus; recurrent and running abscesses
- Indicated when an abscess has broken, or has been lanced and is discharging
- Mucous discharges are yellow, thick, lumpy and mixed with blood
- Conditions where pus has found a vent, in the third stage of inflammation
- Scald head of children with purulent discharge or purulent crusts
- Catarrhal conditions of the head associated with gastric complaints
- Inflammation of eyes, ears, nose, throat with purulent discharge
- **Appetite lost or ravenous, with waterbrash; indigestion with nausea, vertigo; vomiting when moving the head**
- Abscesses around the anus; purulent diarrhoea
- **Menses late, long lasting, with headache, twitching and great weakness**
- Pustular pimples on the face
- Pimples, pustules, felons and furuncles

CONSTITUTION

- Suits an allergic constitution. Purulent, yellow, thick discharges from septic conditions
- A connective tissue remedy
- **Temperament:** Nervous, bilious
- **Thermal:** Ambithermal
- **Miasm:** Psora

CLINICAL

- Cystic tumours
- Thyroid nodules
- Varicosities
- Crusta lactea
- Ophthalmia neonatorum
- Conjunctivitis
- Photophobia
- Cataract
- Gumboils
- Cholelithiasis
- Dysentery
- Constipation
- Prolapse of rectum
- Fistula-in-ano
- Post-nasal discharge
- Pneumonia
- Empyema
- Mitral stenosis
- Arteriosclerosis
- Nephritis
- Uterine fibroids
- Arthritis
- Scoliosis
- Exostosis
- Hectic fever
- Abscesses
- Ulcers
- Pustules
- Herpes
- Burns
- Lupus vulgaris
- Pimples
- Eczema

REMEDY RELATIONSHIP

- **Compare:** Hep., Sil., Calen., Kali-m., Nat-s.
- **Follows well:** Kali-m, Nat-s, Sil.

CALENDULA OFFICINALIS

INTRODUCTION

- **Common name:** Marigold
- **Family:** *Compositae*
- **Source:** Vegetable kingdom
- **Part used:** Fresh flowering tops and leaves

SPHERE OF ACTION

- Mucous membranes
- Gastrointestinal system
- Respiratory system
- Nervous system
- Female genital system
- Skin

MIND

- Frightened easily, fears something horrible or terrible will happen
- Delusion of fainting or falling from a height
- Nervousness
- Anxiety
- Irritability, worse contradiction

MODALITIES

- **Aggravation:** In damp, heavy, cloudy weather, during chill
- **Amelioration:** Walking about, lying perfectly still, warmth

KEYNOTE SYMPTOMS

- **Great homoeopathic antiseptic and healing agent**
- Indicated in all external wounds, in surgeries
- Excessively painful, open, torn, cut, lacerated, ragged, or suppurating wounds
- Old, neglected wounds, threatening gangrene
- Haemostatic, especially after tooth extraction
- **It restores the vitality of an injured part, making it impregnable against the forces of putrefaction**
- Rupture of muscles or tendons
- Wounds penetrating articulations with loss of synovial fluid
- Traumatic neuritis or neuroma
- Inflamed, sloughing, varicose ulcers – purulent
- Makes acrid discharges healthy and prevents suppuration
- **Can be prescribed during cancer as an intermittent**
- Tendency to take cold, especially in damp weather
- Skin appears yellow; goose flesh, especially with heartburn
- Wild delirium in burns
- Unconsciousness in burns or with flesh wounds
- Lacerated scalp wound
- **Hoarseness; green expectoration**
- Coryza in one nostril with profuse green discharge
- Uterine hypertrophy; warts on the external os. Chronic endometritis
- **Laceration and perineal tear during labour**

CONSTITUTION

- **Used as a healing agent; applied locally, promotes healthy granulation tissue**
- Constitutional tendency to erysipelas
- **Temperament:** Nervous, bilious, irritable
- **Thermal:** Chilly
- **Miasm:** Psora, Sycosis, Syphilis

CLINICAL

- Wounds
- Injuries
- Suppurating wounds
- Superficial burns
- Superficial scalds
- Ulcers
- Neuroma
- Pyaemia
- Surgical cuts
- Cuts
- Injury to eyes
- Ear drum rupture
- Deafness
- Bulimia
- Nausea
- Vomiting
- Heartburn
- Ulcers of os uteri
- Menorrhagia
- Endocervicitis
- Prolapse of uterus
- Erysipelas
- Warts

REMEDY RELATIONSHIP

- **Compare:** Ham., Hyper., Symph., Arn., Staph., Bry., Led., Rhus-t., Ruta
- **Antidote:** Chel., Rheum
- **Complementary:** Hep.
- **Incompatible:** Camph.

Calendula officinalis

CAMPHORA OFFICINALIS

INTRODUCTION

- **Common name:** Camphor
- **Group:** Hydrocarbon
- **Source:** Mineral kingdom
- **Formula:** $C_{10}H_{16}O$

SPHERE OF ACTION

- Mind
- Gastrointestinal system
- Muscular system
- Respiratory system
- Urinary system
- Skin

MIND

- Pains are better by thinking of them
- Religious despair
- Loquacious with hasty speech, speech incoherent, wandering
- **Attacks of terror at night, afraid to go to sleep at night. Desire for company at night; anguish at night, as if dying; relieved when she finds herself alive**
- Great anxiety and extreme restlessness

MODALITIES

- **Aggravation:** Motion, night, contact, cold air, drafts
- **Amelioration:** Warmth, free discharges

KEYNOTE SYMPTOMS

- **Collapsed condition with coldness**
- Great weakness, sinking of strength, pulse small, weak, slow
- **Patient is icy cold yet he is averse to covering or wants them off and on alternately with internal burning heat and anxiousness**
- Very sensitive to cold air or takes cold easily
- Inhaled air seems cold; skin and breath cold. Internal heat and external coldness. Feeling as if, cold wind was blowing over the body.
- Bad effects of shock
- Painfully sensitive to slightest touch
- Scantiness or retention of discharges
- Dry collapse with little vomiting and purging
- Cholera with cramps in the calves; scantiness of discharges, yet great weakness, coldness of the body and anxiety
- Cramps in the stomach and bowels. Stools blackish, involuntary
- Fluent coryza; first stage with chillness and sneezing
- **It antidotes almost all drugs of the vegetable kingdom including tabacco, opium, etc.**

CONSTITUTION

- For scrofulous children and irritable, weak blondes
- Surface of the body cold, face pale, blue lips, livid profound prostration; hippocratic face
- **Temperament:** Sanguinous
- **Thermal:** Chilly
- **Miasm:** Psora, Sycosis

CLINICAL

- Delusions
- Chronic fatigue syndrome
- Sepsis
- Collapse with chills
- Fainting
- Convulsions
- Epilepsy
- Tetanic spasms
- Sunstroke
- Dysentery
- Cholera
- Influenza
- Pneumonia
- Asphyxia neonatorum
- Asthma
- Urinary tract infections
- Anuria
- Nephritis
- Gonorrhoea
- Nocturnal emission
- Priapism
- Inflammatory fevers
- Malaria
- Varicose veins
- Erysipelas
- Sequelae of measles
- Insomnia

REMEDY RELATIONSHIP

- Camph. antidotes or modifies the action of nearly every vegetable medicine—tobacco, opium, worm medicines, etc. Luffa actangula. Camphoricum acidum.
- **Incompatible:** Kali-n.
- **Complementary:** Canth.
- **Antidoted by:** Op., Nit-s-d., Phos.
- **Compare:** Carb-v., Cupr., Ars., Verat., Aloe, Canth., Dulc., Sec., Lyc.

SPHERE OF ACTION

- Mucous membranes
- Central nervous system
- Gastrointestinal system
- Genitourinary system

MIND

- Stammering and stuttering
- Weeping, worse laughter
- Fear of going to bed
- Sensation as if intoxicated; as if in a dream
- Mind is too active, crowded with ideas
- Clairvoyance
- Frightful dreams
- Sensation as from pinching with the fingers
- Makes mistakes in writing, omits words, repeats words
- Sadness, better in the afternoon
- Vanishing of senses, confusion of thoughts
- Speech hasty, wandering, incoherent. Loquacity, laughs immoderately
- Time passes too slowly
- Voices, including self's seem to be coming from a distance

MODALITIES

- **Aggravation:** lying down, going upstairs, urinating, darkness, night, coffee, tobacco, liquor
- **Amelioration:** Fresh air, cold water, rest

INTRODUCTION

- **Common** name: Indian hemp
- **Family:** *Cannabiaceae*
- **Source:** Vegetable kingdom
- **Part used:** Flowering tops of both male and female plant

CANNABIS SATIVA

KEYNOTE SYMPTOMS

- **Trickling sensation, as if drops of hot water were poured over him, or as if drops of cold water was falling on the head, or from the anus, or from the heart, while sweating, better uncovering**
- Sensation of water dropping on the head
- Delusion that drops of blood are falling from the heart
- Misty sight
- Dryness of mouth
- **Desires sweets and cold drinks**
- **Abuse of alcohol, tobacco**
- Great fatigue as from overexertion, weary after meals
- Fear arising from stomach
- Cystitis with burning at urethral meatus, while and at the end of micturation
- **Scanty urine, turbid, white or reddish, as if mixed with blood.** Retained urine with constipation
- Paralytic tearing pains. Affections of the foot

CONSTITUTION

- For old people with sexual excitement; urethral stricture
- **Temperament:** Nervous, bilious
- **Thermal:** Chilly
- **Miasm:** Psora, Sycosis, Syphilis

CLINICAL

- Stuttering
- Stammering
- Corneal opacity
- Cataract
- Gonorrheal ophthalmia
- Constipation
- Pericarditis
- Urinary tract infection
- Urethritis
- Cystitis
- Acute gonorrhoea
- Urethral carbuncle
- Urethral stricture
- Leucorrhoea
- Amenorrhoea
- Phimosis
- Prostatitis
- Rheumatism
- Torticollis

REMEDY RELATIONSHIP

- **Antidotes:** Camph., lemon juice, Merc.
- **Compare:** Hedy. gonorrhoea and inflammation of penis, balanitis; Canth., Apis, Cop., Thuj., Kali-n., Cann-i., Med., Petros., Sars.

CANTHARIS VESICATORIA

SPHERE OF ACTION

- Gastrointestinal system
- Central nervous system
- Genitourinary system
- Skin

INTRODUCTION

- **Common name:** Spanish fly, Deger, Fabricus
- **Family:** *Cantharideae*
- **Source:** Animal kingdom
- **Part used:** Whole dried fly
- **Prover:** Hahnemann

CONSTITUTION

- For inflamed sexual organs causing frenzied delirium
- For any condition where urine is scanty, burning and accompanied by constant urging
- **Temperament:** Nervous, bilious
- **Thermal:** Chilly
- **Miasm:** Sycosis, Syphilis

MIND

- Confused
- Excitement, delirious
- Sudden loss of consciousness with a red face
- Irritation, disposition to fly into a rage
- Acute mania, generally of a sexual type; amorous frenzy; fiery sexual desire
- Fits of rage with crying, barking, striking, renewed by the sight of bright, dazzling objects and of water, and by touching the larynx
- Moaning and violent cries, interspersed with barking
- Convulsions and howling like a dog, ending in a stupor
- Tries to do some thing but accomplishes nothing

KEYNOTE SYMPTOMS

- Violent and aggressive action on tissues, especially mucous membranes of the urinary tract. Rapid inflammation followed by severe, destructive pathology
- Inflammations are violently acute and generally associated with irritation of the bladder
- Oversensitiveness of all parts
- **Pains are cutting, smarting, biting, burning, as if part is raw**
- Burning in every part of the body, both internal and external, with severe weakness
- Tendency to haemorrhages from all orifices
- **Tongue covered with vesicles and deeply furred**
- Constriction and aphthous ulceration of the throat; difficulty in swallowing liquids
- All gastric or abdominal complaints aggravated by drinking coffee
- Tenesmus of rectum and bladder
- Great tenesmus; stools mucoid and bloody with scrapings of the intestines
- Urinary tract infection; urinary tract is in a state of inflammation with a tendency to develop gangrene
- **Burning, scalding urine, with cutting, intolerable urging and fearful tenesmus or dribbling. Constant urge to urinate**
- When dysuria is present as a concomitant to any complaint
- Acute and severe cystitis; intolerable tenesmus
- Sexual organs inflamed resulting in frenzied delirium. Sexual excitement during pains
- Sexual desire increased in both sexes, preventing sleep
- Burns and scalds, before and after blister formation

CLINICAL

- Hydrophobia
- Meningitis
- Conjunctivitis
- Stomatitis
- Aphthous ulceration
- Colitis
- Bronchitis
- Pleurisy
- Pericarditis
- Urinary tract infection
- Urethritis
- Urethral stricture
- Cystitis
- Nephritis
- Pyelitis
- Pyelonephritis
- Retained placenta
- Ovarian cyst
- Nymphomania
- Gonorrhoea
- Priapism
- Balanitis
- Spermatorrhoea
- Prostatitis
- Eczema
- Burns
- Scalds
- Vesicles
- Erysipelas

MODALITIES

- **Aggravation:** Touch or approach, micturation, drinking cold water or coffee, bright objects
- **Amelioration:** Rubbing, warmth, rest

REMEDY RELATIONSHIP

- **Antidotes:** Acon., Camph., Puls.
- **Compare:** Canthin., Apis., Ars., Merc-c., Bell., Staph., Cann-s., Merc.
- **Complementary:** Camph.
- **Incompatible:** Coff.

INTRODUCTION

- **Common name:** Cayenne pepper
- **Family:** *Solanaceae*
- **Source:** Vegetable kingdom
- **Part used:** Ripe fruit
- **Prover:** Hahnemann

CAPSICUM ANNUUM

SPHERE OF ACTION

- Head
- Ears
- Gastrointestinal system
- Mucous membranes
- Spinal cord
- Musculoskeletal system
- Urinary system

MIND

- Homesickness with red cheeks, sleeplessness and a disposition to commit suicide (melancholic)
- Awkward, runs into everything. Dipsomania, delirium tremens
- Joyful, sings; yet gets angry at slightest cause
- Obstinacy, capriciousness
- Very sensitive, feels easily insulted
- Insecure without social relationships, tries to be more sociable to hide insecurity
- Fear of censure, of ghosts
- **Nostalgia, very sentimental emotions goes back to past events with such force, as if head would fly to pieces, holds head with hands**
- Desires to be left alone
- Averse to go outside routine, dreads any kind of exercise

MODALITIES

- **Aggravation:** Open air, uncovering, draught of air, dampness, bathing, cold air, drinking
- **Amelioration:** While eating, heat, continuous motion

KEYNOTE SYMPTOMS

- **A general unclean appearance**
- Circulation sluggish
- Burning, smarting pains, worse from cold water. Burning in mouth, throat, rectum, bladder, etc.
- Affects mucous membranes which become dark, red, spongy, ooze bloody mucous, producing a sensation of constriction, soreness and burning; smarting as if pepper was sprinkled on the part
- Sensation of soreness and constriction in various parts – throat, chest, bladder, urethra, rectum, etc.
- Tendency to suppuration in every inflammatory process; with foul discharges
- General chilliness with burning, smarting pains; better from heat
- Complaints in alcoholics when abstaining; delirium tremens
- Inflammation of the mastoid
- **Much thirst, but drinking causes shuddering or shivering. Thirsty after stools**
- Dysentery with burning and tenesmus
- **Sore throat of smokers and drinkers**
- Pain in distant parts on coughing

CONSTITUTION

- For fat, clumsy, dirty children who are always chilly and are disinclined to think or work
- For persons of lax fibre who are weak, lazy, indolent, fat, red, clumsy, awkward and of unclean habits
- Suits relaxed, sluggish people opposed to physical exertion having diminished vital heat
- For elderly people exhausted by mental work and poverty
- **Temperament:** Phlegmatic
- **Thermal:** Chilly
- **Miasm:** Sycosis, Syphilis

CLINICAL

- Disposition to suicide
- Delirium tremens
- Mastoiditis
- Halitosis
- Lack of appetite
- Dyspepsia
- Flatulence
- Vomiting
- Dysentery
- Pharyngitis
- Tonsillitis
- Whooping cough
- Cystitis
- Phimosis
- Gonorrhoea
- Herpes labialis
- Myalgia
- Sciatica
- Eczema

REMEDY RELATIONSHIP

- **Antidote:** Cina, Calad.
- **Compare:** Puls., Lyc., Bell., Arn., Psor., Lach., Nat-m., Carb-v., Meny., Ph-ac., Merc., Cent.

Capsicum annuum

CARBO ANIMALIS

SPHERE OF ACTION

- Mind
- Gastrointestinal system
- Respiratory system
- Female genital system
- Musculoskeletal system
- Glands

INTRODUCTION

- **Common name:** Animal charcoal, Leather charcoal
- **Group:** Organic carbon
- **Source:** Animal kingdom

CONSTITUTION

- Adapted to scrofulous and venous constitutions. Old people with debilitating diseases, feeble circulation and blue cheeks and lips
- For women who weak are with lowered vitality after nursing
- **Temperament:** Nervous, bilious, scrofulous
- **Thermal:** Ambithermal
- **Miasm:** Psora, Sycosis, Syphilis

MIND

- Sad and reflective, especially in the morning
- Homesickness in the morning; longing for the past
- Desires to be alone, avoids conversation; aversion to company
- Weeps when eating
- Alternate gaiety and despondency
- Fearful, easily frightened
- **Afraid of the dark, worse closing eyes**
- Anxiety at night, with orgasm of blood
- Confused and dull, does not know where the sound comes from
- Stupefaction with vertigo

KEYNOTE SYMPTOMS

- For diseases which have an insidious onset, are chronic and sluggish in development
- Feeble circulation; enlargement of veins in different parts of the body, blueness of the skin with weak circulation and lowered vitality
- Indurated, swollen, painful glands – neck, mammae, groin, axillae, etc. Induration after inflammation
- All discharges are putrid and exhausting causing excoriation of the skin like leucorrhoea, diarrhoea, menses, etc.
- Ulceration, decomposition, offensiveness; haemorrhages and gangrene
- Tendency to malignancy; of mammae, uterus, etc.
- **Local congestions without heat**
- Eating tires the patient
- Bad effects of ptomaine poisoning; eating spoiled fish and decayed vegetables
- Weak digestion with flatulence
- Stitch remaining after pleurisy; ulceration of lungs
- Menses too early, frequent, long lasting, followed by severe exhaustion, cannot even speak; offensive lochia
- Nausea of pregnancy; burning in vagina and labia; cancer of uterus
- Limbs easily strained from over lifting. Weak joints; ankles turn easily; easy dislocation
- Burning rawness and fissures on skin

CLINICAL

- Marasmus
- Cancer
- Glandular indurations
- Flatulence
- Eructations
- Ptomaine poisoning
- Hookworms
- Deafness
- Bronchitis
- Pneumonia
- Pleurisy
- Metrorrhagia
- Menorrhagia
- Leucorrhoea
- Carcinoma of breasts
- Cancer of uterus
- Bubo
- Syphilis
- Arthritis
- Rheumatism
- Typhoid
- Gangrene
- Ulceration
- Acne rosacea
- Fissures

MODALITIES

- **Aggravation:** After shaving, loss of animal fluids, cold dry air, menses, loss of vital fluids, sprains, over lifting, cold
- **Amelioration:** Warm room, laying hand on affected part

REMEDY RELATIONSHIP

- In the Carbon group, all have putrid discharges and exhalations. All act on the skin, causing intertrigo and excoriations.
- **Complementary:** Calc-p.
- **Antidoted by:** Ars., Nux-v., vinegar
- **Compare:** Bad., Sep., Sulph., Plb-i., Thymol., Calc-p., Chin. in loss of fluids; Puls, Sil., Calc.

SPHERE OF ACTION

- Mind
- Gastrointestinal system
- Respiratory system
- Musculoskeletal system
- Urinary system
- Skin

INTRODUCTION

- **Common name:** Vegetable charcoal, Carbo ligni, Wood charcoal
- **Group:** Organic carbon
- **Source:** Vegetable kingdom
- **Prover:** Hahnemann

CARBO VEGETABILIS

CONSTITUTION

- Suits people who are sluggish, fat, lazy with a tendency to chronicity of complaints
- For puffy, cyanosed, pale, hippocratic, old persons, or prematurely old people with coldness of the body
- **Temperament:** Nervous, bilious
- **Thermal:** Chilly
- **Miasm:** Psora, Sycosis, Syphilis

MIND

- Much sluggishness mentally as well as physically; much laziness, slowness of thoughts, comprehension, dullness; sudden loss of memory
- Concentration difficult. Weakness of memory – sudden
- Indifference, hears everything without any feelings about it; indifference to music which he loved
- Great irritability, especially directed to the family. Harsh and cutting remarks
- Haughtiness
- Anxiety in the evening accompanied by shuddering
- Anxiety on closing the eyes
- Sees frightful images in the dark
- Child bites, strikes and kicks
- **Confusion better mental exertion**

KEYNOTE SYMPTOMS

- Disintegration and imperfect oxidation
- People who have never recovered from the previous illness
- Ailments from the loss of vital fluids or haemorrhages from any mucous surface; oozing of dark blood
- Lowered vitality; almost lifeless; body cold, head hot; cool breath; must have air – must be fanned constantly; lack of reaction
- **Very debilitated; collapse, anaemia, coma, weak, exhausted and cold – cyanosed**
- General venous stasis resulting in blueness, coldness and ecchymosis. Coldness with prostration. **State of collapse**
- Fainting from indigestion, flatus, sunstroke, infection
- For septic conditions with blueness and decomposition
- **Aversion to milk, meat and fatty things**
- Epigastric region very sensitive; simplest food disagrees; heaviness, fullness and sleepiness after eating
- Simplest food distresses; digestion is slow, rancid, sour belching; food putrifies
- Abdomen tense with flatus, relieved temporarily by belching; flatulent colic
- Spasmodic cough with bluish discolouration of the face and burning in the chest. Hoarseness, worse in the evening
- Discharge from ear or otorrhoea due to suppressed measles, catarrhal condition, parotiditis
- Asthma in elderly with cyanosis
- Limbs go to sleep; joints are weak, want of muscular power. Legs cold from below the knees
- Blue, cold, bruised skin; moist with hot perspiration
- Tendency to varicose ulcers with an offensive discharge

CLINICAL

- Chronic fatigue syndrome
- Collapse
- Syncope
- Fainting
- Coma
- Obesity
- Anaemia
- Dropsy
- Cyanosis
- Post-surgical syncope or shock
- Pyorrhoea
- Dyspepsia
- Gastritis
- Gastralgia
- Diarrhoea
- Constipation
- Epistaxis
- Asphyxia
- Pneumonia
- Tuberculosis
- Asthma
- Chronic aortitis
- Congestive heart failure
- Varicose veins
- Arthritis
- Gangrene

MODALITIES

- **Aggravation:** From butter, pork, fat food, abuse of quinine bark and mercury, from singing or reading aloud, in warm damp weather, high living
- **Amelioration:** From eructation, being fanned, cool air

REMEDY RELATIONSHIP

- **Complementary:** Kali-c., Chin., Dros.
- **Compare:** Chin., Sulph., Plb. in neglected pneumonia Ant-t. in threatened paralysis from inability to expectorate loosened mucous; Opium with lack of reaction after wellselected remedies fail to permanently improve (Valer.); Phos. in easily bleeding ulcers; Puls. in bad effects from fat food and pastry

CARBOLICUM ACIDUM

INTRODUCTION
- **Common name:** Phenol, Carbolic acid
- **Group:** Hydrocarbon
- **Source:** Mineral kingdom
- **Formula:** C_6H_5OH
- **Prover:** Berridge

SPHERE OF ACTION
- Nose
- Gastrointestinal system
- Respiratory system
- Central nervous system
- Urinary system
- Female genital system
- Extremities
- Skin

MIND
- Mental prostration, but desire for mental work
- Mental exhaustion, brain fag; mental exertion aggravates
- Loss of memory for what he was about to do
- Dreams usually not remembered; or amorous dreams, of fire, of journey, of an embalmed body part
- Delusion as if he had taken opium in the morning
- Languid, painless, foul, destructive remedy

MODALITIES
- **Aggravation:** Mental exertion, jar, reading, combing hair, pregnancy
- **Amelioration:** Smoking, drinking a strong cup of tea, rubbing

KEYNOTE SYMPTOMS
- It is an irritant, anaesthetic
- Profound prostration, collapse; surface pale and covered with cold sweat
- Terrible pains, come suddenly, last for a short time and disappear suddenly
- Physical exertion brings on abscesses anywhere in the body, especially in the right ear
- Malignant and septic conditions
- **Offensive discharges** – foul, burning, putrid from nose, mouth, throat, rectum, vagina, etc.
- Increased olfactory sensibility
- **Craving for stimulants like whisky and tobacco**
- **Excessive thirst**
- Very offensive breath with constipation; burning from mouth to stomach; fermentative dyspepsia
- Passes mucous from the anus when urinating
- **Bloody stools like scrapings of intestines with tenesmus**
- Painful swelling in left ovary; cervical erosion with foetid, acrid discharge
- Leucorrhoea – thick, causing itching and burning; leucorrhoea in children
- Palpitation of the heart at night
- Urine dark, black or olive green in colour; alkaline
- Severe pain in lumbo sacral region; muscles of back and limbs sore
- Cramps in fore part of the leg, close to tibia, while walking
- Anaphylaxis to bee stings; swelling of face and tongue

CONSTITUTION
- For weak, anaemic, prostrated people with brain fag having sunken eyes and yellow complexion
- **Temperament:** Nervous, bilious
- **Thermal:** Ambithermal
- **Miasm:** Psora, Sycosis, Syphilis

CLINICAL
- Prostration
- Anaphylactic shock
- Hydrocephalus
- Stomatitis
- Loss of appetite
- Dyspepsia
- Vomiting
- Diarrhoea
- Constipation
- Influenza
- Ozaena
- Laryngitis
- Diphtheria
- Cystitis
- Diabetes
- Leucorrhoea
- Ovarian neuralgia
- Cervical erosion
- Puerperal fever
- Arthritis
- Lumbago
- Paralysis
- Ulcers
- Burns
- Pustules

REMEDY RELATIONSHIP
- **Compare:** Chrysarobinum (locally in ringworm of the scalp, 5-10 percent in glycerine and alcohol. Equal parts). Ars., Kreos., Carb-v., Chin., Apis, Gels., Merc., Sulph; Pic-ac., in burns, ulcers and offensive discharges; Guan.
- **Antidote:** Alcohol, vinegar, chalk, Iod. Glauber's salt in watery solution
- **Incompatible:** Glycerine and vegetable oils

SPHERE OF ACTION

- Mind
- Gastrointestinal system
- Respiratory system
- Muscular system
- Nervous system
- Skin

INTRODUCTION

- **Common name:** Cancer nosode, Carcinosin
- **Group:** Nosode
- **Source:** Animal kingdom
- **Part used:** Nosode from breast cancer
- **Prover:** Foubister

CONSTITUTION

- For brownish, 'café au late' complexion having blue sclerotics and numerous moles or multiple warts anywhere on the body; fair complexion
- **Thermal:** Ambithermal
- **Miasm:** Syphilis

CARCINOSINUM

MIND

- **For ailments observed in people who have lived under severe fear for too long**
- History of emotional suppression and guilt; person is emotionally closed; better by weeping
- Suits those who have been sexually abused or are in a abusive relationship
- Fastidious, sensitive to reprimands or reproaches
- Artistic disposition
- **Desire music, dancing and travel**
- Anticipatory anxiety; fear of unknown
- Anxiety about health – of getting an incurable disease, of getting cancer
- Affectionate and sympathetic, yielding nature
- Autism; mental retardation. Attention deficit syndrome
- Dislikes consolation; worse consolation

KEYNOTE SYMPTOMS

- When even well indicated nosodes fail to cure
- Chronic, excessive fatigue and weariness; low blood sugar also causes fatigue
- Family history of cancer, syphilis, tuberculosis, diabetes mellitus
- Cancer of lungs, breast, uterus, cervix, stomach, prostate
- **Great desire to lie on the abdomen or in knee-chest position**
- Haemorrhagic tendency from all orifices; haemophilia, thalassemia
- **Craving or aversion to eggs, fat, milk, meat. There may be craving at one time now and aversion at another time in the same patient**
- Indigestion, accumulation of gas in stomach and bowels
- Tendency to diarrhoea, constipation or acidosis in children
- **Burning pain as if there is fire in the colon; chronic ulcerative colitis**
- Recurrent attacks of bronchitis, pneumonia, measles, mumps, tonsillitis
- Carcinoma of the uterus with offensive discharges, haemorrhage and pain
- Carcinoma of the mammary gland with great pain and induration of glands
- Tendency for insomnia in children

CLINICAL

- Fatigue
- Haemophilia
- Thalassemia
- Mononucleosis
- Polyps
- Cancerous cachexia
- Mumps
- Acidosis
- Flatulence
- Ulcerative colitis
- Diarrhoea
- Constipation
- Tonsillitis
- Bronchitis
- Asthma
- Pneumonia
- Diabetes
- Mastitis
- Uterine cancer
- Breast cancer
- Prostatic cancer
- Rheumatism
- Measles
- Keloids
- Insomnia

MODALITIES

- **Aggravation:** Warmth, extremes of weather, full or new moon
- **Amelioration:** Open air, during thunderstoms

REMEDY RELATIONSHIP

- **Compare:** Bufo, Con., Phyt., Ast-r., Tub., Thuj., Med., Syph., Nat-m., Sep., Psor., Phos., Ars., Calc-p.

CARDUUS MARIANUS

SPHERE OF ACTION
- Gastrointestinal system
- Liver
- Respiratory system
- Cardiovascular system
- Portal system

MIND
- Alcoholism, dipsomania
- Loss of memory for what he was about to do or say
- Despondency
- Forgetful
- Apathetic, melancholic
- Hypochondriacal

MODALITIES
- **Aggravation:** Lying on left side, motion, touch, eating
- **Amelioration:** Bleeding

INTRODUCTION
- **Common name:** St. Mary's thistle, Blessed thistle
- **Family:** *Compositae*
- **Source:** Vegetable kingdom
- **Part used:** Seeds
- **Prover:** Rademacher

KEYNOTE SYMPTOMS
- Haemorrhagic diathesis associated with liver complaints
- Venous stasis and dropsical conditions due to portal congestion
- Chilliness; on awakening, at night
- **Vertigo with a tendency to fall forward, better nosebleed**
- Nausea, retching, vomiting of green, acrid fluid
- **Pain in liver most marked when lying on left side, worse deep inspiration and motion**
- **Liver engorged, especially left lobe,** swollen laterally in the transverse direction, painful on pressure
- Liver disease affects lungs and heart
- Influenza when liver is affected
- Diseases of miners, associated with asthma
- Disturbs sugar metabolism
- Varicose veins and varicose ulcers; broken or hard, thrombosed veins

CONSTITUTION
- Suits old people with heart complaints haemorrhagic diathesis, suffering from the abuse of alcohol, especially beer
- **Temperament:** Nervous, bilious, haemorrhagic
- **Thermal:** Ambithermal
- **Miasm:** Sycosis, Syphilis

CLINICAL
- Debility
- Haemorrhages
- Vertigo
- Liver disorders
- Hepatomegaly
- Cirrhosis
- Hyperaemia of liver
- Jaundice
- Gall stones
- Diarrhoea
- Constipation
- Haemorrhoids
- Epistaxis
- Hypertension
- Arteriosclerosis
- Bradycardia
- Varicose veins
- Varicose ulcers

REMEDY RELATIONSHIP
- **Compare:** Card-b., which has a strong action upon the eyes, and sensation of contraction in many parts; stomach symptoms are similar; Chel., Chion., Merc., Podo., Bry., Aloe., Nux-v., Lyc.

CAULOPHYLLUM THALICTROIDES

SPHERE OF ACTION

- Gastrointestinal system
- Female genital system
- Small joints
- Skin

INTRODUCTION

- **Common name:** Blue cohosh, Papoose root
- **Family:** *Berberidaceae*
- **Source:** Vegetable kingdom
- **Part used:** Rhizome
- **Prover:** Dr Burt

CONSTITUTION

- Suits the hydrogenoid constitution with sallow complexion, dark hair and rigid muscular fibre; patients are very weak and emaciated
- Mostly suited to women, during pregnancy and labour
- **Temperament:** Rheumatic
- **Thermal:** Chilly
- **Miasm:** Psora, Sycosis

MIND

- Memory weak, prostration of mind after abortion
- Irritability after abortion
- Anger, irritability during menses
- Delusion that she is pregnant
- Hysterical
- Fretful
- Apprehensive
- Restless; nervous and excitable
- Displeased easily

KEYNOTE SYMPTOMS

- Pain changes place every few minutes
- **Heavy upper eyelids, has to raise them with a finger**
- Cardialgia, spasm of stomach, dyspepsia with spasmodic symptoms
- Habitual abortions from uterine debility; lack of uterine toxicity
- **Spasmodic, rigid os, unable to dilate. Labour pains delayed due to rigid os. Weakness, exhaustion, want of uterine tonicity.** Pains intermittent, paroxysmal, spasmodic and erratic, change place every ten minutes
- After pains, across lower abdomen, extending to the groins
- **False labour pains, erratic, changing place every ten minutes**
- Passive haemorrhages. Blood oozes out with want of tonicity
- Leucorrhoea in little girls
- Needle-like pricking pains in cervix
- Dysmenorrhoea, with pain flying to other parts
- Rheumatism, small joints affected
- Stiffness of back; sensitive spine. Erratic pains, flying from one place to another; cramping, shooting, rheumatic in character, ending in the neck which then feels stiff

CLINICAL

- Thrush
- Dyspepsia
- Cardialgia
- Diarrhoea
- Haemorrhoids
- Vaginitis
- Leucorrhoea
- Metrorrhagia
- Menorrhagia
- Dysmenorrhoea
- Abortions
- Infertility
- Uterine atony
- Labour arrested
- False labour pains
- Premature labour
- Lochia
- Rigid os
- Vaginal thrush
- Arthritis
- Rheumatoid arthritis
- Rheumatism of wrist
- Neck stiffness
- Discolouration of skin

MODALITIES

- **Aggravation:** Pregnancy, suppression of menses, coffee, open air

REMEDY RELATIONSHIP

- **Compare:** Cimic., Bell., Lil-t., Sec., Thlas., Vib.; Puls. in labour pains, but mental condition opposite; Sep., in moth patches and reflex symptoms from uterine irregularities
- **Incompatible:** Coff.

CAUSTICUM HAHNEMANNI

SPHERE OF ACTION

- Mind
- Eyes
- Gastrointestinal system
- Respiratory system
- Female genital system
- Musculoskeletal system
- Skin

INTRODUCTION

- **Common name:** Hahnemann's tinctura acris sine kali; Caustic potash
- **Source:** Mineral kingdom
- **Part used:** Obtained by distilling a mix of slaked lime and a solution of potassium sulphate
- **Prover:** Hahnemann

CONSTITUTION

- Hydrogenoid constituion
- Adapted to dark haired persons, of rigid fibre with yellow, sallow complexion
- **Temperament:** Nervous, bilious, lymphatic
- **Thermal:** Chilly
- **Miasm:** Psora, Sycosis, Syphilis

MIND

- Melancholic, sad, hopeless from taking care of someone, grief, sorrow
- Weepy, least thing makes the child cry
- **Intensely sympathetic; great sympathy for the sufferings of others**
- Insanity after suppressed skin eruptions, with mental confusion
- Anxious, forebodings, fear of impending doom
- **Cannot stand injustice, sensitive to authority, opposition; is idealistic, fights for a better world**
- Restlessness at night
- Ailments from long lasting grief, sudden emotions, loss of sleep, nursing loved ones
- Thinking of complaints causes an aggravation of symptoms
- Absentminded; weak memory

KEYNOTE SYMPTOMS

- Predominantly, right sided complaints
- Paralysis of single parts – expectoration slips back; urethra or rectum insensible; urine spurts on coughing; aphonia, etc.
- Weakness, progressive loss of muscular strength causing uncertainty in control over muscles, finally ending in paralysis of single organs or parts
- Paralysis from exposure to cold. Post-diphtheritic paralysis, from lead
- **Aversion to sweets; worse eating fresh meat**
- Burning, rawness and soreness of scalp, respiratory tract, rectum, anus, vagina, urethra
- The patient shows improvement for some time and then the case comes to a standstill
- History of sexual abuse or violence in the family
- Vision is foggy, lids agglutinated; double vision; cornea ulcerated; ptosis, drooping of upper eyelids
- **Sensation of a ball rising in the throat**
- Hoarseness; soreness in chest; cough with scanty expectoration – mucous under the sternum which patient cannot quite reach
- **Left sided sciatica with numbness; unsteady gait**
- Children slow in learning to walk. Unsteady while walking and easy falling in little children
- **Large, jagged, itching warts, bleeding easily; on fingertips, lids, brows and nose**
- Deep burns; ill-effects of old burns which do not heal

CLINICAL

- Neuro-degenerative disorders
- Bell's palsy
- Sclerosis
- Parkinson's disease
- Tremors
- Seizure
- Paralysis
- Meningitis
- Cataract
- Facial paralysis
- Stammering
- Dyspepsia
- Colitis
- Paralysis of rectum
- Coryza
- Laryngitis
- Hoarseness
- Bronchitis
- Asthma
- Retention of urine
- Urinary incontinence
- Cystitis
- Urethral stricture
- Urethritis
- Rheumatism
- Tendonitis
- Sciatica
- Cramps
- Writer's cramps
- Torticollis
- Burns
- Warts
- Eczema
- Insomnia

MODALITIES

- **Aggravation:** Dry, cold winds, in clear fine weather, cold air, twilight, carriage riding, stooping, new moon, while perspiring, coffee, fats
- **Amelioration:** In damp, wet weather, warmth of bed, cold drinks, washing, gentle motion

REMEDY RELATIONSHIP

- **Antidotes:** Paralysis from lead poisoning, Asaf., Chin., Coloc., Euphr., Plb.
- **Complementary:** Carb-v., Petros., Staph., Coloc.
- **Compare:** Rhus-t., Ars.; Am-p. in facial paralysis; Calc., Nat-m., Sep. in cough with spurting of urine; Eup-per, Staph., Coloc., Sep., Sars.

CEANOTHUS AMERICANUS

SPHERE OF ACTION
- Head
- Cardiovascular system
- Gastrointestinal system
- Spleen
- Female genital system
- Respiratory system

INTRODUCTION
- **Common name:** New Jersey tea
- **Family:** *Rhamnaceae*
- **Source:** Vegetable kingdom
- **Part used:** Leaves
- **Prover:** I.C. Fahnestock

CONSTITUTION
- For those with a yellow complexion and anaemia with liver and spleen disorders
- Sanguine constitution
- **Temperament:** Nervous, bilious
- **Thermal:** Chilly
- **Miasm:** Psora, Sycosis, Syphilis

MIND
- Sadness, depression, mental dejection
- Fear he will become unfit for work
- Makes gestures of grasping or reaching at something
- **Children put fingers in the mouth**
- Dreams of snakes and robbers
- Apathy
- Great nervous excitement

KEYNOTE SYMPTOMS
- Left sided remedy
- Chilliness; rigors, shivering especially down the back
- Periodical neuralgia
- Anaemic patient, where liver and spleen are at fault
- Enormous enlargement and tenderness of the spleen. Consciousness of the spleen
- Splenitis, pain all up the left side, cannot lie on left side; stitching pains
- Headache with sensation as if brain was too large; sensation as if head pulsates synchronously with the heart
- **Desire for something sour, acids**
- **Dirty, yellow discolouration of tongue, white in the centre**
- Swelling of liver. Sensation of fullness in liver; worse after eating, lying on the right side
- Pain in left hypochondrium with dyspnoea, diarrhoea, profuse or suppressed menses, leucorrhoea
- Diarrhoea with bearing down pain in abdomen and rectum
- Tendency to chronic bronchitis with increased secretion; lungs feel congested
- **Thick, yellow, profuse, debilitating leucorrhoea with pain under left ribs**
- Locally, it can be used as a hair tonic

CLINICAL
- Anaemia
- Leukaemia
- Enlarged glands
- Hypertrophy of spleen
- Splenitis
- Jaundice
- Diarrhoea
- Tonsillitis
- Diphtheria
- Pharyngitis
- Dyspnoea
- Diabetes
- Leucorrhoea
- Metrorrhagia
- Menorrhagia
- Malaria
- Intermittent fever

MODALITIES
- **Aggravation:** Motion, lying on left side, cold weather
- **Amelioration:** Rest, open air

REMEDY RELATIONSHIP
- **Compare:** Tinas. for chronic cases of fever with splenomegaly; Polym.; Cean-tr., in pharyngitis, tonsillitis, nasal catarrh, diphtheria; Berb., Myric., Cedr., Agar. in spleen
- **Antidote:** Nat-m.,
- **Follows well:** Berb., Querc., Myric.

Ceanothus americanus

CEDRON

SPHERE OF ACTION
- Mind
- Eyes
- Musculoskeletal system
- Nervous system

INTRODUCTION
- **Common name:** Rattlesnake bean
- **Family:** *Simarubaceae*
- **Source:** Vegetable kingdom
- **Part used:** Seeds
- **Prover:** Patroz, Metcal and Douglas

CONSTITUTION
- Suits lean thin individuals of voluptuous disposition suffering from malarial affections of damp, warm, marshy countries
- **Temperament:** Nervous, excitable
- **Thermal:** Chilly
- **Miasm:** Sycosis

MIND
- **Fear of female friend, of bed; aversion to bed**
- Restlessness, nervousness drives the patient from place to place
- Nervousness generally followed by depression
- Numbness
- Anxiety
- Mania
- Aggravation of mental symptoms at night

KEYNOTE SYMPTOMS
- **Exact periodicity is most characteristic. Symptoms return at exactly the same hour every day, especially at 9 am; clock-like periodicity**
- Antidotes the effects of snakebites and stings of insects
- Curative for neuralgias. Neuralgias occurring at exact periodicity is a marked feature
- Useful for people in tropical, warm, marshy areas
- **Severe burning pain in eyeball with radiating pain around the eye, shooting into the nose**
- Valuable in menstrual epilepsy; many symptoms appear during menses or after sex like chorea in women and neuralgia in men
- Curative in malarial affections; regular paroxysms of fever; coming at the same hour
- Excitement before chill
- Chill in the evening with frontal headache extending to the parietal region; chill with congestion of head, feet, hands; nose is icy cold; with shivering. Chill is followed by profuse perspiration
- Hot stage with dryness, heaviness of the head, redness of the face and burning in palms

CLINICAL
- Mania
- Trembling
- Neuralgia
- Dropsy
- Migraine
- Meningitis
- Iritis
- Choroiditis
- Supraorbital neuralgia
- Gout
- Malaria
- Recurrent fever
- Intermittent fever
- Snakebite

MODALITIES
- **Aggravation:** Open air, before a storm, lying down, after sleep, periodically
- **Amelioration:** Standing erect

REMEDY RELATIONSHIP
- **Antidotes:** Lach.
- **Compare:** Ars., Chin., Aran., Bell., Cedr., Sabad.

CHAMOMILLA

SPHERE OF ACTION
- Head
- Ears
- Gastrointestinal system
- Central nervous system
- Respiratory system
- Female genital system

INTRODUCTION
- **Common name:** Bitter chamomile, German chamomile
- **Family:** *Compositae*
- **Source:** Vegetable kingdom
- **Part used:** Dried whole plant during flowering or the whole fresh plant

CONSTITUTION
- Suits people, especially children, with one cheek red and hot, the other pale and cold
- **Suits irritable, colicky babies with teething troubles and earache; who are hypersensitive to pain**
- **Temperament:** Nervous, bilious, excitable, rheumatic
- **Thermal:** Hot
- **Miasm:** Psora, Sycosis, Syphilis

MIND
- Child wants many things, which he refuses when offered with discourtesy
- Piteous moaning because child cannot have what he wants
- **Child becomes quiet only when carried about or petted constantly**
- **Ugly in behaviour; cross, uncivil, quarrelsome. Snappish, cannot return a civil answer**
- Peevish; whining restlessness, impolite, capricious, impatient; vexed at every trifle; cannot be appeased
- Impatient; intolerant of being spoken to or interrupted when spoken to
- Throws things away. Striking in children
- Frightened dreams; weeps during sleep
- Irritable when spoken to during menses

KEYNOTE SYMPTOMS
- Complaints from anger and vexation; also dentition; colic from anger
- Patient is sensitive, irritable, thirsty, hot and numb
- Sleeplessness, restlessness and nervous disorders in children and women
- Unendurable pain with numbness of parts affected; extremely sensitive to every kind of pain
- Oversensitiveness from abuse of coffee, narcotics; to open air
- After a fit of anger in mother, convulsions of children after nursing
- Hyperaesthesia of sentient nerve fibres
- **Toothache worse after a warm drink**
- **One cheek red and hot, other pale and cold**
- Parotid and submaxillary glands are swollen
- Excessive acidity; bilious vomiting; flatulent colic; abdominal colic during dentition
- Portal congestion; haemorrhoids
- **Hot, green, slimy stools, very offensive; from cold, anger, during dentition**
- Earache, swelling and heat driving the patient frantic
- Otitis media with fever and pain; ears sensitive to touch, sore and swollen
- Uterine haemorrhage of dark blood with labour-like pains; menstrual cramps with marked irritability
- Voilent labour with intolerable pains; sends nurse, doctor away
- Mammary glands are swollen and hard; nipples are inflamed and sensitive to touch
- Ankles give way in the afternoon
- Burning of soles at night
- Insomnia due to colic, dentition or ear infection

CLINICAL
- Anxiety states
- Obesity
- Epilepsy
- Vertigo
- Blepharospasm
- Blepharitis
- Earache
- Otitis media
- Toothache
- Dentitional ailments
- Mumps
- Parotiditis
- Flatulence
- Gastric ulcer
- Peptic ulcer
- Colitis
- Jaundice
- Cancer of pancreas
- Diarrhoea
- Hoarseness
- Laryngitis
- Asthma
- Cardiac disorders
- Valvular heart disease
- Abortion
- Labour disorders
- Dysmenorrhoea
- Malaria

MODALITIES
- **Aggravation:** Anger, open air, wind, night, touched, looked at, during dentition, coffee, cold winds
- **Amelioration:** From being carried, warm wet weather, heat, sweating

REMEDY RELATIONSHIP
- **Compare:** Cina., Calc-p., Cypr., Bry., Anth., Acon., Puls., Coff., Bell., Staph., Ign.
- **Follows well:** Bell. in diseases of children and after abuse of Op.
- **Antidotes:** Camph., Nux-v., Puls.
- **Complementary:** Bell., Mag-c.

CHELIDONIUM MAJUS

SPHERE OF ACTION
- Mind
- Liver
- Gastrointestinal system
- Respiratory system
- Musculoskeletal system
- Genitourinary system
- Skin

INTRODUCTION
- **Common name:** Celandine, Greater calandine
- **Family:** *Papaveraceae*
- **Source:** Vegetable kingdom
- **Part used:** Whole plant
- **Prover:** Hahnemann

CONSTITUTION
- Suits light complexioned, thin, spare people with dark rings around the eyes and with a pale, hot face
- **Temperament:** Nervous, bilious
- **Thermal:** Chilly
- **Miasm:** Psora, Sycosis, Syphilis

MIND
- Aversion to mental exertion, despondency
- Anxiety as if she had committed a crime; sudden anxiety with palpitations
- Fear of insanity, of going crazy
- Causeless weeping, restlessness – moves from place to place
- Irritability; upset easily
- Sadness, melancholy
- Patient is cross; vexed about trifles

KEYNOTE SYMPTOMS
- Adapted to persons with a bilious temperament with hepatic, gastric and abdominal complaints
- Predominantly a right sided remedy
- **General lethargy with no inclination to make any effort**
- Serous effusions; hydrocoele
- Sick headache with nausea and bilious vomiting; right sided headache, better after eating
- Dirty yellow colour of eyes
- Stiching pain or neuralgia over right eye
- **Bruised, sharp, aching, constant in inferior angle of right scapula**
- Prefers hot food and drinks. Eating relieves temporarily
- Jaundice. Bilious complaints during gestation. Liver enlarged
- **Stool is pale, clay coloured, floats in water.** Diarrhoea alternates with constipation
- **Constipation; stools round, hard, like sheep's dung**
- Small lumps of mucous fly from the mouth when coughing
- **Urine profuse, foaming like beer**
- Icy coldness of finger tips. Wrists sore
- Rheumatism of hip and thigh
- Yellow or jaundiced discolouration of the skin
- Painful pimples and pustules, especially on face, old spreading ulcers
- Old, spreading ulcers with a history of liver disease

CLINICAL
- Paralysis
- Neuralgia
- Bilious headache
- Orbital neuralgia
- Flatulence
- Gastralgia
- Gall stones
- Hepatomegaly
- Hepatitis
- Jaundice
- Biliary colic
- Cholecystitis
- Diarrhoea
- Dysentery
- Constipation
- Dyspnoea
- Whooping cough
- Pneumonia
- Uterine colic
- Agalactia
- Hydrocoele
- Arthritis
- Rheumatism
- Pruritus
- Pimples

MODALITIES
- **Aggravation:** Right side, motion, touch, change of weather, very early in the morning
- **Amelioration:** After dinner, from pressure, eating, lying on abdomen, bending backwards, hot food

REMEDY RELATIONSHIP
- Sulph. often completes its work
- **Complementary:** Lyc., Bry.
- **Antidotes:** Cham.
- **Compare:** Nux-v., Sulph., Bry., Lyc., Op., Podo., Sang., Ars., Chin., Calc., Chen-a.

CHIMAPHILA UMBELLATA

INTRODUCTION

- **Common name:** Pipsissewa
- **Family:** *Ericaceae*
- **Source:** Vegetable kingdom
- **Part used:** Whole plant
- **Prover:** Jeanes

SPHERE OF ACTION

- Genitourinary system
- Glands
- Breasts

MIND

- Anxiety
- Nervousness
- Irritability, worse contradiction
- Restlessness

MODALITIES

- **Aggravation:** In damp weather, from sitting on cold stones or pavements, left side
- **Amelioration:** Walking, cold water

KEYNOTE SYMPTOMS

- Inward trembling without mental disturbances
- Especially affects lymphatic and mesenteric glands
- Dropsy from kidney and liver diseases
- For incipient and progressive cataract
- **Toothache, as if teeth were being gently pulled**
- Cannot close jaws at night; jaws feel stiff, sleeps with mouth open during toothache
- **Thirst with a desire to cool the tongue**
- Sensation of a ball in the perineum
- **Urine scanty, loaded with ropy, muco-purulent sediment. Must strain before passing urine**
- **Unable to urinate without standing with feet wide apart and body inclined forward**
- Forked stream of urine. Burning and scalding during micturition and straining afterwards
- Acute and chronic catarrh of bladder; also of prostate with mucous, pus and blood
- Rapid atrophy of breasts; tumours of breasts in women with large breasts
- Prostatic enlargement with irritation; urinary retention in benign prostatic enlargement

CONSTITUTION

- For scrofulous and broken down constitution
- Suits plethoric women with large breasts and hepatic and renal dropsies
- Suits chronic alcoholics
- **Temperament:** Nervous, bilious
- **Thermal:** Chilly
- **Miasm:** Psora, Sycosis, Syphilis

CLINICAL

- Chronic alcoholism
- Cataract
- Toothache
- Jaundice
- Hepatic or renal dropsies
- Bladder disorders
- Cystitis
- Kidney ailments
- Nephritis
- Urethritis
- Retention of urine
- Incontinence of urine
- Haematuria
- Diabetes
- Vaginismus
- Breast tumour
- Atrophy of breasts
- Prostatitis
- Prostatic enlargement
- Ulcers

REMEDY RELATIONSHIP

- **Compare:** Chim-m. in intense gnawing hunger; burning fever; sensation of swelling in arm pits; Uva, Led., Epig., Apoc., Sabal.

CHININUM ARSENICOSUM

SPHERE OF ACTION

- Mind
- Nervous system
- Gastrointestinal system
- Respiratory system
- Musculoskeletal system

INTRODUCTION

- **Common name:** Arsenite of quinine, Quinine arsenite
- **Group:** Hydrocarbon
- **Source:** Mineral kingdom
- **Formula:** $(C_{20}H_{24}N_2O_2)_3H_3AsO_3 \cdot 4H_2O$
- **Prover:** Muhr

CONSTITUTION

- For weak, cold, emaciated people, with despair during chill, heat and suffering
- **Temperament:** Nervous, bilious
- **Thermal:** Chilly, ambithermal
- **Miasm:** Psora, Sycosis, Syphilis

MIND

- Complaining, confusion of mind in the morning on waking
- Overconscientious about friends
- Delirious at night, many imaginations; fear of evil, of ghosts with anxiety
- Easily angered and refuses to talk and to answer questions
- Prostration, irritability; disinclined to do any work
- Great anxiety on waking, desires things but does not care after he gets them
- Anxiety with unquenchable thirst must sit bent forward in front of a window
- Dullness of mind
- Thinking of complaints aggravates
- Very forgetful; memory impaired
- Depressed, wants to sit in one place and be quiet

KEYNOTE SYMPTOMS

- Weakness and prostration; hence, used as a tonic
- Increasing anaemia, especially after prolonged malaria, prolonged suppuration, after haemorrhage
- Dropsy in sacs or oedema
- Periodicity of complaints, especially in neuralgias
- Stitching, tearing pains
- Dull, heavy frontal and occipital headache
- **Tongue thickly furred; yellow, slimy coating. Bitter, metallic, saltish taste**
- **Egg and fish produces diarrhoea**
- **Appetite diminished; gone; violent thirst for cold water; desires sweets, aversion to meat**
- Alternation of hyperacidity and decrease of acid
- Constipation; stools – hard, knotty
- Sensation as if heart had stopped; suffocative attacks
- Shortness of breath on ascending; palpitations
- Weak limbs; cold hands, feet, knees and limbs; tearing pains
- Chronic rheumatism of joints without swelling
- Intermittent fever with great prostration and periodicity
- Sleeplessness due to nervous causes

CLINICAL

- Neuralgia
- Vertigo
- Photophobia
- Anorexia nervosa
- Gastralgia
- Dyspepsia
- Diarrhoea
- Asthma
- Cardiac dyspnoea
- Myocardial degeneration
- Angina pectoris
- Arthritis
- Rheumatism
- Hectic fever
- Insomnia

MODALITIES

- **Aggravation:** On an empty stomach, looking up, motion, ascending
- **Amelioration:** Motion, eating, pressure, bending forward, sitting up

REMEDY RELATIONSHIP

- **Compare:** Chinin-s., also Ferr-ci; Chinin-m. (in severe neuralgic pains around the eyes, with chills; exaggerated sensitiveness to alcohol and tobacco; prostration and restlessness); Oeno. in effortless diarrhoea with nervous exhaustion; incipient hydrocephalus; Macroz-s; extreme debility after illness; collapse; Nat-m.

SPHERE OF ACTION

- Mind
- Ears
- Gastrointestinal system
- Musculoskeletal system
- Urinary system
- Skin

INTRODUCTION

- **Common name:** Sulphite of quinine, Quinine sulphate
- **Group:** Hydrocarbon
- **Source:** Mineral kingdom
- **Formula:** $(C_{20}H_{24}N_2)_2 H_2SO_4 \cdot 2H_2O$
- **Prover:** Bohler

CONSTITUTION

- Indicated for marked periodicity and spinal sensitiveness
- For prostration of mind or mental exhaustion with periodicity of symptoms
- **Temperament:** Nervous, bilious
- **Thermal:** Chilly
- **Miasm:** Sycosis, Syphilis

CHININUM SULPHURICUM

MIND

- Fear of impending evil
- Anxiety about the future
- Fear of misfortune, of animals
- **Weakness of mind, abundant ideas at night**
- Memory muddled, thoughts not clear; difficulty in thinking and comprehending
- Makes mistakes, uses wrong words, putting right for left or vice versa
- Dullness and sluggishness
- Indolence on waking in the morning
- Indifference during fever, in typhus
- Discouraged
- Delirium during fever, while lying quietly on the back at night. Delirium; jumps out of bed, escapes, cries and shrieks
- Sadness, despondency, dejection, mental depression, gloomy, melancholy in the afternoon, in smallpox

KEYNOTE SYMPTOMS

- Inflammatory state of tissues and nerves
- Intermittent neuralgic pains in various parts
- Periodicity; symptoms return periodically on alternate days
- Always indicated when there is marked periodicity and spinal sensitiveness
- **Noises in ears; violent ringing, buzzing and roaring in ears**
- Hardness of hearing, sometimes with violent headache
- Flatulence and distention of abdomen
- Pain in the hepatic and splenic region when coughing, bending or taking a deep breath
- Splenomegaly with pain after intermittent fever
- **Great sensitiveness of cervico-dorsal vertebrae; fifth cervical to third dorsal vertebrae very sensitive to pressure and on lying down**
- Acute articular rheumatism. Joints are sensitive. Joints and limbs heavy and achy
- Weeping in spinal irritation

CLINICAL

- Anaemia
- Neuralgia
- Meniere's syndrome
- Tinnitus
- Retrobulbar neuritis
- Amaurosis
- Chronic interstitial nephritis
- Albuminuria
- Haematuria
- Rheumatism
- Polyarticular
- gout
- Lumbago
- Cervico-dorsal spine aches
- Spinal sensitivity
- Recurring fever
- Malaria
- Pruritus
- Erythema nodosum
- Pustules
- Urticaria
- Erythema

REMEDY RELATIONSHIP

- **Compare:** Chin-sal., Ars., Eup-per., Methylene blue. Camph-mbr. is said to intensify the action of quinine and render it more permanent. Baja, an East Indian drug, said to be almost infallible in intermittent fever, quartan type; pulsating headache, injected eyes, flushed face, liver and spleen enlarged. Oedema; also Pambto. for intermittent and tropical fevers.
- **Antidotes:** Parth., Nat-m., Lach., Arn., Puls.

MODALITIES

- **Aggravation:** Touch, cold, periodically, 10 am – 11 am
- **Amelioration:** Pressure, yawning, bending forward

CHOLESTERINUM

SPHERE OF ACTION

- Gastrointestinal system
- Gall bladder
- Liver
- Respiratory system

INTRODUCTION

- **Common name:** Cholesterine
- **Source:** Animal kingdom
- **Part used:** Sarcode. prepared by trituration from potentized cholestrol gall stone
- **Formula:** $C_{27}H_{44}O$
- **Prover:** Dr Wilhelm Ameke

CONSTITUTION

- For old people with liver complaints gall stones and gall stone colic
- **Temperament:** Nervous, bilious
- **Thermal:** Chilly, ambithermal
- **Miasm:** Psora, Sycosis, Syphilis

MIND

- Confusion of mind, incoherent delirium
- Shreiking, shouting and screaming on waking
- Irritable
- Anxiety
- Fear of disease
- Moody

KEYNOTE SYMPTOMS

- Vitreous opacities
- Obstinate hepatic enlargements, cancer of the liver, obstinate gall stones and obstinate jaundice
- Cirrhosis of liver, hepatic engorgements, malignant affections **affecting the left lobe of the liver and what lies between it** and the pylorus and the pancreas
- Burning pain on side of abdomen. On walking, holds his hand on the side
- **Liver region is sore, sensitive to touch or jar; worse lying on affected side**
- Gall stone colic, almost specific for it; attacks come and go suddenly; pushing pain in the region of the bile duct
- Cholesterine is the physiological opponent of lecithin, thus both seem to play some unknown part in the growth of tumours

CLINICAL

- Anaemia
- Vitreous opacities
- Corneal opacity
- Hepatitis
- Obstinate jaundice
- Obstinate hepatic enlargement
- Splenomegaly
- Cancer of liver
- Obstinate gall stones
- Gall stone colic
- Cirrhosis
- Liver cancer
- Diarrhoea
- Dysentery
- Pulmonary oedema
- Cheyne-Stokes breathing
- Insomnia

MODALITIES

- **Aggravation:** Touch, jar, lying on side, bending, sudden motion
- **Amelioration:** Rest

REMEDY RELATIONSHIP

- **Compare:** Taurocholate of soda or Nat-taur.

CICUTA VIROSA

INTRODUCTION
- **Common name:** Water hemlock
- **Family:** *Umbelliferae*
- **Source:** Vegetable kingdom
- **Part used:** Root

SPHERE OF ACTION
- Medulla oblongata
- Cerebrospinal system
- Gastrointestinal system
- Skin

CONSTITUTION
- Suits nervous women who are subjected to epileptic or choreic convulsions
- For spasms of children during dentition, or from worms
- **Temperament:** Hysterical
- **Thermal:** Hot
- **Miasm:** Sycosis, Syphilis

MIND
- Delirium with singing and dancing
- Mistrustful, suspicious
- Stupid feeling
- **Lies without recognizing anyone, but when questioned, answers correctly**
- Consciousness returns suddenly and he remembers nothing of what has occurred. Confuses the present with the past. Imagines himself as a young child. Everything is confusing and strange
- Memory blank for hours or days with or without convulsions
- **Afraid of society and company; wants to be alone. Aversion to company**
- Melancholy with indifference
- Vivid dreams
- Anxiety regarding the future
- Sad stories, bad things affect the patient profoundly, cause nightmares

KEYNOTE SYMPTOMS
- Convulsive tendency; convulsions extend from centre to circumference
- **Convulsions extend from above downwards**
- During convulsions, the attack is violent; tonic spasms
- Bending of the head, neck and spine backwards or opisthotonos. Frightful distortions of the face, limbs or whole body during convulsions
- Convulsions from cerebral concussions
- Cerebrospinal meningitis and contraction of cervical muscles; head turned and twisted to one side
- Cerebral diseases after suppressed eruption
- Pupils dilated, insensible; strabismus; diplopia
- Facial distortions; twitching of facial muscles
- **Patient has strange desires, like for coal, chalk and many other strange articles. Eats coal and raw potatoes**
- **Complaints or spasms after swallowing a fish bone or stick that lodges in the throat**
- Indigestion, hiccough, throbbing in the pit of the stomach, flatulence with anxiety, rumbling
- **Haemorrhage from ears. Difficulty in hearing**
- Heat in the chest; chest feel tight, can hardly breathe
- Barber's itch; eczema with exudation which forms hard, lemon coloured crusts

CLINICAL
- Concussion
- Convulsions
- Paralysis
- Epilepsy
- Hysteria
- Numbness
- Twitching
- Spasmodic jerks
- Tetanus
- Injuries
- Meningitis
- Strabismus
- Lock jaw
- Opisthotonos
- Trismus
- Hiccough
- Worm infestation
- Colic
- Cholera
- Eczema
- Impetigo

MODALITIES
- **Aggravation:** From touch, draughts, concussion, tobacco smoke, jar, turning the head, injury to spine and brain
- **Amelioration:** Warmth, thinking of pain

REMEDY RELATIONSHIP
- **Antidotes:** Op., Arn.
- **Compare:** Cic-m., Hydr-ac., Con., Oean., Stry., Bell., Nux-v., Hell.

CINA MARITIMA

INTRODUCTION
- **Common name:** Wormseed
- **Family:** *Compositae*
- **Source:** Vegetable kingdom
- **Part used:** Flower heads
- **Prover:** Hahnemann

SPHERE OF ACTION
- Mind
- Gastrointestinal system
- Respiratory system
- Musculoskeletal system
- Female genital system
- Urinary system
- Skin

CONSTITUTION
- A remedy for big, fatty, rosy and scrofulous children
- Adapted to pale children with dark hair, circumscribed redness of cheeks, dark rings around the eyes; bluish-white discolouration around the mouth
- **Temperament:** Nervous, bilious
- **Thermal:** Chilly, ambithermal
- **Miasm:** Psora, Sycosis, Syphilis

MIND
- **Child is very cross, ugly, does not want to be touched, caressed or carried, wants to be rocked**
- Indifferent to caresses
- Very touchy, petulant, dissatisfied
- Irritability, better by fast rocking
- Cannot bear to be looked at; or touched children become stiff when looked at
- Cannot remain quiet
- **Desires many things, but rejects everything offered; throws things away**
- Violent, screaming attacks at night, while lying on the back. Strikes and kicks with hands
- Screams and talks in sleep
- Irritable, capricious temper
- Causeless weeping

KEYNOTE SYMPTOMS
- Urge for scratching and boring; striking or pinching
- Convulsions from being scolded or disciplined; convulsions from worms
- Epileptiform convulsions, worse lying on the back; violent screams and motion of the face; more at night
- Strabismus due to worm trouble; unable to swallow liquids, grinding of teeth during sleep; choreic movement of face and hands; itching in the anus
- Pulsations of superciliary muscles
- **Bores and picks the nose till it bleeds; irritation of the nose**
- **Child hungry soon after a meal; gnawing; craves sweets. Child eats a lot but does not gain weight**
- Vomiting of ascarides
- Worm remedy. Colic with cutting, punching pains from worms
- Convulsions more at night
- Spasmodic pain in the abdomen; twisting pain around the navel
- Itching of the anus due to roundworms or thread worms
- Gagging, whooping cough; cough ends in spasm
- Nocturnal bed wetting, involuntary urination. Urine white, milky, turbid
- Twitching, jerking, distortion of limbs; stretches one feet spasmodically

CLINICAL
- Behavioural disorders
- Anxiety
- Obesity
- Convulsions
- Spasms
- Paralysis
- Epilepsy
- Strabismus
- Blepharitis
- Colic
- Worms
- Peptic ulcers
- Gastric ulcers
- Vomiting
- Jaundice
- Colitis
- Diarrhoea
- Otitis media
- Laryngitis
- Cough
- Asthma
- Pertussis
- Bed wetting
- Uterine haemorrhage
- Dysmenorrhoea
- Fever

MODALITIES
- **Aggravation:** Looking fixedly at an object, from worms, at night, in the sun, in summers, full moon, at night, during sleep, touch
- **Amelioration:** Lying on abdomen, motion, shaking the head, rocking

REMEDY RELATIONSHIP
- **Compare:** Santon. often preferable in worm affections; same symptoms as Cina; corresponding to the "pain in shocks" produced by Cina; Helminthochortos—Worm moss. Teucr., Ign., Cham., Spig.
- **Antidote:** Camph., Caps.

SPHERE OF ACTION

- Mind
- Gastrointestinal system
- Respiratory system
- Female genital system
- Musculoskeletal system
- Skin

INTRODUCTION

- **Common name:** Peruvian bark, China officinalis
- **Family:** *Rubiaceae*
- **Source:** Vegetable kingdom
- **Part used:** Bark
- **Prover:** Hahnemann

CONSTITUTION

- Suits stout people, once robust but now broken down by debilitating discharges
- Suits those with a swollen face, anaemia and pale continence with a disposition to dropsical disorders
- **Temperament:** Nervous, bilious
- **Thermal:** Chilly
- **Miasm:** Psora, Sycosis

CINCHONA OFFICINALIS

MIND

- Anxious, frightful dreams
- Sensitive, introverted, intense and touchy individuals with a tendency to take offense; especially in teenagers
- Difficulty in expressing feelings; child cannot express affection with words
- Sensitive, cannot speak or look at anyone during the interview
- **Aversion to exercise**
- Disposed to be quarrelsome and angry; very sensitive
- Constant irritation; very touchy
- Mispelling words in later stage
- Great excitability, nervous erethism, fantasies of heroic deeds at night causing sleeplessness
- **Clearness of mind and abundance of ideas in the evening**
- Delirium from loss of fluids

KEYNOTE SYMPTOMS

- Results of vital losses. Profuse exhausting discharges, haemorrhages
- Haemorrhagic diathesis – from every orifice, long lasting with severe weakness
- Haemorrhages profuse with faintness, loss of sight and ringing in the ears
- Periodicity marked
- Drawing, tearing pains, especially in every joint; hard pressure relieves; worse slight touch
- Congestive headache with intense throbbing of the head and carotids
- Catarrhal condition of middle ear; tinnitus
- **Aversion to hot fatty and rich food, meat and fruit; desires highly seasoned food**
- **Acidity or indigestion by taking fruit. Food poisoning from bad meat or impure water**
- **Excessive flatulence, tympanitic; belching gives no relief**
- Post-operative gas pain; severe flatulent colic
- Cold feeling with pulsations and rumbling in the stomach and abdomen. Belching of bitter fluid; regurgitation of foods
- Liver is enlarged, hard and painful; pain in right hypochondrium; chronic liver complaints. Gallstone colic
- Stools lienteric, frothy, bloody, painless; painless diarrhoea
- Pneumonia after haemorrhage or with bilious lymphatics. Rattling in lungs, suffocative catarrh
- Inflammatory condition of ovaries; prolapse of uterus; metrorrhagia, intermenstrual bleeding; menses dark and profuse
- Anaemia, exhaustion and blood loss since child birth
- **Great thirst before chill stage**
- Intermittent fever with drenching sweats at night. Internal chills with icy cold hands and feet
- **Aversion to food alternates with ravenous appetite during fever**

CLINICAL

- Haemorrhage
- Debility
- Dehydration
- Anaemia
- Neuralgia
- Meniere's disease
- Headache
- Toothache
- Hiccough
- Flatulence
- Gastralgia
- Cholecystitis
- Gall stones
- Biliary colic
- Hepatomegaly
- Jaundice
- Hepatitis
- Gastro-duodenal catarrh
- Splenic disorders
- Diarrhoea
- Dysentery
- Constipation
- Tinnitus
- Influenza
- Whooping cough
- Pneumonia
- Pleurisy
- Asthma
- Agalactia
- Hydrocoele
- Rheumatism
- Gout
- Malaria
- Typhoid
- Dermatitis
- Pruritus
- Erysipelas
- Insomnia

MODALITIES

- **Aggravation:** Slightest touch, draught of air, loss of vital fluids, at night, after eating, bending over
- **Amelioration:** Bending double, hard pressure, open air, warmth, loose clothes

REMEDY RELATIONSHIP

- **Antidotes:** Arn., Ars., Nux-v., Ip., Ferr., Iod., Cham
- **Compare:** Ars., Carb-v., Coloc., Cedr., Caps., Psor., Puls., Ph-ac., Lyc., Aloe.
- **Complementary:** Ferr., Calc-p.
- **Incompatible after:** Dig., Sel.

Cinchona officinalis

CINNABARIS

SPHERE OF ACTION
- Mind
- Eyes
- Musculoskeletal system
- Genitourinary system
- Skin

INTRODUCTION
- **Common name:** Mercuric sulphide, Red mercuric sulphide, Mercurius sulphuratus ruber
- **Source:** Mineral kingdom
- **Formula:** HgS
- **Prover:** Hahnemann

CONSTITUTION
- Adapted to mentally prostrated individuals with ciliary neuralgia and ulcerations on a syphilitic base
- **Temperament:** Nervous, bilious
- **Thermal:** Chilly
- **Miasm:** Sycosis, Syphilis

MIND
- Excitement over trifles
- Easily provoked
- Desire to be alone
- Sadness after eating
- Delusion – thinks he is well
- Prostration of mind, mental exhaustion, brain fag, before menses. Indisposition to mental labour
- Disconnected thoughts with headache
- Fullness of the head from mental application

KEYNOTE SYMPTOMS
- **Fiery looking ulcers, especially in mouth, throat**
- Fiery redness of warts, condylomata, ulcers and infections
- **Lack of vital heat, but better in open air from the warmth of the sun**
- Profuse discharges, salivation, urination, etc.
- Bones, scalp, roots of hair are sensitive to touch
- Ciliary neuralgia. Pain in lachrymal duct which radiates around the eyes to the temples, from the inner canthus, across the brows to the ears
- Redness of the entire eye; granulated lids
- Pressive sensation on the nose, as from heavy spectacles
- Pain in long bones when barometer levels lower
- Nodes on shin bones
- Condylomata, especially of rectum, prepuce
- **Warts bleed when touched; warts on prepuce fan shaped**
- Sleepless at night; starting from sleep
- Perspiration gives no relief

CLINICAL
- Headache
- Ciliary neuralgia
- Conjunctivitis
- Blepharitis
- Eye infection
- Stomatitis
- Post-nasal catarrh
- Leucorrhoea
- Vaginismus
- Bubo
- Condylomata
- Rheumatism
- Warts
- Boils
- Blisters
- Ulcers
- Insomnia

MODALITIES
- **Aggravation:** Lying on the right side (feels as if the contents of the body were being dragged over to that side), summer, dampness, walking, night, touch
- **Amelioration:** Rest, open air, sunshine, after dinner

REMEDY RELATIONSHIP
- **Compare:** Hep., Nit-ac., Thuj., Sep., Camph., Lach., Seneg.
- **Antidoted by:** Hep., Sulph., Op., Nit-ac.,

CINNAMOMUM ZEYLANICUM

INTRODUCTION

- **Common name:** Cinnamon, Dalchini
- **Family:** *Lauraceae*
- **Source:** Vegetable kingdom
- **Part used:** Inner bark

SPHERE OF ACTION

- Mind
- Female genital system
- Gastrointestinal system

CONSTITUTION

- Adapted to cancer and haemorrhages in feeble women with languid circulation
- Suits feeble, lymphatic and cachectic women with lax tissues
- **Temperament:** Nervous, bilious
- **Thermal:** Chilly
- **Miasm:** Sycosis, Syphilis

MIND

- **Delusion that left side of the body is diminished or smaller**
- Forgetfulness
- Hysteria from exhaustion, after loss of fluids
- Talking causes hysterical attacks
- Hysteria better eructations, but soon returns
- Paroxysms of hysteria subside as soon as vomiting sets in
- Unconsciousness, coma, stupor in hysteria
- No desire for anything
- Talking causes hysterical attacks
- Irritability, contradiction

KEYNOTE SYMPTOMS

- Cancer, where pain and foetor are present
- Tendency to bright red, clear haemorrhages, especially during pregnancy; worse on physical exertion and followed by weakness
- Haemorrhages, especially post-partum haemorrhage, from the bowels, haemoptysis, etc.
- Flatulence with colic in the uterine region and diarrhoea
- **Long continued constipation; stools like hard balls**
- A strain in the loins, a false step brings on profuse flow of blood
- Menses are early, profuse, prolonged, bright red; menorrhagia; particularly in females troubled with itching of nose and nocturnal restlessness
- **Profuse flow during menses with cold extremities, pallor of surface**
- Uterine haemorrhage caused by overlifting, during puerperal stage; uterus does not contract well. Fingers seem swollen. Bearing down pains

CLINICAL

- Hysteria
- Haemorrhages
- Cancer
- Hiccough
- Flatulance
- Diarrhoea
- Dysentery
- Constipation
- Haemorrhoids
- Epistaxis
- Haemoptysis
- Menorrhagia
- Metrorrhagia
- Puerperal sepsis
- Abortion
- Insomnia
- Post-partum haemorrhage

MODALITIES

- **Aggravation:** Post delivery, false step, strain, over lifting, while riding, talking
- **Amelioration:** Rest

REMEDY RELATIONSHIP

- **Compare:** Ip., Sil., Tril-p., Phos.
- **Antidoted by:** Acon.
- **Antidotes:** Op.

CISTUS CANADENSIS

SPHERE OF ACTION
- Head
- Nasopharynx
- Mouth
- Gastrointestinal system
- Glands
- Respiratory system
- Skin

INTRODUCTION
- **Common name:** Rock rose, Frost weed
- **Family:** *Cistaceae*
- **Source:** Vegetable kingdom
- **Part used:** Whole plant
- **Prover:** Bute

CONSTITUTION
- For scrofulous subjects who are very sensitive to cold air
- **Temperament:** Nervous, bilious, scrofulous
- **Thermal:** Chilly
- **Miasm:** Psora, Sycosis, Syphilis

MIND
- Restlessness at night
- Mental excitement aggravates complaints
- Anger; feels as if paralyzed
- Anxiety, fear
- Bad effects of vexation

KEYNOTE SYMPTOMS
- **Extremely sensitive to cold and cold inspired air. Sensation of coldness in various parts**
- Cold air causes pain wherever it comes in contact; sore throat from least cold air; mammae sensitive to cold air; etc.
- Glands inflamed and indurated
- **Mucous discharges are thick, yellow, foul, leaving painful rawness; suppurations**
- Internal and external itching, sensation of formication all over the body; burning sensation
- **All orifices and anus itch; patient rubs them until they become raw and bleed**
- Headaches on missing the noon meal, better eating
- Mouth feels cold; pyorrhoea. Scorbutic, receding gums. It hurts to protrude the tongue.
- Malignant diseases or suppuration of the glands of the neck
- Cold feeling in the stomach and abdomen
- Asthma after lying down. Larynx and trachea feels cool on inhaling air
- **Bad smelling leucorrhoea**
- Small painful pimples, mercurio-syphilitic ulcers; itching preventing sleep

CLINICAL
- Malignancy
- Cancer
- Glandular affections
- Lymphosarcoma
- Haemorrhage
- Hemicrania
- Ophthalmia
- Scorbutic gums
- Pyorrhoea
- Parotiditis
- Pharyngitis
- Asthma
- Mastitis
- Mammae induration
- Syphilis ulcers
- Herpes
- Lupus
- Poisoned wounds

MODALITIES
- **Aggravation:** Slightest exposure to cold air, mental exertion, excitement, touch, motion, cold inspired air
- **Amelioration:** After eating, swallowing

REMEDY RELATIONSHIP
- **Antidoted by:** Rhus-t., Sep.
- **Compare:** Arg-n., Bell., Con., Carb-v., Calc., Sulph.

CLEMATIS ERECTA

SPHERE OF ACTION
- Mind
- Gastrointestinal system
- Musculoskeletal system
- Genitourinary system
- Skin

INTRODUCTION
- **Common name:** Virgin's bower
- **Family:** *Ranunculacea*
- **Source:** Vegetable kingdom
- **Part used:** Leaves and stem
- **Prover:** Hahnemann

CONSTITUTION
- Suits rheumatic, scrofulous, gonorrhoeal, syphilitic patients with great emaciation
- For light haired people with tendency to swelling and induration of the glandular system
- **Temperament:** Nervous, bilious
- **Thermal:** Chilly
- **Miasm:** Syphilis, Sycosis

MIND
- Homesickness
- Confused feeling, better in open
- Restless, dreamy sleep and vibratory sensation throughout the body
- Fear of being alone; desires company
- General sadness and dread of misfortune
- Melancholic, pre-occupied by sad thoughts
- Weak memory
- **Aversion to reading, wants to be read to**

KEYNOTE SYMPTOMS
- It affects the glands, especially those of testes, mammae, ovaries, which become very hard, painful, swollen and hot
- Burning, itching, stinging, crawling pains
- Pains drive the patient to despair; neuralgic; relieved by perspiration
- Marked emaciation; muscles relaxed or twitching
- Affects mucous membrane of eye; sensitive to cold air
- **Toothache worse at night, from tobacco, better holding cold water in the mouth; decayed molar tooth. Least contact is very painful**
- Pain on right side of face, radiating to eye, ear and temple; better holding cold water in the mouth
- Affects mucous membrane of urethra; feels constricted; commencing stricture
- **Urine flow interrupted. Frequent, scanty micturition**
- Testicles indurated with a bruised feeling; ailments after suppressed gonorrhoea
- Pruritus, worse washing in cold water, in the scalp, around the occiput
- Great sleepiness with vibratory sensation throughout the body

CLINICAL
- Conjunctivitis
- Blepharitis
- Iritis
- Styes
- Exophthalmos
- Toothache
- Rectal abscess
- Otitis media
- Sinusitis
- Laryngitis
- Pharyngitis
- Tonsillitis
- Pleurisy
- Pneumonia
- Urethral stricture
- Urethritis
- Gonorrhoea
- Mastitis
- Prostatitis
- Varicose ulcers
- Acne
- Vesicles
- Ulcers
- Eczema
- Paronychia
- Herpes

MODALITIES
- **Aggravation:** At night, warmth of bed, washing in cold water, new moon (monthly aggravation) increasing moon, touch, motion
- **Amelioration:** In open air, perspiration, waning moon

REMEDY RELATIONSHIP
- **Compare:** Clem-vit., Sil., Staph., Petr., Old., Sars., Canth., Ph-ac., Puls., Ars., Ant-c., Hep.
- **Antidoted by:** Bry., Camph.
- **Compatible:** Sil.

COBALTUM METALLICUM

INTRODUCTION

- **Common name:** Cobalt
- **Group:** Metal
- **Source:** Mineral kingdom
- **Formula:** Co
- **Prover:** Hering

SPHERE OF ACTION

- Mind
- Eyes
- Gastrointestinal system
- Musculoskeletal system
- Male genital system
- Skin

CONSTITUTION

- For neurasthenic states of spinal origin with disturbances on the sexual sphere
- For fatigue and neurasthenia with a constant interchange of moods
- **Temperament:** Nervous, bilious
- **Thermal:** Chilly
- **Miasm:** Psora, Sycosis, Syphilis

MIND

- Any mental excitement increases the suffering
- Constant change in mood
- Thinks too little of himself; has to be faultless
- Emotional strength, unbreakable will
- Fatigue and neurasthenia
- Dreams – amorous with pollutions
- Feeling of guilt; thinks he is a criminal
- Desire for mental work; patient is disposed to study

KEYNOTE SYMPTOMS

- Vertigo, worse stool, with sensation as if head is growing large
- Weakness during and after headache with nausea. Headache, worse bending head backwards
- Photophobia during spring; spring catarrh
- Lachrymation in cold air or on coming into sunshine
- Itching at the tip of the nose
- **Pain in hollow tooth, which feels too long, sensitive to touch**
- **Cracks across middle of tongue; tongue coated white**
- Sour taste in mouth, pyrosis
- Insatiable thirst, would like to drink the whole day
- **Constant desire for stool while walking**
- Constant dropping of blood from anus, no blood with the stools
- Pain in right testicle and urethra
- Emissions without erection. Lewd dreams with impotence
- Arthritis; severe pain in back and sacrum, worse sitting and after emissions; agitating bone pains
- Weak knees; weakness in legs, trembling
- **Sour foot sweat, especially between toes**
- Itching pimples on chin, hairy scalp and buttocks
- Wakes at night from dryness, soreness of lips

CLINICAL

- Alternating moods
- Fatigue
- Alopecia
- Photophobia
- Toothache
- Stomatitis
- Sexual disturbances
- Gonorrhoea
- Impotence
- Emissions
- Bone pains
- Lumbago
- Rheumatism
- Foot sweat
- Acne
- Insomnia

MODALITIES

- **Aggravation:** Sexual excesses, lying down, sitting, in the morning, warmth of bed
- **Amelioration:** Hawking mucous, continuous motion, walking

REMEDY RELATIONSHIP

- **Compare:** Cann-i., Sep., Zinc., Agn., Sel.

COCA

INTRODUCTION
- **Common name:** Bolivian coca, Coca erythroxylon
- **Family:** *Erythroxylaceae*
- **Source:** Vegetable kingdom
- **Part used:** Leaves, recently dried and carefully selected preserving their characteristic odour
- **Prover:** Mueller

SPHERE OF ACTION
- Mind
- Heart
- Respiratory system
- Musculoskeletal system
- Skin

MIND
- Melancholy from nervous exhaustion
- Nervousness with nocturnal restlessness
- Mental prostration alternating with brightness
- Bashful, timid, ill at ease in society
- Craves solitude and obscurity
- Sense of impending death
- Loquacoius excitement, with blissful visions
- Exhilaration before menses
- Overpowered by indescribable anxiety
- Insomnia
- Irritability
- Delight in solitude
- Sense of right and wrong lost

MODALITIES
- **Aggravation:** Ascending, high altitudes, climbing mountains, exertion – mental or physical, salty food, cold air
- **Amelioration:** From wine, riding, fast motion in open air, lying on face, after dinner

KEYNOTE SYMPTOMS
- Altitude sickness
- Complaints incidental to mountain climbing – palpitation, excessively rapid pulse, dyspnoea, violent sweating, anxiety, insomnia
- Muscle exhaustion, mental prostration. Patient is dizzy, dyspnoeic
- Physical and mental strain of a busy life; who suffer from exhausted nerves and brain. Need of nourishment and sleep even during heavy work. Remarkable vigour
- **Headache with vertigo. Tight headaches of high altitudes as if a rubber band were stretched across the forehead**
- Emphysema and dyspnoea from slight exertion. Incessant dyspnoea, especially in elderly patients. Spasmodic asthma
- Want of breath. Short breath especially in aged, athletes and alcoholic users and those who use tobacco
- Angina and severe palpitation due to mountain climbing or over exertion; with weak heart and dyspnoea
- **Sensation as if worms or small foreign bodies (grains of sand) were under the skin, moving away when touched; formication**
- Chronic sleeplessness; awakes with a shock in the brain

CONSTITUTION
- **A mountaineers remedy; for people under physical and mental strain due to a busy life. They complain of nervous and brain fag**
- Suits weak, nervous, fat, plethoric people who are always short of breath
- **Temperament:** Nervous, bilious
- **Thermal:** Chilly, ambithermal
- **Miasm:** Psora, Sycosis, Syphilis

CLINICAL
- Nervous exhaustion
- Headache
- Vertigo
- Caries of teeth
- Morning sickness
- Tinnitus
- Epistaxis
- Hoarseness
- Instantaneous voice producer
- Loss of voice
- Asthma
- Dyspnoea
- Emphysema
- Angina pectoris
- Palpitations
- Nocturnal enuresis
- Muscular fatigue
- Formication
- Sleeplessness

REMEDY RELATIONSHIP
- **Compare:** Ars., Paull., Cypr., Cham., Calc., Arn., Stram., Coff., Tab., Cann-i.
- **Antidoted by:** Gels.

COCCINELLA SEPTEMPUNCTATA

SPHERE OF ACTION
- Gastrointestinal system
- Musculoskeletal system
- Urinary system

INTRODUCTION
- **Common name:** Lady bug, Lady bird beetle, Lady-cow, Sun chafer
- **Family:** *Coccinellidae*
- **Source:** Animal kingdom
- **Part used:** Live insects

CONSTITUTION
- **For hydrophobia with profuse accumulation of saliva**
- For symptoms that appear in the teeth, and nerves of face and mouth
- **Temperament:** Nervous, bilious
- **Thermal:** Chilly
- **Miasm:** Psora, Sycosis, Syphilis

MIND
- Hydrophobia
- Irritability
- Nervousness
- Anger
- Anxiety

CLINICAL
- Hydrophobia
- Neuralgia
- Migraine
- Facial neuralgia
- Toothache
- Hiccough
- Diarrhoea
- Renal colic
- Arthritis
- Rheumatism

MODALITIES
- **Aggravation:** On seeing any bright object

KEYNOTE SYMPTOMS
- Pains extend from one part to another, may jump from side to side, recur periodically, often of brief duration, but recurring quickly
- Pain, worse any bright object, better sleep
- Profuse accumulation of saliva in the mouth, is awakened by it
- Rush of blood to face
- **Neuralgia of teeth, gums, mouth, worse at night, accompanied with icy cold extremities; cold sensation in teeth and mouth; right side mostly affected**
- Pain in forehead over right eye, sensitive to touch, from superior molars to forehead
- Periodical attacks of facial neuralgia. Cannot open eyes during paroxysm of facial neuralgia
- Uvula feels too long
- Pain in region of kidneys and loins

REMEDY RELATIONSHIP
- **Compare:** Canth., Mag-c., Spig., Thuj.

COCCULUS INDICUS

INTRODUCTION

- **Common name:** Indian cockle
- **Family:** *Menispermaceae*
- **Source:** Vegetable kingdom
- **Part used:** Seeds, fruits

SPHERE OF ACTION

- Mind
- Gastrointestinal system
- Nervous system
- Musculoskeletal system
- Female genital system

CONSTITUTION

- Adapted to bookworms
- For sensitive, romantic girls with irregular menses
- Ailments of drunkards or persons debilitated by sexual excesses
- For women and children with light hair and eyes who suffer severely during rheumatism, pregnancy
- Suits unmarried and childless women
- **Temperament:** Nervous, bilious
- **Thermal:** Chilly
- **Miasm:** Psora, Sycosis, Syphilis

MIND

- Angry at trifles
- Angry from least contradiction
- Time passes too quickly; slow in activities
- Profound sadness, grief; weeping during menses
- Sensitive to voices, rudeness
- Sentimental, serious
- Confusion after eating or drinking
- Introspection
- Starting when touched, at trifles
- Capricious
- Slowness of comprehension
- Mind benumbed
- Anxiety from night watching, after menses
- **Dwells on past, disagreeable occurrences**
- **Bad effects from grief, anger or from nursing a sick loved one; loss of sleep**
- Over sensitive to everything

KEYNOTE SYMPTOMS

- **Motion sickness, especially seasickness; causes nausea and vomiting**
- Empty, hollow, feeling. Sensation of emptiness in various organs of the body; sensation as if two stones are rubbing against each other or as if parts had gone off to sleep
- Extreme weakness, especially during menses, is hardly able to stand
- Headache of occiput, nape of neck with sensation as of a cord tightly bound, worse lying down on back of head, must lie down on a side
- **Lack of appetite with a metallic taste; aversion to food**
- **Nausea on just looking at food or at the thought of food**
- Sensation as if abdomen is full of stones, better lying on sides
- Menses too early, clotted with spasmodic colic
- Debilitating leucorrhoea, in place of menses or between menses
- Spinal weakness. Painful contractions of trunk and limbs
- Paralysing pain in lumbosacral region; trembling; cracking in knees on walking
- Painful stiffness of all joints

CLINICAL

- Motion sickness
- Sea sickness
- Chronic fatigue syndrome
- Hysteria
- Alcoholism
- Paralytic pain
- Convulsions
- Paralysis
- Chorea
- Neurodegenerative disorders
- Multiple sclerosis
- Sick headache
- Vertigo
- Hair lice
- Dysphagia
- Morning sickness
- Hernia
- Leucorrhoea
- Amenorrhoea
- Dysmenorrhoea
- Osteoarthritis

MODALITIES

- **Aggravation:** Motion of cars, train, ship, etc.; eating, after loss of sleep, open air, smoking, riding, swimming, touch, noise, jar, afternoon, menstrual period, after an emotional disturbance, nursing others
- **Amelioration:** Sitting, lying quiet on a side, in a warm room

REMEDY RELATIONSHIP

- **Antidotes:** Coff., Nux-v.
- **Compare:** Picro. in epilepsy, attacks in the morning on leaving horizontal position, hernia, locomotor ataxia, night sweats; Sym-r., in morning sickness; Petr., Puls., Ign., Calad.

COCCUS CACTI

SPHERE OF ACTION
- Mind
- Gastrointestinal system
- Respiratory system
- Musculoskeletal system
- Urinary system
- Female genital system

INTRODUCTION
- **Common name:** Cochineal, Grana fina cochineal insect
- **Family:** *Coccidae*
- **Source:** Animal kingdom
- **Part used:** Dried female insect
- **Prover:** Wachtel et. al

CONSTITUTION
- Suits a respiratory and urinary catarrhal condition, with a gouty, rheumatic diathesis
- **Temperament:** Nervous, bilious, rheumatic, gouty
- **Thermal:** Chilly
- **Miasm:** Psora, Sycosis, Syphilis

MIND
- Anxiety after eating, after midnight
- Sadness early in the morning, on waking, or in the afternoon
- Confusion of mind, better in open air
- Absentmindedness in albuminuria
- Thinking is difficult
- Migraine with sadness
- Apprehensive
- Irritable, fretful
- Talkative mood

KEYNOTE SYMPTOMS
- Catarrhal inflammation of the eyes, throat, respiratory and genitourinary organs
- Sensation of heat and pulsations in various organs
- **Sensation of a foreign body between the upper eyelid and the eyeball**
- **Chronic bronchitis complicated with cough; paroxysms from tickling or irritation in the larynx, ending in vomiting; worse 6 am, 11 or 11:30 pm; better drinking, especially cold drinks**
- Regular paroxysms of violent, tickling, racking cough, ending in vomiting or raising much clear, ropy mucous; intolerable internal itching
- Menses too early, profuse, dark black, thick with large clots. Flow only in the evening and at night
- Labia inflamed. Vulva sensitive when urinating

CLINICAL
- Anasarca
- Migraine
- Conjunctivitis
- Blepharitis
- Vomiting
- Ascites
- Coryza
- Cough
- Croup
- Pertussis
- Bronchitis
- Renal colic
- Urinary calculi
- Dysuria
- Anuria
- Haematuria
- Metrorrhagia
- Gonorrhoea
- Menorrhagia

MODALITIES
- **Aggravation:** Left side, after sleep, touch, pressure of clothing, brushing teeth, slightest exertion
- **Amelioration:** Walking, cold drink, washing in cold water

REMEDY RELATIONSHIP
- **Compare:** Canth., Cact., Sars., Oci., Kali-bi.

COFFEA CRUDA

INTRODUCTION
- **Common name:** Unroasted coffee
- **Family:** *Rubiaceae*
- **Source:** Vegetable kingdom
- **Part used:** Seeds
- **Prover:** Hahnemann

SPHERE OF ACTION
- Mind
- Gastrointestinal system
- Respiratory system
- Central nervous system
- Heart
- Female genital system
- Skin

MIND
- Nervous palpitations, especially from drinking coffee
- Bad effects of sudden emotions, surprises, joy, etc.
- Weeping from delight; alternate laughing and weeping. All ill-effects of fear, fright, disappointed love, over fatigue, long journey, excessive laughing, too much wine
- Unusual activity of mind and body
- Impressionable, especially to pleasurable ones. Full of ideas, quick to act
- Irritable and wakeful
- Now joyous, now gloomy; alternately laughing and crying
- Resents sympathy
- Memory active until midnight. Clearness of mind in the evening, at night
- Mental excitement
- Weeps, laments and tosses about over trifles

MODALITIES
- **Aggravation:** Sudden mental emotion, excessive joy, cold, open air, narcotic medicines, excessive excitement, noise, strong odours, touch
- **Amelioration:** Warmth, sleep, lying down, holding ice in mouth

KEYNOTE SYMPTOMS
- Drinking coffee stimulates the functional activity of all organs; in aged it increases uric acid production
- Patient faints after strong emotions
- Oversensitive to all stimuli. Over-reactive; all the senses are very acute
- Sensitive to sight, hearing, smell, taste, touch
- Restlessness; unusual mental and physical activity
- Neuralgia in various parts, always with great nervous excitability and intolerance of pain, driving to despair
- **Severe headache, as if a nail was driven into the head, drawing the patient to despair**
- **Toothache, better by holding ice cold water in the mouth**
- Short, dry, hacking, constant cough like whooping cough, particularly during inspiration
- Violent irregular palpitation, especially after excessive joy, surprise
- Sudden rise in blood pressure and suppression of urine
- **Vulva and vagina are very sensitive; aversion to sex**
- Profuse menses with oversensitive organs and voluptuous itching; dysmenorrhoea with large clots of dark blood
- Skin is very sensitive, itching, scratches until it bleeds
- Insomnia on account of mental excitability; from excessive use of coffee
- Wakefulness and improved alertness
- Wakes up with a start; sleep disturbed by dreams

CONSTITUTION
- Suits tall, lean, stooping dark complexioned people with increased nervous and vascular capacity and a hypersensitive skin
- **Temperament:** Nervous, sanguine, choleric
- **Thermal:** Chilly
- **Miasm:** Psora, Sycosis, Syphilis

CLINICAL
- Chronic fatigue syndrome
- Neuralgia
- Unconsciousness
- Migraine
- Toothache
- Dentitional problems
- Colic
- Asthma
- Angina pectoris
- Anuria
- Vaginismus
- Abortion
- Dysmenorrhoea
- Pruritus
- Insomnia

REMEDY RELATIONSHIP
- **Compare:** Acon., Cham., Ign., Sulph., Coff-t., Cypr., Bry.
- **Incompatible:** Canth., Caust., Cocc., Ign.
- **Complementary:** Acon.
- **Antidotes:** Coff., Tab., Nux-v.
- Strong black coffee antidotes several poisons, especially narcotics

COLCHICUM AUTUMNALE

INTRODUCTION
- **Common name:** Meadow saffron
- **Family:** *Liliaceae*
- **Source:** Vegetable kingdom
- **Part used:** Corn
- **Prover:** Hahnemann

SPHERE OF ACTION
- Mind
- Gastrointestinal system
- Heart
- Musculoskeletal system
- Urinary system

CONSTITUTION
- Suits rheumatic and gouty diathesis; robust, vigorous constitutions with oedematous swelling
- Adapted to diseases of old people or asthmatic people
- **Temperament:** Nervous, bilious, gouty, rheumatic
- **Thermal:** Chilly
- **Miasm:** Psora, Sycosis, Syphilis

MIND
- Very depressed and irritable
- Ailments from grief, misdeeds of others
- Sensitive to strong odours, bad manners, contact
- Very irritable with pains; troubles seem intolerable. Intolerable to pain
- Sensitive to extreme impressions, like bright light, strong odours, touch, mis-behaviour of others; sensitive to all external impressions
- Mind generally distracted
- Mind befogged but answers correctly
- Cannot tolerate misdeeds of others
- **Dreams of mice**
- Memory weak from fatigue

KEYNOTE SYMPTOMS
- **Cold, weak, sensitive and restless; profuse cold sweat; emaciate rapidly; tendency to collapse; marked prostration and internal coldness**
- All functions – mental and physical, are slow
- Tendency to collapse, particularly after dehydration
- Sensitive to impressions – light, noise, odours, contact, bad manners
- Extreme relaxation of muscular system; head falls forwards or backwards when lifted
- **Smell painfully acute; nausea and faintness from the odour of cooking food, fish; loathes the sight of food**
- Burning, or icy coldness of the stomach or abdomen
- **Stools contain white, shreddy particles and white mucous. Agonizing pain remains long after stool**
- Gouty diathesis; red, hot and swollen parts; with tearing pains, worse evening and touch
- Markedly affects the muscles, fibrous tissues, serous membranes and joints, especially small joints
- Rheumatic complaints, especially chronic ones; tearing pains; drawing pains in muscles, periosteum and joints worse autumn, change of weather, motion, evening, any mental or physical exertion
- Tingling in many parts as if frostbitten; pins and needle sensation in hands, wrists and fingers; tingling in finger nails

CLINICAL
- Prostration
- Cataract
- Asthenopia
- Gingivitis
- Dyspepsia
- Flatulence
- Nausea of pregnancy
- Diarrhoea
- Autumnal dysentery
- Gastroenteritis
- Prolapse of rectum
- Intussuception
- Ascites
- Colic
- Endocarditis
- Nephritis
- Albuminuria
- Diabetes mellitus
- Pericarditis
- Arthritis
- Rheumatism
- Gout
- Lumbago
- Typhoid

MODALITIES
- **Aggravation:** Mental emotion or exhaustion, effects of hard study, odour of cooking food, motion, cold, autumn, getting wet, bathing, living in damp dwelling
- **Amelioration:** Warmth, rest, doubling up, sitting, lying quietly, open air

REMEDY RELATIONSHIP
- **Compare:** Bry. in rheumatic gout with serous effusions, in rheumatism in warm weather; Carb-v., Arn., Lil-t., Ars., Cocc., Kali-c., Verat.
- **Antidotes:** Thuj., Camph., Nux-v., Puls., Cocc.
- Often cures dropsy after Apis and Ars. fail

COLLINSONIA CANADENSIS

INTRODUCTION
- **Common name:** Stoneroot
- **Family:** *Labiatae*
- **Source:** Vegetable kingdom
- **Part used:** Rhizome
- **Prover:** Burt in tincture and Dowla in trituration

SPHERE OF ACTION
- Mind
- Gastrointestinal system
- Respiratory system
- Heart
- Musculoskeletal system
- Female genital system
- Skin

CONSTITUTION
- Adapted to cases with pelvic and portal congestion, and general muscular atony, especially in women
- For chronic nasal, gastric and pharyngeal catarrh due to portal congestion
- **Temperament:** Nervous, bilious
- **Thermal:** Chilly, ambithermal
- **Miasm:** Psora, Sycosis, Syphilis

MIND
- Delirium with open eyes; during pregnancy, from itching of genitals
- Delusion that body parts do not belong to her
- Ailments from excitement
- Excitement causes palpitations
- Depressed
- Irritability
- Confusion
- Restlessness
- Palpitation after passing stool
- Anxiety
- Gloomy and sullen

KEYNOTE SYMPTOMS
- Congestion in pelvic organs especially anus, rectum and uterus
- Sensation of constriction and feeling of enlargement felt in various parts and organs of the body like limbs, vulva, clitoris, etc. Sense of weight and constriction; pelvic engorgement
- **Tongue coated yellow; constipation in children due to intestinal atony**
- Chronic gastric catarrh due to portal obstruction
- Constipation and diarrhoea alternate. Indicated in most obstinate cases of constipation
- Itching in anus
- **Sensation of sharp sticks in the rectum; bleeding, painful piles. Rectal prolapse, sense of constriction in rectum.**
- Flushes of heat with piles, oppressed breathing. Chronic haemorrhoids, alternating with heart, chest, or rheumatic symptoms
- Cough due to excessive use of voice
- Chest pain alternates with haemorrhoids. When heart symptoms are relieved, bleeding piles or suppressed menses return
- Cardiac congestion
- Haemorrhoids, constipation especially in females with dysmenorrhoea
- Prolapse of uterus with itching of vulva
- Pruritus of pregnancy with haemorrhoids
- Ovaries enlarged, cancerous
- Female genitals are swollen and inflamed
- Sensation as if limbs were enlarged; gait unsteady

CLINICAL
- Dropsy
- Chorea
- Epilepsy
- Ptosis
- Cataract
- Enteritis
- Appendicitis
- Dysentery
- Constipation
- Haemorrhoids
- Proctitis
- Rectal fissure
- Rectal carcinoma
- Hoarseness
- Murmurs
- Mammary gland hard and indurated
- Dysmenorrhoea
- Menorrhagia
- Metrorrhagia
- Vulvitis
- Fibroids
- Prolapse of uterus
- Impotence
- Spermatorrhoea
- Urticaria

MODALITIES
- **Aggravation:** From the slightest mental emotion or excitement, cold, at night, during pregnancy
- **Amelioration:** Heat, morning

REMEDY RELATIONSHIP
- **Antidote:** Nux-v.
- **Compare:** Aesc., Aloe, Ham., Lycps-v., Neg., Sulph., Nux-v.

COLOCYNTHIS

INTRODUCTION
- **Common name:** Bitter cucumber
- **Family:** *Curcurbitaceae*
- **Source:** Vegetable kingdom
- **Part used:** Pulp excluding seeds
- **Prover:** Hahnemann

SPHERE OF ACTION
- Mind
- Nerves – trigeminal, facial, sciatic
- Gastrointestinal system
- Musculoskeletal system
- Urinary system
- Female genital system

MIND
- Ailments after anger and silent grief
- Greatly affected by the misfortune of others
- Angered easily, vexed during pain, want of religious feelings. Screams with pain; disinclined to talk, to answer. Impatient.
- Does not want to meet friends
- Morose; becomes offended at everything; depressed, joyless
- Irritable; throws things out of his hand
- Mortification, caused by offense
- Confusion after beer, wine
- Anger with indignation
- Depressed and joyless

MODALITIES
- **Aggravation:** From anger, indignation, vexation, chagrin, drafts, cold, evening and night
- **Amelioration:** Doubling up, hard pressure, warmth, lying with head bent forward, lying on abdomen

KEYNOTE SYMPTOMS
- Neuralgic pains – cutting, pinching, cramping, gnawing, boring, colicky. Pains come suddenly, go suddenly
- Cutting, twisting, grinding, contracting, bruised sensation, as if clamped with iron bands
- **Left sided drug, except sciatica which is on the right side. Worse 4-9 pm, better pressure**
- **Agonising pain in the abdomen, causing patient to bend double**
- Pains are radiating, coming in waves; sensation as if intestines are squeezed between stones
- **Diarrhoea or dysentery due to anger. Stools thick, bloody, jelly-like, white mucous, watery and scanty; aggravated by least food or drink**
- Dysuria; tenesmus of bladder; viscid, scanty urine. Pain in the bladder, radiating all over the abdomen
- Ovarian cyst; boring pain in ovarian region with great restlessness; must bend
- Menses suppressed from anger, chagrin
- Cramps, contractions, twitching, shortening of muscles
- Sciatic pain, better heat and pressure

CONSTITUTION
- Suited to irritable people, especially women with sedentary habits and copious menses, who are easily angered with ill-effects thereafter
- For those with an anxious expression on the face and a tendency to neuralgias
- Tendency to corpulency
- **Temperament:** Nervous
- **Thermal:** Chilly
- **Miasm:** Sycosis

CLINICAL
- Obesity
- Neuralgia
- Glaucoma
- Rheumatic iritis
- Dyspepsia
- Enteritis
- Dysentery
- Diarrhoea
- Peritonitis
- Cystitis
- Dysuria
- Ovarian cyst
- Menstrual colic
- Dysmenorrhoea
- Paraphimosis
- Rheumatism
- Sciatica
- Insomnia

REMEDY RELATIONSHIP
- **Antidoted by:** Coff., Staph., Cham., Op., Camph., Caust.
- **Coloc. is the best antidote for lead poisoning**
- **Compare:** Lob-e. in violent corkscrew-like pains in abdomen; Dip. in writhing, twisting like a dying snake; Dios., Cham., Cocc., Merc., Plb., Mag-p.

CONIUM MACULATUM

INTRODUCTION
- **Common name:** Poison hemlock
- **Family:** *Umbelliferae*
- **Source:** Vegetable kingdom
- **Part used:** Whole plant
- **Prover:** Hahnemann

SPHERE OF ACTION
- Mind
- Nervous system
- Glandular system
- Gastrointestinal system
- Respiratory system
- Female genital system
- Musculoskeletal system

CONSTITUTION
- For ailments of old men or maids with light hair, rigid muscular fibre and sedentary habits
- 'Balm of Gilead' for diseases of old maids and women during and after climacteric
- For hypochondriasis; cancerous diathesis
- **Temperament:** Nervous, cancerous, scrofulous
- **Thermal:** Chilly
- **Miasm:** Sycosis, Syphilis

MIND
- Memory weak, unable to sustain any mental effort
- Domineering
- Morose
- Indolent
- Indifferent
- Quarrelsome
- Scolding
- Cannot bear contradiction
- Mental depression
- Memory weak
- Dread of being alone, yet avoids society
- Sluggish
- Debility
- Timid, averse to society

KEYNOTE SYMPTOMS
- Enlarged glands with cancerous diathesis; especially of ovaries and breasts
- Cancerous tendency, especially after bruises and injuries
- Prostrated, exhausted mentally and physically; trembling
- Ailments from suppressed sexual desires
- Ascending paralysis ending in death by paralysis of respiration
- **Sweats day and night with offensive odour**
- Vertigo, especially when lying down or turning in bed
- Soreness around root of tongue; heartburn, acridity, burning; nausea
- Acrid heartburn with acrid eructation, worse on going to bed
- Abdomen hard, sensitive and swollen
- **Burning or coldness in rectum during stool; cold flatus and stool. Weakness after every stool**
- **Great difficulty in voiding urine, flow intermits – stops and starts**
- Axillary glands painful with a numb feeling down the arm
- Glandular induration or stony hardness of mammae
- Breasts sore, hard and painful; before and during menstruation; stitching pain in breasts and nipples
- **Leucorrhoea ten days after menses, acrid. Discharge milky, profuse, thick, intermittent**
- Ovary and uterus enlarged; induration of os and cervix
- Muscular weakness of lower extremities; paralytic weakness, trembling, sudden loss of strength while walking

CLINICAL
- Enlarged glands
- Cancer
- Tumours
- Debility
- Ascending paralysis
- Muscular weakness
- Chorea
- Polypus
- Paroxysms
- Vertigo
- Styes
- Heartburn
- Jaundice
- Hepatomegaly
- Peritonitis
- Whooping cough
- Asthma
- Arteriosclerosis
- Breast cancer
- Leucorrhoea
- Prolapse of uterus
- Vaginismus
- Dysmenorrhoea
- Ovaritis
- Cancer of prostate
- Impotency
- Chronic ulcers
- Urticaria

MODALITIES
- **Aggravation:** Lying down, turning or rising in bed, celibacy, before and during menses, from taking cold, physical or mental exertion, alcohol, jar
- **Amelioration:** While fasting, in the dark, from letting the limbs hang down, motion, pressure, stooping

REMEDY RELATIONSHIP
- **Compare:** Scir. or Cancer nosode in cancerous diathesis, enlarged glands, cancer of breast, worms; Bar-c., Hydr., Iod., Kali-p., Hyos., Cur.

Conium maculatum

CORALLIUM RUBRUM

INTRODUCTION
- **Common name:** Red coral
- **Family:** *Gorgoriaceae*
- **Source:** Animal kingdom
- **Prover:** Attomyr

SPHERE OF ACTION
- Mind
- Head
- Pneumogastric nerve
- Respiratory system
- Male genital system
- Skin

MIND
- Weak memory
- Sad, fearful; fear of suffering
- Irritable, ill-humoured
- Anguish
- Hysterical, fear of impending diseases with diarrhoea
- Dreams – frightful; nightmares; full of cares
- Work shyness; aversion to work
- Confused, after drinking beer, from spirituous liquors; stupefaction after wine

MODALITIES
- **Aggravation:** In open air, changing from a warm to cold room, eating, touch, uncovering, inhaling air
- **Amelioration:** Covering

KEYNOTE SYMPTOMS
- **Deep seated frontal headache with pain at the back of eyeballs**
- Pneumogastric nerve affections; nausea and violent vomiting
- Pain during articulation in the lower jaw
- **Food tastes like saw dust or straw; beer tastes sweet**
- **Craves salt**
- Inspired air feels cold on deep inspiration
- Epistaxis from one nostril at a time
- Profuse secretion of mucous dropping through posterior nares
- Dry coryza, nose stopped up, ulcerated; painful ulcers in the nostrils
- Throat sensitive, especially to cold air which causes coughing
- **Minute gun cough during the day and whooping cough at night**
- Dry, spasmodic, suffocative, continuous, hysterical cough
- Cough followed by vomiting of stringy mucous and exhaustion
- Cough with a purple face and expectoration of blood
- Ulcers on glans and inner prepuce which are very sensitive to touch
- Involuntary seminal emissions during sleep
- Sensation as if needles pricking in the frenum
- Psoriasis of palms and soles

CONSTITUTION
- Suits exhausted people with a purple face and weakened sexual power
- **Patient is too cold when uncovered and too hot when covered; better by artificial heat**
- **Temperament:** Nervous
- **Thermal:** Chilly
- **Miasm:** Psora, Syphilis

CLINICAL
- Migraine
- Epistaxis
- Sinusitis
- Post-nasal catarrh
- Hoarseness
- Laryngismus stridulus
- Whooping cough
- Hysterical cough
- Asthma
- Gonorrhoea
- Chancroids
- Emissions
- Eczema
- Vesicular pustular eruptions
- Ulcers
- Psoriasis

REMEDY RELATIONSHIP
- **Complementary:** Sulph.
- **Compare:** Bell., Dros., Meph., Caust.

CRATAEGUS OXYACANTHA

SPHERE OF ACTION
- Mind
- Cardiovascular system
- Respiratory system
- Urinary system
- Skin

INTRODUCTION
- **Common name:** Hawthorn berries, Hedge thorn
- **Family:** *Rosaceae*
- **Source:** Vegetable kingdom
- **Part used:** Berries
- **Prover:** Dr Greene

CONSTITUTION
- For old people with a weak, anaemic, oedematous condition
- **Temperament:** Nervous, bilious
- **Thermal:** Chilly, ambithermal
- **Miasm:** Psora, Sycosis

MIND
- Despair of recovery; feels weak and fragile
- Ailments from grief, sorrow, care
- Anxiety with palpitation
- Apprehensive, despondent
- Very nervous and irritable
- Mental dullness
- Sadness, depression, melancholy
- Anxiety of heart disease
- Hurried feeling with rapid action of the heart

KEYNOTE SYMPTOMS
- **Heart tonic for muscular weakness of the heart**
- Valvular murmurs with a history of rheumatism
- Fatty degeneration of the heart; chronic heart disease with marked weakness
- Myocarditis; irregular action of the heart; failing compensation
- Angina pectoris with dysphagia and nervous prostration
- **Low pulse and low blood pressure with air hunger**
- Weak heart muscles with oppression, worn out heart
- **Weak first heart sound with intermittent, irregular, weak pulse**
- Has the ability to dissolve calcareous deposits in arteries – arteriosclerosis
- Insomnia of aortic sufferers
- In cross, irritable cardiac symptoms it acts as a sedative
- Severe dyspnoea, worse least exertion
- Diabetes in children
- Cutaneous chilliness; cyanosis of extremities
- Skin eruptions with profuse perspiration

CLINICAL
- Anaemia
- Dropsy
- Prostration
- Vertigo
- Dyspnoea
- Hypotension
- Hypertension
- Weak pulse
- Cardiac dropsy
- Arteriosclerosis
- Myocarditis
- Pericarditis
- Angina pectoris
- Valvular incompetence
- Fatty degeneration of heart
- Rheumatism
- Eczema
- Insomnia

MODALITIES
- **Aggravation:** In a warm room, on least exertion, night
- **Amelioration:** Fresh air, quiet, rest

REMEDY RELATIONSHIP
- **Compare:** Stroph-h., Dig., Iber., Naja, Cact., Alf., Aven.

SPHERE OF ACTION

- Mind
- Eyes
- Gastrointestinal system
- Respiratory system
- Female genital system

INTRODUCTION

- **Common name:** Saffron
- **Family:** *Iridaceae*
- **Source:** Vegetable kingdom
- **Part used:** Dried stigma
- **Prover:** Stapf and Gross

CONSTITUTION

- Suits women and hysterical men with extreme changeability of mental symptoms.
- Haemorrhagic diathesis
- **Temperament:** Nervous, hysterical
- **Thermal:** Chilly
- **Miasm:** Syphilis

CROCUS SATIVUS

MIND

- Changeability of mental symptoms; laughter quickly followed by tears
- Hysterical, laughing mania
- Pleasant mania, keeps singing and laughing
- Vivid recollection from music
- Frequent and extreme change in sensation from hilarity to melancholy
- Patient is excessively happy and affectionate
- **Wants to kiss everybody, but the very next moment is in a rage; anger with violence, rapidly followed by repentance**
- Lassitude and drowsiness better by literary labour
- Childish behaviour; mentally very distracted

MODALITIES

- **Aggravation:** Lying down, motion, hot weather, warm room, in the morning, fasting, before breakfast, looking fixedly at an object
- **Amelioration:** In open air, after eating breakfast

KEYNOTE SYMPTOMS

- **Haemorrhage from any and every orifice of the body which is dark, viscid, clotted, drawn in long black strings, hanging from the bleeding surface**
- Sensation in eyes as after crying bitterly or as if smoke in eyes
- Epistaxis dark, stringy, clotted; string of dark blood hangs down the nose
- Wheezing cough with frothy expectoration. Sensation of elongated uvula in hysterical women
- Sensation as if something alive and moving in the stomach, abdomen, uterus, arms, chest, breasts, etc.
- Portal stagnation leads to severe and obstinate constipation
- Menses – dark, viscid, frequent, copious. Menorrhagia. Uterine haemorrhage, clots with long strings.
- Dysmenorrrhoea, flow – black, stringy, clotted; slimy
- Threatened abortion with dark, stringy discharge
- Surging of blood to genitals
- Pain, weakness, cracking in knees
- Spasmodic contraction and twitching of a single set of muscles

CLINICAL

- Hysteria
- Haemorrhage
- Chorea
- Brain affections
- Migraine
- Headache
- Ciliary neuralgia
- Ophthalmia neonatorum
- Lachrymation
- Conjuctivitis
- Constipation
- Epistaxis
- Ozaena
- Menstrual disorders
- Dysmenorrhoea
- Threatened abortion

REMEDY RELATIONSHIP

- **Antidote:** Op., Bell.
- **Compare:** Ip., Tril-p., Plat., Chin., Sabin., Phos., Ust.

CROTALUS HORRIDUS

SPHERE OF ACTION

- Eyes
- Nervous system
- Gastrointestinal system
- Respiratory system
- Female genital system
- Skin

INTRODUCTION

- **Common name:** Rattlesnake
- **Family:** *Crotalidae*
- **Source:** Animal kingdom
- **Part used:** Venom, procured by compressing the gland when the serpent is either pinioned in a frame or under the influence of chloroform
- **Prover:** Hering

CONSTITUTION

- Suits those in low septic states with disorganization of blood, jaundice and haemorrhages
- For strumous, debilitated, broken down constitutions, in drunkards with a tendency to blood boils
- **Temperament:** Nervous, bilious
- **Thermal:** Hot
- **Miasm:** Sycosis, Syphilis

MIND

- Low forms of delirium
- Great loquacity
- Wants to talk all the time with a desire to escape from bed
- Delirium with drowsiness and stupor
- **Symptoms worse during sleep**
- Nervous; anxious and pale
- Irritable, cross, provoked on least stimulus
- Mental dullness
- Apprehensive, melancholic
- Despondent, lachrymose mood, clouded perception, memory weak
- Delusion of cerebral decay
- Dreams of dead people

KEYNOTE SYMPTOMS

- Right sided affections
- Profound nervous shock, deathly sickness, trembling and prostrations
- Tired on slightest exertion; fainting
- Putrid and malignant conditions; low septic states – typhoid or malarial fever; bubonic plague
- Haemorrhagic diathesis. Decomposition of blood. Haemorrhages are slow, oozing, of dark thin blood from all the orifices or surfaces, especially pharynx. Bloody pus and sweat. Dark or bluish parts; purpurea haemorrhagica
- Pains – alternate rapidly with each other, frequently recur, also appear and disappear suddenly after lasting for some time, except for headache
- Swelling of affected parts
- Low septic conditions – tonsils, ulcers, abscesses; tendency to carbuncles, malignant conditions
- Epilepsy with trembling, toamine, violent cries and delirium
- **Tongue is fiery red, smooth and polished; swollen**
- **Desires stimulants, alcohol. Aversion to meat**
- **Cancer of stomach; gastric ulcers, gastritis; especially in alcoholics with black or coffee ground vomiting**
- **Stool black, thin, offensive like coffee ground**
- Malignant condition of uterus with marked tendency to haemorrhages
- Miscarriage during septic fever. Menopausal sweating and flushes
- Malignant fevers of haemorrhagic tendency
- Swelling and yellowish discolouration of the body; boils, eruptions, etc. surrounded by purple mottled skin and oedema

CLINICAL

- Delirium
- Epilepsy
- Stroke
- Apoplexy
- Convulsions
- Paralysis
- Streptococcal infection
- Septicaemia
- Plague
- Lymphangitis
- Haemorrhage
- Cancer
- Oedema
- Cerebrospinal meningitis
- Ciliary neuralgia
- Intraocular haemorrhages
- Dyspepsia
- Gastric ulcer
- Cancer of stomach
- Jaundice
- Cirrhosis
- Diarrhoea
- Diphtheria
- Menopause
- Phlegmasia alba dolens
- Yellow fever
- Abscesses
- Ecchymosis
- Purpurea haemorrhagica
- Ulcers
- Chilblains
- Carbuncles
- Boils
- Blood boils
- Insomnia

MODALITIES

- **Aggravation:** Right side, open air, evening and morning, in spring, coming on in warm weather, yearly, on awaking, damp and wet, jar
- **Amelioration:** Rest, motion, light

REMEDY RELATIONSHIP

- **Compare:** Both., Naja; Lach.; Elaps, Crot-c, Bung-fa.
- **Antidote:** Lach., Alco., radiant heat, Camphor

CROTON TIGLIUM

SPHERE OF ACTION
- Mind
- Gastrointestinal system
- Respiratory system
- Genitourinary system
- Skin

INTRODUCTION
- **Common name:** Croton oil seed, Purging nut
- **Family:** *Euphorbiaceae*
- **Source:** Vegetable kingdom
- **Part used:** Oil from seeds
- **Prover:** Herman

CONSTITUTION
- Used in pregnancy and nursing women with skin complaints or for summer complaints in general
- **Temperament:** Nervous, bilious
- **Thermal:** Ambithermal
- **Miasm:** Psora

MIND
- Grumbling, discontented humour
- Dreams are frightful; nightmares
- Work shyness; aversion to work, fritters away his time; would rather dance than attend to business
- Self-esteem, cannot think of anyone else besides himself
- Confusion, worse bread
- Feeling of anxiety as though some personal misfortune would befall him
- Weak memory
- Morose, dissatisfied

KEYNOTE SYMPTOMS
- Left sided affections
- Great affinity for the skin external genitals and face
- Feeling as if parts were drawn backwards; like nipples (pain from the nipples goes to the back), eyes (eyes feel drawn backwards; feeling as if a string were pulling the eyeball back into the head)
- Weight of hat causes headache
- **Watery, profuse stools shooting out forcibly; worse least food or drink**
- **Gurgling or swashing, as of water in the intestines, especially on the left side**
- It is a hepatic stimulant, increasing the secretion of bile
- Hoarseness, as from a cold or with a desire to hawk with tickling in the larynx
- **Asthma with cough, as soon as patient's head touches the pillow, must sit up, cannot expand lungs**
- Eruptions, especially on the face and genitals; intense itching but scratching is painful
- Eczema, vesicular and pustular
- Skin symptoms alternate with internal symptoms, diarrhoea
- Gastrointestinal complaints, mucous membranes of the intestines affected. Abdominal colic before stools. **Constant urging, worse eating or drinking. Colic is better hot milk and warm drinks.**
- **Antidotes Rhus poisoning**

CLINICAL
- Violent inflammations
- Keratitis
- Corneal ulcer
- Nausea
- Oesophagitis
- Violent vomiting
- Colic
- Diarrhoea
- Cholera morbus
- Asthma
- Eczema
- Pruritus
- Pustules
- Scabies
- Vesicles
- Vesicular erysipelas
- Herpes zoster
- Urticaria
- Chilblains

MODALITIES
- **Aggravation:** Least food or drink, during summers, touch, at night and in the morning, washing
- **Amelioration:** After sleep, gentle rubbing

REMEDY RELATIONSHIP
- **Compare:** Mom-ch. has marked, drastic properties, producing colic, nausea, vomiting and cholera-like symptoms, abdomen seems full of fluid which is discharged explosively, thin, watery, yellow, great thirst; Rhus-t., Anag., Anac., Sep.
- **Antidote:** Ant-t.

CUPRUM METALLICUM

INTRODUCTION

- **Common name:** Copper
- **Group:** Metal
- **Source:** Mineral kingdom
- **Formula:** Cu
- **Prover:** Hahnemann

SPHERE OF ACTION

- Nervous system
- Gastrointestinal system
- Respiratory system
- Muscular system
- Skin

CONSTITUTION

- Suits carbo-nitrogenoid constitution in fair people with a bluish face
- Suits women who have borne several children
- **Temperament:** Bilious, anaemic
- **Thermal:** Hot
- **Miasm:** Sycosis

MIND

- Fixed ideas
- Malicious and morose
- Fearful
- Closed and withdrawn; nervous and uneasy
- Dullness and slowness; thoughts move slowly
- Strong desire to make grimaces
- Empty feeling
- Sensation as if water was poured over the head
- Attacks of unconquerable anxiety
- Irritability worse contradiction
- Chorea due to fright
- Uses words which were not intended
- Attacks of rage, wants to bite and strike

KEYNOTE SYMPTOMS

- Mental and physical exhaustion from overexertion
- Complaints begin on the left side
- **Convulsions – tonic and clonic; especially in children**
- Spasmodic affections; violent cramps and clonic spasms beginning in the fingers and toes
- **Epilepsy, aura begins in knees and ascends**
- Epilepsy at night, during menses; after fright, suppressed eruption and foot sweat
- Stammering speech. **Protrusion and retraction of the tongue like a snake; paralysis of the tongue**
- **Metallic, coppery taste in the mouth**
- On drinking, fluid descends with a gurgling sound
- **One of the trios of cholera**
- Vomiting is relived by drinking cold water; with hiccough, colic, diarrhoea and spasms
- Cough in three attacks successively. Cough has a gurgling sound
- Coldness of hands; cramps in palms, calves and soles
- Bluish discolouration of the skin; ulcers, itching in spots, pimples, especially in folds of joints

CLINICAL

- Unconsciousness
- Convulsions
- Cramps
- Spasms
- Neuralgia
- Paralysis
- Epilepsy
- Chlorosis
- Meningitis
- Tongue paralysis
- Cholera morbus
- Asiatic cholera
- Intussusception
- Tapeworms
- Laryngeal spasm
- Whooping cough
- Asthma
- Angina pectoris
- Leprosy
- Psoriasis
- Ringworm

MODALITIES

- **Aggravation:** At night, getting wet, vomiting, contact, emotions, fright, suppressions, mental or physical over work, before menses
- **Amelioration:** During perspiration, drinking cold water, being mesmerized, putting pressure over heart

REMEDY RELATIONSHIP

- **Compare with:** Calc., Plb., Nux-v., Verat, Cupr-s.
- **Antidotes:** Bell., Hep., Camph.
- **Antidoted by:** Bell., Cham., Nux-v.

CYCLAMEN EUROPAEUM

INTRODUCTION

- **Common name:** Sow bread
- **Family:** *Primulaceae*
- **Source:** Vegetable kingdom
- **Part used:** Roots
- **Prover:** Hahnemann

SPHERE OF ACTION

- Eyes
- Gastrointestinal system
- Respiratory system
- Female genital system
- Skin

MIND

- Weeps when alone, thinks she is alone in the world and is prosecuted by everyone
- Depressed, desires to be alone
- Silent weeping
- **Hallucination as if two people are lying in her bed**
- Tearful over imaginary grief, restlessness and morose during menses
- Irritable on waking
- Offended easily
- Weeping during menses which doesn't help
- Ailments from suppressed grief and terrors of conscience
- Dullness of senses

MODALITIES

- **Aggravation:** Open air, cold water, cold, cold bathing, menses worse sitting and lying at night
- **Amelioration:** In a warm room, indoors, menses, walking, moistening diseased parts, bathing, rubbing parts, weeping

KEYNOTE SYMPTOMS

- Easily fatigued, thus, not inclined to any kind of labour
- Sleepiness, moroseness, lassitude
- Drawing or tearing pain of parts where bone lies near the surface
- Vertigo – things turn in a circle or look pale
- Headache in anaemic persons with flickering before the eyes, fiery sparks; prolonged migraine
- Dim vision. **Flickering of colours before the eyes; sees countless stars. Disturbed vision.**
- **Salty taste, salty saliva; hiccough-like eructations, worse fatty foods**
- **Distaste for meat, pork, bread and butter; desires lemonade, sardines and indigestible things**
- Hiccough during pregnancy with yawning; also vomiting of pregnancy
- Diarrhoea after a cup of coffee; pain around anus and perineum
- Nocturnal cough, especially in children, when asleep, without waking them up
- Menses profuse, black clotted, membranous with labour-like pains
- Feels better during menstrual flow

CONSTITUTION

- For leucophlegmatic constitutions with anaemia or chlorosis; with feeble functions of organs and senses, and a tendency to fatigue
- For those with a blue face and clenched thumbs, anaemic, chlorotic women with scanty menses, amenorrhoea
- **Temperament:** Bilious, nervous
- **Thermal:** Hot
- **Miasm:** Sycosis, Syphilis

CLINICAL

- Delirium
- Enlarged glands
- Cancer
- Convulsions
- Epilepsy
- Diplopia
- Hemiopia
- Convergent strabismus
- Hiccoughs
- Dysentery
- Diphtheria
- Cough
- Asthma
- Arteriosclerosis
- Menorrhagia
- Dysmenorrhoea
- Sterility
- Gonorrhoea
- Pruritus
- Ecchymosis
- Acne
- Chilblains
- Carbuncles

REMEDY RELATIONSHIP

- **Compare:** Puls., Chin., Ferr., in chlorosis and anaemic affections; Croc., Thuj. as if something alive in abdomen; also Ign., Ambr., Kali-bi., Rhus-t., Iris.

DIGITALIS PURPUREA

SPHERE OF ACTION
- Mind
- Gastrointestinal system
- Heart
- Urinary system
- Male genital system
- Skin

INTRODUCTION
- **Common name:** Foxglove
- **Family:** *Scrophulariaceae*
- **Source:** Vegetable kingdom
- **Part used:** Leaves of the second year's growth
- **Prover:** Hahnemann

CONSTITUTION
- Suits cyanosed, nervous, lymphatic constitutions who are sad with a weak heart and pale face
- Suits scrofulous children with very pale complexion
- **Temperament:** Nervous
- **Thermal:** Ambithermal
- **Miasm:** Sycosis, Syphilis

MIND
- Lascivious thoughts in old men with enlarged prostate
- Forgetfulness, dullness of senses
- Excessive desire to be alone. Indisposed to speak; tearful, morose
- Symptoms, especially sense of guilt better by weeping
- Despondent, fearful, anxious about future. Great anxiety, as from a troubled conscience
- Remorse. Sadness with sleeplessness, from unhappy love, grief; deep sighing
- Melancholia, worse from music
- Anxious, desires solitude
- Suspicious
- Fear of suffocation, especially at night

KEYNOTE SYMPTOMS
- **Thirsty, especially for acidic drinks; loss of appetite**
- Excessive nausea with faintness and sinking feeling in stomach; not better after vomiting
- Liver enlarged and painful; jaundice. Tenderness of epigastrium with heart disease
- White, chalk-like, pasty stool; constipation. Diarrhoea during jaundice
- Cough associated with heart trouble; dyspnoea, deep sighing, gasps for breath
- Heart slow; feels it will stop on motion. Weak, irregular heart with faint-like weakness. Constant pain or anguish in cardiac region
- Must walk about with praecordial anxiety
- **Heart troubles with slow, intermittent, weak and irregular pulse. Pulse intermits every third, fifth or seventh beat**
- Weakness and dilatation of myocardium. Mitral valve disease.
- Failure of compensation; very effective when auricular fibrillation sets in; auricular fibrillation or flutter, especially after rheumatic fever
- Heart block; cardiac muscular failure; organic heart disease, cardiac irritability
- Dropsical swelling of genitals; balanitis with oedema of prepuce
- Spermatorrhoea, inflammatory condition of urethra; prostate enlarged in elderly
- Fingers go to sleep frequently. Coldness of hands and feet
- Blueness of skin; cyanosis. Skin itching and jaundiced
- Starts from sleep in alarm, as if falling from a height

CLINICAL
- Weakness
- Faintness
- Dropsy
- Cyanosis
- Cholera
- Nausea
- Gastralgia
- Liver complaints
- Deafness
- Haemoptysis
- Pneumonia
- Respiration irregular
- Dyspnoea
- Hectic fever of phthisis
- Heart trouble
- Angina pectoris
- Pericarditis
- Cardiac failure
- Intermittent pulse
- Valvular complications
- Bradycardia
- Anuria
- Albuminuria
- Nocturnal emissions
- Gonorrhoea
- Balanitis
- Enlarged prostate
- Urethritis

MODALITIES
- **Aggravation:** Sitting erect, after meals, music, motion, exertion, sexual excess, alcohol, smell of food, at night, cold air, cold weather
- **Amelioration:** When stomach is empty, in open cool air, rest, weeping, lying flat on the back

REMEDY RELATIONSHIP
- **Antidotes:** Camph., Chin.
- **Incompatible:** Chin.
- **Compare:** Olnd., Adon., Crat., Kalm., Spig., Liat., Digox., Conv.
- **Compatible:** Bell., Bry., Cham., Lay.c, Nux-v.

Digitalis purpurea

DIOSCOREA VILLOSA

INTRODUCTION

- **Common name:** Wild yam, Colic root
- **Family:** *Dioscoreaceae*
- **Source:** Vegetable kingdom
- **Part used:** Rhizome
- **Prover:** Cushing

SPHERE OF ACTION

- Gastrointestinal system
- Respiratory system
- Genitourinary system
- Nervous system

CONSTITUTION

- For persons of feeble digestive powers – old or young, who drink a lot of tea and have a lot of flatus as a consequence
- **Temperament:** Nervous, bilious
- **Thermal:** Chilly, ambithermal
- **Miasm:** Psora, Sycosis, Syphilis

MIND

- Memory poor, calls things by wrong names, uses wrong words, putting right for left or vice versa
- Loss of memory in spermatorrhoea
- Dreams of women, of amorous people all night
- Appears cheerful, jovial, but looks down when walking on the street
- Loss of memory cells
- Weak concentration
- Cross, nervous
- Depression after seminal emission
- Restlessness, better walking

KEYNOTE SYMPTOMS

- Pains, colic especially abdominal and pelvic – unbearable, sharp, cutting, twisting, griping, grinding; radiates to distant parts
- Pain moves upwards or downwards, in paroxysms; suddenly ceases in one part then starts in another
- Nervous shuddering from pain; labour-like pains
- **Colic, worse bending forward and lying, better standing erect**
- Dull pain in both temples as if squeezed in a vise, better pressure, but worse afterwards
- Sinking at the pit of the stomach
- Gastric disorders during pregnancy and menses
- Flatulent colic after meals, better belching; worse from fasting or eating in excess, hiccough
- **Gall stone colic; radiates to chest, back and arms**
- Haemorrhoids, look like a bunch of grapes, cherries. Morning diarrhoea
- Pain along the sternum extending into the arms
- **Severe dysmenorrhoea with spasmodic uterine colic; pains fly to distant parts**
- Relaxation and coldness of male genitalia, with strong smelling sweat. Emissions in sleep with weak knees

CLINICAL

- Neuralgia
- Hiccough
- Gastralgia
- Jaundice
- Abdominal colic
- Gall stone colic
- Haemorrhoids
- Angina pectoris
- Renal colic
- Renal stone
- Uterine colic
- Menstrual colic
- Sterility
- Spermatorrhoea
- Early emission
- Sciatica
- Paronychia
- Whitlow
- Felon

MODALITIES

- **Aggravation:** Evening and night, lying down, doubling up, eating, drinking tea
- **Amelioration:** Standing erect, motion in open air, pressure, stretching out, bending backwards, hard pressure

REMEDY RELATIONSHIP

- **Antidotes:** Cham., Camph.
- **Compare: Coloc. differs in modalities;** Nux-v., Cham., Bry., Podo., Stann., Sulph.

DIPHTHERINUM

INTRODUCTION
- **Common name:** Diphtheria nosode
- **Group:** Nosode
- **Part used:** Trituration of diphtheritic membrane
- **Source:** Diphtheretic microbe

SPHERE OF ACTION
- Mind
- Gastrointestinal system
- Respiratory system
- Throat

CONSTITUTION
- Suits scrofulous people prone to catarrhal affections of the throat and respiratory mucous membranes, prostrated with an exhausted vitality
- **Temperament:** Nervous, bilious
- **Thermal:** Chilly
- **Miasm:** Psora, Sycosis, Syphilis, Tubercular

MIND
- Unconsciousness, answers but stupor returns quickly after answering
- Talks in sleep with eyes open
- Desire to be held which ameliorates
- Nervousness anxiety
- Prostrated but restless without any pain
- Carphology

KEYNOTE SYMPTOMS
- Weak and restless; profound prostration with an exhausted vitality
- Glands swollen
- Malignancy, from the start
- Flushed with centre of cheeks purple
- **Moist tongue with red tip or a dark red spot at the back of the tip; red papillae**
- Fanning of alae nasi, with snoring
- Yellow, thick nasal discharge; epistaxis
- Marked tendency to take cold and bronchitis. Severe sore throat and inflammation of tonsils. Obstinate tonsillitis.
- Swallows without pain; horribly offensive breath
- **Thick grey membrane on left tonsil with foetor; painless diphtheria**
- A dynamic diphtheria when the patient from the first seems doomed and the most carefully selected remedies fail to relieve or permanently improve
- **Diphtheria with prostration, sopor or stupor, but easily aroused when spoken to**
- Prophylactic in diphtheria and post-diphtheric complications, like paralysis

CLINICAL
- Malignancy
- Glands swollen
- Snoring
- Stomatitis
- Dysentery
- Diarrhoea
- Epistaxis
- Ozaena
- Diphtheria
- Post-diphtheritic paralysis
- Laryngeal paralysis
- Tonsillitis
- Cough
- Toxic bronchitis

MODALITIES
- **Aggravation:** Movement, lying down
- **Amelioration:** Heat, in bed, taking sips of milk

REMEDY RELATIONSHIP
- **Compare:** Diphtox. in chronic bronchitis with rales; Cartier suggests it in the vago-paralytic forms of bronchitis in the aged or in toxic bronchitis after influenza

DOLICHOS PRURIENS

SPHERE OF ACTION
- Mouth
- Gastrointestinal system
- Throat
- Skin

INTRODUCTION
- **Common name:** Cowhage
- **Family:** *Leguminosae*
- **Source:** Vegetable kingdom
- **Part used:** Hair is carefully scraped from the epidermis of the pod and then a trituration or tincture of the whole pod is made
- **Prover:** Jeans

CONSTITUTION
- For old people with hepatic derangement and pruritus
- Adapted to psoric and allergic constitutions
- **Temperament:** Nervous, bilious
- **Thermal:** Chilly, ambithermal
- **Miasm:** Psora

MIND
- Despair or suicidal thoughts from unbearable itching at night
- Increased nervous sensibility

CLINICAL
- Abdominal colic
- Hepatomegaly
- Jaundice
- Hepatitis
- Constipation
- Haemorrhoids
- Pharyngitis
- Itching
- Senile pruritus
- Eczema
- Herpes zoster

KEYNOTE SYMPTOMS
- Right sided medicine with pronounced liver and skin symptoms
- General intense itching without eruptions; worse across shoulders, elbows, knees, hairy parts
- Itching, especially as a concomitant to affections of liver, or gall bladder, or to constipation
- **Upper gums extremely sensitive during dentition; gums seem to itch, wants them continually rubbed; worse at night, prevents sleep**
- Haemorrhoidal diathesis with burning sensation in rectum
- **Pain in the throat, below the right angle of jaw, as if a splinter was embedded vertically, worse swallowing**
- Pruritus during pregnancy or in old people
- Skin, yellow in spots
- Herpes zoster, when the itching of neuralgic pain persists
- Senile pruritus; itching excessive at night. Skin burns at night in bed or after scratching
- Cold water relieves itching but it burns the skin and causes trembling

MODALITIES
- **Aggravation:** At night, scratching, right side

REMEDY RELATIONSHIP
- **Compare:** Rhus-t., Bell., Hep., Nit-ac., Fago., Arg-n., Lyc., Cann-i.
- **Antidoted by:** Acon.
- Dolichos follows Rhus-t. in herpes

DROSERA ROTUNDIFOLIA

SPHERE OF ACTION

- Mind
- Gastrointestinal system
- Respiratory system

INTRODUCTION

- **Common name:** Sundew
- **Family:** *Droseraceae*
- **Source:** Vegetable kingdom
- **Part used:** Whole plant
- **Prover:** Hahnemann

CONSTITUTION

- For phthisical patients; young consumptives who suffer from spasmodic cough
- **Temperament:** Tubercular
- **Thermal:** Chilly
- **Miasm:** Tubercular

MIND

- Sadness when alone, anxiety in solitude. Wants company
- Peevish, a trifle puts him out of humour
- Inclination to drown himself; depressed
- Delusions of persecution. Imagines he was being deceived by spiteful, envious people
- Anxiety, worse at night, on waking, when alone. Restlessness. Anxiety as if his enemies would not leave him quiet.
- Very restless and uneasy

KEYNOTE SYMPTOMS

- Vertigo when walking in open air, with an inclination to fall
- Colicky pain in the abdomen after taking sour food
- **Sensation of a feather in the larynx**
- Constriction in the larynx; hoarseness, bloody or purulent expectoration. **Clergyman's store throat**
- Laryngeal phthisis post whooping cough
- Paroxysms of cough following each other very rapidly with bleeding from the nose and mouth, retching, gagging and vomiting
- **Prolonged, periodical fits of choking cough, compels him to hold sides of chest; as soon as head touches the pillow at night**
- Whooping cough; barking with hoarseness; worse, lying down, eating, drinking, talking, after midnight; nocturnal cough
- Convulsions due to violent cough
- Cough with profuse sweating
- Asthma, dyspnoea on talking

CLINICAL

- Vomiting
- Tubercular glands
- Coryza
- Aphonia
- Hoarseness
- Laryngitis
- Laryngeal phthisis
- Cough
- Whooping cough
- Bronchitis
- Emphysema
- Asthma
- Tuberculosis
- Cystitis
- Sciatica

MODALITIES

- **Aggravation:** After midnight, lying down, getting warm in bed, drinking, singing, laughing, talking after measles, during rest, weeping
- **Amelioration:** Open air, pressure, motion, remaining quiet

REMEDY RELATIONSHIP

- **Antidoted by:** Camph.
- **Compare:** Chel., Cor-r., Cupr., Cast., Arg-met., Meny., Bell., Hyos., Ip., Samb., Meph., Op., Coc-c., Caust., Sep., Kali-c., Flf.

Drosera rotundifolia

DUBOISINUM

INTRODUCTION
- **Common name:** Cork wood tree alkaloid
- **Family:** *Solanaceae*
- **Source:** Vegetable kingdom
- **Part used:** An alkaloid prepared from the extract of leaves of *Duboisia myopoides*

SPHERE OF ACTION
- Central nervous system
- Eyes
- Gastrointestinal system
- Respiratory system

CONSTITUTION
- Suits old people with an unsteady gait, vertigo and a pale face
- **Temperament:** Nervous, bilious
- **Thermal:** Chilly, ambithermal
- **Miasm:** Psora, Sycosis, Syphilis

MIND
- **Glances suspiciously under bedclothes and behind the back. Left to himself, upsets room in a few moments – towels, brushes, shoes are placed on the bed, boots on the dressing table; throughout, there is an air of fun and humour**
- On recovery, remembers nothing of what he had done; memory impaired
- Silly, non-sensical
- Delusion, that there is no life in him
- Irritability
- Absentminded

KEYNOTE SYMPTOMS
- **Sensation as if he was stepping on an empty space; unsteady gait, catches himself for fear of falling**
- Feeling of largeness in eyes, tongue
- Vertigo with pale face; impossible to stand with eyes closed, tendency to fall backwards
- **Red spots float in field of vision, moving with the eye**
- Conjunctivitis, red spot floats in the field of vision
- Dim vision; weakness of accomodation; pupils dilated
- Dryness of mucous membranes, especially of mouth, throat; checks perspiration
- Great difficulty in empty swallowing
- Pharyngitis with black, stringy mucous

CLINICAL
- Anaemia
- Locomotor ataxia
- Vertigo
- Headache
- Presbyopia
- Mydriasis
- Conjunctivitis
- Constipation
- Laryngitis
- Dryness of throat
- Pharyngitis
- Bronchitis
- Asthma

MODALITIES
- **Aggravation:** Heat, ascending stairs

REMEDY RELATIONSHIP
- **Antidotes:** Morph., Pilo.
- **Compare:** Bell., Stram., Hyos., Dulc., Atro.
- **Antidoted by:** Coffee, lemon juice

DULCAMARA

INTRODUCTION
- **Common name:** Bitter-sweet
- **Family:** *Solanaceae*
- **Source:** Vegetable kingdom
- **Part used:** Whole plant excluding the root. Plants growing with rootlets running into water are preferable
- **Prover:** Hahnemann

SPHERE OF ACTION
- Eyes
- Gastrointestinal system
- Respiratory system
- Serous membranes
- Mucous membranes
- Muscular system
- Urinary system
- Skin

CONSTITUTION
- For complaints of scrofulous, phlegmatic constitutions, who are exposed to a constant change of temperature or working in damp, cold basements
- **Temperament:** Nervous, bilious
- **Thermal:** Chilly
- **Miasm:** Psora, Sycosis, Syphilis

MIND
- Confusion, cannot concentrate his thoughts
- Impatient in the morning
- Depression
- Scolds without being angry
- Rejects things asked for
- Easily becomes delirious; with pain
- Restless, irritable
- Scolds or quarrels without being angry
- Speech difficult as patient cannot find the right word

KEYNOTE SYMPTOMS
- **Ailments resulting from damp weather, in hot days and cold nights towards the close of summer.** Results from sitting on cold, damp ground, living or working in damp, cold basements. Complaints of workers in an ice factory
- Every cold settles in the eyes, nose, throat, bladder, respiration, stools, neuralgias, joints, etc., all worse from cold and damp
- Persons who are prone to catarrhal, rheumatic and herpetic affections on account of exposure to cold, damp weather, sudden change in hot weather
- Paralysis of single parts, vocal cord, tongue, etc; paralysed part icy cold
- Anasarca after suppressed sweat, eruptions, or exposure to cold, or after rheumatism
- **Increased secretion from mucous membranes but suppression of sweat from cold**
- **Watery, slimy, green mucoid stool in summers,** when the weather suddenly changes to cold
- Nose stopped up every time there is a rain. Every cold settles in the eyes. **Hay fever with profuse, watery discharge**
- Cough – loose, rattling, after physical exertion
- Tonsillitis from every changes in weather. Constant hawking of tough saliva
- Nephritis from cold. Urine thick, mucoid with purulent sediment
- Stiffness, numbness, aching, soreness of muscles on every exposure to cold, especially of back. Rheumatism on exposure to wet weather
- **Skin rash, before menses. Ringworm of hair in children**
- Large, fleshy warts especially on face, back of hands and fingers
- Glands swollen and indurated; hypertrophy of glands, adenitis

CLINICAL
- Enlarged glands
- Convulsions
- Paralysis
- Headache
- Scald head
- Ringworm of scalp
- Tinea capitis
- Facial neuralgia
- Diarrhoea
- Rhinitis
- Middle ear catarrh
- Adenitis
- Hay fever
- Whooping cough
- Asthma
- Albuminuria
- Nephritis
- Rheumatism
- Eruptions
- Eczema
- Erythema
- Pemphigus
- Pruritus
- Urticaria
- Warts
- Herpes zoster

MODALITIES
- **Aggravation:** At night, from cold in general, damp, rainy weather, damp ground, from being chilled while hot, sudden changes of temperature
- **Amelioration:** From moving about, external warmth, lying on side

REMEDY RELATIONSHIP
- **Antidoted by:** Camph., Cupr.
- **Complementary:** Bar-c.
- **Incompatible:** Bell., Lach.
- **Compare:** Pimp. for respiratory mucous membrane sensitive to draughts, pain and coldness in the occiput and nape; Rhus-t., Cimic., Calc., Puls., Bry., Nat-s., Acon., Ars., Cham., Hell., Nit-ac., Staph., Sulph.

SPHERE OF ACTION

- Mind
- Gastrointestinal system
- Respiratory system
- Musculoskeletal system
- Female genital system
- Skin

MIND

- Becomes angry when corrected, doesn't wish to be contradicted
- Cannot exert mind, worse mental exertion. Mental prostration, brain fag
- Does not wish to think or study, aversion to thinking
- Confused, depressed

MODALITIES

- **Aggravation:** Mental or physical exertion, injury, surgery, cold air, evening
- **Amelioration:** Lying down, rest, pain better by bending double

INTRODUCTION

- **Common name:** Purple cone flower
- **Family:** *Compositae*
- **Source:** Vegetable kingdom
- **Part used:** Whole plant
- **Prover:** Dr J.C. Fahnestock and T.C. Duncan

ECHINACEA ANGUSTIFOLIA

KEYNOTE SYMPTOMS

- Septic conditions, blood poisoning and septic conditions. Corrects blood dyscrasias
- Snake bites or venomous infections. Boils, gangrene, ulcers, lymphangitis
- **Slowness in every action** – speech, replying, walking, etc.
- **Foetid and foul secretions** – catarrh, flatus, diarrhoea, leucorrhoea, lochia, etc.
- Weak, tired. Aching in muscles. Unable to sit up from weakness. Weakness is felt more in stomach, bowels, heart, knees, and is accompanied by vertigo.
- Tendency to malignancy, in acute and subacute cases
- Eases pain of cancer in last stages
- **White coating of tongue with red edges. Tongue swollen and dry, despite increased salivation. Corners of mouth and lips cracked. Gums recede and bleed easily**
- Nausea, with loss of appetite and chilliness. **Desires cold drinks.** Sleepiness after eating
- Tendency for ear infections and septic throat, foetid oezena
- Excoriating leucorrhoea; puerperal septicaemia

CONSTITUTION

- Suits dark complexioned people suffering from blood dyscrasias
- Adapted to weak, broken down constitutions
- **Temperament:** Nervous, bilious
- **Thermal:** Chilly
- **Miasm:** Psora, Sycosis, Syphilis

CLINICAL

- Septic conditions
- Pustules
- Blood disorders
- Blood poisoning
- Malignancy
- Lymphangitis
- Goitre
- Cerebrospinal meningitis
- Diarrhoea
- Appendicitis
- Peritonitis
- Piles
- Puerperal infection
- Gonorrhoea
- Typhoid
- Malarial fever
- Ulcers
- Snake bites
- Sepsis
- Boils
- Gangrene
- Insect bites
- Erysipelas

REMEDY RELATIONSHIP

- **Compare:** Cench., Both., Ars., Lach., Bapt., Rhus-t., Cist., Hep., Calen.

ELATERIUM

SPHERE OF ACTION
- Mind
- Eyes
- Gastrointestinal system
- Musculoskeletal system
- Urinary system
- Skin

INTRODUCTION
- **Common name:** Squirting cucumber
- **Family:** *Cucurbitaceae*
- **Source:** Vegetable kingdom
- **Part used:** Sediment of the juice of the green mature fruit
- **Prover:** Mathews and Cooper

CONSTITUTION
- Suits old people with chilliness, yawning and stretching
- For the effects of damp weather or standing on damp ground
- **Temperament:** Nervous, bilious
- **Thermal:** Chilly
- **Miasm:** Psora, Sycosis, Syphilis

MIND
- Fear of disaster
- Starting during sleep
- Mania and madness during fever with suppressed chill
- Desire to stretch
- Irresistible desire to wander away from home at night
- Depression

KEYNOTE SYMPTOMS
- Urticaria and mental symptoms appearing after suppressed malaria
- Chilliness and prostration
- **Sensation of a splinter in the left eye**
- Scurvy, where a gushing diarrhoea is a prominent symptom
- Violent vomiting and purging of copious watery evacuations
- Stools – copious, watery, frothy, forceful and explosive
- **Squirting diarrhoea; frothy, olive green; preceded by violent cutting pains in the abdomen; chilliness and prostration**
- Sensation as if posterior nares and upper part of oesophagus were enlarged. Vomiting of greenish, bilious matter, forcibly ejected
- Pains in extremities darting to fingers and toes. Sciatica with pain darting to the toes
- **Pain extending from shoulders to ends of fingers**
- Chill preceded by attacks of yawning and stretching, continuing during chill
- Opening of abscesses, boils
- **Dropsical, orange coloured skin**

CLINICAL
- Beriberi
- Scurvy
- Dropsy
- Vomiting
- Jaundice of newborns
- Diarrhoea
- Cholera
- Bladder affections
- Arthritic nodules
- Bilious fever
- Malaria
- Urticaria
- Burns
- Yawning

MODALITIES
- **Aggravation:** From exposure to damp weather, standing on damp ground

REMEDY RELATIONSHIP
- **Compare:** Bry., Crot-t., Gamb., Coloc., Verat.

ELECTRICITAS

INTRODUCTION
- **Common name:** Electricity
- **Source:** Imponderabilia
- **Prover:** Caspri and his co-workers had first published the symptoms caused by electricity natural (thunderstorm) and artificial static electricity and electric current

SPHERE OF ACTION
- Mind
- Eyes
- Gastrointestinal system
- Respiratory system
- Musculoskeletal system
- Urinary system

CONSTITUTION
- Suits people who are powerfully affected by the approach of a thunderstorm
- **Temperament:** Nervous, bilious
- **Thermal:** Chilly, ambithermal
- **Miasm:** Psora, Sycosis, Syphilis

MIND
- **Dreads the approach of thunderstorm.** Anxiety during a storm
- Severe nervous anxiety, nervous tremors. Sighs and screams from nervous fear
- Timid, sighing
- Fearful, weeping in paroxysms
- Restlessness, anxiety, anguish
- Violent agitation; the patient cries aloud
- Confused, disquietening dreams
- General depression and weariness
- Loss of memory

KEYNOTE SYMPTOMS
- General relaxation of nerves and muscles
- Glaucoma with blindness
- **Tongue is sensitive to touch, especially the tip; swelling of the tongue**
- **Increased secretion of saliva, foam in the mouth**
- Vomiting with sore throat. Difficult deglutition
- Cutting pain in abdomen, at approach of a storm; with diarrhoea
- Asthma with constriction or oppression of the chest, palpitation of heart
- Palpitation of the heart, with fever, headache or restlessness; especially at the approach of a storm
- Pulse – rapid and intermittent
- Burning and incontinence of urine; sensation as if bladder would burst
- Discharge of blood and mucous with urine, frequent micturition, complaints aggravated before and during a thunderstorm
- **Leucorrhoea first thin and then thick. Black, thick menstrual blood; profuse menses**
- Pain in nape of neck, cervical spondylosis
- Stiffness and sensation of heaviness of limbs; swelling of parts

CLINICAL
- Delirium
- Paralysis
- Hemiplegia
- Parkinsonism
- Cataract
- Glaucoma
- Blindness
- Gastritis
- Inability to articulate
- Loss of speech
- Asthma
- Haematuria
- Arthritis
- Sciatica
- Cervical spondylosis
- Ecchymosis

MODALITIES
- **Aggravation:** Approach of thunderstorm
- **Amelioration:** Fine, clear weather

REMEDY RELATIONSHIP
- **Compare:** Phos., Rhod.
- **Antidoted by:** Morph-act.
- **Antidotes:** Merc.

EQUISETUM HYMALE

SPHERE OF ACTION
- Mind
- Gastrointestinal system
- Urinary system
- Skin

INTRODUCTION
- **Common name:** Scouring rush, Horsetail
- **Family:** *Equisetaceae*
- **Source:** Vegetable kingdom
- **Part used:** Aerial part of the rush

CONSTITUTION
- Suits people with tendency for bladder and kidney irritation
- **Temperament:** Nervous, bilious
- **Thermal:** Chilly, ambithermal
- **Miasm:** Sycosis

MIND
- Dreams of people, crowds, many things
- Disposed to frown
- Delusion that he is falling
- Irritability marked
- Easily fatigued

KEYNOTE SYMPTOMS
- Incontinence or dribbling of urine in old women, with involuntary stools
- Severe dull pain and feeling of fullness in bladder, not better by urination – cystitis
- **Frequent, intolerable urging to urinate with severe burning pain at the close of urination;** dysuria
- More urging when bladder is nearly empty, and less urging and less dysuria when there is more urine
- Constant desire to urinate, passes large quantities of clear, light coloured urine without relief. Much mucous in urine; cloudy urine
- **Nocturnal enuresis, especially during first sleep,** without cause in children, habitual enuresis
- **Incontinence, in children with dreams of crowds or nightmares**
- Retention and dysuria during pregnancy and after delivery

CLINICAL
- Dropsy
- Diarrhoea
- Dysentery
- Constipation
- Pleuritic effusion
- Weakness of bladder
- Cystitis
- Enuresis
- Incontinence
- Polyuria
- Dysuria
- Retention of urine
- Calculus
- Albuminuria
- Diabetes
- Eczema
- Nightmares

MODALITIES
- **Aggravation:** Right side, movement, pressure, touch, sitting down, close of urination
- **Amelioration:** Better, in the afternoon, from lying down, continuous motion

REMEDY RELATIONSHIP
- **Compare:** Hydrang., Ferr-p., Apis, Canth., Lina., Chim. Equis-h., Sars., Berb., Cann-i., Puls.

Equisetum hymale

ERIGERON CANADENSE

SPHERE OF ACTION
- Head
- Gastrointestinal system
- Blood vessels
- Urinary system
- Female genital system

INTRODUCTION
- **Common name:** Fleabane
- **Family:** *Compositae*
- **Source:** Vegetable kingdom
- **Part used:** Whole fresh plant when in bloom
- **Prover:** Burt

CONSTITUTION
- Suits pregnant women with weak uterus and haemorrhagic diathesis
- **Temperament:** Nervous, bilious
- **Thermal:** Chilly
- **Miasm:** Psora, Sycosis, Syphilis

MIND
- Severe despondency
- Wearisome, with an aversion to mental work
- Anxiety
- Restlessness
- Weeping while urinating
- Very tired, especially in the morning with depression

KEYNOTE SYMPTOMS
- Haemorrhages with vesico-rectal tenesmus
- Haemorrhages – profuse, bright red, gushing, brought on by least motion
- Congestions, smart and burn
- **Sensation as if something is lodged in the upper part of the oesophagus**
- Severe pain in umbilical region, with feeling as if anus is torn
- Bleeding haemorrhoids; with hard lumpy stools
- Dysentery with soreness and burning in the bladder
- Urination painful or suppressed. **Sharp, stinging pain in left kidney region**
- Pain in left ovary and hip
- Pregnant women with a weak uterus; have a bloody discharge on the slightest exertion
- **Bloody lochia after least exertion; abortion due to exertion**
- Profuse leucorrhoea with urinary irritability
- Metrorrhagia with vesico-rectal tenesmus; after abortion; with uterine prolapse
- **Nosebleed instead of menses**
- Chronic gonorrhoea with soreness and burning during micturition; gleet; continuous dribbling

CLINICAL
- Haemorrhages
- Epistaxis
- Tympanitis
- Dysentery
- Constipation
- Haemorrhoids
- Urinary tract infection
- Cystitis
- Gonorrhoea
- Sterility
- Weak uterus
- Ovaritis
- Leucorrhoea
- Menorrhagia
- Metrorrhagia
- Placenta previa
- Lochia
- Wounds
- Bruises

MODALITIES
- **Aggravation:** Left side, exertion, rainy weather, every movement aggravates the flow or lochia
- **Amelioration:** Rest

REMEDY RELATIONSHIP
- **Similar:** Ter.
- **Compare:** Phos., Ham., Ip., Cop., Canth., Arn., Sabin., Ter.

EUCALYPTUS GLOBULUS

SPHERE OF ACTION

- Gastrointestinal system
- Respiratory system
- Musculoskeletal system
- Urinary system
- Female genital system

INTRODUCTION

- **Common name:** Blue gum tree
- **Family:** *Myrtaceae*
- **Source:** Vegetable kingdom
- **Part used:** Leaves
- **Prover:** Roder

CONSTITUTION

- For affections of mucous membranes, catarrhal processes, malasi and intestinal disturbances
- **Temperament:** Nervous, bilious
- **Thermal:** Chilly
- **Miasm:** Psora, Sycosis, Syphilis

MIND

- Mental exhilaration
- Desire to exercise, to move about
- Industrious; mania for work
- Delusions, imagines she is too lazy to move

KEYNOTE SYMPTOMS

- It is a strong antiseptic and an efficient diaphoretic
- Symptoms of exhaustion with toxaemia and haemorrhage; no desire for mental work or any motion
- Haemorrhages – local and internal
- Affects mucous membranes producing profuse, catarrhal discharges which are acrid and foul
- **Effects of old malarias; suits fevers of a relapsing or intermittent character**
- Slow and difficult digestion and much foetid gas; atonic dyspepsia
- Gastrointestinal irritation. **Pain in stomach and upper intestines, several hours after eating; gastric and intestinal catarrh**
- Acute diarrhoea; stool thin, watery, preceded by sharp pains
- Dysentery with rectal heat, tenesmus and haemorrhage
- Stuffed up sensation in nose; thin, watery coryza; nose doesn't stop running, tightness across the bridge
- Bronchial asthma and bronchitis, especially of aged; profuse expectoration of offensive muco-pus
- Acute nephritis; suppurative inflammation of kidneys. Catarrh of bladder
- Aching stiffness is arms and legs; also weariness, as from taking cold. Prickling sensation in limbs followed by aching
- Nodular swelling of joints, especially metacarpal and metatarsal joints

CLINICAL

- Haemorrhages
- Malignant diseases
- Haematemesis
- Spleen affections
- Cancer of stomach
- Dysentery
- Sinusitis
- Tinnitus
- Influenza
- Bronchitis
- Bronchorrhoea
- Asthma
- Emphysema
- Aneurysm
- Aortitis
- Acute nephritis
- Pyelonephritis
- Hydronephrosis
- Gonorrhoea
- Rheumatism
- Malaria
- Typhoid
- Herpetic eruptions

MODALITIES

- **Aggravation:** At night, periodically

REMEDY RELATIONSHIP

- **Compare:** Ol-eucal., Eucol., Eucal-t., Anac., Hydr., Kali-s.
- Eucal. neutralizes ill-effects of Stry., Ango., Eucal-r.

Eucalyptus globulus

EUGENIA JAMBOS

INTRODUCTION
- **Common name:** Rose apple
- **Family:** *Myrtaceae*
- **Source:** Vegetable kingdom
- **Part used:** Tincture of fresh seeds

SPHERE OF ACTION
- Mind
- Eyes
- Gastrointestinal system
- Heart
- Skin

CONSTITUTION
- For bad effects of alcoholism
- **Temperament:** Nervous, bilious
- **Thermal:** Chilly
- **Miasm:** Psora, Sycosis, Syphilis

MIND
- Lazy and loquacious
- Remarkably changed, especially mentally after urination; quite talkative but indolent; things appear brighter but after 15 minutes everything is gloomy again
- Sadness, better after urination
- Sense of intoxication, better after urination
- Delusion; all things seem beautiful after micturition
- Prefers to do nothing but smoke all day
- Everything seems wrong
- Forgetfulness of business, creeps into a corner and must sleep, but cannot sleep, still, stays lying down
- Talkative but indolent
- Restlessness

KEYNOTE SYMPTOMS
- State like alcoholism – everything appears beautiful and larger; but excitement soon changes to depression
- Vertigo with whirling in head while sitting
- Darkness before eyes and double vision. On looking intently, double vision disappears
- **Hot lachrymation and sensation as if fire were passing out of eyes. Burning in eyes, as if from pepper, worse closing the eyes, preventing sleep at night**
- Abundant accumulation of frothy and viscid saliva in the mouth especially before a meal and when talking
- **Great thirst from dryness low down in the throat at night, especially during headache, after coition**
- **Great desire for tobacco. Nausea, better by smoking**
- Nocturnal cramps in soles of feet
- Skin cracks around toes; fissures between toes
- Acne – simple and indurated on the face; area around pimples painful

CLINICAL
- Vertigo
- Cramps
- Diplopia
- Hot lachrymation
- Nausea
- Haemorrhoids
- Cramps in soles
- Acne
- Pimples
- Comedones
- Paronychia
- Onychia
- Panaritium
- Tinea pedis
- Fissures

MODALITIES
- **Aggravation:** Evening, night
- **Amelioration:** After urination, especially mentally, nausea is better by smoking

REMEDY RELATIONSHIP
- **Compare:** Myrt-ch., Ant.-t., Berb-a., Puls.
- **Antidoted by:** Coffee, smoking, tobacco

EUPATORIUM PERFOLIATUM

INTRODUCTION

- **Common name:** Agueweed, Boneset, Thoroughwort
- **Family:** *Compositae*
- **Source:** Vegetable kingdom
- **Part used:** Flowering tops

SPHERE OF ACTION

- Gastrointestinal system
- Respiratory system
- Spinal cord
- Musculoskeletal system
- Skin

CONSTITUTION

- Suits old people with a worn out constitution due to excessive abuse of alcohol
- **Temperament:** Nervous, bilious
- **Thermal:** Chilly
- **Miasm:** Psora, Sycosis, Syphilis

MIND

- Moaning and groaning with chill and restlessness; nervousness with heat
- Fear of losing reason
- **Delusion that she will go insane or out of her mind, especially at night**
- Homesickness; nostalgia, desires to go home
- Weakness
- Irritability
- Headache ameliorated by conversation
- Sluggishness

KEYNOTE SYMPTOMS

- Marked periodicity
- Bruised feeling, as if broken all over the body. Bone pains
- Vertigo with sensation as if falling to the left
- Soreness in eyeballs
- **Cracks in the corner of mouth; tongue yellow coated**
- **Vomiting of bile; vomiting preceded by thirst**
- Constipation with soreness over liver region
- Stools frequent, green, watery with cramps
- Coryza with sneezing, hoarseness and cough; with aching in every bone and muscle
- Cough with extreme soreness down the trachea
- Violent aching in bones of extremities with soreness of flesh
- Aching pain in the back, arms and wrist
- Chill between 7 to 9 am; insatiable thirst before and during chill and fever
- Cachexia, from frequent or prolonged attacks of bilious or intermittent fever
- Intermittent fever preceded by thirst, with great soreness and aching in the bones
- **Perspiration relieves all symptoms except headache**

CLINICAL

- Cachexia
- Cramps
- Vertigo
- Stomatitis
- Hiccough
- Gastro-hepatic ulcer
- Hepatitis
- Constipation
- Coryza
- Influenza
- Cough
- Bone pains
- Arthritis
- Rheumatism
- Gout
- Dengue
- Malaria
- Bilious fever

MODALITIES

- **Aggravation:** Cold air, periodically, 7 am – 9 am, motion, coughing
- **Amelioration:** Conversation, getting on hands and knee position, sweating, vomiting bile

REMEDY RELATIONSHIP

- **Compare:** Bry., Sep., Chel., Nat-m, Nyct.

EUPHRASIA OFFICINALIS

INTRODUCTION
- **Common name:** Eyebright
- **Family:** *Scrophulariaceae*
- **Source:** Vegetable kingdom
- **Part used:** Whole plant

SPHERE OF ACTION
- Eyes
- Gastrointestinal system
- Respiratory system
- Genitourinary system
- Skin

MIND
- Sadness, melancholy
- Fear of being alone
- Weak memory
- Disinclined to talk; aversion to answering
- Indolent
- Hypochondriacal mood

MODALITIES
- **Aggravation:** In the evening, indoors, warmth, winds, from light, sunlight, after sleep
- **Amelioration:** From coffee, in the dark, winking, open air, wiping the eyes

KEYNOTE SYMPTOMS
- Ill-effects of falls, mechanical and external injuries
- Catarrhal conjunctivitis with violent inflammation; with measles; instead of menses. Sensation of sand in the eyes
- **Abundant, hot, acrid, smarting lachrymation with bland coryza.** Eyes water all the time
- **Nausea and bitter taste after smoking**
- Prolapse of anus; pressure down the anus; worse while sitting; constipation
- Fluent, profuse, bland coryza with violent cough. Hay fever and allergies
- Cough, with hawking up of offensive, profuse mucous
- Whooping cough, worse during daytime with profuse lachrymation
- Nocturnal irritability of bladder with dribbling of urine
- Spasmodic retraction of genitals
- Amenorrhoea with ophthalmic symptoms
- **Menses lasting only an hour or day**
- Eruptive fevers like measles
- Suitable in first stage of measles where eye symptoms are marked. Measles with watery eyes and fluent coryza
- Yawning when waking in open air; sleepy during the day

CONSTITUTION
- Suits children with catarrhal affections of mucous membranes, especially that of eyes and nose
- **Temperament:** Nervous, bilious
- **Thermal:** Chilly
- **Miasm:** Psora, Sycosis, Syphilis

CLINICAL
- Allergy
- Conjunctivitis
- Iritis
- Chemosis
- Blepharitis
- Cataract
- Photophobia
- Amblyopia
- Injury to the eye
- Dysentery
- Constipation
- Anal prolapse
- Rhinitis
- Hay fever
- Whooping cough
- Pertussis
- Bronchitis
- Prostatitis
- Measles
- Injuries

REMEDY RELATIONSHIP
- **Antidoted by:** Camph., Puls.
- **Compare:** Hydro. catarrhal inflammation of the eyes, hot lachrymation with itching, swollen lids, dull headache, also for effects of Poison oak; All-c., Ars., Gels., Kali-i., Sabad., Apis., Arg-n., Puls., Acon., Merc., Hep., Sil.
- **Compatible:** Acon., Con., Calc., Nux-v., Phos., Puls., Rhus-t., Sil., Sulph.

FAGOPYRUM ESCULENTUM

INTRODUCTION

- **Common name:** Buck wheat
- **Family:** *Polygonaceae*
- **Source:** Vegetable kingdom
- **Part used:** Whole plant
- **Prover:** Hitchcock

SPHERE OF ACTION

- Gastrointestinal system
- Respiratory system
- Genitourinary system
- Skin

MIND

- Depressed
- Cross
- Irritable
- Inability to fix attention
- Excessively happy
- Inability to study or remember
- Fearfulness
- Restless when trying to study

MODALITIES

- **Aggravation:** In the afternoon, from sunlight, scratching, motion, ascending, stooping, walking
- **Amelioration:** Cold water, coffee, cold applications, pressure

KEYNOTE SYMPTOMS

- Marked general pruritus, with or without eruptions; pruritus senilis. Itching in eyes, vulva, arms, legs, knees, elbows, hairy parts, especially deep in the hands; better by bathing in cold water
- Visible pulsation of arteries, especially in carotids
- Pulse – irregular, intermittent, rapid. Throbbing in arteries after retiring
- Offensiveness of all discharges
- **Pains in streaks**
- Headache. Pain deep in head with upward pressure, better bending backward
- Stiffness, bruised sensation in the muscles as if neck could not support head
- Bad taste in the mouth with persistent nausea in the morning
- **Eructations scalding, hot, acrid, watery, better by coffee**
- Post-nasal catarrh with dry crusts and itching in posterior nares
- Soreness and feeling of excoriation deep down the pharynx.
- Itching, smarting, swelling and soreness of ears
- Fluent coryza with sneezing
- **Severe pruritus vulvae with yellow leucorrhoea, which leaves yellow stains**

CONSTITUTION

- Suits weak constitutions presenting with skin and gastrointestinal symptoms
- **Temperament:** Nervous, bilious
- **Thermal:** Chilly
- **Miasm:** Psora, Sycosis, Syphilis

CLINICAL

- Cerebral hyperaemia
- Constipation
- Diarrhoea
- Tonsillitis
- Angina pectoris
- Palpitation
- Ovaritis
- Leucorrhoea
- Pruritus vulvae
- Arthritis
- Rheumatism
- Cervical spondylosis
- Pruritus
- Senile pruritus
- Dermatitis– vesicular, pustular and phlegmonous
- Eczema
- Boils
- Pustules
- Ulcers

REMEDY RELATIONSHIP

- **Compare:** Dol., Bov., Urt-u., Sulph., Psor., Rhus-t., Lyc., Puls., Polyg., Seneg.

SPHERE OF ACTION

- Blood
- Glands
- Gastrointestinal system
- Urinary system
- Female genital system
- Skin

INTRODUCTION

- **Common name:** Ferrum iodide
- **Group:** Salt
- **Source:** Mineral kingdom
- **Formula:** FeI_2
- **Prover:** Muller

CONSTITUTION

- Suits pale, anaemic, chlorotic young girls whose body is emaciated, face is alternately pale and red and flushes after drinking wine; scrofulous affections
- **Temperament:** Nervous, sanguine, scrofulous
- **Thermal:** Chilly
- **Miasm:** Tubercular, Sycosis, Syphilis

MIND

- Irritability when movement is restricted
- Sensation as if lying in a cramped position
- Vivid dreams of bed being small, of things seen small
- Many dreams long past events
- Dreams of thieves

FERRUM IODATUM

CLINICAL

- Anaemia
- Tumours
- Glandular enlargements
- Exophthalmic goitre
- Coryza
- Hoarseness
- Haemoptysis
- Bronchorrhoea
- Albuminuria
- Acute nephritis
- Incontinence of urine
- Uterine displacements
- Retroversion of uterus
- Uterine prolapse
- Leucorrhoea
- Uterine haemorrhage
- Impetigo
- Boils

KEYNOTE SYMPTOMS

- Scrofulous affections, glandular enlargements and tumours
- Anaemia, emaciation and marked debility
- Physical restlessness, physical exertion aggravates
- Lancinating, sharp and cutting pains in eyes, ears, root of nose to occiput
- Fullness, even after a little food; stuffed feeling, feels she can not lean forward
- **Food seems to push up into the throat, as if it had not been swallowed**
- Sensation as if anus was compressed; as if worms in anus; or as if something twisted around the anus
- Crawling sensation in urethra and rectum
- **Urine dark, deposits white sediments, smells sweet**
- Feeling as if something pressing upwards in vagina on sitting
- Uterine displacements – prolapse or retroversion
- Exophthalmic goitre following suppression of menses
- Impetigo of cheeks; tendency to crops of boils. Skin eruptions are short lasting

MODALITIES

- **Aggravation:** Touch, warmth, motion, at night and in the morning
- **Amelioration:** Open air

REMEDY RELATIONSHIP

- **Compare:** Alum. in anaemia, leucorrhoea and prolapse; Alumn. in prolapsed uterus; Helon., Hydr., Graph., Iod., Kali-bi., Thyr., Ferr-br., Ferr-a.

FERRUM METALLICUM

INTRODUCTION
- **Common name:** Iron
- **Group:** Metal
- **Source:** Mineral kingdom
- **Formula:** Fe
- **Prover:** Hahnemann

SPHERE OF ACTION
- Mind
- Blood
- Gastrointestinal system
- Respiratory system
- Heart
- Musculoskeletal system
- Urinary system
- Female genital system

CONSTITUTION
- For anaemia and chlorotic young persons with flushed cheeks but pale lips
- Suits delicate girls who are constipated with low spirits, weakness, pallor of skin.
- Suits red faced old men
- **Temperament:** Sanguine
- **Thermal:** Chilly
- **Miasm:** Psora

MIND
- **Slightest noise is unbearable, especially rustling of paper**
- Confusion, brainfag; cannot collect thoughts
- Anxiety from slightest cause; regarding family
- Desire for solitude; conversation aggravates; marked indifference
- Irritability, peevishness, quarrelsomeness
- Aggressive and domineering
- Changeable mood. Restlessness driving him out of bed but walks about slowly
- Anxiety as after committing a crime
- Despondent after menses
- Forceful, determined and strong preoccupation with business matters
- Anger from contradiction
- Occupation relieves

KEYNOTE SYMPTOMS
- General weakness, emaciation; weakness just from talking, must lie down; with anaemia
- Excited, irregular surgings and wandering orgasms. Pulsations, false erethism or plethora
- It relaxes the blood vessels causing haemorrhages, which are bright red and easily coagulable or with small clots, especially in rapidly growing youth; or the veins dilate, during neuralgia, menses or fever. Pulse small, weak
- **Red parts become white, bloodless. Pallor**
- Extremely pale skin; flushes easily on least pain, exertion or emotion
- Dropsy, especially of feet with shooting pains; after loss of vital fluids
- **Vertigo on seeing flowing water**
- Eructation of food; spits out food by the mouthful
- **Intolerance of egg.** Vomiting after midnight; while eating, leaves table suddenly and with one effort, vomits everything eaten; can sit down and eat again
- Painless, undigested stools, at night or while eating or drinking; diarrhoea during pregnancy
- Stool hard, followed by backache; constipation from iron pills
- Cough only during the daytime; dry, tickling; from tobacco. Chest oppressed with difficult breathing.
- Least movement increases menstrual flow; suppressed menses with extreme nervousness
- Tendency to miscarriages. Very dry vagina
- Softening of bones; cracking in joints
- Nocturnal pain in limbs with restlessness; feels best when walking about slowly

CLINICAL
- Chronic fatigue syndrome
- Haemorrhages
- Blood disorders
- Anaemia
- Dropsy
- Obesity
- Vertigo
- Migraine
- Nausea
- Vomiting
- Flatulent dyspepsia
- Gastritis
- Diarrhoea
- Constipation
- Photophobia
- Epistaxis
- Hoarseness
- Haemoptysis
- Palpitation
- Arrhythmia
- Involuntary urination
- Nephritis
- Albuminuria
- Diabetes
- Menorrhagia
- Arthritis
- Sciatica
- Rheumatism
- Bursitis

MODALITIES
- **Aggravation:** At night, midnight, at rest, especially while sitting still, loss of vital fluids, emotions, exertion, during menses conversations
- **Amelioration:** Walking slowly, in summer, solitude, gentle motion

REMEDY RELATIONSHIP
- **Complementary:** Alum., Chin., Ham
- Chin., the vegetable analogue follows well in nearly all diseases, acute or chronic
- Should never be given in syphilis; always aggravates the condition
- **Antidotes:** Ars., Hep.
- **Compare:** Rumx., Graph., Mang., Cupra, all ferrums

FERRUM PHOSPHORICUM

INTRODUCTION

- **Common name:** Phosphate of iron, Ferroso-ferric phosphate
- **Group:** Salt
- **Source:** Mineral kingdom
- **Formula:** $Fe_3(PO_4)_2 \cdot 8H_2O$
- **Prover:** Schussler

SPHERE OF ACTION

- Eyes
- Ears
- Gastrointestinal system
- Respiratory system
- Musculoskeletal system
- Urinary system
- Female genital system
- Skin

MIND

- **Fear of going into a crowd**
- Anger, becomes violent. Apathy
- Aversion to company
- **Guilty mind**
- Changeable
- Confusion
- Hilarious, talkative, excited
- Anticipation of failure
- Indifference to pleasurable things
- Anxious dreams
- Likes to keep quiet

MODALITIES

- **Aggravation:** At night, 4 to 6 am, touch, jar, motion, right side, noise
- **Amelioration:** Cold applications, lying down, rest, bleeding, gentle motion

KEYNOTE SYMPTOMS

- Generally **right sided complaints**
- For first stage of all inflammatory conditions. Non-specific inflammation at the onset of inflammation, before exudation sets in.
- Haemorrhagic diathesis; blood is bright red and easily coagulable. Passive congestion and haemorrhage due to hyperaemia
- Anaemia, false plethora and easy flushing
- Great prostration, can hardly move about. Mental and physical lassitudes.
- **Pains wandering; appear and disappear suddenly, migrating from below upwards. Burning rawness**
- Headache – stinging, pressing, throbbing; worse motion of head
- **Discharges are blood streaked or like washing of meat**
- Vomiting of undigested food; blood. Sour eructations
- Susceptibility to chest complaints. Paroxysmal cough, especially when asleep
- Palpitation; pulse rapid
- First stage of dysentery with a lot of blood
- First stage of otitis media, prevents suppuration
- Expectoration of pure blood, especially in pneumonia; bronchitis in children
- Menses with bearing down sensation; dysmenorrhoea with frequent urging to micturition
- High fever due to exposure to cold air or cold drinks, over exertion
- Congestion with cold extremities. Palms hot. Hands swollen and painful.
- Skin – capillary congestion with burning of skin

CONSTITUTION

- For pale, anaemic subjects with violent local congestion, with tendency to haemorrhages
- For those who are tall, irritable, graceful with delicate transparent skin
- **Temperament:** Sanguine, leuco-phlegmatic, nervous, oxygenoid
- **Thermal:** Chilly
- **Miasm:** Psora, Sycosis, Syphilis

CLINICAL

- Emaciation
- Debility
- Haemorrhages
- Anaemia
- Conjunctivitis
- Photophobia
- Ophthalmia
- Styes
- Headache
- Vertigo
- Facial neuralgia
- Ranula
- Gastritis
- Dysentery
- Haemorrhoids
- Tinnitus
- Otitis media
- Epistaxis
- Influenza
- Rhinitis
- Sinusitis
- Laryngitis
- Pharyngitis
- Tonsillitis
- Hoarseness
- Diphtheria
- Asthma
- Pneumonia
- Pleurisy
- Polyuria
- Incontinence
- Dysmenorrhea
- Vaginismus
- Bursitis
- Articular rheumatism
- Fevers
- Insomnia
- Ulcers

REMEDY RELATIONSHIP

- **Compare:** Acon., Chin., Ars., Graph., Petr.; Ferr-py. in congestion of brain and headache following great loss of blood, tarsal cysts; Gels., Chin., Caust., Puls., Kali-m., Ant-t.

FERRUM PICRICUM

INTRODUCTION
- **Common name:** Picrate of iron, Iron picrate
- **Group:** Salt
- **Source:** Mineral kingdom
- **Prover:** Cooper

SPHERE OF ACTION
- Ears
- Gastrointestinal system
- Respiratory system
- Urinary system
- Male genital system
- Skin

CONSTITUTION
- Suits people with dark hair and eyes, bilious looking, plethoric patients with a sensitive liver
- **Temperament:** Nervous, bilious
- **Thermal:** Chilly
- **Miasm:** Sycosis

MIND
- Mentally prostrated
- Irritability, worse contradiction
- Sadness, anxiety
- Oversensitiveness
- Restless sleep with unpleasant dreams

MODALITIES
- **Aggravation:** Fatigue

KEYNOTE SYMPTOMS
- Failure of an organ to function under exertion, for example, voice fails after public speaking
- Liver and bilious disorders. Liver is weak and sensitive
- Almost specific remedy for epistaxis
- Deafness before menses. Deafness in young people cutting wisdom teeth
- **Humming in the ears as from telegraph wires**
- **Smarting pain in neck of bladder and penis; meatus dry**
- Senile hypertrophy of prostate with frequent micturition at night and a full feeling and pressure in the bladder
- **Dirty appearance about the joint due to deposition of bile pigments**
- Corns with yellowish discolouration
- Sensation as if a wart is growing on the thumb. For old, pedunculated warts accompanying chronic deafness

CLINICAL
- Epithelial overgrowths
- Pseudo-leukaemia
- Dental neuralgia
- Indigestion
- Jaundice
- Liver disorders
- Constipation
- Chronic deafness
- Vascular deafness
- Tinnitus
- Epistaxis
- Urethritis
- Retention of urine
- Senile hypertrophy of prostate
- Locomotor ataxia
- Gout
- Warts
- Corns

REMEDY RELATIONSHIP
- **Compare:** Pic-ac., Nit-ac., Thuj., Am-pic., Calc-pic., Sulph., all ferrums

Ferrum picricum

FICUS RELIGIOSA

SPHERE OF ACTION
- Eyes
- Gastrointestinal system
- Respiratory system
- Circulatory system
- Urinary system
- Female genital system

INTRODUCTION
- **Common name:** Ashwathva, Pipal
- **Family:** *Moraceae*
- **Source:** Plant kingdom
- **Part used:** Tender leaves
- **Prover:** Dr S.C. Ghose

CONSTITUTION
- Suits very weak and restless people
- In haemorrhagic diathesis
- **Temperament:** Nervous, bilious
- **Thermal:** Chilly, ambithermal
- **Miasm:** Psora, Sycosis, Syphilis

MIND
- Sad, melancholic
- Quiet and disinclined to move
- Restlessness
- Anxiety

CLINICAL
- Prostration
- Haemorrhages
- Vertigo
- Headache
- Dim vision
- Nausea
- Vomiting
- Haematemesis
- Diarrhoea
- Dysentery
- Constipation
- Epistaxis
- Haemoptysis
- Asthma
- Breathlessness
- Haematuria
- Menorrhagia
- Metrorrhagia
- Typhoid

KEYNOTE SYMPTOMS
- **Active haemorrhages** – haematemesis, menorrhagia, haemoptysis, nose bleed, etc. **Blood is bright red, profuse and from every orifice of the body**
- Generalized weakness and restlessness
- Headache, nausea and vertigo
- Headache with haemorrhages, and burning at the vertex
- Vision diminished; dim sight
- Nausea, pain and sick feeling in stomach
- Vomiting of bright red blood
- Dysentery with menorrhagia; dysentery of bright red blood
- Difficult breathing. Inclination to cough causing patient to spit blood, pulse very weak
- **Frequent desire to micturate, urine contains much blood**
- Bearing down pain in lower abdomen with haemorrhage from the uterus; menorrhagia of bright red blood

MODALITIES
- **Aggravation:** Drinking cold water, morning
- **Amelioration:** Cold application, lying down, pressure, warm drinks, warm application

REMEDY RELATIONSHIP
- **Compare:** Acal., Ip., Arn., Mill., Phos., Thlasp., Ferr., Cact.

SPHERE OF ACTION

- Mind
- Eyes
- Gastrointestinal system
- Respiratory system
- Circulatory system
- Genitourinary system
- Skin

INTRODUCTION

- **Common name:** Hydrofluoric acid
- **Group:** Acid
- **Source:** Mineral kingdom
- **Formula:** HF
- **Prover:** Dr Hering

CONSTITUTION

- Used in chronic diseases with a history of syphilis; cancerous diathesis
- In premature old age – young people look too old with weak, distended blood vessels
- Suits pale, flabby, miserable, broken down patients with dropsy of limbs
- **Temperament:** Bilious
- **Thermal:** Hot
- **Miasm:** Psora, Syphilis

FLUORICUM ACIDUM

MIND

- Materialistic man, enjoys life in its full extent
- Insensitive and aggressive
- Develops a feeling of superiority; dominating behaviour
- Anxiety about own health; anxious; apprehensive
- Indifference towards those loved most, towards business, towards own family
- Inability to realise responsibility
- Hasty, impulse to walk faster
- Abuses and reproaches others
- Cheerful when walking in open air, during menses
- Absentminded; forgetful, especially in the evening

KEYNOTE SYMPTOMS

- Profound weakness and debility runs through the whole remedy
- Patient has increased ability to exercise; constant, irresistible desire to walk in open air which does not fatigue
- Burning pains in small spots on skin. Violent, jerking, burning pains confined to a small spot
- Tissues are putty, dropsical, indurated and fistulous
- **Rapid caries of teeth; fistula dentalis; fistula lacrymalis**
- **Deficient enamel on teeth; teeth black, rough, unsightly**
- Exostoses of bones of the face and head; glabella region bloated
- Varicose veins, caries and necrosis, especially of long bones
- Frequent, sour, stale eructations and flatulence
- Soreness over the liver. Degeneration of liver or ascites in alcoholics
- Sore throat, intensely red and very swollen, with foetid breath, nasal voice, worse inspiring cold air
- Burning in the urethra during and after urination
- Sexual passion and desire increased, with erection at night, during sleep; scrotum swollen
- Old cicatrices become red around the edges and threaten to become open ulcers
- Red blotches on the skin which tend to desquamate. Old scars become red and itch

CLINICAL

- Bone affections
- Dropsy
- Oedema
- Alcoholism
- Goitre
- Hairfall
- Alopecia
- Headache
- Eye affections
- Dental caries
- Teeth decay
- Dental fistulae
- Ascitis
- Liver affections
- Bilious diarrhoea
- Haemorrhoids
- Sore throat
- Hydrothorax
- Dyspnoea
- Urethritis
- Gonorrhoea
- Hydrocoele
- Osteomyelitis
- Varicose veins
- Varicose ulcers
- Abscesses
- Ulcers
- Felon
- Naevi
- Fistula
- Cicatrices
- Whitlow

MODALITIES

- **Aggravation:** Warmth, morning, warm drinks, heat of the room, rest, rising
- **Amelioration:** Cold, while walking, cool bathing, rapid motion, eating, open air

REMEDY RELATIONSHIP

- **Compare:** Thiosina. in action on cicatricial tissues, adhesions, strictures, tumours; Calc-f., Sil.
- **Complementary:** Coca, Sil.
- **Follows well:** After, Ars. in ascites of drunkards; after, Kali-c., in hip disease; after, Coff., Staph. in sensitive teeth; after, Ph-ac., in diabetes; after, Sil., Symph. in bone diseases; after, Spong.

FORMICA RUFA

INTRODUCTION
- **Common name:** Wood ant, Red ant, Myrnexine
- **Family:** *Formicidae*
- **Source:** Animal kingdom
- **Part used:** Living, unfeathered female workers
- **Prover:** Lippe and Hering

SPHERE OF ACTION
- Mind
- Gastrointestinal system
- Respiratory system
- Musculoskeletal system
- Urinary system
- Skin

CONSTITUTION
- For rheumatic and gouty complaints in old people
- **Temperament:** Nervous, bilious
- **Thermal:** Chilly
- **Miasm:** Psora, Sycosis, Syphilis

MIND
- Remarkable and unexpected activity of mind during daytime with absence of usual dullness and sleepiness
- **Cheerfulness, gaiety, happiness, exhilaration mirth after pain**
- Restlessness and nervousness from pain
- Weepy, tearful mood, morose
- Hysterical at night after cough
- Impossible to work at night
- Forgetful in the evening

KEYNOTE SYMPTOMS
- **Right sided affections**
- Complaints from overlifting
- Consequences of suppressed foot sweat
- General aggravation or great liability to complaints from cold and damp; worse before snow storms
- Has a marked deterrent influence on the formation of polypi
- Brain feels too heavy and large
- **Headache with sensation as if a bubble has burst in the forehead, better combing the hair**
- Drawing pain around naval before stool
- Ringing and buzzing in ears
- Indicated in violent, long lasting cough, with vomiting
- Medicine for arthritis, gout and articular rheumatism
- Rheumatism appears suddenly with restlessness
- Chronic gout and stiffness in joints; acute outbursts of gouty poisons especially when assuming a neuralgic form
- **Pains are worse by motion, better from pressure.** Pains start from one side and go to the other side. Pain assumes neuralgic form
- Profuse perspiration without relief
- Atrophy of wounds
- Hives, red, itchy and burning

CLINICAL
- Apoplexy
- Carcinoma
- Polypi
- Spleen painful
- Diarrhoea
- Tapeworm
- Nasal polyp
- Cough
- Sore throat
- Tuberculosis
- Nephritis
- Spinal affections
- Arthritis
- Rheumatism
- Gout
- Dislocations
- Nettle rash
- Lupus

MODALITIES
- **Aggravation:** Cold, cold washing, dampness, before a snow storm, motion
- **Amelioration:** Warmth, pressure, rubbing, combing hair, after midnight

REMEDY RELATIONSHIP
- **Compatible:** After Cham.
- **Compare:** Form-ac., Ars., Bry., Dulc., Urt-u., Frag-v., Tromb., Caps. in burning pains worse cold water.

GAMBOGIA

SPHERE OF ACTION
- Eyes
- Pneumogastric nerve
- Gastrointestinal system
- Kidneys

INTRODUCTION
- **Common name:** Gummi gutti, Gamboge
- **Family:** *Guttiferae*
- **Source:** Vegetable kingdom
- **Part used:** Gum resin
- **Prover:** Nenning, Noack and Trinks

CONSTITUTION
- For old people with profuse, watery diarrhoea; has an intense and definite action on the digestive tract
- **Temperament:** Nervous, bilious
- **Thermal:** Chilly, ambithermal
- **Miasm:** Psora, Sycosis

MIND
- Sadness during diarrhoea or from suppression of diarrhoea
- Irritability in the morning on waking
- Violent on rising
- Cheerful, talkative, feeling of ease, great lightness of all his motions
- Delusion that his work is not moving fast enough
- Restlessness, anxiety
- Gloomy

KEYNOTE SYMPTOMS
- Flushes of heat
- Heaviness in the head with drowsiness and pain in the head
- **Heat rises to the head with perspiration, better in open air**
- Itching of the inner canthi of eyes with discharge of acrid, corrosive tears after rubbing, better in open air
- **Eyes feel sticky and dry; eyelids stick together on sneezing**
- Rumbling, gurgling and rolling in the abdomen with sudden, forcible ejection of bilious stools
- Burning in anus with tenesmus, abdominal distension and flatulence; anus sore and excoriated. Tenesmus after stools
- Profuse, watery diarrhoea in hot weather, particularly in old people
- Burning pain and soreness in coccyx
- **Severe itching in various parts with sensation of formication; burning after scratching**
- Frightful vomiting and purging, with fainting. Burning in liver region

CLINICAL
- Inflammation of eyes
- Vomiting
- Food poisoning
- Anal complaints
- Diarrhoea
- Dysentery
- Typhlitis
- Coccygodynia

MODALITIES
- **Aggravation:** Towards evening, at night, after stools
- **Amelioration:** Open air, after stools, sitting up

REMEDY RELATIONSHIP
- **Compare:** Crot-t., Aloe, Podo., Puls., Apoc.
- **Antidoted by:** Camph., Coff., Coloc., Op., Kali-c.

GELSEMIUM SEMPERVIRENS

SPHERE OF ACTION

- Mind
- Head
- Eyes
- Gastrointestinal system
- Respiratory system
- Heart
- Nervous system
- Urinary system

INTRODUCTION

- **Common name:** Yellow jasmine, Bignonia
- **Family:** *Loganiaceae*
- **Source:** Vegetable kingdom
- **Part used:** Rhizome
- **Prover:** Henry and Douglas

CONSTITUTION

- Suits children, young people and women of nervous, hysterical temperament
- Face is hot, heavy, flushed with a besotted expression
- **Temperament:** Nervous, bilious
- **Thermal:** Chilly
- **Miasm:** Psora, Sycosis, Syphilis

MIND

- Bad effect of fear, bad news, fright, emotional excitement
- Dullness of mental faculties with languor, listless and inability to fix attention. Mental exhaustion
- **Fear of falling; child grabs the crib or seizes the nurse**
- Drowsy, dazed
- Apathy regarding illness
- Doesn't wish to speak or have anyone near her, even if the person is silent
- Confused; fear of loosing self control
- Desire to be left alone
- Nervous dread of appearing in public. Nervousness and fear, after traumatic shock
- **Anticipation of any unusual ordeal like preparing for church, exam, etc.** It brings on complaints. Depression, utter lack of courage.

KEYNOTE SYMPTOMS

- Weakness; mental, emotional and physical
- Paresis of various groups of muscles; gradual paralysis; motor paralysis. Muscles feel heavy, weak, sore and tired
- General depression from heat of sun or summer
- Vertigo spreading from the occiput with diplopia, blurred vision
- **Headache preceded by blindness, relieved by profuse urination**
- Dull, heavy headache; sensation of a band around the head
- Eyelids feel heavy drooping; cannot open eyes
- **Thirstlessness. Empty or weak feeling in stomach**
- **Anticipatory diarrhoea while preparing for exams**
- Earache – neuralgic while swallowing; from cold with closure of eustachian tube
- Influenza with fever, headache and drowsiness
- **Pain from throat to ear, worse swallowing.** Sensation of a lump in throat; spasm of glottis. Aphonia, especially from fright.
- Patient wants to be held during chills because he shakes so much
- **Fears that heart will stop beating unless he moves.** Pulse – slow and weak, as in old age
- Nervous chills during labour
- Insomnia from exhaustion, mental excitement
- Constant desire to urinate; urine profuse, clear, watery, with trembling and chillness
- Excessive weakness, trembling and numbness of all the limbs
- Chills running up and down the back (in waves), without thirst with aching and langour

CLINICAL

- Emotional shock
- Anxiety
- Chronic fatigue syndrome
- Stupor
- Paralysis
- Muscular weakness
- Parkinsons
- Hysterical convulsions
- Tremors
- Pellagra
- Sunstroke
- Headache
- Migraine
- Diplopia
- Ptosis
- Orbital neuralgia
- Glaucoma
- Retinitis
- Choroiditis
- Photophobia
- Amblyopia
- Diarrhoea
- Ascites
- Influenza
- Laryngitis
- Hay fever
- Aphonia
- Post-diphtheritic paralysis
- Fatty degeneration of heart
- Angina pectoris
- Retention of urine
- Multiple sclerosis
- Fever
- Insomnia

MODALITIES

- **Aggravation:** Damp weather, before a thunderstorm; mental emotion or excitement, bad news, tobacco smoking, when thinking of ailments, when spoken of his loss, at 10 am, anticipation, shock, fog
- **Amelioration:** Bending forward, profuse micturition, open air, continuous motion, stimulants, mental exertion, shaking

REMEDY RELATIONSHIP

- **Compare:** Bapt., Ip., Ign., Acon., Bell., Cimic., Mag-p.; Culx.
- **Antidotes:** Chin., Coff., Dig., Atrop., Nux-m., Mag-p.
- Alcoholic stimulants relieve all complaints where Gels. is useful.

GINSENG QUINQUEFOLIA

INTRODUCTION
- **Common name:** Wild ginseng
- **Family:** *Araliaceae*
- **Source:** Vegetable kingdom
- **Part used:** Root
- **Prover:** Jouve and Lembke

SPHERE OF ACTION
- Mind
- Gastrointestinal system
- Heart
- Spinal cord
- Musculoskeletal system
- Genital system
- Skin

CONSTITUTION
- For dark complexioned people; with pallor and pimples on neck and chest
- **Temperament:** Nervous, bilious
- **Thermal:** Chilly
- **Miasm:** Psora, Sycosis, Syphilis

MIND
- Generally calm, but there are impatient impulses; quiet and content
- Fear of accidents. At times, disposition to weep or to be anxious about the future
- Mental and nervous exhaustion from overwork
- Prostration of mind
- Mental exhaustion, brain fag with pain in lumbar region
- Anxiety, especially regarding the future
- Restlessness
- Lachrymose
- Weak memory

KEYNOTE SYMPTOMS
- Neurasthenia after debilitating diseases; paralytic weakness
- General prostration and stiffness of lumbar region
- Great sensitiveness to cold
- Great drowsiness, yawning; awakens with difficulty or else with a start
- Sensitive to light
- Tight clothes intolerable
- Stimulant to secretory glands, especially salivary glands
- **Vertigo on going downstairs.** While standing, the ground seems to be wavy. **Vertigo with grey spots before the eyes**
- **Great dryness of mouth, tongue, lips, palate**
- Oppression of chest with anxiety and pain in the pit of stomach and lumbar region
- Marked affinity for lower part of spinal cord – lumbago, sciatica, rheumatism
- Hands feels swollen; stiff, contracted joints
- Skin feels tight; sensation of constriction
- Severe cutting lancinating pains and stitches in the precordia. Violent heart beats while sitting
- Weakness of genital organs, especially in men; sexual excitement

CLINICAL
- Weakness
- Paralysis
- Vertigo
- Hiccough
- Perityphlitis
- Pharyngitis
- Tonsillitis
- Sexual excitement
- Impotency
- Orchitis
- Arthritis
- Rheumatism
- Lumbago
- Backache
- Sciatica
- Pimples

MODALITIES
- **Aggravation:** Night, open air, talking, descending, bending, sitting
- **Amelioration:** At dinner

REMEDY RELATIONSHIP
- **Compare:** Aral., Coca., Hed.- in mental depression and skin irritation; Gels., Nat-s., Hera. in drowsiness with headache; Bry., Nux-m., Sulph.

GLONOINUM

INTRODUCTION

- **Common name:** Nitroglycerine
- **Group:** Organic compound
- **Source:** Mineral kingdom
- **Formula:** $C_3H_5N_3O_9$
- **Prover:** Hering

SPHERE OF ACTION

- Head
- Central nervous system
- Gastrointestinal system
- Respiratory system
- Circulatory system
- Genitourinary system

CONSTITUTION

- For children getting sick on sitting before an open fire
- Plethoric, florid, sensitive women with a flushed face, who are hot, livid and dusky with a tendency to sudden and violent irregularities in circulation
- **Temperament:** Nervous, bilious, sanguine
- **Thermal:** Hot
- **Miasm:** Psora, Sycosis, Syphilis

MIND

- **Confusion as to location. Lost in well known places. Well known streets seem strange**
- Disinclined to speak, would hardly answer
- Confusion on waking at night. Confusion from inhaling fumes
- Frantic, attempts to run away or jump out of the window
- **Exalted ideas. Thinks she is the almighty and others are inferior**
- Fear she has been poisoned
- Fear from sensation of swelling in throat
- Time passes too slowly
- Thinks as if in a dream, doesn't know where he is
- Very irritable
- Dwells on past, disagreeable events

KEYNOTE SYMPTOMS

- Sensitive women, especially during climacteric or children during dentition with congestion of head and heart
- Warm blooded; a peculiar sensation of warmth throughout the body with pulsations. Flushes of heat
- **Bad effects of sunstroke, carries an umbrella all the time; sun headache**
- Sudden irregularities in circulation; sensation of bursting. Sudden vascular congestion, surges of blood
- Pulsations throughout the body, especially heart and head; violent ebullitions. Surging of blood upwards, to head and heart. Threatened stroke
- Congestive headaches. Every throb of cerebral arteries seems to be synchronous with beats of the heart; pulsating headache with bursting and expanding sensation
- Headache with protrusion of eyeballs
- Angiospastic neuralgia of head and face
- Convulsions, especially in children, from cerebral congestion
- Severe vertigo on assuming an upright posture
- Neck feels full. **Choking and swelling under the ears**
- Abnormal hunger. Gastralgia with anaemia and feeble circulation
- Constipation with itching, painful haemorrhoids
- Diarrhoea – copious, blackish, lumpy stools
- Hypertension with headache; least exertion causes rush of blood to heart with fainting
- **Palpitations with an accelerated pulse; laborious action of the heart**
- Acute or chronic nephritis due to hypertension
- Sudden cessation of menses with congestion of head and chest
- Cardiac neuralgia with radiating pains

CLINICAL

- Sunstroke
- Convulsions
- Cerebral congestion
- Headache
- Vertigo
- Meningitis
- Apoplexy
- Toothache
- Bulimia
- Nausea
- Vomiting
- Gastralgia
- Diarrhoea
- Constipation
- Haemorrhoids
- Meniere's disease
- Dyspnoea
- Angina pectoris
- Palpitation
- Heart affections
- Nephritis
- Climacteric flushing
- Menopausal disturbances
- Amenorrhoea
- Dysmenorrhoea
- Backache
- Rheumatism
- Sciatica

MODALITIES

- **Aggravation:** In the sun, gas-light, overheating, jar, stooping, ascending, hair cut, peaches, stimulants, lying down, from 6 am to noon, left side
- **Amelioration:** Brandy, open air, cold things and applications

REMEDY RELATIONSHIP

- **Compare:** Op., Stram., Verat-v., Aml-ns., Bell., Ferr., Gels., Meli., Cimic., Hyos., Sec.
- **Antidoted by:** Acon., Camph., Nux-v., Coff.

SPHERE OF ACTION

- Metabolism
- Central nervous system
- Gastrointestinal system
- Respiratory system
- Cardiovascular system
- Urinary system
- Skin

MIND

- Mental dullness
- Confused
- Forgetful
- Mental weakness
- Anxiety, apprehension
- Restlessness
- Desires company

MODALITIES

- **Aggravation:** Exertion – mental and physical, motion
- **Amelioration:** Rest

INTRODUCTION

- **Common name:** Glycerine, Glycerol
- **Group:** Organic compound
- **Source:** Mineral kingdom
- **Formula:** $C_3H_8O_3$

GLYCERINUM

KEYNOTE SYMPTOMS

- A long and deep acting remedy for building up tissues, especially during marasmus, debility, etc. Improves the state of nutrition
- Useful in children, young girls with recurrent stomatitis and gingivitis
- Physical and mental weakness; neurasthenia
- General sense of exhaustion; debilitated, feels tired almost to the state of utter prostration
- **Disturbed nutrition; balances general metabolism**
- Burning in stomach and oesophagus
- Acute catarrhal condition of the nasopharyngeal mucous membrane
- Hacking cough with weakness. Chest feels full
- **Profuse and frequent micturition with traces of sugar; diabetes**
- Dysmenorrhoea; profuse, long lasting flow with a bearing down heaviness in the uterus
- Feet painful and hot, feel enlarged
- Sleep restless and dreamy

CONSTITUTION

- Suited to anaemic young girls who are physically and mentally weak and have a tendency for blisters in the mouth
- **Temperament:** Nervous, bilious
- **Thermal:** Ambithermal
- **Miasm:** Psora, Sycosis, Syphilis

CLINICAL

- Senile debility
- Weakness
- Marasmus
- Pernicious anaemia
- Alopecia
- Dandruff
- Constipation
- Sneezing
- Coryza
- Influenza
- Postnasal dripping
- Cough
- Pneumonia
- Diabetes
- Rheumatism
- Acne
- Dry eczema
- Cracks
- Fissures
- Psoriasis

REMEDY RELATIONSHIP

- **Compare:** Lac-ac., Gels., Calc., Lec.

GNAPHALIUM POLYCEPHALUM

INTRODUCTION
- **Common name:** Cudweed, Old balsam
- **Family:** *Compositae*
- **Source:** Vegetable kingdom
- **Part used:** Whole plant
- **Prover:** Banks, Fuller and Woodbury

SPHERE OF ACTION
- Mind
- Gastrointestinal system
- Respiratory system
- Sciatic nerve
- Musculoskeletal system
- Genitourinary system
- Skin

MIND
- Very irritable for two or three days after the diarrhoea
- Sad
- Gloomy
- Restlessness
- Anxiety

MODALITIES
- **Aggravation:** Walking, cold damp weather, lying down
- **Amelioration:** Sitting on a chair, flexing limbs

KEYNOTE SYMPTOMS
- Neuralgic affections
- Colic, pain in the abdomen, vomiting
- First stage of cholera. Morning diarrhoea
- Dysmenorrhoea with painful, scanty menses; sensation of weight and heaviness in pelvis
- Irritated prostate
- **Sciatica – right side more affected than left.** Intense pain along the sciatic nerve; pain alternates with numbness
- Lumbar backache, better resting on the back
- **Lumbago is rheumatic in origin, worse cold, damp weather; accompanied by numbness in the lower part of back**
- **Pain in joints, as if they lacked oil**
- Gouty pain in big toe
- Anterior crural neuralgia
- Cramps in calves and feet

CONSTITUTION
- For pale, anaemic patients with intermittent pain in superior maxillary bone of both side
- Used mainly for disorders of the sciatic nerve
- **Temperament:** Nervous, bilious
- **Thermal:** Chilly
- **Miasm:** Psora, Sycosis, Syphilis

CLINICAL
- Neuralgia
- Cramps
- Nausea
- Vomiting
- Borborygmus
- Morning diarrhoea
- Cholera
- Asthma
- Polyuria
- Dysmenorrhoea
- Enlarged prostate
- Arthritis
- Rheumatism
- Gout
- Sciatica
- Backache
- Lumbar spondylosis

REMEDY RELATIONSHIP
- **Compare:** Xan., Cham., Puls., Lyc., Caul., Merc., Ip., Coloc.

GRAPHITES

INTRODUCTION

- **Common name:** Black lead
- **Group:** Carbon
- **Source:** Mineral kingdom
- **Prover:** Hahnemann

SPHERE OF ACTION

- Mind
- Eyes
- Ears
- Gastrointestinal system
- Musculoskeletal system
- Female genital system
- Skin

CONSTITUTION

- Suited to women who are inclined to get obese, who suffer from habitual constipation with delayed menstruation
- For affections of skin, glands and mucous membranes at the orifices
- Defective animal heat from defective oxygenation
- Cancerous diathesis
- **Temperament:** Nervous, bilious
- **Thermal:** Chilly
- **Miasm:** Psora, Sycosis, Syphilis

MIND

- Simple, basic, earthy and unrefined patients
- Slow thinking, irresolution, poor concentration. Dullness, slowness. Inability to think from weakness of the brain
- Sad, tearsome, irresolute, hesitates at trifles, absentminded
- Timid, dread of work
- **Sensation of a cobweb on the forehead, tries hard to brush it off**
- Fidgety or restless while working
- Feels miserable and unhappy
- Weeps without cause, from music. Sensitive to music. Weeping ameliorates symptoms
- Forgetful, makes mistakes in speaking and writing
- Child impudent, teasing. Laughs at reprimands
- Irritable and fretful
- Obstinate and moody

KEYNOTE SYMPTOMS

- Left sided complaints
- Sudden weakness. Cataleptic – conscious but does not have the power to move or speak. Emaciation of affected parts
- Sour taste, eructations, stools, urine, teeth, etc.
- Scaliness of scalp with severe itching, forms scurf – milk crusts, eczema capitis
- Eyelids red, swollen, fissured; blepharitis, eczema of lids
- Opthalmia with intolerance of artificial light
- **Hears better when in noise, riding a carriage**
- Inner ear very dry. Moisture and eruptions behind the ears; cracks and fissures behind the ears
- **Digestive and skin symptoms alternate**
- Palpitations of heart with anxiety from least exertion
- Morning sickness during menses
- Sexual debility from sexual abuse
- Menses late and scanty; sighing during menses
- **Acrid leucorrhoea – gushing, thin excoriating with marked weakness of the back;** especially before and after menses
- Every little injury suppurates – unhealthy skin; dry, rough skin
- Skin lumpy, thick, hard. Moist, crusty eruptions. Gluey moisture.
- **Watery, transparent, sticky, honey-like fluid discharged from the eruptions and tissues. Sweat leaves yellow stains**
- Removes tendency for erysipelas
- Tendency for cracks and fissures at mucocutaneous junctions of eyes, nose, anus, nipples, labial commissures, etc. and ends of fingers
- Absorption of cicatricial tissue; cancerous diathesis in old scars
- Thickening and induration of skin. Tendency to callous formation, cystic tumours and wens
- Nails thick and ingrown; brittle and crumbling

CLINICAL

- Anaemia
- Obesity
- Atony
- Malignancy
- Indurations
- Flushes
- Blepharitis
- Styes
- Otitis media
- Gastritis
- Peptic ulcer
- Duodenal ulcer
- Cancer of pylorus
- Constipation
- Leucorrhoea
- Moist, sticky eruptions
- Phlegmonous erysipelas
- Eczema
- Fissures
- Psoriasis
- Corns
- Impetigo
- Keloids
- Wens
- Scars

MODALITIES

- **Aggravation:** At night, during and after menstruation, cold drafts, suppression of secretions or eruptions, light
- **Amelioration:** In the dark, from wrapping up, walking, in open air, hot drinks especially milk, eating, belching, weeping

REMEDY RELATIONSHIP

- **Complementary:** Caust., Hep., Lyc., Arg-n. (follows well in gastric derangements); Ars., Tub.
- **Follows well:** Lyc., Puls.; Calc. in obesity of young women with a large amount of unhealthy adipose tissue; Sulph. in skin affections; Sepia in gushing leucorrhoea.
- **Compare:** Petr., Sep., Sulph., Fl-ac.
- **Antidoted by:** Nux-v., Acon., Ars.

Graphites

SPHERE OF ACTION

- Head
- Eyes
- Gastrointestinal system
- Musculoskeletal system
- Female genital system

INTRODUCTION

- **Common name:** Hedge hyssop, Herb of Grace
- **Family:** *Scrophulariaceae*
- **Source:** Vegetable kingdom
- **Part used:** Whole plant before flowering
- **Prover:** Nenning, Hartlaub and Trinks

CONSTITUTION

- **For mental troubles from overweening pride, especially in women**
- **Temperament:** Nervous, bilious
- **Thermal:** Chilly
- **Miasm:** Psora, Sycosis, Syphilis

GRATIOLA OFFICINALIS

MIND

- Ailments from overweening pride of others
- Aversion to everything at 1 pm
- Haughty
- Irresolute, want of perseverance
- Sadness, despondency. Severe depression, does not want to do anything. Gloomy.
- Ill-humour, tired of life
- Apprehensive regarding the future; hypochondriasis
- Loquacity and gaiety
- Restlessness
- Nymphomania
- Confusion on lying down
- Violent anger on contradiction

MODALITIES

- **Aggravation:** Drinking too much water or coffee, dinner, summers, warm room, motion
- **Amelioration:** Rest, open air, eating

KEYNOTE SYMPTOMS

- Left side is more affected than the right
- Paralytic pains and feeling of coldness, especially in the abdomen
- Rush of blood to the head with vanishing of sight
- Sensation as if the brain was contracting and the head was becoming smaller
- Tightness in forehead, with wrinkles on the skin
- Myopia on reading, sees distant objects better than near ones, better on closing the eyes
- **Eyes, dry and burn; sensation as if sand were in them**
- Dysphagia for liquids
- Dyspepsia – cramps after eating at night with swelling of the abdomen and constipation. Chronic gastrointestinal catarrh
- **Frothy, green, watery diarrhoea, evacuated forcibly**
- Haemorrhoids with hypochondriasis
- Menses too profuse and long lasting, premature
- Irritability and congestion of sexual organs, lymphomania

CLINICAL

- Delirium tremens
- Cramps
- Vertigo
- Sick headache
- Myopia
- Dyspepsia
- Dysphagia
- Colic
- Diarrhoea
- Constipation
- Haemorrhoids
- Asthma
- Gonorrhoea
- Nymphomania
- Metrorrhagia
- Menorrhagia
- Leucorrhoea
- Rheumatism
- Ulcers
- Insomnia

REMEDY RELATIONSHIP

- **Compare:** Dig., Euph., Tab., Cham., Am-pic., Nux-v., Apis., Bell., Elat., Heil., Podo.,
- **Antidotes:** Iod.

GRINDELIA ROBUSTA

INTRODUCTION

Common name: Rosinwood
Family: *Compositae*
Source: Vegetable kingdom
Part used: Leaves and flowering tops
Prover: Bundy and Hale

SPHERE OF ACTION

- Eyes
- Gastrointestinal system
- Respiratory system
- Heart
- Female genital system
- Skin

CONSTITUTION

- For cardio-pulmonary affections, as it produces paralysis of the pneumogastric nerve producing respiratory symptoms
- **Temperament:** Nervous, bilious
- **Thermal:** Chilly
- **Miasm:** Psora, Sycosis, Syphilis

MIND

- **Fears going to sleep; fear of suffocation, owing to arrested respiration on falling asleep**
- Fear of darkness
- **Longing for sunshine, light and company**
- Startled during sleep
- Irritability, worse contradiction
- Melancholic
- Gloomy
- Forgetful

KEYNOTE SYMPTOMS

- Head feels full, as from quinine
- **Pain in the eyeballs, running back to the brain; worse moving the eyes; pupils dilated**
- Purulent ophthalmia and iritis
- Nausea and retching of gastric ulcer
- Enlarged spleen. Cutting pain in splenic region, radiating to the hips
- Asthma with profuse tenacious expectoration. Expectoration difficult but relieves
- Asthma or emphysema with a dilated heart
- **Sibilant rales, disseminated with foamy mucous, very difficult to detach**
- Cannot breathe when lying down, must sit up; cheyne-stokes respiration
- Stops breathing (smothering feeling) when falling asleep, wakes with a start, and gasps for breath, must sit up
- Weak heart and respiration. Raises the blood pressure
- Severe pruritus in vaginal and vulvar region, from leucorrhoea or aphthae
- Vesicular and papular eruptions; itching and burning
- Ulcers with swollen, purplish skin

CLINICAL

- Hyperaemia
- Ophthalmia
- Conjunctivitis
- Iritis
- Nausea
- Hyper-chlor-hydria
- Splenomegaly
- Diarrhoea
- Constipation
- Pertussis
- Chronic bronchitis
- Asthma
- Cheyne-Stokes breathing
- Bronchorrhoea
- Heart affections
- Diabetes
- Pruritus vulvae
- Malaria
- Erythema
- Herpes zoster
- Ulcers
- Blisters
- Burns

MODALITIES

- **Aggravation:** From motion, in the dark, from falling asleep
- **Amelioration:** Sitting position

REMEDY RELATIONSHIP

- **Compare:** Ant-t., Erw., Lach., Sang., Am-m., Kali-bi., Gels., Stram., Op.

GUAIACUM OFFICINALE

INTRODUCTION
- **Common name:** Resin of Lignum vitae
- **Part used:** Resin
- **Source:** Vegetable kingdom
- **Prover:** Hahnemann

SPHERE OF ACTION
- Mind
- Eyes
- Gastrointestinal system
- Respiratory system
- Musculoskeletal system
- Urinary system
- Female genital system
- Skin

MIND
- Obstinate, disobedient
- Strong desire to criticise and to despise everything
- Indolence and dread of movement
- Weakness of memory and excessive forgetfulness, especially of names
- Slow to comprehend
- Dreams of falling
- Nightmares cause weeping
- Screaming during sleep
- Aversion to mental work
- Fixed look and absence of ideas, especially in the morning
- Depressed, sad

MODALITIES
- **Aggravation:** From motion, heat, cold wet weather, pressure, touch, from 6 pm to 4 am
- **Amelioration:** External pressure, eating apples, yawning and stretching

KEYNOTE SYMPTOMS
- Patient is sensitive and aggravated by local heat
- General ill feeling, progressive emaciation, better yawning and stretching
- **Unclean odour from whole body. Free foul secretions**
- Promotes suppuration of abscesses
- All pains generally end in a stitch
- Pupils dilated. Eyelid inflamed; feels too short; pimples around the eye
- **Desires apples, aversion to milk**
- **Tongue furred; burning in the stomach; excessive flatulence**
- Acute tonsillitis; throat feels dry, swollen, burns and has stitches towards the ears
- Dry cough with pleuritic stitches
- Violent, spasmodic inflammation of wind pipe and larynx with palpitation and inability to cry out for help
- Feels suffocated; shortness of breath, relieved by expectoration
- **Constant desire to urinate, even after urinations.** Sharp stitch in neck of bladder after urinating
- Ovaritis in rheumatic complaints, irregular menses, dysmenorrhoea; irritable bladder
- Joints swollen, painful, stinging pain in the limbs; affected limb feels hot. Acute rheumatism
- Aching pain in nape of neck. Stiff neck, sore shoulders
- Limbs feel contracted and stiff; immobility. Patient feels he must stretch
- Sensation of heat in affected limbs

CONSTITUTION
- Suits arthritic diathesis – main action is on fibrous tissues. Growing pains
- **Temperament:** Gouty, rheumatic
- **Thermal:** Hot, ambithermal
- **Miasm:** Psora

CLINICAL
- Growing pains
- Intestinal fermentation
- Diarrhoea
- Cholera infantum
- Constipation
- Laryngitis
- Pharyngitis
- Tonsillitis
- Pleuritic stitches
- Pleurodynia
- Asthma
- Cystitis
- Secondary syphilis
- Arthritis
- Rheumatism
- Cervical spondylosis
- Lumbago
- Backache
- Sciatica
- Gout
- Abscesses
- Pimples
- Eczema

REMEDY RELATIONSHIP
- **Antidoted by:** Nux-v.
- **Follows:** Sep.
- **Compare:** Merc., Rhus-t., Mez., Rhod, Ph-ac., in growing pains; Cimic., Colo., Caust., Bry. in chronic rheumatism
- **Antidotes:** Caust., Rhus-t.

HAMAMELIS VIRGINIANA

SPHERE OF ACTION

- Mind
- Circulatory system
- Hepato-biliary system
- Veins
- Female genital system

INTRODUCTION

- **Common name:** Witch-hazel
- **Family:** Hamamelaceae
- **Source:** Vegetable kingdom
- **Part used:** Bark and leaves
- **Prover:** Dr Constantine Hering

CONSTITUTION

- Acts as an antihaemorrhagic remedy
- Suits anaemic women with history of threatened abortions
- Haemorrhagic diathesis
- **Miasm:** Tubercular, Syphilitic
- **Thermal:** Chilly
- **Temperament:** Nervous

MIND

- Irritability, sensitivity, fear
- Forgetful
- No desire to study
- Irritable, doesn't want anyone to speak to him
- Depressed; lowness of spirits, very gloomy
- Wants due respect to her opinions. Feels unappreciated.

KEYNOTE SYMPTOMS

- Great lassitude and a feeling of weariness
- Haemorrhage passive, profuse, dark, grumous, incoagulable, from every orifice of the body
- Incised, lacerated, contused wounds from falls; chronic effects of mechanical injuries
- Haemorrhoids bleed profusely, with burning, soreness and fullness of affected parts. Acts upon the coats of the veins causing relaxation with consequent engorgement.
- Painful weakness; sore pain in the eyes; bloodshot appearance; inflamed vessels greatly injected. Hastens absorption of intraocular haemorrhage.
- **Tongue feels burnt, blisters on the sides**
- Haematemesis of black blood. Throbbing and pain in stomach.
- **Stools are bluish; anus feels raw and sore to touch**
- Ovarian congestion and neuralgia; feels very sore
- Uterine haemorrhage active or passive with bearing-down pain in back
- Menses dark, profuse, with soreness in abdomen after a blow on ovary, or a fall
- Metrorrhagia, occurring midway between menstrual periods
- Pain in spermatic cord, running into testes
- Haemoptysis; tickling cough
- Chest feels sore and constricted
- Varicose veins in lower extremities enlarged and very marked. Varicose veins during pregnancy, taking cold easily
- Neuralgia of internal saphenous nerve
- **Prostration out of proportion to the amount of blood lost**

CLINICAL

- Phlebitis
- Venous congestion
- Haemorrhages
- Varicose veins
- Milk-leg
- Haemorrhoids
- Sore nipples
- Metrorrhagia
- Profuse leucorrhoea
- Vaginismus
- Ovaritis
- Orchitis
- Epididymitis
- Headaches
- Epistaxis
- Vicarious menstruation
- Chilblains
- Purpura
- Varicose veins and ulcers
- Burns
- Ecchymosis
- Rheumatism
- Traumatic inflammations
- Post-operative conditions

MODALITIES

- **Aggravation:** Warm moist air, rainy weather, motion, mental strain, touch, physical strain, bending forward, menstrual period
- **Amelioration:** Rest, outdoor, open air

REMEDY RELATIONSHIP

- **Compare:** Arnica; Calend.; Trillium; Bellis; Sulph.-ac.; Puls., Calc. fluor.; Aloe; Mur.-ac.
- **Antidote by:** Arn., Comph., Chin., Puls
- **Complementary:** Ferr.

HECLA LAVA

SPHERE OF ACTION
- Mind
- Gastrointestinal system
- Skeletal system
- Skin

INTRODUCTION
- **Common name:** Lava scoriae from Mt Hecla
- **Source:** Mineral kingdom
- **Prover:** Morris
- **Part used:** Volcanic ash from Mt Hecla

CONSTITUTION
- For arresting many types of bone diseases
- Cases where cervical glands are enlarged and indurated; for tendency to bone necrosis, nodosities
- **Temperament:** Nervous, bilious
- **Thermal:** Chilly
- **Miasm:** Psora, Sycosis, Syphilis

MIND
- Intense nervousness in the morning
- Outburst of violent anger
- **Very calm and poised person, but when provoked, bursts out into violent anger.** No self-control, shouting at others, whoever they may be, using words that offend
- Suppresses anger
- Gentle disposition and highly sensitive to admonitions, criticisms and injustice done to him and to others, leading to irritability
- Suppresses the anger, yet when his anger is beyond control, he becomes violent
- Irritability
- Gloomy, reserved

KEYNOTE SYMPTOMS
- **Right side is predominantly affected**
- Symptoms come suddenly and go suddenly
- Affections of bones, include brittle bones, exostosis, necrosis, caries, nodosities, injuries, inflammation, abscesses, fistulae, sinuses, tumours, ulcerations, enlargements, etc.
- Tendency to suppuration and fistulae
- Tendency to enlargement of bones or for bony growths especially of the maxillary bone; osteosarcoma, osteitis, exostosis
- Tendency for tumours in general
- **Swelling and induration of glands; especially cervical glands, which appear like a row of pearls in the neck; cervical lymphadenopathy**
- Caries of teeth, with facial neuralgia; toothache with swelling around jaws
- **Exostosis of lower jaw, tibia**
- Neuralgic pains remaining after tooth extraction
- Periodontitis, periostitis, chronic gingivitis, abscess of gums
- Delayed or difficult dentition in undernourished children
- Ulceration of nasal bones

CLINICAL
- Tumours
- Neuralgic pains
- Toothache
- Facial neuralgia
- Teething troubles
- Tooth extraction
- Caries of teeth
- Gum abscess
- Enlargement of maxillary bone
- Diarrhoea
- Dysentery
- Constipation
- Bone fistulae
- Bone sinuses
- Bony spurs
- Exostosis
- Osteosarcoma
- Periostitis
- Osteitis
- Rachitis
- Bone necrosis
- Cervical lymphadenopathy
- Abscesses
- Nodosities
- Whitlow

MODALITIES
- **Aggravation:** Touch, pressure, left side, beginning motion

REMEDY RELATIONSHIP
- **Compare:** Sil., Merc., Phos., Calc-f., Calc., Sulph., Symph., Ruta.; Conch. in diaphysis of bones, parts extremely sensitive to touch; Amph., great affinity for the jaw bones, worse by air and dampness; Slag for great itching of parts

HELLEBORUS NIGER

SPHERE OF ACTION

- Mind
- Head
- Nerves
- Gastrointestinal system
- Respiratory system
- Urinary system

INTRODUCTION

- **Common name:** Snow rose, Christmas rose
- **Family:** *Ranunculaceae*
- **Source:** Vegetable kingdom
- **Part used:** Rhizome
- **Prover:** Hahnemann

CONSTITUTION

- Adapted to pale, weak, delicate, psoric children prone to brain troubles, with serous effusions; have sunken face and cold sweat
- **Temperament:** Nervous
- **Thermal:** Chilly
- **Miasm:** Psora

MIND

- Ailments from disappointment in love
- Complete unconsciousness; on arousal, talks about spirits and devils
- Picks clothes, lips, ends of fingers, etc., or bores into nose with his finger
- Irritability
- Dull, stupid, slow perception, apathetic
- Answers slowly, in a confused manner, as though thinking of something else
- Indifference towards loved ones, pleasures, relations, sufferings
- Involuntary sighing
- Must concentrate his mind on what he is doing or the muscles do not act properly
- Answers slowly and with great effort due to weak memory
- Slowness of perception, apathetic.
- Melancholic mania, woeful, sensorial depression; gloomy
- Jealous on seeing others happy

KEYNOTE SYMPTOMS

- Stupefaction with all complaints
- Sensorial depression – all senses are dulled and responses are sluggish
- General muscular weakness which proceeds to complete paralysis with dropsy
- **Twitching and convulsions of muscles. Automatic motion of one arm and one leg**
- Thinking of complaints aggravates
- Concussion of brain from a blow to the head
- Epilepsy with consciousness, followed by deep sleep
- Forehead wrinkled in folds
- Headache stupefying, culminates in vomiting
- Rolls head from side to side, day and night; moaning. Sudden screams during sleep, soporous, cannot be aroused
- **Bores head into pillow and beats it with hands**
- Chewing motion of the mouth
- Horrible smell from the mouth; lips dry, cracked
- **Tongue red, dry; falling of lower jaw**
- **Greedily swallows cold water, when unconscious;** child nurses greedily
- Sense of suffocation; sighing respiration; gasps for breath but cannot inhale. Breathes better on lying down
- Urine suppressed, scanty, dark with coffee ground sediment, albuminous; suppressed during pregnancy, in brain troubles and dropsy

CLINICAL

- Dementia
- Alzheimer's disease
- Ataxia
- Coma
- Neuralgia
- Dropsical effusion
- Oedema
- Angioneurotic oedema
- Tetanus
- Head injury
- Epilepsy
- Meningitis
- Encephalitis
- Criencephalique
- Hydrocephalus
- Headache
- Migraine
- Night blindness
- Diarrhoea
- Dysentery
- Constipation
- Hydrothorax
- Involuntary urination

MODALITIES

- **Aggravation:** From evening till morning, from uncovering, cold air, 4 to 8 pm, suppressions, exertions, motion, thinking of ailments
- **Amelioration:** When the mind is diverted, warm air, wrapping up

REMEDY RELATIONSHIP

- **Antidote:** Camph., Chin.
- **Compare:** Apis, Apoc., Ars., Bell., Bry., Dig., Lach., Sulph., Tub., Zinc. in brain or meningeal affections; Tub., Apis, Zinc., Op., Chin., Cic., Iodof. in threatening effusion.

HELODERMA

INTRODUCTION
- **Common name:** Gila monster
- **Family:** *Helodermatidae*
- **Source:** Animal kingdom
- **Part used:** Venom
- **Prover:** Boocock

SPHERE OF ACTION
- Mind
- Eyes
- Gastrointestinal system
- Heart
- Nervous system
- Musculoskeletal system

CONSTITUTION
- For many diseases which are characterized by intense coldness – arctic coldness
- **Temperament:** Nervous
- **Thermal:** Chilly
- **Miasm:** Psora, Sycosis, Syphilis

MIND
- Easily startles and then trembles
- Indolence, aversion to work; especially in the morning
- Loss of memory, words; makes mistakes in spelling, even of simple words, when talking
- Very depressed, gloomy, melancholic and lachrymose
- Restless
- Cannot confine mind on one subject
- Passively indifferent

KEYNOTE SYMPTOMS
- Benumbing paralysis, like paralysis agitans and locomotor ataxia
- **Cock's gait, staggering gait – lifts feet higher than usual and puts down heel hard while walking**
- **Turns to the right when walking. Cannot balance while walking, staggers**
- Intense icy coldness, as if frozen from within outwards
- Cold waves from occiput to feet or ascending. Generalized coldness; arctic coldness
- Breath and tongue cold. Cold crawling feeling on face as if facial muscles were tight
- Cold feeling in lungs, back, across scapulae
- **Headache. Sensation as if would fall on the right side. Cold band around the head. Pain beginning in right ear, extending around back of head to left ear.**
- Eyelids heavy, eye balls are prominent; exophthalmos due to pressure of blood behind the eyeballs
- **Tongue cold, tender and dry. Very thirsty. Swallowing difficult.**
- Slow, laboured, thumping of the heart; palpitations and dysponea

CLINICAL
- Coldness
- Cyanosis
- Tetanus
- Locomotor ataxia
- Paralysis agitans
- Paralysis
- Headache
- Corneal opacities
- Exophthalmos
- Iritis
- Dysphagia
- Nausea
- Vomiting
- Arthritis
- Backache
- Vesicles

MODALITIES
- **Aggravation:** Thinking of ailments, exposure to cold, stormy weather, after sleep
- **Amelioration:** Warmth, stretching

REMEDY RELATIONSHIP
- **Compare:** Lacer. skin eruptions, vesicles under the tongue; Camph., Lach., Crot-h.; Arg-n., Alum. in locomotor ataxis; Ant-t., Merc., Gels., Con.

HELONIAS DIOICA

SPHERE OF ACTION
- Mind
- Musculoskeletal system
- Urinary system
- Female genital system
- Skin

INTRODUCTION
- **Common name:** Unicorn root
- **Family:** *Liliaceae*
- **Source:** Vegetable kingdom
- **Part used:** Rhizome and root
- **Prover:** Proved by Tully and introduced by Parr

CONSTITUTION
- Suits women, worn out from mental or physical work; overtaxed muscles; with uterine prolapse. Women feel so tired that they cannot sleep
- **Temperament:** Nervous, bilious
- **Thermal:** Chilly, ambithermal
- **Miasm:** Psora, Sycosis, Syphilis

MIND
- Always better when doing something, when the mind is occupied or engaged
- Restless, must move constantly
- Melancholy, desire to be left alone. Deep gloom
- Irritable, cannot endure least contradiction, fault finding
- Hysteria

KEYNOTE SYMPTOMS
- Exhaustion from least physical or mental work
- Ill-effects of miscarriages and abortions
- Initial stages of diabetes with polyuria, polydipsia, restlessness and emaciation
- Kidneys sore and tender; ache all the time
- Nephritis of pregnancy. Albuminuria; patient is unusually tired, drowsy
- Unduly exhausted females from repeated pregnancies, multiple abortions or uterine haemorrhages
- Uterine prolapse from atony, enervated by luxury and indolence. Relaxation of pelvic ligaments
- **Great consciousness of the womb.** Feels uterus at all times, feels that it moves and shifts with her movements
- Heavy, sore, tender, ulcerated or prolapsed uterus. Heavy dragging in pelvis; sense of weight; misplacement
- Fatigue or hysteria with prolapse or other uterine complaints
- Menses too early, profuse, from uterine atony. Loss of blood more than that is made during the intermenstrual period

CLINICAL
- Atony
- Debility
- Anaemia
- Nephritis
- Diabetes mellitus
- Diabetes insipidus
- Albuminuria
- Uterine affections
- Dysmenorrhoea
- Leucorrhoea
- Pruritus vulvae
- Vaginitis
- Malposition of uterus
- Prolapse of uterus
- Fibroids
- Sterility

MODALITIES
- **Aggravation:** Motion, touch, pressure especially on breasts, nipples or kidneys
- **Amelioration:** When doing something (mental diversion), holding abdomen, when busy

REMEDY RELATIONSHIP
- **Compare:** Alet., Ferr., Lil-t., Ph-ac., Agri., in painful kidneys, impaired digestion, menstrual problems; bronchorrhoea and dysuria; Puls., Senec., Stann.
- **Similar to:** Alet. in debility from prolapsus, protracted illness, defective nutrition

Helonias dioica

HEPAR SULPHURIS CALCAREUM

SPHERE OF ACTION
- Mind
- Ears
- Mucous membranes
- Gastrointestinal system
- Respiratory system
- Larynx
- Musculoskeletal system
- Skin

INTRODUCTION
- **Common name:** Hahnemann's calcium sulphide, Impure calcium sulphide
- **Source:** Mineral kingdom
- **Formula:** CaS
- **Prover:** Hahnemann

CONSTITUTION
- Adapted to blondes, with a sluggish character, who are slow to act and have weak, flabby muscles
- For debilitated subjects with scrofulous, lymphatic constitution and a tendency to suppuration
- **Temperament:** Tubercular
- **Thermal:** Chilly
- **Miasm:** Psora

MIND
- Severe irritability and dissatisfaction with oneself and others
- Critical, impatient, quarrelsome
- **Hasty in speech and drinking**
- Peevish, gets angry at trifles
- Starting soon after falling asleep
- **Strong, violent impulses; impulse to stab or kill; impulsive**
- Anguish in the evening and at night, with thoughts of suicide
- Dejected, melancholic
- Restlessness, wants a constant change
- Bad tempered; least upset irritates immensely
- Cross children; hit, kick and scream

KEYNOTE SYMPTOMS
- Oversensitiveness to all impressions – mental and physical; to cold, pain, touch, noise, odours, draught of air
- Skin sensitive to touch; pain often causes fainting
- Intolerant to drafts; chilliness; sensation as if wind was blowing on some part
- **Cannot bear to be uncovered; wants warm wrapping**
- Catarrh of mucous membrane with a tendency to suppuration. Catarrh is mostly of the throat, stomach, uterus and urethra.
- Splinter-like sensation or pricking in affected parts
- **Easy, profuse perspiration without relief – sour, offensive**
- Sourness of all discharges – sweat, stool, etc.
- Discharges are thick, ropy, acrid and yellow, like leucorrhoea, expectoration, etc.
- Vertigo and headache on shaking the head or riding
- Middle and lower lip cracked. **Craves sour and strong things like acids and wine.**
- Hepatitis, liver abscess, chronic abdominal affections
- Diarrhoea, especially of children; clay coloured foetid stools
- Deafness after scarlet fever
- Sensation of a splinter in the throat, burning pains – when suppuration threatens; hoarseness; aphonia
- Pneumonia in suppurative stage; empyema; bronchiectasis
- Urine voided slowly without force, falls vertically; bladder weak
- Menses late, scanty. **Leucorrhea smells like old cheese.**
- Discharge of blood, from the uterus; ulcers in the uterus
- Unhealthy skin, slightest injury causes suppuration, which develops rapidly
- Chronic, recurring urticaria. Deep cracks on hands and feet
- Ulcers, suppurating, surrounded by small pimples, very sensitive to contact

CLINICAL
- Abusive
- Agoraphobia
- Pellagra
- Suppuration
- Adenopathy
- Blepharitis
- Corneal ulcer
- Hypopion
- Iritis
- Constipation
- Rectal abscess
- Cold
- Ear affections
- Otitis media
- Laryngitis
- Pharyngitis
- Sinusitis
- Tonsillitis
- Hay fever
- Ozaena
- Croup
- Bronchitis
- Tuberculosis
- Pneumonia
- Asthma
- Pleurisy
- Urethral stricture
- Urethritis
- Balanitis
- Mastitis
- Prostatitis
- Ulcers
- Boils
- Carbuncles
- Abscesses
- Acne
- Eczema
- Urticaria-recurring
- Herpes circinatus
- Paronychia

MODALITIES
- **Aggravation:** Lying on painful side, dry cold air, uncovering, eating or drinking cold things, touching affected parts, abuse of mercury, night, motion
- **Amelioration:** Warmth in general, wrapping up warmly especially the head (Psor., Sil.), in damp, wet weather, after eating

REMEDY RELATIONSHIP
- **Complementary:** Calen. in injuries of soft parts
- **Compare:** Sulph. for dry, itching, better by scratching, and not sensitive to touch; Acon., Spong., Staph., Sil., Calc-s., Myris.
- **Antidotes:** Bell., Cham., Sil. Bad effects of mercury and other metals; iodine, iodide of potash, cod-liver oil

HYDRASTIS CANADENSIS

INTRODUCTION

- **Common name:** Golden seal
- **Family:** *Ranunculaceae*
- **Source:** Vegetable kingdom
- **Part used:** Rhizome and root
- **Prover:** Hale

SPHERE OF ACTION

- Eyes
- Gastrointestinal system
- Respiratory system
- Mucous membranes
- Musculoskeletal system
- Urinary system
- Female genital system
- Skin

CONSTITUTION

- Suits old, cachectic, easily tired, debilitated persons. For emaciation, prostration and muscular weakness with mucoid discharges
- **Malignant dyscrasia with hepatic and gastric derangement, especially due to alcoholism**
- **Temperament:** Nervous, bilious
- **Thermal:** Chilly
- **Miasm:** Sycosis, Syphilis

MIND

- Irritability after dinner
- Weakness of memory, absent-minded
- Depressed; sure of death; desires death
- Indifference to everything
- Malicious, desire to strike
- Sadness, gloomy, taciturn, disagreeable
- Anxious
- Suspicious
- Nervous and sensitive
- Very restless
- Aversion to conversation

KEYNOTE SYMPTOMS

- **For constitutions broken down by excessive use of alcohol**
- Tendency to haemorrhages and ulceration
- Cancerous and pre-cancerous states with pain before ulceration starts; retards growth of cancer
- Catarrhal processes everywhere – mouth, throat, stomach, urethra, uterus, etc. with a mucoid discharge
- **Secretions – thick, yellow, ropy and tenacious**
- Stomatitis of nursing mothers or weak children; bitter taste
- **Loss of appetite with a sensation of emptiness or goneness in the region of stomach, worse after eating. Improves appetite**
- Cancer of stomach with emaciation; gastric ulcers, weak digestion
- Obstinate constipation, especially during pregnancy, with sinking sensation in the stomach; with foetid flatus
- Gargle in septic state of throat, in malignant scarlet fever
- Post-nasal dripping; hawking of thick, yellow mucous from posterior sinuses
- Catarrh of bladder with thick, yellow, gleety discharge. Difficult, painful micturition
- Goitre of pregnancy and puberty
- **Leucorrhoea, worse after menses; acrid, corroding, shreddy, tenacious, hanging from the os in long strings**
- Tumour or cancer of breast; retraction of nipple
- Pain across lumbar region. Must use arms in raising himself from the seat
- Excoriation of skin in infants
- Erysipelatous rash with severe, burning heat followed by exfoliation of the skin

CLINICAL

- Malnutrition
- Emaciation
- Prostration
- Cancer
- Ulceration
- Goitre
- Conjunctivitis
- Stomatitis
- Gastritis
- Constipation
- Haemorrhoids
- Eustachian catarrh
- Ozaena
- Sinusitis
- Bronchitis
- Gonorrhoea
- Prolapse
- Menorrhagia
- Arthritis
- Lumbago
- Leucorrhoea
- Cervical erosion
- Ingrown toe nails
- Pruritus vulvae
- Erysipelas
- Nettle rash
- Ulcers
- Lupus

MODALITIES

- **Aggravation:** Cold dry winds, inhaling air, open air, night, washing, touch
- **Amelioration:** Dry weather, warm coverings, rest, pressure

REMEDY RELATIONSHIP

- **Antidote:** Sulph.
- **Compare:** Xanrhi., Kali-bi., Con., Ars-i., Phyt., Gali., Aster., Stann., Puls; also Manz., Hydrinin-m., Hydrainin-s., Marr.

Hydrastis canadensis

HYDROCOTYLE ASIATICA

SPHERE OF ACTION

- Connective tissues
- Genitourinary system
- Female genital system
- Skin

INTRODUCTION

- **Common name:** Thankuni, Indian pennywort
- **Family:** *Umbelliferae*
- **Source:** Vegetable kingdom
- **Part used:** Whole plant
- **Prover:** Dr Andouit

CONSTITUTION

- Suits people with a dark dusky complexion, and a tendency to Acne, psoriasis, pustules, profuse sweating and difficulty in maintaining an upright posture
- **Temperament:** Nervous, bilious
- **Thermal:** Chilly, ambithermal
- **Miasm:** Psora, Sycosis, Syphilis

MIND

- Fearful
- Anxiety
- Restlessness
- Supression of desire
- Forgetfull, weak memory and concentration
- Loquacity
- Indifference

KEYNOTE SYMPTOMS

- Interstitial inflammation and cellular proliferation
- Hypertrophy and induration of connective tissue
- Neuralgia of supra and infra orbital nerves
- **Aversion to liquid food, tobacco smoking. Strong desire for lime juice**
- Cramping pain in stomach without nausea; rumbling in abdomen; wind colic
- Irritation and inflammation of neck of bladder. Profuse and frequent urination
- Heat at the bottom of the vagina, and pricking and itching at its orifice
- Intolerable itching of vagina; profuse leucorrhoea
- Pains of cervical cancer, cervical redness
- Granular ulceration of the womb, partly fungoid
- Acute and secondary gonorrhoea; suppressed gonorrhoea
- Back – difficulty in maintaining an upright posture
- Copious perspiration
- Great thickening of the epidermoid layer and exfoliation of scales
- **Copper coloured eruptions at various sites,** especially face
- In leprosy and lupus when ulceration has not set in various parts
- Intolerable itching, especially in soles of feet

CLINICAL

- Flatulence
- Wind colic
- Connective tissue disorders
- Orbital neuralgia
- Cervical cancer
- Uterine ulcers
- Syphilitic affections
- Leucorrhoea
- Gonorrhoea
- Exfoliation
- Leprosy
- Lupus
- Psoriasis
- Pemphigus
- Pustules
- Acne
- Dry eruptions
- Pruritus
- Abscesses
- Ichthyosis
- Elephantiasis

MODALITIES

- **Aggravation:** Heat
- **Amelioration:** Rest, cold

REMEDY RELATIONSHIP

- **Compare:** Elae. in scleroderma, elephantiasis, leprosy, skin thickened, itching and hardened, anaesthesia; Hura; Strych-g. in bites of serpents, ulcers and cutaneous affections generally; Chaulmoogra oil from seeds of Tarakiogenos; Hydr., Ars., Aur., Sep.

HYDROCYANICUM ACIDUM

INTRODUCTION

- **Common name:** Prussic acid, Hydrocyanic acid
- **Group:** Organic acid
- **Source:** Mineral kingdom
- **Formula:** HCN
- **Prover:** Jorg

SPHERE OF ACTION

- Brain
- Nervous system
- Gastrointestinal system
- Respiratory system
- Heart

CONSTITUTION

- It is an extremely toxic agent, producing a state of convulsions, paralysis, cyanosis, hysteria and epilepsy
- **Temperament:** Nervous, bilious
- **Thermal:** Chilly
- **Miasm:** Psora, Sycosis, Syphilis

MIND

- Anxiety and fretfulness
- **Confusion, better in open air**
- Inability to think
- Delusion, he is surrounded by friends, shaking hands and calling them by name; makes involutary motions and gestures
- **Fear of imaginary troubles**
- Fear of animals, horses, cars, street vehicles and falling of houses
- Sometimes rises in bed, gazes around vacantly and then throws self upon a pillow
- Wild delirium, laughs loudly
- Hydrophobia
- Insanity from excessive excitement; sometimes screams out suddenly and does not know why
- Thoughtless staring, violent sighing
- Morose, cross, fretful, peevish
- Fear of imaginary problems
- Vivid, incoherent dreams
- Depressed and discouraged
- Marked irritability, peevish temper

KEYNOTE SYMPTOMS

- Convulsions and paralysis, body becomes stiff and is thrown back
- Epileptic and hysterical convulsions; epilepsy preceded by nausea and vomiting
- Spasmodic constriction in the larynx, suffocation, palpitations, pain, tightness in the chest, etc.
- Suddenness of complaints such as collapse, spasms, apoplexy, unconsciousness, with coldness
- Cyanosis of lips and nails; bluish tinge of skin
- Collapse due to some pulmonary condition, in cholera
- **Violent, stupefying headaches. Brain feels as if on fire**
- Intense cerebral congestion; sudden and severe cases of meningitis
- Supraorbital neuralgia with flushing on the same side of the face
- Eyes turn towards the right and upwards followed by general spasms
- **Aversion to meat; drinks rumble through the throat and stomach**
- Sinking at the pit of the stomach; gastralgia and dyspepsia
- Cholera, during stage of collapse, with coldness. Stools are involuntary and accompanied with severe prostation and hiccoughs
- Asphyxia; asthma with contraction of the throat. Lung paralysis. Noisy and agitated breathing.
- Dry, spasmodic, suffocative cough, especially in tuberculosis and asthma
- **Clutches the heart, as if in distress. Pulse is weak and irregular**

CLINICAL

- Hydrophobia
- Collapse
- Convulsions
- Paralysis
- Hemiplegia
- Epilepsy
- Catalepsy
- Cyanosis
- Tetanus
- Meningitis
- Risus sardonicus
- Supraorbital neuralgia
- Gastralgia
- Cholera
- Asiatic cholera
- Contraction of larynx
- Whooping cough
- Asthma
- Angina pectoris
- Drowsiness

MODALITIES

- **Aggravation:** Full moon, suppressions, storms

REMEDY RELATIONSHIP

- **Compare:** Cic., Oena., Camph., Laur., Helo., Nux-v., Lach., Tab.
- **Antidoted by:** Camph., Coff., Ip., Nux-v., Op., Verat.

HYOSCYAMUS NIGER

INTRODUCTION
- **Common name:** Henbane, Black henbane
- **Family:** *Solanaceae*
- **Source:** Vegetable kingdom
- **Part used:** Whole plant of second year's growth
- **Prover:** Hahnemann

SPHERE OF ACTION
- Mind
- Eyes
- Ears
- Central nervous system
- Gastrointestinal system
- Respiratory system
- Musculoskeletal system
- Genitourinary organs

CONSTITUTION
- For irritable, nervous, hysterical people with a pale face and protruding eyes; have increased cerebral activity and absence of morals
- **Temperament:** Nervous, bilious, sanguine
- **Thermal:** Chilly, ambithermal
- **Miasm:** Psora, Sycosis, Syphilis

MIND
- Bad effects of unfortunate love, with anger, rage, jealousy
- **Lascivious mania, obscene mania uncovers body, sings obscene songs; nymphomania**
- Restlessness; delirium – low muttering
- Talkative; loquacious, laughs at everything, speaks rapidly and changes subject
- Very suspicious; scared to eat or drink, to take what is offered
- Fear of being alone, being pursued, of water, of being poisoned, of being bitten, of syphilis, of being betrayed, of being sold
- Desire for company
- Depression
- Quarrelsome mania
- Absence of morals
- Flamboyant stage of exhibitionism or mania

KEYNOTE SYMPTOMS
- Increased, non-inflammatory cerebral activity
- Convulsions and spasmodic affections frequently
- Tremulous weakness and twitching of tendons. Every muscle of the body twitches from eyes to toes without consciousness
- Makes ridiculous gestures, picks at bed clothes with fingers; carphology
- Epileptic attacks ending in deep sleep
- **Tongue, dry, red, cracked, stiff, immovable; difficult speech**
- **Teeth yellow, covered with sordes; toothache, after taking cold or in open air**
- Colic as if the abdomen would burst, distention, tympanites
- Spasms from worms. Before attack – vertigo, sparks before eyes, ringing in the ears and gnawing hunger
- Elongated uvula. Dry, spasmodic constriction of the throat; difficulty in swallowing
- Dry, spasmodic, hacking cough; worse lying down, at night; suffocating attacks
- Increased sexual desire. Tendency for masturbation
- Spasms in pregnant women
- Impotence, plays with genitals during fever. Tendency to expose genitals
- Intense sleeplessness, with restlessness twitching and startings; coma, sopor with convulsions

CLINICAL
- Behavioural disorders
- Mania
- Schizophrenia
- Senility
- Alzheimer's diseases
- Lasciviousness
- Cerebral accidents
- Epilepsy
- Seizures
- Twitching
- Chorea
- Tetanus
- Delirium tremens
- Meningitis
- Strabismus
- Diplopia
- Hiccough
- Vomiting
- Colic
- Toxic gastritis
- Diarrhoea
- Constipation
- Faecal impaction
- Cough
- Haemoptysis
- Enuresis
- Puerperal mania
- Typhoid
- Typhus
- Biting nails
- Insomnia

MODALITIES
- **Aggravation:** At night, during menses, mental affections, jealousy, unhappy love, when lying down, after eating, touch
- **Amelioration:** Stooping, sitting up, warmth, motion

REMEDY RELATIONSHIP
- **Compare:** Bell., Stram., Agar., Gels., Verat.; Phos. often cures lasciviousness when Hyos. fails.; Nux-v. or Opium in haemoptysis of drunkards
- **Follows well:** Bell. in deafness after apoplexy.
- **Antidotes:** Bell., Camph., Stram.

HYPERICUM PERFORATUM

SPHERE OF ACTION

- Mind
- Nervous system
- Gastrointestinal system
- Respiratory system
- Musculoskeletal system
- Female genital system
- Skin

INTRODUCTION

- **Common name:** St John's wort
- **Family:** *Hypericaceae*
- **Source:** Vegetable kingdom
- **Part used:** Whole plant
- **Prover:** Dr Muller

CONSTITUTION

- Suits nervous constitutions
- For nerve injuries, especially of fingers, toes and nails
- **Temperament:** Nervous, bilious
- **Thermal:** Chilly, ambithermal
- **Miasm:** Psora, Sycosis, Syphilis

MIND

- Ailments from fright; mental effects of injury, frights, shock
- Feels as if lifted high in air, or patient has anxiety lest he falls from a height
- Makes mistakes in writing; omits letters
- Makes mistakes in speaking; uses wrong words, saying right for left or vice versa
- Neurasthenia; brain fag
- Forgets what she wants to say
- Drowsiness
- Melancholic, depressed
- Restlessness
- Anxiety
- Irritability, speaks sharply
- Delirium, talks nonsense

KEYNOTE SYMPTOMS

- **Complaints from fright, shock, injury to head, following wounds, surgical operations, spinal taps or injections**
- **Remedy for injury to nerves especially of finger, toes and nails; crushing injury of finger tips**
- Nerve injury from animal bites. Punctured and penetrating wounds; infected wounds
- Neuritis, burning, tingling and numbness
- Where nerve trunks have been handled, stretched or bruised and when partial paralysis exists. Postural paresis. Paresis caused by entanglement of nerves in scars
- Neuralgia of leg with profuse sweating
- Excessive pain with injury
- Tetanus – after traumatic injuries. Prevents lock jaw.
- Convulsions after concussion; blows to head; spasms after injury. Brain and spinal cord injuries
- **Injury to coccyx, from a fall. Spine very sensitive to touch,** after a fall
- Vertigo. Head feels elongated to a point, extending upward like a conical hat; throbbing in the vertex. Falling out of hair
- Facial neuralgia and toothache; nerve pain after dental procedure
- **Thirst, nausea, tongue coated white at base, tip clean**
- Attack of asthma with changes of weather or before storms, or during foggy weather; better perspiration, after expectoration
- Cramps in calf muscles. Crawling in hands and feet
- Skin rough, feels as if full of small knots
- Nails groove or become deformed after the removal of a splinter or foreign body

CLINICAL

- Nerve injuries
- Traumatic neuralgia
- Post-operative pains
- Neuritis
- Venous system – capillary paralysis
- Congestion
- Punctured wounds
- Lymphangitis
- Tetanus
- Lock jaw
- Facial neuralgia
- Facial paralysis
- Tooth extraction
- Haemorrhoids
- Rheumatoid inflammation
- Coccygodynia
- Bunions
- Corns
- Crushed fingers

MODALITIES

- **Aggravation:** In cold, dampness, in a fog, in a closed room, least exposure, touch, injury, puncture, bites, stings, surgery, jar, pressure
- **Amelioration:** Bending head backwards, rubbing, lying on face, lying quietly

REMEDY RELATIONSHIP

- **Compare:** Arn., Calen., Ruta, Staph., Led. in punctured wounds and bites of animals; Coff.
- In wounds where formerly Acon. and Arn. were given alternately, Hyper. cures
- **Antidotes:** Ars., Cham., Led.

IBERIS AMARA

SPHERE OF ACTION
- Mind
- Cardiovascular system
- Gastrointestinal system
- Musculoskeletal system
- Skin

INTRODUCTION
- **Common name:** Bitter candytuft
- **Family:** *Cruciferae*
- **Source:** Vegetable kingdom
- **Part used:** Seeds
- **Prover:** Hale and Sabin

CONSTITUTION
- For cases with hypertrophy of the heart; conciousness of heart's action
- **Temperament:** Nervous, bilious
- **Thermal:** Chilly
- **Miasm:** Psora, Sycosis, Syphilis

MIND
- Anxiety with trembling; fearful
- Irritable, especially in the morning. Bad tempered
- Restless sleep with frightful dreams
- Sentimental
- Weakness or loss of memory, trouble in remembering recent events
- Excited, frightened feeling with cold sweat on the face
- Diminished intelligence
- Sad with a desire to sigh
- Fear of taking a lot of medicines

KEYNOTE SYMPTOMS
- Whole body sore, lame and trembling
- Desires to lie down due to trembling, weakness and nervousness
- **Vertigo begins in nape of neck or occiput; as if occiput were turning around; eyes feel forced outwards**
- Desires alcoholic stimulants
- Liver region full and painful. Heavy, full sensation gastric and liver region
- Cough causes redness of face
- Constant hawking of thick and stringy mucous
- **Controls vascular excitement in cardiac hypertrophy with thickening of the walls of the heart**
- Cardiac debility after influenza
- Cardiac dyspnoea. Conscious of heart's action
- Sharp, stinging pains from before backwards, on least exertion, even on coughing or laughing
- Palpitations with vertigo and choking in the throat
- Pulse full, irregular, intermittent; tachycardia

CLINICAL
- Dropsy
- Numbness
- Vertigo
- Headache
- Hepatomegaly
- Jaundice
- Enlarged heart
- Cardiac dyspnoea
- Cardiac dilatation
- Cardiac hypertrophy
- Palpitations
- Tachycardia
- Angina pectoris

MODALITIES
- **Aggravation:** Lying down, on the left side, motion, exertion, warm room, on rising
- **Amelioration:** Eating, belching, passing flatus

REMEDY RELATIONSHIP
- **Compare:** Cact., Dig., Aml-ns., Bell., Crat., Spig., Lepi.

IGNATIA AMARA

INTRODUCTION

- **Common name:** St Ignatius bean
- **Family:** *Loganiaceae*
- **Source:** Vegetable kingdom
- **Part used:** Seeds
- **Prover:** Hahnemann

SPHERE OF ACTION

- Mind
- Blood vessels
- Gastrointestinal system
- Respiratory system
- Musculoskeletal system
- Female genital system

CONSTITUTION

- Especially suited to sensitive, easily excited women with dark hair and skin, having a mild disposition but are quick to perceive and rapid in execution
- For those who are mentally and physically exhausted by long, concentrated grief
- **Temperament:** Nervous, bilious, mild
- **Thermal:** Chilly
- **Miasm:** Psora, Sycosis, Syphilis

MIND

- Hysteria. Rapid change of physical and mental state
- Acute grief, acute disappointments makes patient bitter and hardened
- **Depth of sorrow and grief stuck deep within, cannot be surfaced**
- Romantic, idealistic, emotional, oversensitive, easily hurt
- Alert, oversensitive and nervous individuals
- Incredible change of moods, jesting and laughter changing to sadness and tears, or weeping alternating with laughing
- Great defensiveness and touchiness; easily offended. Cramping of emotions leads to defensiveness
- Jealous suspicious and doubtful
- Rigid. Quarrelsome, rude. At times rapid alternation of moods (Sep., Lil-t.)
- Ailments from silent grief and disappointment in love
- Broods over imaginary troubles
- Involuntary sighing and sobbing

KEYNOTE SYMPTOMS

- **Changeable, erratic symptoms**
- **Remedy for contradiction** – pain in ears better by music, piles better by walking, haemorrhoids and prolapsus ani with loose stool, sore throat better by swallowing, thirst during chill but no thirst during fever, empty feeling in stomach not better by eating, etc.
- Oversensitiveness to pain; pain in small, circumscribed spots
- **Cannot bear tobacco, smoking – aggravates headache, toothache, vomiting**
- Tendency to clonic spasms; twitching of muscles of face, lips whenever patient attempts to talk; spasms and convulsions ending in long sighs; convulsions in children
- Headache, as if a nail was driven out of the side of head terminating with profuse flow of urine
- Face changes colour, when at rest
- Deep, involuntary sighing – takes deep breaths for ameliorating sinking in the stomach. Craving for acids
- Sour taste and constant salivation; bites inside of cheeks while talking or chewing
- Stitching pain between acts of swallowing. Globus hystericus
- Spasms and cramps in abdomen. Extreme flatus and flatulent colic with hysteria; fullness and distention causes difficulty in breathing
- Constipation – from cold, carriage riding; urge felt in upper intestines. Stool soft but difficult to expel
- Itching, stitching pains in rectum; rectal prolapse
- Hoarse, hacking, dry, irritating cough – the more the patient coughs, more the cough is aggravated
- Reflex cough from remote affections like that of the womb, ovaries, worms, etc.
- Dyspnoea, must take a deep breath for relief
- Menses suppressed or uterine haemorrhage from grief. Threatened miscarriage from grief
- Sighing before menses; menstrual cramps

CLINICAL

- Hysteria
- Depression
- Chronic fatigue syndrome
- Spasms
- Tetanus
- Chorea
- Obesity
- Plague
- Hirsuitism
- Alopecia
- Congestive headache
- Migraine
- Encephalitis
- Blepharospasm
- Asthenopia
- Toothache
- Bulimia
- Hiccough
- Globus hystericus
- Hysterical vomiting
- Rectal cramps
- Constipation
- Rectal fissures
- Rectal prolapse
- Laryngismus stridulus
- Follicular tonsillitis
- Cough
- Asthma
- Catamenia
- Premenstrual syndrome
- Metrorrhagia
- Dysmenorrhoea
- Leucorrhoea
- Lumbago

MODALITIES

- **Aggravation:** From tobacco, coffee, brandy, contact, motion, strong odours, mental emotions, grief, shock, in the morning, open air
- **Amelioration:** Warmth, hard pressure (Chin.); swallowing, walking, change of position, while eating, lying on back or affected part

REMEDY RELATIONSHIP

- **Compare:** Zinc., Kali-p., Sep., Cimic., Nat-m., Ph-ac. in chronic grief; Bell., Caust., Hyos, Lach., Lyc., Phos., in difficulty in swallowing liquids; Apis., Lach., Hyos. in jealously; also Cupr. Plat., Asaf., Sep., Staph., Op.
- **Complementary:** Nat-m.
- **Incompatible:** Coff., Nux-v., Tab.
- **Antidoted by:** Puls. (chiefly), Cham., Cocc., Coff., Arn., Camph.

INSULINUM

SPHERE OF ACTION
- Pancreas
- Liver
- Gastrointestinal system
- Musculoskeletal system
- Skin

INTRODUCTION
- **Common name:** Insulin
- **Group:** Hormone from pancreas
- **Source:** Animal kingdom
- **Prover:** William F. Baker and S.K. Ghosh

CONSTITUTION
- Suits constitutions broken down by suppurative and infectious diseases
- **Temperament:** Nervous, bilious
- **Thermal:** Chilly
- **Miasm:** Psora, Sycosis, Syphilis

MIND
- Easily discouraged; sad
- Very tired feeling
- Irritability, worse contradiction
- Angry
- Anxious
- Suspicious

KEYNOTE SYMPTOMS
- Restores the lost ability to oxidize carbohydrates and store glycogen in the liver
- After effects of acute infectious diseases with a disordered liver like – ulcers, boils, bed sores
- Emaciation, debility, when well selected remedies fail to act; with loose bowels
- **Craving for sweets**
- Chronic intestinal complaints with diarrhoea and an enlarged liver
- **Chronic, painless liver enlargement with all complaints**
- Enlarged liver with a suppurative condition
- Intestinal complaints with chronic diarrhoea; chronic diarrhoea in children with debility and an enlarged liver
- Case of persistent skin irritation, acne, boils or varicose ulceration with polyuria. Diabetes
- Acne, carbuncles, chronic erythema, eczema
- Skin – pale, yellow

CLINICAL
- Acute infections
- Weakness
- Prostration
- Chronic enlarged liver
- Hepatitis
- Diarrhoea
- Dysentery
- Constipation
- Asthma
- Polyuria
- Diabetes
- Glycosuria
- Gout
- Typhoid
- Acne
- Boils
- Carbuncles
- Erythema
- Eczema
- Varicose ulcers
- Bed sores

MODALITIES
- **Aggravation:** After typhoid or pneumonia

REMEDY RELATIONSHIP
- **Compare:** Chin., Phos., Caps., Calc-ar.

IODIUM

INTRODUCTION
- **Common name:** Iodine
- **Group:** Metal
- **Source:** Mineral kingdom
- **Formula:** I
- **Prover:** Hahnemann

SPHERE OF ACTION
- Glandular system – lymph glands, thyroid, salivary
- Gastrointestinal system
- Respiratory system
- Circulatory system
- Connective tissues
- Mucous membranes
- Female genital system
- Male genital system

CONSTITUTION
- For extremely thin persons of dark or black hair, eyes with low cachectic condition, profound debility and general emaciation, overgrown body with hypertrophy and induration of glands
- Suits tubercular and scrofulous diathesis
- **Temperament:** Irritable
- **Thermal:** Hot
- **Miasm:** Sycosis, Tubercular

MIND
- Very weak mentally, lachrymose
- Great anxiety when quiet with depression. Must keep himself busy. Sudden impulse to do violence and to kill.
- Wants to do everything hurriedly. Mentally exhausted, but continues to work
- Melancholic, suicidal tendency
- Forgetful, forgets what he was about to say
- Irritability; cross and restless

KEYNOTE SYMPTOMS
- Acute excerbations of chronic inflammations
- Emaciation and weight loss despite a good appetite, with glandular atrophy
- All glands are hypertrophied and enlarged except mammary glands, which dwindle and become flabby
- Profound debility – least effort induces sweating; loss of breath from going upstairs
- **Emaciation of single parts**
- Locally, it is used as a disinfectant and microbicide; and as a paint in all swellings
- Acts prominently on all connective tissues
- Pulsations in large arterial trunks, all over the body
- Profuse lachrymation. Pain in eyes, pupils dilated. Acute dacryocystitis.
- Ravenous hunger; relieved while eating and after eating; however, loses flesh while eating well; anxious if does not eat
- Liver, spleen and mesenteric glands are sore and enlarged
- Haemorrhage with stool; constipation, better by drinking cold milk; constipation alternates with diarrhoea
- Pneumonia, especially right sided with high temprature. Hepatization spreads rapidly. Pleuritic effusion.
- Croupy, wheezy cough with difficult respiration; raw, tickling feeling all over chest provoking dry cough
- Tuberculosis – pulmonary, tabes-mesenterica, in rapidly growing, thin, dark people
- **Painful compression felt around the heart, as if grasped by an iron hand**
- **Urine dark, yellow-green, thick, acrid, copious and frequent**
- Leucorrhoea – acrid, corroding, slimy and thick; with ovaritis
- Wedge – like pain from ovaries to uterus
- Dwindling of breasts; atrophy of mammary glands
- Testicles swollen and indurated; painless swelling with offensive sweat
- **Acrid foot sweat**

CLINICAL
- Atrophy
- Malnutrition
- Debility
- Tremors
- Glandular affections
- Nodosities
- Lead poisoning
- Plague
- Goitre
- Headache
- Appetite disorders
- Pancreatitis
- Jaundice
- Diarrhoea
- Constipation
- Anosmia
- Eustachian deafness
- Adenoids
- Laryngitis
- Diphtheria
- Throat affections
- Cough
- Lung affections
- Pneumonia
- Pleuritic effusion
- Heart affections
- Myocarditis
- Palpitations
- Tachycardia
- Ovaritis
- Uterine haemorrhage
- Acrid leucorrhoea
- Sterility
- Orchitis
- Hydrocoele
- Atrophied testis
- Arthritis deformans
- Rheumatism
- Rickets

MODALITIES
- **Aggravation:** Warmth, wraping up the head, when quiet, in a warm room, right side, sitting up, exertion, touch, pressure, fasting
- **Amelioration:** Walking in open air, cold bathing, eating

REMEDY RELATIONSHIP
- **Complementary:** Lyc., Bad.
- **Compare:** Acet-ac., Brom., Con., Kali-bi., Spong.; Hep., Merc., Phos., Abrot., Nat-m., Sanic., Tub.
- Pathogenesis is similar to that of Carb-ac.
- **Follows well:** Hep., Merc.; is followed by Kali-bi. in croup.
- **Antidotes:** Merc.

IPECACUANHA

SPHERE OF ACTION
- Pneumogastric nerve
- Gastrointestinal system
- Respiratory system
- Musculoskeletal system
- Female genital system

INTRODUCTION
- **Common name:** Ipecac root
- **Family:** *Rubiaceae*
- **Source:** Vegetable kingdom
- **Part used:** Roots and rhizome
- **Prover:** Hahnemann

CONSTITUTION
Adapted to fat children and adults who are feeble; who catch a cold in a relaxing atmosphere or warm, moist weather. Face blue, cyanosed. Disposed to haemorrhages.
- **Temperament:** Nervous, bilious
- **Thermal:** Chilly
- **Miasm:** Psora, Sycosis, Syphilis

MIND
- Ailments from anger, mortification, vexation and indigestion
- Holds everything in contempt and desires that others should also do the same
- Cries, screams, howls and is hard to please
- Full of desires, but does not know for what
- Faints suddenly during summer or in a hot room
- Intolerance to noise
- Tranquility after anger
- Anxiety during fever
- Censorious, critical
- Delusion, he is unfortunate
- Haughty, irritable

KEYNOTE SYMPTOMS
- **All complaints are accompanied with constant nausea and persistent vomiting; nausea is not better by vomiting**
- Discharges are adhesive, sticky, stringy, yellow, tough, lumpy or thick
- **Pain can be covered with a point of finger; spotty pain**
- Tendency for active or passive haemorrhages – bright red from all orifices with nausea
- Migraine or gastric headache with intense nausea and vomiting
- **Tongue clean, moist. Saliva increased**
- Nausea from looking at moving objects or at food
- **Craving for sweets, dainties. Aversion and disgust to all food**
- Indulgence in beer and malt liquors
- Vomiting during pregnancy. Gastroenteritis; food posioning
- Stomach feels relaxed, as if hanging down. Pain – clutching, squeezing, griping – as from a hand, each finger sharply pressing into the abdomen, around the naval
- **Stool green, grass-like, frothy molasses**
- Amoebic dysentery with tenesmus. While straining, there is so much pain that it nauseates. Little thirst.
- Autumnal dysentery and first stages of Asiatic cholera where nausea and vomiting predominate
- Whooping cough with epistaxis and bleeding from the mouth
- Dyspnoea with constant constriction of the chest
- Violent cough, chest feels full of phlegm which does not yield to coughing. Rattling of mucous in bronchi during inspiration
- Menses too early, too profuse, haemorrhagic – active or passive, bright red
- Rheumatism alternates with gastric symptoms or dysentery
- **Ulcers deep, perforating, round, punched with overhanging edges or thick crusts**

CLINICAL
- Neuralgia
- Haemorrhages
- Cyanosis
- Cramps
- Tetanus
- Migraine
- Photophobia
- Conjunctivitis
- Hypermetropia
- Periorbital neuralgia
- Hiccough
- Nausea
- Vomiting
- Gastric ulcer
- Haematemesis
- Dysentery
- Epistaxis
- Coryza
- Hoarseness
- Aphonia
- Cough
- Croup
- Haemoptysis
- Dyspnoea
- Bronchitis
- Asthma
- Phthisis
- Bubbling rales
- Haematuria
- Menorrhagia
- Metrorrhagia
- Miscarriage
- Recurring fevers

MODALITIES
- **Aggravation:** Winter and dry weather; warm, moist, south winds, slightest motion, from veal, lying down
- **Amelioration:** Open air, rest, pressure, cold drinks, closing eyes

REMEDY RELATIONSHIP
- **Complementary:** Cupr., Arn.
- **Followed well:** Bry, Ars. in influenza, chills, croup, debility, cholera infantum; Ant-t. in foreign bodies in the larynx
- **Similar:** Puls., Ant-c., gastric troubles.
- **Compare:** Ip., Lob., Blatta, in asthma; Ars., Tab., Cham., Puls, Ant-t., Squil., Conv.
- **Antidoted by:** Ars., Chin., Tab., Arn., Dulc., Ferr., Op., Sul-ac.

IRIS VERSICOLOR

SPHERE OF ACTION
- Salivary glands
- Pancreas
- Liver
- Intestinal mucous membrane
- Skin

INTRODUCTION
- **Common name:** Blue flag
- **Family:** *Iridaceae*
- **Source:** Vegetable kingdom
- **Part used:** Rhizome
- **Prover:** Rowland

CONSTITUTION
- For those with an anxious expression on the face and vesicular and pustular eruptions on face, around nose, lips and cheeks
- **Temperament:** Nervous, bilious
- **Thermal:** Chilly
- **Miasm:** Psora, Sycosis, Syphilis

MIND
- Discouraged, low spirited, dull. Great depression with headache. Sad, despondent.
- Nervous debility; more tired in the morning than in the evening
- Fear of an approaching illness
- **Dreams of falling into a grave, of snakes, of suffocation**
- Tired feeling
- Irritability
- Memory weak
- Restless at night
- Cannot fix mind on any subject; mind wanders while writing

KEYNOTE SYMPTOMS
- Right sided, especially for headache and supraorbital neuralgia
- Pains are erratic, generally shoot from right to left
- Profuse secretions which are sour, acrid and burning
- Sourness; whole person smells sour
- **Periodicity of complaints as in headache, pains; diarrhoea and dysentery recur every spring and autumn, diarrhoea and pain everyday at 2 or 3 am**
- Pustular eruptions on the scalp
- Sick headache, generally induced by eating anything sweet – dull, throbbing or shooting, especially right side, with nausea and profuse salivation
- Facial neuralgia, after breakfast every morning with a stupefying, stunning headache; right side affected
- **Profuse ropy saliva, drops while talking**
- **Taste first sweetish or insipid, later burning. Tongue and gums feel as if covered by a greasy substance in the morning**
- Appetite reduced; nausea and empty eructations; continuous nausea
- Bilious, watery, sour, acrid or sweetish vomitus with burning along the whole digestive system. Mouth and stomach feels as if on fire, mouth and tongue feel scalded; cancer of pylorus
- Pain in stomach before breakfast. Burning of entire alimentary canal
- Everything in the stomach turns to vinegar
- **Sweat smells strongly of vinegar during fever**
- Fine eruptions; severe itching at night

CLINICAL
- Goitre
- Headache
- Hemicrania
- Infraorbital neuralgia
- Deafness
- Meniere's disease
- Nausea
- Vomiting
- Diarrhoea
- Dysentery
- Cholera
- Constipation
- Pancreatitis
- Diabetes
- Gonorrhoeal rheumatism
- Sciatica
- Pustules
- Eczema
- Psoriasis
- Herpes zoster

MODALITIES
- **Aggravation:** In the evening, at night, from rest, mental exhaustion
- **Amelioration:** From continuous gentle motion

REMEDY RELATIONSHIP
- **Compare:** Iris-fl., Iris-fa., Iris-g., Iris-te., Pancr., Peps., Ip., Podo., Sang., Ars., Ant-c.
- **Antidote:** Nux-v.

Iris versicolor

JALAPA

INTRODUCTION
- **Common name:** Jalap, Iponoea purga
- **Family:** *Convolvulaceae*
- **Source:** Vegetable kingdom
- **Part used:** Root
- **Prover:** Noack and Trinks

SPHERE OF ACTION
- Mind
- Gastrointestinal system
- Respiratory system
- Musculoskeletal system
- Skin

CONSTITUTION
- Suits the child who is good all day, but screams, and is restless and troublesome at night
- **Temperament:** Tubercular
- **Thermal:** Chilly, ambithermal
- **Miasm:** Sycosis

MIND
- Irritability only at night
- Restlessness and anxiety
- Restlessness day and night with every complaint
- Anxiety with stools
- Wants to be carried
- Inconsolable
- Desire to be occupied during the day, prefers to read, to study, no desire to play with toys
- Precocious, curious
- Very clever children
- Shrieking, screaming and shouting at night with diarrhoea

KEYNOTE SYMPTOMS
- Fainting fits, weakness, excessive uneasiness and tossing about of limbs
- Complaints worse at night
- General coldness with infantile diarrhoea and a blue face
- **Tongue smooth, glazed, dry, smarting**
- **Craving for chocolate, salt, vinegar, oil**
- **Aversion to mother's milk; vomits after milk**
- Cutting colic before and during stools. In adults with cutting pains, especially in the sigmoid colon with coldness and prostration
- Pinching and griping in the abdomen, as if it would be cut into pieces. Stools worse at night
- Watery, muddy, bloody, sour smelling stools with a weak pulse
- Child shrieks, screams, shouts and tosses about during diarrhoea or any other complaint
- Aching in limbs; marked uneasiness and tossing about of limbs
- **Perspiration, especially on head and upper part of the body**

CLINICAL
- Summer complaints
- Weakness
- Fainting fits
- Enterocolitis
- Gastrocolitis
- Colic
- Diarrhoea
- Dysentery
- Cholera
- Constipation
- Haemorrhoids
- Sinusitis
- Cough
- Tuberculosis

MODALITIES
- **Aggravation:** Night
- **Amelioration:** Pain in stomach relieved by belching a frothy matter and by passing flatus

REMEDY RELATIONSHIP
- **Compare:** Camph., Coloc., Bell., Merc., Phytol., Iris-t.
- **Antidotes:** Elat., Cann-s., Merc.

KALIUM BICHROMICUM

INTRODUCTION

- **Common name:** Bichromate of potash, Potassium bichromate
- **Group:** Mineral salt
- **Source:** Mineral kingdom
- **Formula:** $K_2Cr_2O_7$
- **Prover:** Dr. J. Drysdale

SPHERE OF ACTION

- Gastrointestinal system
- Respiratory system
- Musculoskeletal system
- Mucous membranes
- Heart
- Urinary system
- Skin

MIND

- Low spirited; ill humoured
- Aversion to mental and physical exertion
- Talks to himself
- Vanishing of thoughts
- Sadness after annoyance. Gloomy; indifference to business affairs
- Irritability, better after eating
- Easily gets attached

MODALITIES

- **Aggravation:** Heat of summer; hot weather, beer, morning, undressing, stooping, cold damp open air
- **Amelioration:** Skin symptoms are better in cold weather otherwise better from heat, wrapping up, pressure, motion

KEYNOTE SYMPTOMS

- Adapted to the subacute stages of disease
- **Pain – in spots – can be covered with the tip of a finger – wandering, periodic, occurs at the same hour each day, come and go suddenly**
- Dilatation of stomach; round ulcer of stomach
- Thick, lumpy, gluey, stringy, viscid, **adherent discharges; can be drawn into long strings. Yellow or yellow-green in colour.**
- The mucous membranes of the air passages, nose, pharynx, stomach, duodenum have a tendency for deep perforation and ulceration
- **Punched out, perforating ulcers, on skin, mucous membranes and bones**
- **Tongue yellow or glistening, cracked, red, dry and shiny; sensation of a hair on the tongue**
- Alternating and shifting conditions – pain travels from one part to another, rheumatic pain alternates with gastric complaints, etc.
- Uvula is oedematous, relaxed. Formation of false membrane in diphtheria and croup with hoarse, metallic cough.
- Profuse, watery nasal discharge. Post-nasal discharge with hawking
- Coryza with nasal obstruction and violent sneezing; discharge of plugs or clinkers. Chronic ozaena
- Perforation of nasal septum; chronic catarrh and ozaena. **Foetid smell. Thick, ropy, greenish-yellow discharge.**
- **After urine, a drop seems to remain which cannot be discharged**
- Ropy mucous in urine; bloody urine with backache
- Copious, viscid, ropy leucorrhoea; vulval pruritus with burning and excitement

CONSTITUTION

- Suits fair, fat, light haired persons who suffer from catarrhal, syphilitic or psoric affections
- Suits fat, chubby children with a short neck having a tendency for croupy affections
- **Temperament:** Nervous, bilious
- **Thermal:** Chilly
- **Miasm:** Psora, Sycosis, Syphilis

CLINICAL

- Obesity
- Migraine
- Trachoma
- Colic
- Gastritis
- Peptic ulcer
- Cirrhosis
- Diarrhoea
- Dysentery
- Constipation
- Nasal polyp
- Anosmia
- Coryza
- Chronic ozaena
- Sinusitis
- Laryngitis
- Pharyngitis
- Diphtheria
- Post nasal discharge
- Croup
- Bronchitis
- Hypertension
- Nephritis
- Albuminuria
- Diabetes
- Ovarian cyst
- Dysmenorrhoea
- Arthritis
- Rheumatism
- Sciatica
- Backache
- Ulcers

REMEDY RELATIONSHIP

- **Follows well:** Canth. or Carb-ac. has removed the scrapings in dysentery. Iod. in croup, when hoarse cough, with tough membrane, general weakness and coldness are present; Calc. in acute or chronic nasal catarrh. Ant-t. in catarrhal affections and skin diseases.
- **Compare:** Ant-t., Brom., Hep., Ind., Calc., Ant-c., Caust., Sul-ac., Ip. in production of false membrane; Puls., Kali-c., Hydr., Sil., Phyt.
- **Antidotes:** Ars., Lach.

SPHERE OF ACTION

- Mind
- Central nervous system
- Cardiovascular system
- Mucous membranes
- Anus
- Throat
- Genital system

INTRODUCTION

- **Common name:** Bromide of Potash, Potassium bromide
- **Group:** Mineral salt
- **Source:** Mineral kingdom
- **Part used:** KBr

CONSTITUTION

- Suits fleshy people inclined to obesity, especially children and nervous women with tendency to crops of boils
- **Temperament:** Nervous
- **Thermal:** Chilly
- **Miasm:** Sycosis

KALIUM BROMATUM

MIND

- Nervous, restless; cannot sit still, must move about or keep occupied
- Restlessness, sleeplessness and brain fag due to worry, grief, sexual excess, loss of property or reputation, from business embarrasments. Weakness, anxiety, brain fag
- Stammering; slow and difficult speech
- Complete loss of memory; forgets how to talk and walk. Absentmindedness.
- Amnesic aphasia; has to be told the word before he can speak it
- Paranoia, schizophrenia, thinks he is being pushed, paranoid delusions
- Night terrors in children, cannot be comforted
- Profound melancholic depression with religious delusions and depression. Uncontrollable weeping
- Delusion in pregnant women that they have or will commit a crime
- Fear of breaking down under stress; loss of self confidence

KEYNOTE SYMPTOMS

- **Marked periodicity in symptoms**
- Acts upon the mind and nerves producing failure of mental power
- General numbness and anaesthesia – of mucous membranes, of fauces, larynx, pharynx, urethra, other parts of the body
- Lowered temperature, coldness of extremities
- Weakens the heart. **Feeble heart, action slow and fluttering.** Cardiac neurosis from uterine or spinal irritation
- **Pulse first accelerated, later slower and small**
- Vasomotor capillary spasm
- Numb feeling in brain; brain fag
- Epilepsy during new moon, at menstrual period.
- **Can pronounce any word told, but cannot speak otherwise**
- **Foetid breath; has a peculiar sickening odour**
- Cholera infantum with reflex irritation of the brain
- Vomiting with intense thirst; persistant hiccough
- Daily colic of infants at 5 am
- Excessive sexual desire, increased during menses. Nymphomania
- Impotency with debility, melancholy, loss of memory; effect of sexual excesses, incoordination of muscles; numbness; and tingling in limbs. Effects of sexual excesses
- Hands and fingers in constant motion. Fidgety; busy hands. Twitching of fingers
- Removes tendency to boils and unsightly marks in fleshy persons
- Skin eruptions, acne, psoriasis, at puberty or menstrual period
- Acne in young people; itching pimples and pustules leaving scars
- Somnambulism, especially in children

CLINICAL

- Cerebral accidents
- Schizophrenia
- Seizures
- Convulsions
- Sensory and motor paralysis
- Incoordination of muscles
- Ataxia
- Tabes dorsalis
- Delirium tremens
- Giddiness
- Hiccough
- Cholera infantum
- Diabetes mellitus
- Incontinence
- Ovarian tumours
- Ovarian cysts
- Ovarian neuralgia
- Uterine fibroids
- Puerperal nymphomania
- Puerperal mania
- Impotency
- Spermatorrhoea
- Chronic gout
- Psoriasis
- Acne
- Boils
- Drowsiness

MODALITIES

- **Aggravation:** Mental exertion, emotions, anger, grief, at night, sexual excess, summers, before during and after menses
- **Amelioration:** When occupied mentally or physically

REMEDY RELATIONSHIP

- **Antidoted by:** Vegetable acids, oils, Camph., Nux-v., Zinc
- **Follows well:** Acon., Spong. in croup; Eug. in acne
- **Compare:** Brom., Camph-br., Am-br., Aur-br., Kali-i, Kali-p., Calc., Hyos., Plat., Arg-n., Glon. Staph., Gels., Con., Bov., Stram., Ip., Zinc., Tarent.

KALIUM CARBONICUM

INTRODUCTION
- **Common name:** Carbonate of potassium, Potassium carbonate
- **Group:** Mineral salt
- **Source:** Mineral kingdom
- **Formula:** K_2CO_3

SPHERE OF ACTION
- Gastrointestinal system
- Respiratory system
- Heart
- Mucous membranes
- Musculoskeletal system
- Urinary system
- Female genital system

CONSTITUTION
- Suits people with dark skin and hair, lax fibre and an inclination to obesity
- For diseases of old people who are fleshy with a dropsical and paretic condition. Puffiness of upper eyelids and paretic tendencies
- Tubercular diathesis
- **Temperament:** Nervous, bilious
- **Thermal state:** Chilly
- **Miasm:** Psora

MIND
- Great aversion to being alone, desire for company, but treats them badly
- Alternating moods
- Obstinate, has strong rigid beliefs
- Anxiety arising from chest
- Afraid of imaginary things; full of fears and imagination
- Dreams of thieves, ghosts, diseases, dead people, etc.
- Easily frightened, kleptomania
- Indifference to surroundings with physical exhaustion
- Marked irritability and peevishness
- Severe depression, with want of self confidence
- Weakness of memory
- Mental dullness

KEYNOTE SYMPTOMS
- Ailments from loss of fluids or vitality, especially anaemia
- **Sweat, backache and weakness are the three cardinal symptoms**
- Oversensitiveness; cannot bear to be touched, even lightly, especially on feet
- Pains are sharp stitching, cutting and darting, worse during rest and on lying on the affected side; nearly all pains are better on motion. Hypersensitive to pain
- Inclined to take cold; intolerance to cold weather
- Exhaustion, weakness – to the point of fainting, with trembling
- **Tendency to dropsy. Bag-like swelling between the upper eyelid and eyebrow**
- Eyes weak after coition, pollution, abortion, measles
- **Toothache only when eating, worse touch**
- Sour eructations; nausea; sensation as if stomach is full of water; burning acidity
- Chronic liver problems; soreness and stitches in liver region
- Painful distension of the abdomen with flatus; everything eaten seems to turn to gas; sensation as if it will burst
- Cough – dry, paroxysmal, spasmodic with gagging; and vomiting of ingesta; affects the right side of the lung. Pale, flushed during a fit of coughing
- **Asthma relieved by sitting up, worse bending forward, 2 to 4 am**
- Fatty degeneration of heart and muscles. Weak, rapid pulse; intermits
- Sharp pain in kidney region; nocturnal bed wetting in adults
- Labour pains insufficient; complaints after childbirth
- Sweating, weakness after abortion, metrorrhagia
- **Backache – pains stitching and after abortion, labour pains shoot down gluteus muscle. Small of back feels weak. Pain from hip to knee**
- During sleep, they start to grinding their teeth, talk and cry; wakes up between 3 to 4 am and then cannot sleep

CLINICAL
- Haemorrhages
- Paralysis
- Hypothyroidism
- Dropsical effusions
- Anaemia
- Hallucinations
- Vertigo
- Headache
- Migraine
- Eye affections
- Toothache
- Dyspepsia
- Biliousness
- Jaundice
- Constipation
- Diarrhoea
- Haemorrhoids
- Ear affections
- Epistaxis
- Cold
- Cough
- Catarrh
- Whooping cough
- Bronchitis
- Hydrothorax
- Pneumonia
- Asthma
- Pleurisy
- Tuberculosis
- Angina pectoris
- Urinary troubles
- Pre menstrual syndrome
- Menstrual disorders
- Pregnancy disorders
- Arthritis
- Rheumatism
- Backache
- Sciatica
- Insomnia

MODALITIES
- **Aggravation:** After coition, in cold weather, from soup and coffee, in the morning around three o'clock, lying on the left and painful side, 2 am to 4 am, exertion, touch, after childbirth or miscarriage
- **Amelioration:** In warm weather, during the day, while moving around, in open air

REMEDY RELATIONSHIP
- **Complementary:** Carb-v., in low vitality; Nux-v. in stomach and bladder problems.
- **Compare:** Calc., Am-p., Phos., Lyc., Bry., Nat-m., Stann., Sep. and Kalium group remedies
- **Antidotes:** Camph., Coff.
- **Follows well:** Kali-s., Phos., Stann. in loose, rattling cough
- Will bring on the menses when Nat-m., though apparently indicated, fails

Kalium carbonicum

KALIUM MURIATICUM

INTRODUCTION

- **Common name:** Chloride of potassium, Potassium chloride
- **Group:** Mineral salt
- **Source:** Mineral kingdom
- **Formula:** KCl
- **Prover:** Martin

SPHERE OF ACTION

- Mind
- Gastrointestinal system
- Respiratory system
- Musculoskeletal system
- Female genital system
- Skin

MIND

- Irritable at trifles
- Imagines he must starve
- Discontented, discouraged; sits in silence
- Anxiety
- Restlessness
- Desires company
- Affectionate
- Nervous

MODALITIES

- **Aggravation:** Rich foods, fats, pastries, motion, open air, dampness, at night
- **Amelioration:** Cold drinks, rubbing

KEYNOTE SYMPTOMS

- Anti-infective and antiviral remedy
- **Catarrhal conditions where discharges are thick, white or greyish-white, tenacious, soapy and can be pulled into long threads. Exudation is sticky**
- Whiteness of all secretions, exudations
- For subacute inflammatory states, fibrinous exudations and glandular swellings; scrofulous enlargement of glands
- Hard deposits. Scorbutic infiltration of subcutaneous tissue
- Habitual loss of appetite or refuses food
- **Tongue has a white-grey coating at the base. Salty and bitter taste**
- Indigestion, diarrhoea – aggravation from fatty foods, pastries
- Chronic catarrhal condition of the middle ear. Blockage of eustachian tube. Deafness. Snapping and noises in the ear.
- Earache, deafness due to swelling or congestion of middle ear or external ear
- Frontal sinus catarrh with headache and thick white discharge
- **Hawks out thick, white, cheesy mucous; catarrhal pneumonia**
- Menses with excessive discharge which is dark, clotted, tough or tar-like
- Exudation and swelling around joints
- Acne, eczema, pimples, erythema with vesicles having thick white contents

CONSTITUTION

- For people with dark complexion, rigid musculature and fibrinous exudations
- For catarrhal disorders in subacute inflammatory states
- **Temperament:** Nervous, bilious
- **Thermal:** Chilly
- **Miasm:** Psora, Sycosis, Syphilis

CLINICAL

- Swelling of glands
- Hodgkin's disease
- Crusta lactea
- Aphthae
- Indigestion
- Liver enlargement
- Peritonitis
- Diarrhoea
- Dysentery
- Constipation
- Haemorrhoids
- Deafness
- Catarrhal otitis media
- Earache
- Laryngitis
- Laryngeal croup
- Tonsillitis
- Cough
- Diphtheria
- Pneumonia
- Asthma
- Pleuritis
- Chronic rheumatism
- Bursitis
- Pimples
- Acne
- Vesicles
- Eczema
- Erythema

REMEDY RELATIONSHIP

- **Compare:** Bell. which Kali-m. follows well in catarrhal and hypertrophic conditions. Kino; also Bry., Merc., Puls., Sulph.
- **Follows well:** Ferr-p., Calc-p., Calc-fl.

KALIUM PHOSPHORICUM

SPHERE OF ACTION

- Mind
- Nerves
- Gastrointestinal system
- Heart
- Musculoskeletal system
- Genitourinary system

INTRODUCTION

- **Common name:** Phosphate of potassium, Potassium hydrogen phosphate
- **Group:** Mineral salt
- **Source:** Mineral kingdom
- **Formula:** K_2HPO_4
- **Prover:** Allen

CONSTITUTION

- For dark complexioned, lean, thin people with extreme sensitiveness, general anaemia and weakness; especially suited to young people
- **Temperament:** Nervous, bilious
- **Thermal:** Chilly
- **Miasm:** Psora, Sycosis, Syphilis

MIND

- Mental fatigue
- Irritable, restless and anxious, from mental exertion
- Nervous dread. Feels unable to cope; despondency
- Mental breakdown after enormous mental exertion with nervousness and oversensitiveness
- Brain fag, hysteria
- Slightest labour seems like a heavy task
- Indisposition to meet people or to talk with them. Extreme lassitude and depression
- Very nervous, starts easily from least noise or when touched. Hypersensitivity to all stimuli
- Night terrors. Somnambulism
- Hysterical fits of laughing and crying

KEYNOTE SYMPTOMS

- Conditions arising from want of nerve power, neurasthenia, mental and physical depression. Nervous prostration
- Exhaustion of nerve cells, prostration; from overwork, worry, excessive excitement or shock
- Nervous, sensitive, weak and easily fagged by slightest cause, like pain, worry, mental fatigue
- General depletion, weakness after chemotherapy or cancer or surgery; helps in convalescence after exhausting diseases
- Adynamia. Condition of decay as in gangrene
- Numb sensations; muscular weakness after acute diseases
- **Discharges are golden yellow, copious or orange-yellow, as in urine, expectoration, leucorrhoea discharge from and old pelvic abscess, etc.**
- **Putrid, carrion-like odour from secretion; foul odour from the body. Breath is also foul**
- Oversensitive to sudden noises like banging of the door
- Intense sexual desire after menses
- **Night terrors of children, wake up from sound sleep, screaming and in fright**
- Severe prostration after coitus
- Nervousness from excessive sexual excitement, either indulged or suppressed, resulting in seminal losses and impotence
- Paralytic weakness or pain; sensation of paralysis. Infantile paralysis during dentition
- Nervous restlessness; feet fidgety; trembling sensation in leg muscles

CLINICAL

- Mental depression
- Anxiety
- Chronic fatigue syndrome
- Neurasthenia
- Anaemia
- Weakness
- Cancer
- Leukaemia
- Multiple sclerosis
- Headache
- Indigestion
- Dyspepsia
- Diarrhoea
- Cholera
- Constipation
- Tuberculosis
- Nocturnal enuresis
- Vaginitis
- Rheumatism

MODALITIES

- **Aggravation:** Excitement, worry, mental and physical exertion, eating, cold, early morning, pain
- **Amelioration:** Warmth, rest, nourishment, sleep, gentle motion

REMEDY RELATIONSHIP

- **Compare:** Kali-hp., Macroz., Genist., Zinc., Gels., Cimic., Lach., Mur-ac.

Kalium phosphoricum

KALIUM SULPHURICUM

INTRODUCTION

- **Common name:** Potassium sulphate
- **Group:** Mineral salt
- **Source:** Mineral kingdom
- **Formula:** K_2SO_4
- **Prover:** Bayard

SPHERE OF ACTION

- Mind
- Gastrointestinal system
- Respiratory system
- Musculoskeletal system
- Genitourinary system
- Skin

CONSTITUTION

- For ailments accompanied by marked desquamation
- Suits conditions with catarrh of mucous membranes and profuse yellow discharges
- **Temperament:** Nervous, bilious
- **Thermal:** Hot
- **Miasm:** Psora, Sycosis, Syphilis

MIND

- Nervous dread. Feels unable to cope, despondent
- Mental breakdown after enormous mental exertion with nervousness and oversensitiveness
- Hysteria
- Slightest labour seems a heavy task. Mental exertion aggravates
- Mental depression
- Always hurried
- Confused
- Restless
- Anxiety, worse in evening, better in open air

KEYNOTE SYMPTOMS

- Yellow mucous and serous discharges, profuse and intermittent. Ailments accompanied by profuse desquamation
- Applicable to later stages of inflammation; suppuration
- Shifting, tearing wandering pains; wandering rheumatism
- Ringworm of scalp or beard with abundant scales
- **Moist, sticky, yellow dandruff; scald head**
- Colicky pain. Abdomen feels cold to touch, tympanitic; yellow, slimy diarrhoea
- Constipation with haemorrhoids or black, thin, offensive stools
- Engorgement of naso-pharyngeal mucous membrane. Oral breathing, snoring, after removal of adenoids
- **Cold, with yellow, shiny discharge and nasal obstruction**
- Post-grippe cough, especially in children. Cough worse in the evening and in hot atmosphere
- **Ratting of loose, yellow mucous in the chest which is expectorated with difficulty**
- Metrorrhagia. Menses too late, scanty, with feeling of weight in abdomen
- Gonorrhoea, discharge slimy, yellowish-green. Orchitis, gleet
- Desquamation of skin; tendency to formation of yellow scales
- Eczema with burning, itching and papular eruptions
- **Rise of temperature at night. Intermittent fever with a slimy tongue**

CLINICAL

- Mental depression
- Neurasthenia
- Multiple sclerosis
- Cancer
- Dandruff
- Scald head
- Seborrhoea
- Vomiting
- Dyspepsia
- Indigestion
- Diarrhoea
- Constipation
- Anosmia
- Polypi
- Deafness
- Sinusitis
- Cold
- Tuberculosis
- Oxaluria
- Vaginitis
- Gonorrhoea
- Orchitis
- Rheumatism
- Intermittent fever
- Epithelioma
- Eczema
- Psoriasis
- Ringworm
- Scabies

MODALITIES

- **Aggravation:** In the evening, heated room, warmth, warm wraps
- **Amelioration:** In cool, open air, walking, discharge of flatus, fasting

REMEDY RELATIONSHIP

- **Compare:** Puls., Kali-bi., Nat-m., Kali-s., Chr., Hydr.
- **Antidotes:** Rhus poisoning

KALMIA LATIFOLIA

SPHERE OF ACTION
- Mind
- Gastrointestinal system
- Respiratory system
- Heart
- Musculoskeletal system
- Urinary system
- Skin

INTRODUCTION
- **Common name:** Mountain laurel, Broad leaved laurel
- **Family:** *Ericaceae*
- **Source:** Vegetable kingdom
- **Part used:** Leaves
- **Prover:** Hering

CONSTITUTION
- Adapted to delicate subjects suffering from gout, rheumatism or acute neuralgia with a tendency to emaciation
- **Temperament:** Nervous, bilious
- **Thermal:** Chilly
- **Miasm:** Psora, Sycosis, Syphilis

MIND
- Confusion and dullness from motion
- On lying down, the mental faculties and memory are perfect but there is vertigo on motion
- Aversion of being spoken to
- Talk of others
- Very irritable
- Harsh, passionate, cross
- Sad, weepy
- Anxiety with palpitations

KEYNOTE SYMPTOMS
- **A rheumatic remedy; pains shift rapidly, shooting outward, along the nerves with nausea and a slow pulse**
- Neuralgic pains shoot downwards and is accompanied or succeeded by numbness, tingling, trembling or paralytic weakness
- Aches and pains in limbs accompany most symptoms
- **Left sided in heart and circulation complaints and right sided in monologues**
- Palpitation with constriction in the throat; worse leaning forward
- Fluttering of the heart with anxiety. Pains – sharp, burning, shooting, stabbing, radiating to the left. Sharp pains take the breath away
- **Hypertrophy of the heart. Tumultus, rapid and visible action of the heart**
- Cardiac symptoms, especially as a sequele of rheumatism or gout
- Tingling and numbness of left arm
- Sudden, severe and acute arthritis. Joints are red, hot and swollen
- Pains affect a large part of a limb, or affects several joints
- Aching, bruised, stiff feeling. Weakness and numbness of painful parts as if paralysed
- Fulgurating pains of locomotor ataxia
- **Urine shows presence of albumin – albumunuria with pain in lower limbs and dropsy**
- Frequent urination of large quantities of yellow urine with sharp pains in the lumbar region
- Sleepless, turns frequently, wakes up very early in the morning

CLINICAL
- Neuralgia
- Vertigo
- Headache
- Migraine
- Hydrocephalus
- Cerebral congestion
- Orbital neuralgia
- Iritis
- Facial neuralgia
- Diarrhoea
- Constipation
- Sinusitis
- Dyspnoea
- Intercostal neuralgia
- Angina pectoris
- Valvular heart disease
- Bradycardia
- Cystitis
- Albuminuria
- Arthritis
- Rheumatism
- Bursitis
- Gout
- Fibrositis
- Locomotor ataxia
- Rheumatic fever

MODALITIES
- **Aggravation:** Leaning forward, looking down; motion, open air, heat of sun
- **Amelioration:** Eating, cloudy weather

REMEDY RELATIONSHIP
- **Compare:** Spig., Puls., Der.
- **Complementary:** Benz-ac.
- **Similar to:** Led., Rhod., Spig., in rheumatic affections and gout.
- **Follows well:** Spig., Thyr., Nux-v.

Kalmia latifolia

KREOSOTUM

INTRODUCTION

- **Common name:** Beechwood kreosote
- **Source:** Vegetable kingdom
- **Part used:** Distillation of wood tar from *Fagus sylvaticus*
- **Prover:** Meredith

SPHERE OF ACTION

- Teeth
- Gastrointestinal system
- Mucous membranes
- Female genital system
- Skin

CONSTITUTION

- People who have a dark complexion and are lean
- Children are old looking, wrinkled and emaciate rapidly or overgrown and poorly developed children with marasmus
- Haemorrhagic diathesis
- **Temperament:** Nervous, leucophlegmatic
- **Thermal:** Ambithermal
- **Miasm:** Sycosis, Syphilis

MIND

- Restlessness with frequent desire to draw a long breath
- Music causes palpitations and weeping
- Vanishing of thoughts; forgetful and peevish; weak memory
- Cross, willful and obstinate
- Apprehensive; starts from fright
- Ill-humour. Dwells on past disagreeable occurrences; morose, melancholic
- Child wants everything, but throws it away when given

KEYNOTE SYMPTOMS

- Haemorrhagic diathesis. Passive bleeding of brown blood
- Corrosive, foetid, ichorous, burning discharge from mucous membranes
- Rapid decomposition of fluids and secretions; ulceration, gangrene and cancerous affections, especially of gastrointestinal tract or uterus
- **Teeth begin to decay as soon as they appear. Gums bluish, red, soft, spongy, bleeding, inflamed and ulcerated**
- Ailments of teething children; very painful dentition
- Vomiting of pregnancy with salivation
- Malignant affections of stomach
- **Incontinence of urine, must hurry, when desire to urinate comes**
- Can urinate only when lying; copious, pale urine. Urging, during first sleep
- Pain during coition
- Violent corrosive itching of pudenda with swelling of labia
- Menstrual flow intermits; ceases on sitting or walking; reappears on lying down. Discharge of blood clots with a foul smell
- Severe headache before and during menses
- **Leucorrhoea acrid, corrosive, offensive, worse between periods, has odour of green corn, stiffens like starch, stains the linen yellow**
- Ulceration of neck of the uterus with stringy, foetid discharge. Cancer of the uterus. Puffiness of vagina, cervical erosion
- Post-climacteric ailments
- Lienteric, greyish or whitish stools; have cadaverous smell, very foetid

CLINICAL

- Haemorrhages of urine
- Cancer
- Collapse
- Painful dentition
- Dental caries
- Epistaxis
- Nausea
- Vomiting
- Vomiting of pregnancy
- Diarrhoea
- Cholera
- Constipation
- Incontinence
- Haematuria
- Leucorrhoea
- Vaginitis
- Lochia
- Miscarriage
- Cancer of uterus
- Arthritis
- Rheumatism
- Typhoid
- Ulceration
- Eruptions
- Gangrene

MODALITIES

- **Aggravation:** In the open air, cold weather, from washing or bathing with cold water, rest, especially when lying, after menses, from dentition
- **Amelioration:** Warmth, warm diet, motion, pressure

REMEDY RELATIONSHIP

- **Followed by:** Ars., Phos., Sulph., in cancer and diseases of a malignant tendency; also Bell., Calc., Lyc., Nit-ac., Rhus-t., Sep.
- **Antidote:** Nux-v., Acon.
- **Inimical:** Carb-v.
- **Complementary:** Ars., Phos., Sulph. in malignant diseases
- **Compare:** Fuli., Carb-ac., Iod., Lach., Kali-c.,

LAC CANINUM

INTRODUCTION
- **Common name:** Bitch's milk
- **Family:** *Mammalia*
- **Source:** Animal kingdom
- **Prover:** Reisig

SPHERE OF ACTION
- Mind
- Breasts
- Gastrointestinal system
- Respiratory system
- Musculoskeletal system

CONSTITUTION
- Suits nervous, restless, highly sensitive people, who can't bear anything touching them
- **Temperament:** Nervous, bilious
- **Thermal:** Chilly
- **Miasm:** Psora, Sycosis, Syphilis

MIND
- Restlessness, nervousness
- Alternation of moods
- Forgetful, absentminded – makes purchases and walks away without taking them
- **Forgets own name, cannot find proper word during conversation; cannot concentrate on studies**
- Fear of being alone, of dying, of going insane
- Hopeless, despondent. Very pessimistic
- **Sensation of walking or floating in air**
- Cross, irritable; gets angry, curses and swears on least provocation. Cries and screams all the time
- **Dreams of snakes**
- Illusions, delusions, imaginations of snakes
- Thinks himself of little consequence

KEYNOTE SYMPTOMS
- Severe weakness, prostration and lassitude
- **Erratic pains on alternating side; constantly flying from one part to another, changing from side to side every few hours or days**
- Hypersensitiveness of parts, skin; cannot bear one part of her body to touch another, must keep her fingers apart; oversensitiveness to touch
- Foetidness of discharges and exudative tendency
- Headache on one side which ends in vomiting at night – migraine. Violent frontal and occipital headache
- Very hungry but cannot eat enough; hungry after eating
- Curative and prophylactic in diphtheria
- Symptoms of diphtheria and tonsillitis change sides; with silvery shiny or porcelain white deposits
- Glistening parts – inflamed surfaces, especially of throat and ulcerated surfaces of skin appear shiny and glistening
- Menses too early, profuse, bright red and stringy
- Swollen, painful and sensitive breasts, before and during menses
- **Dries up milk in women who cannot nurse their baby**
- Rheumatic pains in joints, extremities and back; shifting from side to side; wandering pains
- **Sciatica – right side; legs feel numb, stiff; cramps in feet; burning in palms and soles**
- While walking seems as if walking in air, while lying does not seem to touch the bed

CLINICAL
- Weakness
- Headache
- Migraine
- Nausea
- Vomiting
- Diarrhoea
- Dysentery
- Obstinate constipation
- Coryza
- Ozaena
- Tinnitus
- Laryngitis
- Pharyngitis
- Tonsillitis
- Diphtheria
- Asthma
- Mastitis
- Galactorrhoea
- Uterine disorders
- Infertility
- Arthritis
- Rheumatism
- Backache
- Sciatica
- Insomnia

MODALITIES
- **Aggravation:** Morning of one day and the evening of next, touch, during menses, rest, jar, empty swallowing
- **Amelioration:** Cold, cold drinks, open air, walking

REMEDY RELATIONSHIP
- **Compare:** Lach., Con., Lac-f., Lac-d., Lac-ac.
- **Similar:** Apis, Con., Murx., Lach., Kali-bi., Puls., Sep., Sulph.

LAC DEFLORATUM

INTRODUCTION
- **Common name:** Skimmed cow's milk
- **Family:** *Mammalia*
- **Source:** Animal kingdom

SPHERE OF ACTION
- Mind
- Head
- Gastrointestinal system
- Heart
- Urinary system
- Female genital system

CONSTITUTION
- Suits pale, anxious patients with faulty nutrition
- For symptoms caused by milk in sensitive people, especially headache and constipation
- **Temperament:** Nervous, bilious
- **Thermal:** Chilly
- **Miasm:** Psora, Sycosis, Syphilis

MIND
- **Despondent, does not care to live, has no fear of death, but is sure that he is going to die**
- Aversion to company, suicidal disposition. Does not want to talk to anybody
- **Great horror of closed places,** car sickness
- Fear of being alone
- Restlessness
- Shy, timid
- Depression with tears, palpitations and fainting
- Vacillation of mind
- Listless–not inclined for physical or mental exertion
- Sad before and during menses
- Imagines all her friends will die or are dead and that she will have to go to a convent
- Loss of memory

KEYNOTE SYMPTOMS
- Useful in diseases with faulty nutrition; for diseases with malnutrition and anaemia
- Great prostration, especially when walking; feels completely exhausted, whether she does anything or not
- Sensation of cold air blowing over her even when covered or as if the sheets are damp
- Faintness from raising the arm above the head
- American sick migraine headaches with intense throbbing, nausea, vomiting, blindness and severe constipation
- Headache, worse light, noise, motion; better pressure, bandaging the head tightly
- Copious, pale urination during headache
- **Aversion to milk and milk allergy in children**
- **Obstinate constipation with ineffectual urging; stools – hard, large, passed after great straining; painful, lacerating the anus and extorting cries**
- Dropsy from organic heart disease or chronic liver complaint. Pressure around heart with dyspnoea; sharp pain in apex of heart
- **Intense thirst and emaciation with diabetes. Constant pain in kidney region**
- **Very dark and thick urine; frequent but scanty**
- Restores the flow of milk in young mothers who have deficient milk
- Milk causes suppression of menses till next period
- **Menses suppressed from putting hands in cold water**

CLINICAL
- Malnutrition
- Nutritional disorders
- Anaemia
- Car sickness
- Motion sickness
- Headache
- Migraine
- Globus hystericus
- Nausea
- Vomiting
- Flatulence
- Milk allergy
- Diarrhoea
- Dysentery
- Constipation
- Haemorrhoids
- Fissure-in-ano
- Albuminuria
- Diabetes
- Nephritis
- Mastitis

MODALITIES
- **Aggravation:** Cold, least draft, milk, morning, motion, walking
- **Amelioration:** Rest, pressure, tying a bandage, profuse discharge of urine

REMEDY RELATIONSHIP
- **Compare:** Colos. in diarrhoea of infants, the whole body smells sour, colic; Nat-m., Lac-c., Lac-v-c., Lac-ac., Vac., Cocc.

SPHERE OF ACTION

- Mind
- Nervous system
- Pneumogastric nerve
- Mucous membranes
- Cardiovascular system
- Female genital system
- Skin

INTRODUCTION

- **Common name:** Surukuku snake, Bushmaster snake
- **Family:** *Ophidia*
- **Source:** Animal kingdom
- **Part used:** Venom of Surukuku snake
- **Prover:** Hering

CONSTITUTION

- Suits women who have never been well since menopause. Pale face, bluish-purple, mottled, puffed look; chlorotic, thin, emaciated during and after climacteric age
- Especially suited to alchoholics
- **Temperament:** Melancholic
- **Diasthesis:** Haemorrhagic
- **Thermal:** Hot
- **Miasm:** Psora, Syphilis

LACHESIS MUTUS

MIND

- **Great loquacity,** constant overflowing of ideas–jumps from one subject to another. Communicative, expansive. Sharp tongued and witty.
- Aggressive. Critical. Sarcasm. Dictatorial
- **Religious mania,** delusion has committed a crime
- Psychosis; **fear of snakes, insanity, heart disease, being poisoned**
- Hysterical reactions over small things
- **Delusion is under superhuman control;** delusion of dead people, talking with; of his own funeral
- Clairvoyance. Anxiety; indolence, apathy
- Long lasting grief, sorrow, fright, disappointment in love, vexation unwarranted jealously and suspiciousness, hides, spits, mocks, revengeful, intolerance to authority
- Violent anger and behaviour
- Maniacal depression; hysteria after suppression of discharges

KEYNOTE SYMPTOMS

- **Left sided remedy. Complaints go from left to right side**
- Haemorrhagic tendency from any orifice; blood dark black; vicarious haemorrhages – epistaxis, bloody urine, petechiae, etc.
- Decomposes blood, making it more fluid; blood is thin, offensive, non-coagulable
- Rapid onset of diseases with marked prostration
- Ill-effects of suppressed discharges
- Tendency to low forms of disease like purpurea, diphtheria, typhoid
- Malignant and septic states with profound prostration from any disease – out of proportion to the condition
- Burning all over the body, hot flushes and hot perspiration, especially during menopause
- Tendency to ulceration, destruction, cancer and gangrene
- All discharges are offensive and acrid
- Increased sensitivity of nerves, especially cutaneous and vasomotor nerves. Epilepsy, catalepsy, delirium tremens
- **All complaints mental and physical are aggravated after sleep and better with the onset of menstrual flow**
- **Sense of constriction, tight feeling everywhere – heart, throat, abdomen, head, etc.**
- **Great desire for fanning, but slowly and from a distance**
- Paralytic conditions with heaviness and stiffness of parts; paralysis after a stroke
- Aphthous and denuded spots in mouth with burning and rawness
- **Tongue black, trembling and difficult to protrude**
- Sensation of a ball rolling in the urinary bladder; sensation of a lump in throat, abdomen, rectum, etc.
- Climateric ailments; has never been well since that time

CLINICAL

Mania	Quinsy
Schizophrenia	Epistaxis
Haemorrhage	Laryngitis
Haemophilia	Tonsillitis
Stroke	Diphtheria
Hypertension	Pneumonia
Pyaemia	Vicarious menses
Cellulitis	Puerperal fever
Paralysis	Menopause
Alcoholism	Typhoid
Delirium tremens	Purpurea
Vertigo	Varicose veins
Congestive headache	Malignant pustules
Trigeminal neuralgia	Wens
	Erysipelas
Aphthous ulcer	Bedsores
Jaundice	Boils
Meniere's disease	Carbuncles

MODALITIES

- **Aggravation:** After sleep, morning, left side, heat, summers, hard pressure, sun heat, extremes of temperature, empty swallowing, suppressed discharges, climacteric, alcohol
- **Amelioration:** Onset of discharges, menses, nasal catarrh, warm application, open air, cold drinks, loosening clothes

REMEDY RELATIONSHIP

- **Antidote:** Ars., Merc., Alum., Bell., Cocc., Coff., Hep., Merc., Nit-ac., Nux-v., Ph-ac.
- **Complementary:** Lyc., Hep., Crot-c.
- **Compare:** Puls., Con., Graph., Anthraci., Ter., Phos., Mur-ac., Kali-bi., Apis., Ph-ac., Lyss., Naja., Elaps., Crot-h.

Lachesis mutus

LAUROCERASUS

SPHERE OF ACTION
- Mind
- Gastrointestinal system
- Respiratory system
- Heart
- Musculoskeletal system

INTRODUCTION
- **Common name:** Cherry laurel
- **Family:** *Rosaceae*
- **Source:** Vegetable kingdom
- **Part used:** Young leaves
- **Prover:** Jorg, Hartlaub, Nenning

CONSTITUTION
- For cyanosed, blue, cold skinned, pale looking people
- **Temperament:** Nervous, bilious
- **Thermal:** Chilly
- **Miasm:** Psora, Sycosis, Syphilis

MIND
- Sudden loss of memory from pain, fright, etc.
- Inability to collect ideas
- Cries on being criticised
- Marked anxiety, agitations and apprehension which does not allow a moments rest
- Mental symptoms, better in open air
- Speech indistinct after every excitement
- Anxious, agitated and troublesome dreams
- Idiocy, dullness and sluggishness
- Want of moral feelings
- Irritability
- Anxiety and fear regarding imaginary evil, insanity
- Dullness of special senses

KEYNOTE SYMPTOMS
- When well indicated remedies fail to act due to a lack of reaction
- **General coldness, not ameliorated by warmth**
- Symptoms with sudden debility and lack of reaction
- Nervous collapse
- Blunted senses, lack of reaction, especially in chest and heart affections; internal burning
- Inclined to loose flesh
- Haemorrhage of thin, bright blood mixed with gelatinous clots, especially from the chest, uterus and rectum
- Falling down sensation in brain, abdomen and heart. Spells of deep sleep
- Coldness and blueness with epileptic form convulsion
- Drink rolls audibly through the oesophagus and intestines
- Spasmodic, tickling cough, in cardiac patients; with jelly-like expectoration dotted with blood
- **Patient keeps hands on chest – gasping for breath.** Cough with valvular disease; cardiac cough. Asphyxia neonatorum.
- Cardiac complaints, especially dyspnoea and cyanosis, worse sitting, better lying with head low
- Toe and finger nails become knotty
- Veins of hands distended
- Skin blue, cold, clammy – cyanosis

CLINICAL
- Debility
- Cyanosis
- Epilepsy
- Gastritis
- Diarrhoea
- Constipation
- Loss of speech
- Dyspnoea
- Asthma
- Asphyxia neonatorum
- Tuberculosis
- Lung paralysis
- Clubbed nails
- Cardiac cough
- Mitral regurgitation
- Fever
- Insomnia

MODALITIES
- **Aggravation:** Sitting up, stooping, exertion, cold, fright
- **Amelioration:** Lying with head low, sleep, open air, eating

REMEDY RELATIONSHIP
- **Compare:** Hydr-ac., Camph., Sec., Am-c., Ambr., Petr., Calc., Sil., Thuj.
- **Compatible:** Phos., Puls., Bell., Verat.

LEDUM PALUSTRE

INTRODUCTION
- **Common name:** Marsh tea
- **Family:** *Ericaceae*
- **Source:** Vegetable kingdom
- **Part used:** Whole plant
- **Prover:** Hahnemann

SPHERE OF ACTION
- Mind
- Gastrointestinal system
- Respiratory system
- Musculoskeletal system
- Skin

CONSTITUTION
- Suits plethoric, robust, full blooded people
- Adapted to gouty and rheumatic constitutions abused by alcohol
- **Temperament:** Nervous, bilious, sanguine
- **Thermal:** Chilly
- **Miasm:** Psora, Sycosis, Syphilis

MIND
- Angry, out of humour. Cross and surly
- Dissatisfied, hates his fellow beings, avoids their company; aversion to friends
- Anxiety, timidity
- Restlessness
- Fear of crowds, desires solitude
- Mental confusion, as if intoxicated
- Difficulty in thinking and comprehending
- Absentminded, sluggish

KEYNOTE SYMPTOMS
- **Animals bites, insect stings, punctured wounds, stab wounds; wounded parts feel cold**
- **Helps prevent tetanus; tetanus with twitching of muscles around the wound**
- Long discolouration after injury
- Venous congestion. Purple discolouration. Passive oedema and haemorrhage.
- People who are cold all the time; lack of animal heat but cannot bear heat of bed
- **Inspite of coldness of the body, symptoms are relieved by cold applications; sometimes amelioration is only obtained by putting feet into ice cold water**
- Extravasation of blood in the lids, conjunctiva and anterior chamber; contusion of eyes and lids
- Anal fissures. Haemorrhoidal pain
- Cough with haemoptysis; haemoptysis alternating with rheumatism
- Chronic rheumatism, better application of ice cold water, though chilly
- Rheumatism begins in lower limbs and ascends
- Gouty pains shoot through the limbs, joints, especially small joints; soles painful, can hardly step on them
- Stones and nodosities in small joints like wrists, fingers, ankles and toes

CLINICAL
- Alcoholism
- Punctured wounds
- Bites
- Stings
- Bruises
- Sprains
- Haemorrhage
- Tetanus
- Vertigo
- Black eye
- Conjunctivitis
- Cataract
- Fissure in ano
- Haemorrhoids
- Epistaxis
- Whooping cough
- Dyspnoea
- Rheumatism
- Gout
- Paronychia
- Carbuncles
- Acne
- Ecchymosis
- Purpura

MODALITIES
- **Aggravation:** At night, in the evening, heat of bed, store, injury, motion
- **Amelioration:** From cold, putting feet in cold water, bathing

REMEDY RELATIONSHIP
- **Compare:** Ruta, Ham., Bell-p., Arn., Crot-t., in traumatism; Con. in long lasting effects of injuries; Kalm.
- **Antidoted by:** Camph., Rhus-t.
- **Compatible:** Acon., Arn., Rhus-t., Puls., Bell., Bry., Nux-v., Sulph.
- Antidotes Rhus poisoning

LEPTANDRA VIRGINICA

INTRODUCTION
- **Common name:** Culver's root
- **Family:** *Scrophulariaceae*
- **Source:** Vegetable kingdom
- **Part used:** Rhizome and root
- **Prover:** Hale and Burt

SPHERE OF ACTION
- Mind
- Gastrointestinal system
- Musculoskeletal system
- Skin

CONSTITUTION
- Suits depressed, drowsy people with weakness and prostration
- Hepato-haemorrhagic diathesis
- **Temperament:** Nervous, bilious
- **Thermal:** Chilly, ambithermal
- **Miasm:** Psora, Sycosis, Syphilis

MIND
- Hopeless, despondent, doubtful of recovery at the thought of disease
- Drowsy, depressed with liver affections
- Gloomy, melancholic
- Delirium in hepatic diseases
- Anxiety on waking and after stool, in abdomen
- Oversensitiveness to noise, it penetrates
- Irritable

CLINICAL
- Vertigo
- Jaundice
- Gall stones
- Diarrhoea
- Constipation
- Haemorrhoids
- Rectal prolapse
- Malaria
- Typhoid

KEYNOTE SYMPTOMS
- Depression, drowsiness and delirium with hepatic disorders
- Right sided affections
- Weakness, hardly able to stand or walk
- Dull frontal headache
- **Craving for cold drinks which aggravate the burning and aching in the stomach**
- **Canine hunger; craves cold food; desires raw food, salads. Meat and vegetables disagree**
- A liver remedy with clay coloured stools
- Stools mushy, muddy, watery, foetid; or tarry, black and foul smelling, especially during typhoid; runs in a stream from the bowels with pain at the naval, worse in the morning
- Sore or dull bursting ache over the gall bladder, liver, travelling down the bowels to the navel, towards the left scapula or along the spine
- Pains in liver, umbilical and hypogastric region after stools
- **Clay coloured stools with jaundice**
- Prolapse of rectum with haemorrhage
- Bilious and typhoid fevers with black, tarry stools

MODALITIES
- **Aggravation:** Exposure to wet weather, motion, cold drinks
- **Amelioration:** Lying on abdomen

REMEDY RELATIONSHIP
- **Compare:** Podo., Iris, Bry., Merc., Ptel., Myric., Dig., Tab., in sinking in the pit of the stomach

LILIUM TIGRINUM

SPHERE OF ACTION
- Mind
- Eyes
- Gastrointestinal system
- Circulatory system
- Female genital system
- Musculoskeletal system

INTRODUCTION
- **Common name:** Tiger Lily
- **Family:** *Liliaceae*
- **Source:** Vegetable kingdom
- **Part used:** Tincture of fresh stalk, leaves and flowers
- **Prover:** W. Payne

CONSTITUTION
- Adapted to plethoric and nervous women at change of life.
- Suits unmarried woman who suffer from uterine troubles
- **Temperament:** Irritable, hysterical
- **Thermal:** Hot
- **Miasm:** Psora

MIND
- Desire for fine things, dissatisfied with her own, envious of others
- Tormented about her salvation
- Profound depression of spirits.
- Inclination to weep
- Aimless hurried manner
- Disposed to curse, strike, thinks obscene things.
- Fear of being alone, prefers society; very low spirited
- Mistakes is speaking; uses wrong words; forgetful

KEYNOTE SYMPTOMS
- **Headache on waking; aggravated in open air, better at sunset, with heaviness, as if full of blood; blowing blood from the nose, desires to support his head with hands**
- Neuralgia over left eye to vertex
- Warm blooded with left sided complaints.
- Bearing down sensation, dragging sensation in the abdomen and pelvis as if all the organs would escape.
- Hungry longs for meat. **Thirsty, drinks often and much. Desire for sour or sweet dairties, alternating with disgust for food**
- Hyperesthesia of the retina, Impaired vision.
- Sensation of a lump in centre of chest; moved up and down by empty swallowing
- Morning diarrhoea; stools loose, bilious; dark, offensive, very urgent, can't wait a moment; preceeded by great tenesmus
- Sensation as if the heart was grasped in a vise. Nervous affection of heart
- Pain in back and spine with trembling, legache, throbbing throughout the body
- Aching and burning pains in ovaries; feeling like live coals; severe pain with sensation as if a knife is ripped from groin and front of thigh
- Severe neuralgic pain in uterus; could not bear to touch; not even the weight of bedclothes or slightest jar
- Congestion of the uterus, prolapse and anteversion
- Leucorrhoea; bright yellow, acrid, excoriating; leaving a brown stain; after menses
- Menses early, scanty, dark, clotted, offensive, flow only when moving about.
- Sexual instinct awakened, pruritus pudenda

CLINICAL
- Angina pectoris
- Asthenopia
- Astigmatism
- Dementia
- Diarrhoea
- Dysentry
- Myopia
- Cardiac affections
- Hysteria
- Pruritus pudendi
- Uterine affections
- Prolapse of uterus
- Menstrual disorders
- Rheumatoid arthritis

MODALITIES
- **Aggravation:** Consolation, warm room, at night
- **Amelioration:** In open fresh air, from keeping busy

REMEDY RELATIONSHIP
- **Compare:** Agar., Cact., Helon., Murx., Sep., Plat., Pall., Nat-p
- **Antidoted by:** Plat., Nux-v, Puls., Helon.

LITHIUM CARBONICUM

SPHERE OF ACTION
- Mind
- Head
- Gastrointestinal system
- Cardiovascular system
- Breasts
- Urinary system
- Skin

INTRODUCTION
- **Common name:** Carbonate of lithium, Lithium carbonate
- **Group:** Salt
- **Source:** Mineral kingdom
- **Formula:** Li_2CO_3
- **Prover:** Hering

CONSTITUTION
- Suits a uric acid or gouty diathesis
- For prostration, weakness and chronic rheumatism in a uric acid diathesis
- **Temperament:** Nervous, bilious
- **Thermal:** Chilly
- **Miasm:** Psora, Sycosis, Syphilis

MIND
- Severe depression, disposed to weep about his lonesome condition; is staring and thoughtless
- Absentminded, has difficulty in concentrating
- Difficulty in remembering names
- Anxiety, and helplessness at night. Despair.
- Confusion of mind while standing
- Restless and nervous
- Shy, timid, want of confidence
- Averse to being touched or spoken to, wants to be alone
- Obsessive compulsive disorders

KEYNOTE SYMPTOMS
- Soreness of whole body; whole body feels sore and heavy; better rising and moving about
- Prostration; paralytic stiffening of the whole body
- **Pressing as of a dull point from within outwards, usually in small spots, worse left side – in head, abdominal ring, chest, perineum**
- Violent, lancinating pain as from hot needles
- Headache from sudden suppression of menses, better while eating
- Acidity, nausea and gnawing, relieved by eating.
- Constriction of the chest. Violent cough when lying down
- Rheumatic soreness in cardiac region; trembling and fluttering in heart, extending to back
- Heart pain associated with bladder pain, better after urinating
- Pains in mammae extend to the arms and fingers
- **Before menses symptoms more violent on left side and after menses on right side**
- Uric acid diathesis; gout and tophi. Rheumatic nodes
- Chronic rheumatism connected with heart lesions and asthenopia. **Pain in joints is relieved by very hot water**
- Paralytic stiffness all over. Itching around joints. Swelling and tenderness of finger and toe joints.
- **Dry skin, itchy; eruptions, rash all over the body; worse hot water**
- Scabby, tettery eruptions. Barber's itch

CLINICAL
- Depression
- Obsessive compulsive disorders
- Uric acid diathesis
- Paralysis
- Headache
- Asthenopia
- Hemiopia
- Photophobia
- Meniere's disease
- Nausea
- Acidity
- Angina pectoris
- Cystitis
- Albuminuria
- Cancer of breast
- Rheumatism
- Gout
- Barber's itch

MODALITIES
- **Aggravation:** In the morning, at night, right side, during menses
- **Amelioration:** Rising and moving about, rest, eating

REMEDY RELATIONSHIP
- **Compare:** Lyc., Am-p., Benz-ac., Calc., Lith-m., Lith-lac., Lith-be., Lith-br.

LOBELIA INFLATA

INTRODUCTION
- **Common name:** Indian tobacco, Red Indian tobacco, Pukeweed
- **Family:** *Lobeliaceae*
- **Source:** Vegetable kingdom
- **Part used:** Whole plant excluding roots
- **Prover:** Jeanes

SPHERE OF ACTION
- Ears
- Pneumogastric nerve
- Vasomotor nerve
- Gastrointestinal system
- Respiratory system
- Heart

CONSTITUTION
- Suited to light complexioned, fleshy people with languor and dyspepsia, especially in asthma and gastric affections
- **Temperament:** Nervous, bilious
- **Thermal:** Chilly
- **Miasm:** Psora, Sycosis, Syphilis

MIND
- Despondent, sobbing like a child
- Anxiety about health
- Serious, closed persons
- Psychogenic dyspnoea – fear of death or feels he is dying with distress in chest
- Fear of death

KEYNOTE SYMPTOMS
- It stimulates the vasomotor and pneumogastric nerves
- Ill-effects of alcoholism in light complexioned, corpulent people
- **Intolerant to tobacco – smell and taste; ailments from excessive use of tobacco**
- Vertigo with fear of death
- Gastric headache with nausea and vomiting and great prostration
- **Profuse salivation and nausea with a good appetite and a mercurial taste**
- Faintness and weakness, felt in the epigastrium
- Prickling and itching of the skin with intense nausea
- Marked nausea and vomiting with dyspepsia, a good appetite, profuse sweat and prostration
- Flatulence, with shortness of breath after eating
- Deafness due to suppression of discharges
- Nausea and vomiting with all lung and stomach disorders
- Asthma with stomach ailments
- Dyspnoea from constriction of chest
- Sensation of pressure or weight on the chest, better walking rapidly
- Spasmodic asthma, threatening suffocation; preceded by prickling all over; hyperventilation, laboured breathing
- Urine, deep orange in colour is copious and contains a red sediment
- Pain in the sacrum. Cannot bear the slightest touch; not even of soft clothes

CLINICAL
- Alcoholism
- Heartburn
- Acidity
- Nausea
- Vomiting
- Morning sickness
- Flatulence
- Globus hystericus
- Catarrhal jaundice
- Deafness
- Sinusitis
- Diphtheria
- Hyper-ventilation
- Cough
- Whooping cough
- Dyspnoea
- Asthma
- Senile emphysema
- Backache

MODALITIES
- **Aggravation:** Slightest motion, touch, cold especially cold washing, tobacco or tobacco smoke, afternoon, exertion, after sleep
- **Amelioration:** Walking rapidly, from warmth, in the afternoon, towards the evening, eating little

REMEDY RELATIONSHIP
- **Compare:** Ant-t., Ars., Ip., Tab., Verat., Rosa., Nux-v., Thuj., Ign., Bry., Abies-n.; other Lobelias, Dig., Tab., in heart affections
- **Antidote:** Ip., Tab.

SPHERE OF ACTION

- Mind
- Gastrointestinal system
- Respiratory system
- Mucous membranes
- Musculoskeletal system
- Genitourinary system

INTRODUCTION

- **Common name:** Club moss
- **Family:** *Lycopodiaceae*
- **Source:** Vegetable kingdom
- **Part used:** Spores
- **Prover:** Hahnemann

CONSTITUTION

- Suits a carbonitrogenoid constitution
- Patient looks older than he is, malnourished and premature baldness
- For people who are intellectually keen but physically weak
- For weak children with a well developed head but puny bodies
- **Temperament:** Nervous, bilious, scrofulous
- **Thermal:** Chilly
- **Miasm:** Psora, Sycosis, Syphilis

LYCOPODIUM CLAVATUM

MIND

- Very tired state of mind. Chronic fatigue
- **Dread of appearing in public, often professional lawyers and ministers, who have to appear in public – there is a feeling of incompetence and inability to undertake the task; stage fright**
- Afraid to be alone; anxiety in the house
- A lawyer cannot think of appearing in court. He delays until he is obliged to appear because he has a fear that he will stumble or make mistakes; loss of self confidences
- Patient dreads the presence of new persons. Wants to keep silent. Great anticipation.
- Easily angered, cannot endure contradiction
- Melancholic, sad
- Ailments from fright, anger, mortification
- Very sensitive
- Fear of breaking down under stress
- Dyslexic, weak memory, spells or writes wrong words
- Headstrong, hauty, domineering

KEYNOTE SYMPTOMS

- For deep seated, progressive, chronic diseases
- **Right sided remedy;** complaints start on the right side and go to the left
- Worse in the afternoon from 4 to 8 pm
- **Upper part of body is emaciated, lower part is semi-dropsical;** malnutrition due to weak digestion
- Half open condition of eyes during sleep
- Fan-like movement of nasal alae
- **Desires sweets; aversion to bread, oysters. Intolerant to cold drinks.** Craves everything warm. Canine hunger, but a few mouthfuls fill upto the throat
- Weak digestion; sour eructations; dyspepsia, much bloating; distention, especially in the lower abdomen. Food allergies.
- Disturbed liver function; ascites, dropsy from liver disease
- Alternate diarrhoea and constipation; stools is small, hard and difficult. Painful haemorrhoids.
- Red sand in urine. Child cries before urinating, polyuria at night
- Vagina dry. Bruning in vagina during coitus
- Impotence from sexual excesses; cold, relaxed penis. Old men with great desire but faulty erection
- Numbness, drawing and tearing pains in limbs; chronic gout. Profuse foot sweat. Cannot lie on painful side.
- Painful callosities on soles, toes and fingers. Cramps in calves. Twitching and jerking.
- **Right foot hot and left foot cold. Sciatica worse right side**
- Drowsy during the day. **Hemiopia: sees only left half**

CLINICAL

Dyslexia	Haemorrhoids
Cancer	Deafness
Presenility	Otorrhoea
Atony	Coryza
Malnutrition	Diphtheria
Emaciation	Tonsillitis
Blepharitis	Cough
Styes	Asthma
Night blindness	Aneurysm
Hiccough	Retention of urine
Eructations	
Biliousness	Diabetes
Dyspepsia	Hypoglycaemia
Hernia	Physometra
Gall stones	Impotence
Hepatitis	Sciatica
Colitis	Eczema
Dysentery	Ulceration
Constipation	Varicose veins

MODALITIES

- **Aggravation:** Nearly all diseases from 4 to 8 pm, right side, from above downward, from heat or in a warm room, hot air, bed, warm applications except throat and stomach which are better from warm drinks
- **Amelioration:** Warm foods and drinks, from uncovering especially the head, loosening the garments, from motion, after midnight

REMEDY RELATIONSHIP

- **Complementary:** Iod., Graph., Lach., Chel.
- **Antidotes:** Camph., Puls., Caust.
- **Compare:** Sulph., Rhus-t., Urt-u., Merc., Hep. Alum. Ant-c., Nat-m., Bry., Nux-v.
- **Follows well:** Calc., Carb-v., Lach., Sulph.
- It is rarely advisable to begin the treatment of a chronic disease with Lyc. unless clearly indicated; it is better to first give another antipsoric

LYCOPUS VIRGINICUS

SPHERE OF ACTION

- Mind
- Gastrointestinal system
- Respiratory system
- Heart
- Genitourinary system

INTRODUCTION

- **Common name:** Bulge weed
- **Family:** *Labiatae*
- **Source:** Vegetable kingdom
- **Part used:** Whole plant
- **Prover:** N.S. Davis

CONSTITUTION

- For diseases with tumultuous action of the heart and praecordial pain
- **Temperament:** Nervous, bilious
- **Thermal:** Chilly
- **Miasm:** Psora, Sycosis, Syphilis

MIND

- Suspiciousness, mistrustful
- Dullness and sluggishness. Slow comprehension with headache
- Irritability, unless spoken to very softly
- Stupefaction, as if intoxicated during menses. Deficiency of ideas during menses
- Desire to be silent. Taciturn
- Instability
- Increased mental and physical activity in the evening
- Restless in the evening

KEYNOTE SYMPTOMS

- **Passive haemorrhages** from nose, piles and lungs
- Shifting pains from heart to eyes, head to heart, heart to wrist, etc., especially rheumatoid pain. Also, shifting of symptoms, as from rectum to heart and head
- Persistent giddiness, commencing in open air and continuing while sitting
- Relieves protrusion of eyes, but has no effect upon the glandular enlargement of thyroid
- Epistaxis, generally due to hypertension
- **Thirst for large quantities of water. Desires cold drinks**
- Pulmonary complaints with loose stools
- Cough with haemoptysis. Haemoptysis due to valvular heart disease
- **Lowers blood pressure, reduces heart rate and increases the length of systole**
- Pulse weak, irregular, intermittent; tremulous and rapid
- Palpitations, worse when thinking of them
- For cardiac irritability with depressed force, with or without organic heart disease
- Profuse flow of limpid, watery urine, especially with an irritable heart
- Pain in testicles
- Wakefulness with marked vigilance and alertness

CLINICAL

- Exophthalmic goitre
- Headache
- Toothache
- Diarrhoea
- Constipation
- Haemorrhoids
- Haemoptysis
- Wheezing
- Asthma
- Cardiac asthma
- Cyanosis
- Hypertension
- Praecordial pain
- Valvular heart disease
- Diabetes mellitus
- Testicular pain
- Rheumatism
- Insomnia

MODALITIES

- **Aggravation:** Motion, exercise, walking, ascending, evening
- **Amelioration:** Rest, after rising

REMEDY RELATIONSHIP

- **Compare:** Eph. in exophthalmic goitre; eyes feel pushed out with tumultuous action of heart; Fuc., Spartin-s., Crat., Adren., Lam. in haemorrhoids; Spig., Cact., Crat., Dig., Laur., Hydr.-ac. in affections of the heart
- **Antidotes:** Cimic.

Lycopus virginicus

LYSSINUM

INTRODUCTION
- **Common name:** Saliva of rabid dog – Lyssin
- **Family:** *Mammalia*
- **Source:** Animal kingdom
- **Part used:** Saliva
- **Prover:** Hering

SPHERE OF ACTION
- Mind
- Nervous system
- Gastrointestinal system
- Respiratory system
- Genitourinary system
- Skin

CONSTITUTION
- Suits complaints from abnormal sexual desires
- Affects the nervous system causing convulsions and trembling
- **Temperament:** Nervous, bilious
- **Thermal:** Chilly
- **Miasm:** Psora, Sycosis, Syphilis

MIND
- Impatience and violent temper; irritable, critical
- Fear of being alone
- Fear something bad will happen
- Fear of suffocation, choking, driving, aeroplanes, of injury, water or running water; claustrophobia
- Agoraphobia
- Feeling of isolation; feels ridiculed or tormented
- Biting when angry, growls, violent temper, does reckless things. Strikes or stabs, curses
- Anger followed by quick remorse
- Lyssophobia – fear of becoming mad
- Emotions and bad news aggravate
- Anxiety and restlessness

KEYNOTE SYMPTOMS
- **Ill-effects of a dog bite**
- Over acute or hypersensitiveness of senses
- Trembling or quivering throughout the whole body
- Cannot bear the heat of the sun
- **Aversion to water. Conscious of water**
- Sight or sound of running water aggravates all the complaints
- Convulsions from dazzling light or seeing running water
- **Froth in the mouth. Thirst with inability to swallow**
- Constant spitting; saliva tough, viscid and ropy
- **Desires chocolate, tobacco and strange things during pregnancy**
- Dysentery with pain and tenesmus on hearing water running from a tap
- Sore throat with a constant desire to swallow, which is difficult. Spasm, gagging on swallowing water; spasmodic contracture of respiratory muscles
- Desire to urinate on seeing running water
- Uterus and vagina sensitive. Uterine prolapse
- Atrophy of testicles. Complaints from abnormal sexual desire
- Priapism with frequent emission
- Bluish discolouration of wounds
- Malignant ulcers from the bite of a dog

CLINICAL
- Hysteria
- Mania
- Phobias
- Agoraphobia
- Lyssophobia
- Hydrophobia
- Rabies
- Convulsions
- Opisthotonus
- Chronic headache
- Diarrhoea
- Constipation
- Haemorrhoids
- Hoarseness
- Sore throat
- Diabetes
- Vaginitis
- Dysparunia
- Chronic prolapsus uteri
- Priapism
- Atrophy of testicles
- Keloids

MODALITIES
- **Aggravation:** Sight or sound of water, pouring water or even thinking of water, bright dazzling light, carriage riding, heat of sun, stooping, bad news, mental exertion
- **Amelioration:** Gentle rubbing, bending backwards, sweating

REMEDY RELATIONSHIP
- **Compare:** Bell., Canth., Hyos., Stram., in hydrophobia. Xanth. is said to be specific for hydrophobia and is recommended for chronic cystitis in women; also Lach., Nat-m.

SPHERE OF ACTION

- Mind
- Head
- Nerves
- Gastrointestinal system
- Female genital system

INTRODUCTION

- **Common name:** Carbonate of magnesia, Magnesium carbonate
- **Group:** Mineral salt
- **Source:** Mineral kingdom
- **Formula:** $(MgCO_3)_4\ Mg(OH)_2 \cdot 5H_2O$
- **Prover:** Hahnemann

CONSTITUTION

- Suits nervous systems that demand soothing
- Especially for children with irritable, nervous dispositions whose body smells sour
- Suits worn out, broken down, nervous, flatulent, flabby women who smell sour, with uterine and climacteric disorders
- **Temperament:** Nervous
- **Thermal:** Chilly
- **Miasm:** Psora, Sycosis, Syphilis

MAGNESIA CARBONICA

MIND

- Mentally exhausted; symptoms worse on mental exertion
- Fear of aggression or violence, that something bad will happen
- Sad, taciturn. Anxiety during the day, as if some accident would happen, of the future; ameliorated in the evening, in bed
- Intolerance to quarrels, confrontations or disharmony
- Inscantity with fear and trembling
- Oversensitiveness – mentally and physically
- Neglected feeling, forsaken feeling
- Mentally confused and dazed, as if intoxicated
- Ill-effects of shock, mental stress, excess of care and worry
- Lachrimose during pregnancy
- Sense of anticipation, restlessness and nervousness in children

KEYNOTE SYMPTOMS

- Remedy for nervous irritation, nerve exhaustion and sleeplessness
- Emaciated, marasmic children despite being well fed. **Milk passes undigested in nursing children**
- Intense neuralgia; lightening pains in various parts. Nerves causing sharp, shooting pain along their course; ameliorated by walking about.
- Restlessness; body feels tired; sensation of numbness
- Sensitiveness – to least touch, noise, draft of cold air
- Sensitive to cold air. Cannot bear to be covered, yet chilled by uncovering
- Sour odour from secretions or discharges – perspiration, menses, vomitus, diarrhoea, especially in women, children or nurslings
- **Toothache during pregnancy; teeth feel too long**
- Catarrh of gastrointestinal tract resulting in severe acidity and in increased mucous secretions
- Sour eructations with vomiting of bitter water
- **Stools frothy, grass green, like water and scum of a frog pond, lienteric with gelatinous or fatty masses**
- Tendency to constipation, especially after nervous strain
- Sore throat, coryza before menses
- Menses tarry, dark, thick, indelibly staining the linen
- **Menstrual flow – late and scanty, only at night or when lying down, ceases when walking**
- Chilly in the evening, fever at night, followed by greasy, sour perspiration
- Unrefreshing sleep, more tired on rising. Has several anxious dreams; starts from sleep

CLINICAL

- Homesickness
- Marasmus
- Chronic fatigue syndrome
- Alcoholism
- Tumours
- Neuralgia
- Trigeminal neuralgia
- Cataract
- Heartburn
- Belching
- Colic
- Stomach disorders
- Dyspepsia
- Vomiting
- Hepatitis
- Diarrhoea
- Dysentery
- Constipation
- Haemoptysis
- Deafness
- Premenstrual syndrome
- Leucorrhoea
- Dysmenorrhoea
- Insomnia

MODALITIES

- **Aggravation:** Change of temperature, every three weeks, rest, milk, during menses, warmth of bed, mental exertion
- **Amelioration:** Warm air, but worse warmth of bed, walking in open air

REMEDY RELATIONSHIP

- **Complementary:** Cham.
- **Antidotes:** Ars., Merc.
- **Compare:** Rheum, Kreos., Aloe, Cheir. in deafness, otorrhea, nose stopped up at night from irritation of cutting wisdom teeth

Magnesia carbonica

MAGNESIA MURIATICA

SPHERE OF ACTION

- Mind
- Nervous system
- Gastrointestinal system
- Heart
- Urinary system
- Skin

INTRODUCTION

- **Common name:** Muriate of magnesia, Magnesium chloride
- **Group:** Mineral salt
- **Source:** Mineral kingdom
- **Formula:** $MgCl_2 \cdot 6H_2O$

CONSTITUTION

- Suits women with spasmodic and hysterical complaints, complicated by uterine diseases, who have suffered from attacks of indigestion or biliousness for years
- For puny, rickety children during dentition
- **Temperament:** Nervous, bilious, irritable
- **Thermal:** Chilly
- **Miasm:** Psora, Sycosis, Syphilis

MIND

- Homesickness; has nostalgias
- Sadness and maniacal depression
- Sensitive to voices; aversion to conversation, is reserved
- Aversion to quarrels. Peace-maker, passivity; dislikes confrontations
- Nervous excitability with a tendency to weep easily
- Difficulty in concentration; confused
- Feels on the verge of a nervous breakdown
- Excessive anxiety, with worries, especially at night
- Aversion to work, but desires to move and keep busy
- Anxiety during night in bed, when not doing anything or when not active
- **Needs peace and peaceful surroundings**
- **Dreams of robbers**
- Irritability, more in the morning

KEYNOTE SYMPTOMS

- Look of long suffering and sourness, tiredness, weakness and fatigue
- Sea shore aggravates chest complaints, constipation and liver complaints. Ill effects of sea bathing
- Neuralgic pains; boring; cramp-like. Paralytic drawing and tearing in limbs
- **Tongue has rhagades with violent burning. Inside of mouth feels as if burnt**
- **Eructations taste like rotten eggs, onions**
- Children, during dentition are unable to digest milk. It causes pain in stomach and is passed undigested
- Hepatic affections; chronic liver disorders with pressing pain and tenderness, worse walking
- Diarrhoea or abdominal pains from milk. Chronic tendency to diarrhoea. Diarrhoea, worse milk, fruits, fats.
- Obstruction of bowels from faeces – extremely obstinate constipation. **Stools hard, knotty, like sheep's dung, crumbling at the verge of anus**
- Cardiac affections with liver enlargement. **Palpitations worse sitting, lying on left side, better moving about**
- Congenital scrotal hernia
- Acne before and during menses, leave behind scars
- Menses dark, black, clotted, causing cramps, hysteria and excitement; metrorrhagia worse at night
- Leucorrhoea, in gushes after exercise, during movement, while passing stools; preceded by cramps in the abdomen

CLINICAL

- Homesickness
- Anxiety
- Chronic fatigue syndrome
- Neuralgia
- Headache
- Gingivitis
- Globus hystericus
- Eructations
- Flatulence
- Hernia
- Hepatomegaly
- Hepatitis
- Cirrhosis
- Diarrhoea
- Constipation
- Sinusitis
- Cough
- Asthma
- Palpitations
- Angina pectoris
- Cystitis
- Metrorrhagia
- Leucorrhoea

MODALITIES

- **Aggravation:** Immediately after eating, lying on the right side, from sea bathing
- **Amelioration:** From hard pressure, motion, open air except headache, hanging down affected part

REMEDY RELATIONSHIP

- **Antidotes:** Camph., Cham.
- **Compare:** Nat-m., Puls., Sep., Am-m., Nast. is useful in scorbutic affections and constipation, related to strictures of the urinary apparatus, supposed to be aphrodisiacal in its action; cirrhosis of liver and dropsy; Cham. in the disease of children
- **Compatible:** Bell., Nat-m., Sulph., Sep., Puls.

MAGNESIA PHOSPHORICA

INTRODUCTION

- **Common name:** Phosphate of magnesia, Magnesium phosphate
- **Group:** Mineral salt
- **Source:** Mineral kingdom
- **Formula:** $MgHPO_4 \cdot 7H_2O$
- **Prover:** Allen

SPHERE OF ACTION

- Mind
- Gastrointestinal system
- Respiratory system
- Heart
- Musculoskeletal system
- Urinary system
- Female genital system

CONSTITUTION

- Suits tall, slender children who are tired, emaciated, languid and exhausted, having a tendency for neuralgic pains
- **Temperament:** Nervous
- **Thermal:** Chilly, ambithermal
- **Miasm:** Psora, Sycosis, Syphilis

MIND

- Irritable and oversensitive with many fears (similar to *Phos.*)
- Oversensitive to pain, noise, excitement
- Illusions of senses
- Forgetful, dull; inability to think clearly
- Indisposition to mental or physical exertion. Indisposition to study or make any mental effort
- Sobbing and lamenting. Laments constantly about the pain with hiccough
- Anxiety from pains
- Weeping during convulsions
- Talks to herself, or sits still in moody silence
- Inability to think clearly; drowsiness on attempting to study
- Sleepless

KEYNOTE SYMPTOMS

- **Right sided affections** of head, ear, face, chest, ovary and sciatic nerve
- Affects muscles and nerves causing spasmodic effects like cramping of muscles with radiating pains
- Languid, tired, exhausted; unable to sit up
- Great dread of cold air, uncovering or touching the affected part
- Pains – cramping, lightening, shooting, sharp, cutting, stabbing, stitching, rapidly changing place. Pains come and go suddenly
- Neuralgic pains; mostly right sided relieved by warmth; dread of touching the affected part
- Neuralgic pains, especially facial neuralgia, supra or infra-orbital
- **Toothache, relieved by heat and hot drinks**
- Flatulent colic, forcing the patient to bend double, relieved by rubbing, warmth, pressure and accompanied by belching of gas, which gives no relief
- **Menstrual cramps, ovarian neuralgia; colicky pain in abdomen, forcing patient to bend double, better by heat, warmth, pressure and when menstrual flow begins**
- Constipation in rheumatic persons
- Spasmodic, whooping cough with soreness and stiffness in the throat
- Involuntary shaking of hands

CLINICAL

- Neuralgias
- Cramps
- Tetanus
- Chorea
- Goitre
- Vertigo
- Facial neuralgia
- Nystagmus
- Strabismus
- Toothache
- Hiccough
- Enteralgia
- Flatulent colic
- Whooping cough
- Asthma
- Angina pectoris
- Enuresis after catheterization
- Ovarian neuralgia
- Menstrual colic
- Membranous dysmenorrhoea
- Writer's cramps
- Sciatica

MODALITIES

- **Aggravation:** Cold air, draft of cold air or cold wind, cold bathing or washing, motion, touch.
- **Amelioration:** Bending double, heat, warmth, pressure, bathing with hot water

REMEDY RELATIONSHIP

- **Compare:** Bell., Caul., Coloc., Lyc., Lac-c., Puls.; Cham. is its vegetable analogue, Kali-p., Sil., Zinc., Dios.
- **Antidotes:** Bell., Gels., Lach.
- Acts best when given in hot water

MALARIA OFFICINALIS

SPHERE OF ACTION
- Gastrointestinal system
- Liver
- Spleen
- Respiratory system
- Urinary system

INTRODUCTION
- **Common name:** Malaria
- **Group:** Nosode
- **Source:** Vegetable kingdom
- **Part used:** From vegetable matter decomposed in a jar of water for 1, 2 and 3 weeks
- **Prover:** G.W. Bowen

CONSTITUTION
- Malarial cachexia; suffering from rheumatic paralysis and emaciation
- **Temperament:** Bilious
- **Thermal:** Chilly
- **Miasm:** Tubercular

MIND
- Feels stupid and sleepy
- Cross
- Morosed
- Peevish
- Ill-humoured
- Fear to drink
- Very forgetful
- Stupor, sleepiness and confusion
- **Great desire to stretch**
- Feels dizzy and drowsy

KEYNOTE SYMPTOMS
- **All symptoms are relieved by eating**
- General sense of weariness from a very short walk, especially through the pelvis, sacral region and upper thighs. Strong desire to lie down
- A kind of simmering all through the body
- Headache with nausea. Dull headache; dizzy and drowsy at all times; worse in the morning
- Itching of right cheek over the malar bone
- Eyes feel heavy, sleepy and burn like fire, making reading difficult
- Sensation of contraction at the root of the nose; as if about to have a severe cold, like hay fever
- **Tongue – coated thickly white with a brown streak down the centre**
- **Sensation of specks of pepper on tip of tongue**
- Aversion to food. Bilious colic, cramps, nausea, diarrhoea and headache
- Splenic disorders and functional hepatic diseases. Distress in the hypochondriac regions
- Sluggish bowels but natural stools
- Diarrhoea – thin, yellow, foul, worse mornings
- Irritation in the larynx, with cough and expectoration of bloody mucous
- Urine – high coloured, scanty, offensive, red
- Rheumatic paralysis and emaciation; right arm becomes numb and has to be rubbed; cold limbs

CLINICAL
- Delirium
- Malarial cachexia
- Parkinsonism
- Spleen affections
- Splenomegaly
- Liver affections
- Hepatitis
- Diarrhoea
- Constipation
- Haemorrhoids
- Bronchitis
- Pneumonia
- Tuberculosis
- Asthma
- Rheumatism
- Malaria
- Bilious fever
- Intermittent fever
- Typhoid
- Insomnia

MODALITIES
- **Aggravation:** Pain in liver region is worse lying down
- **Amelioration:** By eating, stretching, dull ache in liver region is better after urinating and hard pressure over liver region

REMEDY RELATIONSHIP
- **Compare:** Cean.; Bry., Lyc. in bed wetting; Nux-v., Chel., in liver; Cor-r., Coc-c. in half minute gun cough; also Lith-c., Syzyg., Ip., Cedr., Nat-m., Meny. in intermittent fever.

MANGANUM ACETICUM

INTRODUCTION
- **Common name:** Manganese acetate
- **Group:** Mineral salt
- **Source:** Mineral kingdom
- **Formula:** $Mn(CH_3.COO)_2 \cdot 4H_2O$
- **Prover:** Hahnemann

SPHERE OF ACTION
- Mind
- Inner ear
- Larynx
- Gastrointestinal system
- Respiratory system
- Musculoskeletal system
- Urinary system

CONSTITUTION
- For syphlitic and chlorotic patients with anaemia and paralysis
- **Suits mask-like face**
- Great soreness and aching with early stages of tuberculosis
- **Temperament:** Nervous, bilious
- **Thermal:** Chilly
- **Miasm:** Psora, Sycosis, Syphilis

MIND
- Silent and reserved
- Sadness, depression better from hearing sad music
- Constant moaning and groaning
- All mental conditions are better by lying down
- Walks backwards
- Irritability in the morning, while listening to music, while talking
- Anxiety and fear when moving in the room, better lying down
- Anxiety as if something bad is going to happen
- Peevish, fretful, weak and nervous
- Confusion while sitting
- Hates people who offend him

KEYNOTE SYMPTOMS
- Anaemia with destruction of red blood corpuscles
- **Generally all symptoms are ameliorated by lying down**
- Subacute stage of cellulitis; promotes suppuration and hastens regeneration
- Painful, deep, soreness of the whole body; every part of the body feels sore when touched
- Fatty degeneration of the liver. Flatulence and chronic hepatomegaly
- Ear feels stopped. Pains from other parts extend to the ear
- Deafness during damp weather
- Nose – dry and obstructed
- Tuberculosis of the larynx
- Cough better by lying down
- Chronic, rough, hoarse voice on change of weather, raising head, bending forward or bending double; chronic sore throat and hoarseness. Hemming and hawking all the time
- Great accumulation of mucous in the respiratory tract
- Inflammation of bones and joints with nocturnal digging pains
- Periosteum inflamed, of shin bones, joints, ankles and lower limbs
- **Strongly exaggerated reflexes. Progressive paraplegia, wasting. Feeble and staggering gait; walks stooping forward.**
- Progressive muscular atrophy; ascending paralysis
- Paralysis agitans; cock's gait – a peculiar slapping gait – walks on metatarso-phalangeal joints. Tendency to fall forward

CLINICAL
- Growing pains
- Anaemia
- Paralysis agitans
- Parkinson's disease
- Wilson's disease
- Toothache
- Hepatomegaly
- Fatty degeneration of liver
- Jaundice
- Epistaxis
- Tinnitus
- Chronic catarrh
- Deafness
- Hoarseness
- Haemoptysis
- Bronchitis
- Asthma
- Nephritis
- Albuminuria
- Arthritis
- Rheumatism
- Osteomyelitis
- Periostitis
- Gout
- Paraplegia
- Cellulitis
- Eczema
- Ulcers
- Scabies
- Insomnia

MODALITIES
- **Aggravation:** Cold wet weather, damp, touch, night, talking, motion
- **Amelioration:** Lying down, listening to sad music, eating, swallowing, open air

REMEDY RELATIONSHIP
- **Compare:** Mang-coll., Mang-m., Mang-o., Mang-s., Arg-met., Rhus-t., Sulph.
- **Antidotes:** Merc., Coff.

SPHERE OF ACTION

- Mind
- Nervous system
- Gastrointestinal system
- Respiratory system
- Heart
- Musculoskeletal system
- Genitourinary system
- Skin

INTRODUCTION

- **Common name:** The gonorrhoeal virus
- **Group:** Nosode
- **Source:** Animal kingdom
- **Part used:** Urethral discharge from patients having acute gonorrhoea
- **Prover:** Swan

CONSTITUTION

- Constitutional effects of maltreated or suppressed gonorrhoea with trembling, weakness and fatigue. Generally restores the gonorrhoeal discharge
- For women with chronic pelvic disorders like chronic ovaritis, salphingitis, pelvic cellulitis, fibroids, cysts and other uterine and ovarian growths
- Suits a dwarfish baby with stunted growth is idiotic and pale
- **Temperament:** Nervous, bilious
- **Thermal:** Hot
- **Miasm:** Sycosis

MEDORRHINUM

MIND

- Time passes very slowly
- **In impulsive/aggressive phase always thinks about sex; desires sex**
- Great difficulty in stating symptoms; loses thread of talk
- **Predicts future events very correctly**
- Feels as if a delicate hand smoothing or stroking her head from front to back or as if her entire life was unreal like a dream
- Thinks someone is behind her, hears whispering, sees faces that peer at her from behind the bed and furniture
- Absentmindedness, weak memory, loss of mental power
- Confused; forgetfulness – of names and words
- Weeping tendency – cannot speak without crying. Suicidal
- Always in a great hurry. Very impatient
- Irritated at little things

KEYNOTE SYMPTOMS

- Soreness all over the body with burning in hands and feet
- Trembling all over the body with intense nervousness and profound exhaustion. Great disturbance and irritability of the nervous system
- A state of collapse, **wants to be fanned all the time**
- Chronic ailments from suppressed gonorrhoea or a history of gonorrhoea
- Sensation of tightness and constriction all over the body; especially in the head, extending down the spine
- Inordinate craving for liquor, salt, sweets, acids
- Ravenous hunger immediately after eating
- **Ball-like stools due to constriction and inertia of bowels; can pass stool only by leaning far back**
- Dyspnoea relieved by lying on face, protruding tongue; inhalation is easy, exhalation is difficult
- Pain in heart region from apex to base
- Breast and nipples cold, sore and sensitive (during menses)
- Menses profuse, dark, clotted; stains difficult to wash. Metrorrhagia during climacteric or with malignant disease of uterus
- Intensely restless and fidgety legs and feet. Aching in legs – unable to keep them still
- **Backache relieved by profuse urination**
- Finger joints large, puffy. Swelling and stiffness of ankles. Tender heels and balls of feet. Soreness of soles.

CLINICAL

- Mental disorders
- Alcoholism
- Drug abuse
- Mental depression
- Retardation
- Epilepsy
- Necrosis
- Tumours
- Paralysis
- Liver affections
- Pruritus ani
- Sinusitis
- Cough
- Dyspnoea
- Throat affections
- Asthma
- Lung affections
- Renal colic
- Tenesmus
- Cystitis
- Urethritis
- Nocturnal enuresis
- Diabetes
- Masturbation
- Venereal diseases
- Vaginitis
- Suppressed gonorrhoea
- Leucorrhoea
- Metrorrhagia
- Sterility
- Impotence
- Spermatorrhoea
- Rheumatism
- Arthritis
- Gout
- Corns
- Warts
- Condylomata
- Boils

MODALITIES

- **Aggravation:** When thinking of ailments, heat, covering, stretching, thunderstorm, least movement, sweets, from daylight to sunset
- **Amelioration:** At the seashore, lying on stomach, damp weather

REMEDY RELATIONSHIP

- **Compare:** Ip. in dry cough; Camph., Sec., Tab., Verat., in collapse; Pic-ac., Gels. in inability to walk; Aloe, Sulph., morning diarrhoea; Syph., Zinc.
- The burning feet of Sulph. and restless fidgety legs and feet of Zinc. are both found at the same time in Med.

MELILOTUS OFFICINALIS

SPHERE OF ACTION
- Mind
- Blood vessels
- Gastrointestinal system
- Musculoskeletal system
- Female genital system

INTRODUCTION
- **Common name:** Yellow melilot, Sweet clover
- **Family:** *Leguminosae*
- **Source:** Vegetable kingdom
- **Part used:** Flowering tops
- **Prover:** Bowen

CONSTITUTION
- Tendency to congestion and haemorrhages with coldness. Face is flushed, livid and purple
- **Temperament:** Nervous, bilious
- **Thermal:** Chilly
- **Miasm:** Psora, Sycosis, Syphilis

MIND
- **Wants to run away or hide, wants to kill himself or threatens to kill those who approach**
- Religious melancholy with an intensely red face
- Irritability, worse contradiction
- Restlessness, anxiety
- Melancholy
- Early stages of insanity
- Impatient, fault-finding, indolent
- Treacherous memory; cannot fix mind
- Delusion that everyone is looking at her

KEYNOTE SYMPTOMS
- **Tendency for haemorrhages, profuse and bright**
- Pain and debility
- **Congestion, especially of the head. Severe, violent, congestive throbbing headache;** sick headache; **ameliorated by haemorrhage** – epistaxis or menstrual flow. Fullness of the head.
- Vomiting with headache
- Epilepsy from a blow to the head
- Infantile spasms during dentition
- Difficult, painful constriction in the anus
- **Throbbing and fullness of anus with no desire to defecate until there is a large accumulation**
- Nosebleed preceded by intense redness, flushing of face and throbbing of carotids, followed by relief of complaints
- Weight on chest, feels smothered
- Menses – scanty, intermittent with bearing down pain. Dysmenorrhoea
- Wants to stretch the knee, though it does not relieve the pain
- Skin cold; numbness

CLINICAL
- Delusions
- Congestion
- Haemorrhages
- Epilepsy
- Neuralgia
- Headache
- Migraine
- Nausea
- Vomiting
- Diarrhoea
- Constipation
- Haemorrhoids
- Epistaxis
- Haemoptysis
- Pneumonia
- Ovarian neuralgia
- Metrorrhagia
- Dysmenorrhoea

MODALITIES
- **Aggravation:** Approach of a storm, rainy changeable weather, motion, 4 pm
- **Aggravation:** From bleeding, profuse micturition

REMEDY RELATIONSHIP
- **Compare:** Aml-ns., Ant-c. in epistaxis after headache, but does not relieve; Bell., Glon., Sang. in congestive headache, red face, hot head, etc. Meli-a. has practically the same action – haemorrhages, congestive headaches, engorged blood vessels, spasms

Melilotus officinalis

SPHERE OF ACTION

- Mind
- Gastrointestinal system
- Musculoskeletal system
- Urinary system
- Skin

INTRODUCTION

- **Common name:** Buck bean
- **Family:** *Gentianaceae*
- **Source:** Vegetable kingdom
- **Part used:** Whole plant
- **Prover:** Hahnemann

CONSTITUTION

- For weak, nervous, anxious, pale faced people
- Suits jumpy, fidgety women with urinary problems
- **Temperament:** Nervous
- **Thermal:** Chilly
- **Miasm:** Sycosis

MIND

- Vivid dreams but does not remember them, agitated sleep
- Deficiency of ideas with dull headache
- Anxiety in cardiac region, with apprehension, as if something evil will happen
- Indifference

MENYANTHES TRIFOLIATA

KEYNOTE SYMPTOMS

- Sensation of tension and compression
- Jerking of muscles in different parts, especially during repose
- Twitching of the muscles is visible but painless. Icy coldness of parts
- Headache with pressing pain in the vertex, better hard pressure with hand and stooping
- **Dryness of mouth and throat without thirst**
- **Aversion to bread and butter. Craving for meat**
- **Frequent and ineffectual efforts to emit flatus**
- **Frequent desire to urinate with scanty urine**
- Cramps from ankles to calves
- Icy coldness of hands and feet
- Legs jerk and twitch as soon as the patient lies down; shooting and pinching pain in limbs and joints
- Skin feels very tense, as if it were too smelly to accommodate the body

CLINICAL

- Neuralgia
- Twitching
- Jerking
- Headache
- Gingivitis
- Stomatitis
- Cold
- Dyspnoea
- Scanty urine
- Diabetes
- Arthritis
- Rheumatism
- Intermittent fever
- Malaria

MODALITIES

- **Aggravation:** During rest; lying down, ascending
- **Amelioration:** Pressure on affected part, motion, stooping

REMEDY RELATIONSHIP

- **Compare:** Caps., Puls., Calc., Ph-ac., Sang., Cact., Gels., Sep., Mag-m., Par., Glon., Lach.
- **Antidote by:** Camph.
- **Follow well:** Caps., Lach., Lyc., Puls., Rhus-t., Verat.

MEPHITIS PUTORIUS

SPHERE OF ACTION
- Mind
- Gastrointestinal system
- Respiratory system
- Musculoskeletal system

INTRODUCTION
- **Common name:** Skunk
- **Family:** *Mustelide*
- **Source:** Animal kingdom
- **Part used:** Discharge of skunk which is very offensive
- **Prover:** Hering

CONSTITUTION
- A short acting remedy for cough, especially whooping cough
- Bloated face of child, must be raised, gets blue in the face, cannot exhale
- **Temperament:** Nervous
- **Thermal:** Chilly
- **Miasm:** Psora, Sycosis, Syphilis

MIND
- Loquacity. Talkative from too lively an imagination
- Excited, full of fancies; can neither sleep nor work
- Dreams of water, fire, distressing losses; nightmares
- Shy
- Timid
- Restless
- Pain on exertion
- Full of fancies
- Disinclined to work
- Indolence

KEYNOTE SYMPTOMS
- Debility after severe illness; nervous exhaustion
- Internal agitation of the whole body with extreme uneasiness
- **Wants to bath in ice cold water**
- Spasmodic effects, chokes easily, trembling; convulsions
- **Eyes – pain from overexertion, as if there was a foreign body in them.** Conjunctiva red. Blurring of vision, unable to distinguish letters especially small print.
- **Metallic coppery taste in mouth. Desires salted foods.**
- Food goes down the wrong way; cough with vomiting after eating
- Cough – spasmodic, suffocative, whooping, hollow, deep with rawnesss, hoarseness and pains through chest; asthmatic paroxysms
- **Few paroxysms of cough in day time but many at night**
- Suffocative feeling; cannot exhale. Because of cough child gets blue in face, must be raised up, cannot exhale.
- Mucous rales through upper part of chest. Mucous expelled after a bout of coughing in the morning; rattling cough in the morning
- Asthma, as if inhaling sulphur; of drunkards
- **Rheumatic pain – shifting with a desire to urinate.** Sensation of paralysis during the pains

CLINICAL
- Cyanosis
- Conjunctivitis
- Myopia
- Diarrhoea
- Constipation
- Sinusitis
- Laryngitis
- Pharyngitis
- Hoarseness
- Choking
- False croup
- Whooping cough
- Spasm of glottis
- Bronchitis
- Asthma
- Rheumatic pains

MODALITIES
- **Aggravation:** Lying down, after menses, night, day break, rest
- **Amelioration:** Cold icy weather, bathing, motion, sitting up

REMEDY RELATIONSHIP
- **Compare:** Dros., Cor-r., Stich., Rumx., Aur., Plat., Nux-v., in cough; Lach. in easy choking; Lach., Agar. in loquacity
- **Follows well:** Dros.

MERCURIUS CORROSIVUS

SPHERE OF ACTION

- Mucous membranes
- Eyes
- Ears
- Gastrointestinal system
- Respiratory system
- Genitourinary system

INTRODUCTION

- **Common name:** Corrosive sublimate, Mercuric chloride
- **Group:** Salt
- **Source:** Mineral kingdom
- **Formula:** $HgCl_2$

CONSTITUTION

- More indicated in males than females
- Marked action in producing tenesmus of rectum and bladder
- For debility, prostration; second stage of gonorrhoea
- **Temperament:** Nervous, scrofulous
- **Thermal:** Ambithermal
- **Miasm:** Sycosis, Syphilis

MIND

- Anxious, restless; rocks hard; worse at night
- **Stares at persons who talk to him, doesn't understand them; stupid, imbecile**
- Anxiety during sleep, after menses
- Delirium and stupor
- Ill-humour; during which nothing pleases
- Absentminded, confused mentally; difficulty in thinking

KEYNOTE SYMPTOMS

- Prostration, debility, faintness, weakness
- Tormenting tenesmus of rectum and bladder at the same time, not ameliorated by stool or urine
- Stools – hot, scanty, bloody, slimy, offensive, with cutting pains and shreds of mucous membrane; a never get done feeling after stools
- Urine – hot, burning, in drops; scanty or suppressed
- Stitching, tearing pains here and there, especially in the chest
- **Thirst insatiable for cold drinks, yet drinking aggravates; fluids return through the nose. Desire for cold food**
- **Sweats from every motion, partial, foul, at night; worse on forehead, lower parts;** sweats after urination, before and after stools
- Internal burning in the throat, stomach, rectum, bladder, etc. **Burning is most marked in this drug than in any other mercury salt**
- Corrosiveness of all discharges, especially tears and nasal discharge
- Constriction of throat, rectum and bladder
- Second stage of gonorrhoea with continuous tenesmus. Rapidly spreading chancres; phagedenic ulcers
- Throat-sore, red, painful and burning; tonsils swollen and covered with ulcers. Swallowing difficult and painful

CLINICAL

- Delirium
- Photophobia
- Conjunctivitis
- Iritis
- Choroiditis
- Retinitis
- Iridocyclitis
- Keratoiritis
- Phlyctenulae on cornea
- Gum disorders
- Tongue disorders
- Tenesmus
- Colitis
- Crohn's disease
- Peritonitis
- Diarrhoea
- Dysentery
- Constipation
- Ozaena
- Otorrhoea
- Pharyngitis
- Albuminuria
- Cystitis
- Urethritis
- Nephritis
- Bright's disease
- Gonorrhoea
- Syphilis
- Chancre
- Leucorrhoea
- Toxic conditions of pregnancy
- Balanitis
- Phimosis
- Paraphimosis
- Ulceration
- Pustules

MODALITIES

- **Aggravation:** After stool, after micturating, at night, in cold open air, hot days and cool nights
- **Amelioration:** Rest

REMEDY RELATIONSHIP

- **Compare:** Ars., Lach.; Leon., influences pelvic organs, promotes secretion and reduces febrile excitement, valuable in suppressed menses and lochia, dysentery, vomiting, severe pains in the abdomen, violent thirst, tongue dry and cracked; Mons. in dysentery
- **Antidote:** Calc-s.

MERCURIUS CYANATUS

SPHERE OF ACTION

- Gastrointestinal system
- Respiratory system
- Circulatory system
- Musculoskeletal system
- Urinary system
- Skin

INTRODUCTION

- **Common name:** Bicyanide of mercury, Mercuric cyanide
- **Group:** Salt
- **Source:** Mineral kingdom
- **Formula:** $Hg(CN)_2$
- **Prover:** Beck

CONSTITUTION

- For eyes sunken and fixed, face is pale
- Overall, patient has profound prostration, coldness and cyanosis
- **Temperament:** Haemorrhagic, billious
- **Thermal:** Chilly
- **Miasm:** Syphilis

MIND

- Irritability after eating to satiety
- Talkativeness
- Great excitement, fits of passion and fury

KEYNOTE SYMPTOMS

- Toxaemia of acute infections and diseases, especially diphtheria
- **Haemorrhages – dark and persistent, of fluid blood**
- Early, rapid and marked prostration
- **Cyanosis, rapid respiration and heart action**
- Nausea; vomiting – bilious and bloody, incessant hiccough; abdomen painful, tender on pressure
- Redness around the anus. Frequent diarrhoea with tenesmus
- Stools are bloody, black, offensive, slimy, green
- Necrotic destruction of soft parts of palate and fauces. Diphtheria develops rapidly, is putrid, gangrenous and septic accompanied by extreme prostration, tremors, coldness and cyanosis
- Dark blood from nose, profuse, several times a day
- Chronic sore throat of public speakers; intense redness of fauces
- Anxiety from pain in throat on swallowing, from rough, dry cough in diphtheria
- Cutting pain in throat or larynx on swallowing with rawness in spots
- **Malignant diphtheria with impossible swallowing,** cutting pain on swallowing. **Thick, grayish membrane in throat**
- Suppression of urine; amber coloured, scanty, painful and albuminous

CLINICAL

- Haemorrhages
- Toxaemia
- Prostration
- Cyanosis
- Aphthae
- Halitosis
- Nausea
- Dysentery
- Hoarseness
- Laryngitis
- Pharyngitis
- Tonsillitis
- Diphtheria
- Dyspnoea
- Pleural effusion
- Typhoidal pneumonia
- Nephritis
- Phlebitis
- Varicose veins
- Ulceration

MODALITIES

- **Aggravation:** From speaking, after eating, swallowing
- **Amelioration:** Milk

REMEDY RELATIONSHIP

- **Compare:** Arum-t., Caust., Hep., Kali-bi., Phyt., Echi., Lach., Gels.

SPHERE OF ACTION

- Ears
- Gastrointestinal system
- Respiratory system
- Musculoskeletal system
- Genitourinary system
- Skin

INTRODUCTION

- **Common name:** Calomel, Mercurous chloride, Subchloride of mercury
- **Group:** Salt
- **Source:** Mineral kingdom
- **Formula:** HgCl
- **Prover:** Hale

CONSTITUTION

- Suits ill nourished, pale, scrofulous children presenting with swelling of cervical and other glands
- Patient is pallid as a corpse and has flabby bloatedness
- Suits scrofulous children liable to remittent bilious attacks
- **Temperament:** Nervous, bilious
- **Thermal:** Ambithermal
- **Miasm:** Sycosis, Syphilis

MERCURIUS DULCIS

MIND

- Mentally agitated and restless; nervous and apprehensive
- Moody, gloomy, irritable
- Hypochondriasis
- Peculiar whimpering

KEYNOTE SYMPTOMS

- **Marked pallor, patient is pallid as a corpse**
- Inflammation with plastic exudation. Inflammation with peritonitis, meningitis, pleurisy
- Scrofulous inflammation in general, but particular of the eyes
- Swollen glands especially parotid and cervical glands
- **Tongue black, indented and indurated; with aphthae**
- Cyclic vomiting of infants. Nausea and vomiting
- Biliousness. Biliary stasis
- Constant desire for stool with tenesmus
- **Acrid, grass green diarrhoea of infants without tenesmus, with an ulcerated mouth and enlarged glands**
- Anus sore and burning. Dysentery; small stools of mucous and blood, covered with bile
- Deafness, due to a swelling which compresses the eustachian tube
- Catarrhal inflammation of middle ear. Eustachian tube closed, with plastic exudate or catarrh
- Severe ulceration of throat, makes swallowing difficult
- Broad, moist, burning and offensive condylomata around external genitals and anus
- Flabby and ill nourished skin
- Copper coloured eruptions; desquamation of skin

CLINICAL

- Meningitis
- Halitosis
- Gingivitis
- Aphthae
- Peritonitis
- Diarrhoea
- Dysentery
- Eustachian catarrh
- Catarrhal deafness
- Otitis media
- Earache
- Tonsillitis
- Pharyngitis
- Prostatitis
- Condylomatous growth
- Measles

MODALITIES

- **Aggravation:** Acids
- **Amelioration:** Cold drinks

REMEDY RELATIONSHIP

- **Compare:** Kali-m. in catarrhal inflammation of the middle ear; Sul-ac., in stringy stools
- **Antidoted by:** Hep.

MERCURIUS SOLUBILIS

INTRODUCTION

- **Common name:** Quicksilver, Mercurius vivus
- **Group:** Salt
- **Source:** Mineral kingdom
- **Formula:** $2(NH_2Hg_2)NO_3 \cdot H_2O$
- **Prover:** Hahnemann

SPHERE OF ACTION

- Head
- Glands
- Eyes
- Ears
- Nose
- Gastrointestinal system
- Respiratory system
- Genitourinary system

CONSTITUTION

- Suits light haired people with a pale face and lax skin and muscles. Skin has a translucent quality, like marble with blotchiness
- Suits scrofulous children
- **Temperament:** Tremulous, weak, sweaty, nervous, scrofulous
- **Thermal:** Ambithermal, sensitive to heat and cold
- **Miasm:** Syphilis

MIND

- Introverted, reserved, mistrustful
- **Memory is weak; slow in answering questions**
- Poor self-confidence; indifference to everything
- Loss of will power. Weary of life
- Irresolution; changes mind constantly; unstable mental behaviour
- Restlessness; constantly changing position, especially at night
- Hypersensitive to external impressions
- Strong emotions internally but they are rarely given expression; thinks he is losing reason
- Desires to communicate, but has difficulty making contact
- Stammering, nervous with tremors. Hurried speech
- Have violent impulses, to strike or even kill, that frightens them. Tries to restrain impulses. Suicidal, especially during menses. Postpartum mania

KEYNOTE SYMPTOMS

- **Patients are human 'thermometers' – sensitive to both heat and cold**
- A typical antisyphilitic remedy – converts healthy cells into necrotic wrecks; decomposes blood leading to anaemia; destructive inflammation of bones and joints
- Secondary stage of syphilis with febrile anaemia, rhumatoid pains and ulcerations
- All discharges are foul, free, thin, slimy, acrid, burning and yellowish-green
- Tremors everywhere. Trembling, twitching from least exertion
- All complaints are associated with prostration, weariness and trembling
- Glandular enlargement, especially that of lymph glands with easy suppuration
- Tendency to pus formation – thin, greenish, putrid, streaked with thin blood
- Tendency to vesicles, ulcers on mucous membranes, especially of mouth and throat. Ulcers spread superficially and have a lardaceous base
- **Perspiration is profuse, debilitating and oily, which does not relieve**
- **Marked thirst with moist mouth. Increased salivary secretion. Sweetish metallic taste.**
- **Tongue is flabby, indented; furrow in upper surface, length wise;** Aphthae. Gums are spongy, recede and bleed easily. Offensive breath.
- Greenish, bloody, slimy stools accompanied with pain and tenesmus. A never get done feeling
- Chronic ear infections. Otorrhoea with thick yellow discharge; swimmers ear infection.
- Excoriating, greenish, bloody leucorrhoea; Sensation of rawness in parts. Stinging pain in ovaries. Mammae are painful and engorged with milk at menses
- Blood stained nocturnal emissions. Vesicles and ulcers on fore part and sides of penis

CLINICAL

- Phobic disorder
- Hydrophobia
- Malignancy
- Connective tissue disease
- Glandular swelling
- Parkinson's disease
- Eye disorders
- Iritis
- Conjunctivitis
- Mumps
- Parotiditis
- Stomatitis
- Gum disorders
- Glossitis
- Enteritis
- Gastralgia
- Colitis
- Ulcerative colitis
- Diarrhoea
- Constipation
- Dysentery
- Otorrhoea
- Otitis media
- Coryza
- Sinusitis
- Epistaxis
- Pharyngitis
- Tonsillitis
- Asthma
- Arthritis
- Sexual disorders
- Syphilis
- Vaginal abscess
- Vaginitis
- Leucorrhoea
- Balanitis
- Premature ejaculation
- Orchitis
- Bed sores
- Measles

MODALITIES

- **Aggravation:** At night, from wet damp weather, in autumn, during warm days and cold damp nights, lying on right side, perspiring, changing weather, warmth of bed
- **Amelioration:** From moderate temperature, rest

REMEDY RELATIONSHIP

- **Compare:** Mez., its vegetable analogue, Bell., Hep., Puls., Nux-v., Ars., Acon., Kali-i.
- **Follows well:** Bell., Hep., Lach., Sulph., but should not be given before or after Sil. If given in low (weak) potencies hastens rather than aborting suppuration
- **Antidote:** Hep., Aur., Mez.
- **Complementary:** Bad.

MEZEREUM

INTRODUCTION

- **Common name:** Spurge olive, Daphne mezereum
- **Family:** *Thymelaceae*
- **Source:** Vegetable kingdom
- **Part used:** Bark
- **Prover:** Hahnemann

SPHERE OF ACTION

- Mind
- Teeth
- Nerves
- Gastrointestinal system
- Bones
- Skin

CONSTITUTION

- Suits light haired, irresolute persons
- **Temperament:** Phlegmatic, rheumatic, gouty
- **Thermal:** Chilly
- **Miasm:** Psora, Syphilis

MIND

- Indifferent to everything and everyone; looks outside a window for hours without noticing anything
- Angry at trifles and soon sorry for it
- Weak memory. **Vanishing of thoughts while speaking**
- Absentminded and forgetful
- Aversion to talking; uttering even a single word seems like a great task
- Fear, apprehension and faintness, especially felt in the pit of the stomach, as if something would happen
- Faintness caused by shock, pain and hearing bad news
- Nervous, keeps moving about
- Hypochondriacal and despondent

KEYNOTE SYMPTOMS

- Suits complaints that come on in the earliest months of the years. Thus, epidemics occurring in January and February often call for this remedy
- Acrid secretions like pus, leucorrhoea, etc.
- Sudden pains of several kinds with chilliness, numbness and soreness
- Bones, especially long bones inflamed, swollen with burning, boring pains, especially at night. Decay and exostosis of bones
- **The head is covered with thick, leather-like crusts under which thick pus collects. Dandruff. Hair falls by handful.**
- Violent facial neuralgia, especially around teeth, worse at night, and after eating
- Ciliary neuralgia after surgery, especially removal of eyeball
- **Cracks at corner of mouth. Red eruptions around the mouth with coryza. Mouth waters.**
- **Toothache in carious teeth, better by opening the mouth and drawing in air. Teeth feel elongated. Rapid decay of hollow teeth**
- Chronic gastritis with burning pains, better eating and from milk. Ulcer in the stomach
- Constipation after confinement; with uterine or hepatic inertia. Green discharges from the rectum
- Sensation as if tympanum was exposed to cold air – ears feel too open
- Intolerable itching, worse in bed and from a warm bath
- Itching changes location on scratching. Skin cold in areas where there is intense itching
- Eruptions ulcerate and form thick, yellowish-white scabs under which thick yellow pus collects. An acrid, gluey moisture oozes from under the eruptions
- Eczema and itching eruptions after vaccination

CLINICAL

- Vaccination – bad effects
- Neuralgia
- Bone affections
- Exostosis
- Pediculosis
- Tinea capitis
- Ciliary neuralgia
- Facial neuralgia
- Teeth affections
- Caries
- Toothache
- Teeth decay
- Tongue affections
- Gastric ulcer
- Inguinal hernia
- Prolapse of rectum
- Ear affections
- Syphilis
- Skin affections
- Eruptions
- Eczema
- Eczema capitis
- Senile pruritus
- Pityriasis
- Tinia versicolor
- Impetigo
- Herpes zoster
- Ulcers

MODALITIES

- **Aggravation:** Cold air, cold washing, at night, touch or motion, bad effects of mercury or alcohol, warmth of bed, fire, during menses, after vaccinations
- **Amelioration:** Open air, wrapping up, eating

REMEDY RELATIONSHIP

- **Compare:** Merc., Phyt., Rhus-t., Guaj., Syph. Caust.
- **Antidotes:** Kali-i., Merc.; Mez. and Merc. antidote each other

MILLEFOLIUM

INTRODUCTION

- **Common name:** Yarrow, Millefolium achillea
- **Family:** *Compositae*
- **Source:** Vegetable kingdom
- **Part used:** Whole fresh plant
- **Prover:** Nenning, Hartlaub and Trinks

SPHERE OF ACTION

- Mind
- Blood vessels
- Gastrointestinal system
- Urinary system
- Female genital system
- Skin

CONSTITUTION

- Indicated in atonic, anaemic women and children; also suits the aged
- **Temperament:** Haemorrhagic
- **Thermal:** Chilly
- **Miasm:** Tubercular

MIND

- Marked irritability
- Loss of memory. **Seems to have forgotten something, does not know what he is doing or wants to do**
- Sad, hysterical
- Aversion to work
- **Strikes - knocks his head against the wall**
- Excitable during pain in pit of stomach
- Violent and vehement, especially in the evening after dinner
- Anxiety in chest

MODALITIES

- **Aggravation:** Injury, violent exertion, coffee, evening, night, suppression of discharges
- **Amelioration:** From bleeding, re-establishment of discharges, during the day

KEYNOTE SYMPTOMS

- **Haemorrhages - profuse, bright red, florid and painless,** especially from injuries, without fever, without anxiety, without nausea, from various organs
- Haemorrhage after labour, abortion or miscarriage
- Preventive for bleeding before extraction of teeth in people who have a haemorrhagic diathesis. Preventive in postpartum haemorrhages
- **Bad effects of a fall from a height**
- Wounds bleed profusely, especially after a fall
- Useful for resolving blood clots, after injuries, falls or surgeries
- Copious mucous discharges, especially from atony
- Convulsions, after suppression of haemorrhages, menses, milk, discharges
- Very effective for nose bleeds with congestions of head and chest
- Cough with bloody sputum from suppression of menses or haemorrhoids.
- Haemoptysis after injury or in incipient phthisis. Expectoration of bright red blood, without coughing too much or as a consequence of violent exertion
- Menses early, profuse, protracted, with colicky pain in the abdomen. Suppressed menses with epileptic attacks
- Painful varicose veins during pregnancy
- Continuous high temperature; from suppressed lochia or itch

CLINICAL

- Haemorrhage
- Anaemia
- Chlorosis
- Fall, injury
- Sprains
- Wounds
- Bruises
- Post operative for stone-biliary, renal
- Epilepsy
- Convulsions
- Fistula lachrymalis
- Dental extractions
- Incarcerated hernia
- Haemorrhoids
- Epistaxis
- Cough
- Haemoptysis
- Haematuria
- Menorrhagia
- Haemorrhage after abortion
- Confinement haemorrhages
- Postpartum haemorrhage
- Antepartum haemorrhage
- Suppressed menses
- Suppressed lochia
- Varicose veins
- Infertility
- Smallpox

REMEDY RELATIONSHIP

- **Compare:** Erech. in epistaxis and haemoptysis, blood bright red; Fic-v. in haemorrhage from bowels and lungs; Acal. and Helx. in haemoptysis, diseases of the chest, consumption; also, Sec., Ip., Arn., Bell-p., Calen., Ust., Ger., Ham.
- **Follows well:** After, Acon. and Arn. in haemorrhages
- **Incompatible:** Coffee
- **Antidotes:** Ars-i, Arum-m.

MORGAN GAERTNER

INTRODUCTION

- **Common name:** Proteus
- **Group:** A bowel nosode
- **Source:** Prepared from cultures of non-lactose fermenting bacterial flora of the instestinal tract
- **Prover:** John Paterson

SPHERE OF ACTION

- Gastrointestinal system
- Respiratory system
- Urinary system
- Female genital system
- Musculoskeletal system
- Skin

CONSTITUTION

- Suits pale, impatient, claustrophobic persons with fine, brown hair
- **Temperament:** Nervous
- **Thermal:** Chilly
- **Miasm:** Sycosis

MIND

- Irritable, quick tempered
- Impatient
- Tense, nervous, full of apprehensions
- Depressive psychosis
- Jealous
- Gets excited in company
- Bites nails due to nervousness
- Nervous breakdown
- Claustrophobic
- Restless and weepy

KEYNOTE SYMPTOMS

- Chronic inflammation of eyelids – styes, blepharitis, chalazion
- **Desires sweet, salt and prefers hot food. Aversion to fat, eggs and meat. Taste is bad or bitter**
- Flatulent dyspepsia; fulness of the epigastrium. Excessive eructations
- Distention of abdomen and colon. Pain in ileo-caecal region.
- Gall bladder region tender and painful; cholecystitis
- Diarrhoea – stool watery, profuse, involuntary; causes insomnia
- Tendency to constipation – dry, hard stool; mucous is passed per rectum even if patient is not constipated. Bowels sluggish
- Anal fissure, prolapse of rectum, pruritis ani
- Recurrent ulcers in nose and mouth, bleeding
- Otitis, mastoiditis, furuncles in the ear
- Hypersecretion from nasal fossa and maxillary sinus; post-nasal and nasal catarrh
- Intercostal neuralgia, thoracic pain; constriction of the chest radiating to left arm.
- Renal colic due to calculi. Frequent micturition
- **Leucorrhoea – profuse, foul smelling, corrosive; pruritus vulva**
- **Rheumatism of right shoulder, arm, deltoid, elbow or wrist; painful swelling of thumbs**
- Arthritis of knees; knees stiff and painful
- Sensitive skin; psoriasis, urticaria, eczema, pustulous eruptions, herpes
- **Warts on hands – large, flat or jagged**

CLINICAL

- Alopecia areata
- Styes
- Corneal ulcer
- Vitreous opacity
- Blepharitis
- Mastoiditis
- Stomatitis
- Gingivitis
- Cholecystitis
- Diarrhoea
- Constipation
- Haemorrhoids
- Piles
- Sinusitis
- Nasal herpes
- Ulcers in nose
- Renal colic
- Bedwetting
- Nephritis
- Pyelonephritis
- Arthritis
- Rheumatism
- Herpes
- Psoriasis
- Urticaria
- Warts
- Eczema
- Insomnia

MODALITIES

- **Aggravation:** In company, after meals, at night, before menses, right side, heat of bed
- **Amelioration:** Movement, passing flatus, eructations

REMEDY RELATIONSHIP

- **Compare:** Puls., Lyc., Sil., Kali-bi., Nat-m, Nux-v., Sulph., Sep., Calc., Graph.

MORPHINUM

INTRODUCTION

- **Common name:** An alkoloid of Opium
- **Family:** *Papaveraceae*
- **Source:** Vegetable kingdom
- **Formula:** $C_{17}H_{19}NO_3 \cdot H_2O$
- **Prover:** Serturner and Rufus L. Thurston

SPHERE OF ACTION

- Mind
- Eyes
- Nervous system
- Gastrointestinal system
- Respiratory system
- Heart
- Musculoskeletal system
- Genitourinary system
- Skin

CONSTITUTION

- Indicated in people who are extremely susceptible to pain
- Suits people with a dusky red or pale face
- **Temperament:** Nervous
- **Thermal:** Chilly
- **Miasm:** Tubercular

MIND

- Mentally exhausted; difficulty in concentrating; weak memory
- Ailments from fright or fear
- Forgetful – hunts for words while speaking
- Apathy and indifference
- Melancholic delirium; during fever, sleep
- Delusions – sees brilliant coloured birds, hears voices
- Very self-willed and deceitful, want of morality
- Pathological liars; will even fake illness to gain attention in order to manipulate
- They lie and deceive and look you straight in the eye; never speak the truth, does not know what they are saying
- Profound depression; shock induced by terror, cannot describe symptoms because of tears and sobs
- Dream-like state
- Violence; sudden from slight causes
- Suspiciousness, mistrustfulness.

KEYNOTE SYMPTOMS

- Violent and sudden neuralgic pains
- Indicated in neuralgia where pains are so violent that they threaten convulsions; pain causes twitching or jerking of limbs. Extreme susceptibility to pain.
- Hyperaesthesia
- **Sudden spell of fainting, with great anxiety, and a numb feeling all over; thought that she was going to die**
- Vertigo from least movement of the head
- Head is very heavy and hot; giddiness and drowsiness
- Dusky red or pale face; intensely flushed face, puffed, livid and cyanotic
- Vomiting of green matter – bitter or sour greenish matter
- Bloated sensation of abdomen, distended. Excoriating soreness of anus
- Impotency, erections incomplete or absent
- **Restlessness of legs, wants them held; sensation of worms in legs**
- Heaviness, drowsiness; sleepy but cannot sleep or prolonged deep sleep or half sleeping state

CLINICAL

- Delirium
- Depression
- Drug addiction
- Drug overdose
- Coma
- Neuralgia
- Multiple neuritis
- Trismus
- Vertigo
- Eye affections
- Ptosis
- Nausea
- Diaphragmatic paralysis
- Tympanitis
- Diarrhoea
- Constipation
- Sneezing
- Rhinitis
- Asthma
- Tachycardia
- Bradycardia
- Retention of urine
- Uraemia
- Orchitis
- Prostatic hypertrophy
- Impotency
- Arthritis
- Rheumatism
- Lumbosacral backache
- Urticaria
- Insomnia

MODALITIES

- **Aggravation:** On movement, after sleep, in the morning, from vinegar, slightest movement of the head
- **Amelioration:** Coffee, cold

REMEDY RELATIONSHIP

- **Compare:** Op., Cod., Apom.; in excessive sensibility, Acon., Cham.; weep in telling symptoms, Puls.; Nux-v., Heroin., Ign.
- **Antidote to:** Ther.
- **Antidoted by:** Camph.

MOSCHUS MOSCHIFERUS

SPHERE OF ACTION

- Mind
- Respiratory system
- Heart
- Female genital system
- Male genital system

INTRODUCTION

- **Common name:** Musk deer, Musk, Kasturi
- **Family:** *Mammalia*
- **Source:** Trituration of secretion obtained in preputial follicles of Musk deer
- **Part used:** Dried, inspissated secretion
- **Prover:** Hahnemann, Gross and Stapf

CONSTITUTION

- Suits spoiled, sensitive natures, also hysterical men and women
- People with one cheek red and cold, other pale and hot; lips blue
- **Suits girls who are selfish, obstinate, self-willed and much pampered, resort to all kinds of cunning acts to have their whims gratified**
- **Temperament:** Hysterical, nervous
- **Thermal:** Chilly
- **Miasm:** Sycosis

MIND

- Hysterical women and men
- Slightest disturbance of her mental equilibrium or least emotional change brings on a state of fainting
- Awkward, hurried with weakness so that everything falls from the hands.
- **Violent anger, talks excitedly, raves, scolds till mouth becomes dry, lips blue, eyes staring, and she falls unconscious. Desire to break things**
- Imaginary sufferings
- Uncontrollable laughter, alternates with weeping.
- Fears – noise, death, dying, suffocation
- Sexual hypochondriasis, nymphomania
- Talks to himself and gesticulates
- Sudden loss of memory; absentminded
- Frightened easily; anxiety with palpitations

KEYNOTE SYMPTOMS

- Indicated in all complaints that have easy fainting with main indication
- A remedy for hysteria and nervous paroxysms, fainting fits and convulsions, catalepsy
- Spasmodic nervous effects with a feeling of coldness
- **Coldness in general or of single parts, but wants to uncover;** nervous and spasmodic complaints where the patient feels very cold. Pallor accompanies coldness
- Spasms and tension in muscles, skin and mind; laryngeal spasms, hiccups, spasm of chest or heart and general convulsions
- Buzzing, squeezing, plug-like sensation
- Easy fainting in any diseased condition. Faints while eating, during menses, from heart disease
- Epileptic fits with rigors or shuddering, as if patient is felling very cold
- Vertigo with fainting, as if falling from a height; worse least motion
- Headache with coldness, faintings, involuntary stools and polyuria
- Spasmodic, nervous hiccup. Everything tastes flat. Faints while eating.
- **Craving for cheese, black coffee, beer and brandy; aversion to food**
- Globus hystericus, ending in unconsciousness
- Nausea on sight or thought of food
- Asthma with intense anxiety, fear and smothering sensation; chest oppressed, difficult respiration
- Trembling around the heart; hysterical palpitations
- Increased sexual desire in both sexes, even the aged

CLINICAL

- Hysteria
- Violent anger
- Nervous trembling
- Fainting
- Convulsions
- Catalepsy
- Vertigo
- Globus hystericus
- Hiccups
- Post-operative abdominal distention
- Cough
- Croup
- Whooping cough
- Asthma
- Heart failure
- Palpitations
- Arrhythmia
- Diabetes mellitus
- Sexual disorders
- Nymphomania
- Impotence

MODALITIES

- **Aggravation:** From excitement, cold, side lain on, suppressions, menses during or after a meal, pressure, motion
- **Amelioration:** In open air, rubbing, smell of musk

REMEDY RELATIONSHIP

- **Compare:** Asaf., Carb-v., Castor, Ign., Nux-m., Nux-v., Valer., Sumb.
- **Antidoted by:** Camph., Coff.
- **Antidote to:** Ther.

MUREX PURPUREA

SPHERE OF ACTION
- Mind
- Musculoskeletal system
- Urinary system
- Female genital system

INTRODUCTION
- **Common name:** Purple fish
- **Family:** *Muricidae*
- **Source:** Animal kingdom
- **Part used:** The dessicated juice
- **Prover:** Petroz

CONSTITUTION
- Especially suits nervous, lively, affectionate women; menopausal sufferings
- Suits those who are tired, weak and run down; must lie down, which aggravates
- **Temperament:** Sanguine, lymphatic, nervous
- **Thermal:** Chilly
- **Miasm:** Tubercular

MIND
- Great sadness, especially towards evening; marked depression of spirits
- Anxious, apprehensive, better leucorrhoea
- Imagines herself very sick or hopelessly ill
- Repungence to conversation
- Weak memory, cannot find the correct words to express herself
- Sad, unconscious before menses
- Nymphomania from suppressed menses

KEYNOTE SYMPTOMS
- Tendency to excessive haemorrhage from the uterus with large clots; menses – irregular, frequent, profuse, of large clots
- **Chief action is on female sexual sphere producing frantic sexual desire; patient is easily excited; nymphomania, slightest touch reawakens desire**
- **Sinking, all gone sensation in stomach very marked; violent hunger even after eating**
- Constant urge to urinate with excessive secretion; frequent necessity to rise at night to urinate, thus good for diabetes
- **Urine smells like valerian**
- Sensation as if something was pressing on a sore spot in the pelvis
- **Pains are diagonal – right ovary to left breast or visa versa**
- Cutting pains in the cervix and os
- **Consciousness of the womb; prolapsed, must cross legs tightly.** Sore pain in uterus
- **Leucorrhoea green or bloody, alternates with mental symptoms** and pain in sacrum
- Difficulty in walking; all joints are weak during pregnancy

CLINICAL
- Constipation
- Diabetes
- Tumour of breast
- Cervix disorders
- Leucorrhoea
- Menorrhagia
- Metrorrhagia
- Dysmenorrhoea
- Nymphomania
- Uterine prolapse
- Chronic endometritis
- Ailments during pregnancy
- Ailments during menopause

MODALITIES
- **Aggravation:** Exertion, least touch, night, after sleep, sitting, lying down
- **Amelioration:** Before menses, pressure, eating, putting head back

REMEDY RELATIONSHIP
- **Compare:** Plat., Sep. (the latter lacks sexual erethism of Murx.). Lil-t., in nymphomania; Sep. in bearing down sensation, but has no sexual erethism; Sec., Bell., Kreos., Puls., Lach., Helon., Lyss.

MURIATICUM ACIDUM

INTRODUCTION
- **Common name:** Hydrochloric acid
- **Group:** Acid
- **Source:** Mineral kingdom
- **Formula:** HCl
- **Prover:** Hahnemann

SPHERE OF ACTION
- Mind
- Blood
- Gastrointestinal system
- Respiratory system
- Musculoskeletal system
- Genitourinary system
- Skin

CONSTITUTION
- Indicated in persons with black hair and dark eyes; skin is sensitive to sun's rays
- **Temperament:** Nervous
- **Thermal:** Chilly
- **Miasm:** Syphilis

MIND
- Loud moaning, muttering
- Great restlessness
- Sad, taciturn, suffers in silence
- Conscientious about trifles
- Irritable, peevish
- Disposition to be angry
- Weak memory; absentminded

KEYNOTE SYMPTOMS
- Physical debility followed by mental debility
- Great debility, as soon as patient sits down, eyes close, lower jaw hangs down, slides down and he is in bed
- Has a marked affinity for the blood causing septic states
- Muscular prostration from blood poisoning going on to paralysis like that of the heart, bladder, tongue and especially that of the mouth and anus
- Decomposition of fluids with tendency to violent haemorrhages
- Excretions sour and acrid; offensive secretions, offensive breath and body odour. Putridity
- Mucous membranes are dry, bleeding, cracked and ulcerated
- **Burning is a keynote** – in ulcers, especially the margins, piles, varices, stomach, eruptions
- Vertigo, worse lying on right side
- **Tongue is heavy and stiff, makes talking difficult, paralysed. Tongue pale, swollen, dry, leathery, shrunken or burnt looking**
- Malignant affections of the tongue, studded with ulcers, deep, perforating, having a black or dark base, offensive, foul breath, aversion to meat
- **Sordes on teeth;** gums swollen, bleeding and ulcerating
- Sinking sensation in stomach, not better by eating
- Stools very difficult to pass as from inactivity of bowels; involuntary evacuation of liquid and serous faeces when urinating
- **Haemorrhoids like a bunch of grapes, purple; burn on being touched, even by toilet paper; especially during pregnancy**
- **Pulse is feeble and small; drops every third beat**
- Indicated in all types of fevers, especially low grade typhoidal fevers, when the mental and paretic state is present; septic fever

CLINICAL
- Haemorrhages
- Prostration
- Muscular exhaustion
- Septic states
- Malignancy
- Epithelioma
- Fistulae
- Fissures
- Aphthae
- Tongue affections
- Cirrhosis
- Haemorrhoids
- Anal prolapse
- Varices
- Diphtheria
- Menorrhagia
- Metrorrhagia
- Gonorrhoea
- Ulcers
- Carbuncles
- Eczema
- Bedsores
- Typhoid

MODALITIES
- **Aggravation:** Damp weather, before midnight, rest, after sleep, touch, walking, sitting
- **Amelioration:** Motion, warmth, uncovering during fever, lying on left side, after drinking

REMEDY RELATIONSHIP
- **Compare:** Ph-ac., Ars., Bapt., Bry., Rhus-t.
- **Antidote:** Merc., Op.
- **Follows well:** After, Bry., Merc., Rhus-t.
- Cures the muscular weakness following excessive use of Opium and tobacco

MYRICA CERIFERA

INTRODUCTION

- **Common name:** Bayberry, Wax myrtle, Candleberry
- **Family:** *Myricaceae*
- **Source:** Vegetable kingdom
- **Part used:** The bark of the root
- **Prover:** Samuel Thomson

SPHERE OF ACTION

- Mind
- Gastrointestinal system
- Liver
- Heart
- Female genital system
- Sleep

CONSTITUTION

- Suits cases with thick, viscid secretions from mucous membrane of the throat or stomach which is difficult to detach
- Cases with underlying liver disorders, especially jaundice
- **Temperament:** Nervous
- **Thermal:** Ambithermal
- **Miasm:** Sycosis

MIND

- Exhilaration followed by sadness
- Indifference to everything, even to friends
- Irritable with a constant desire to find fault
- Despodent, dejected, gloomy
- Cannot concentrate
- Dull, drowsy state
- **Ugly dreams, as if head is attacked by an enormous bug**

KEYNOTE SYMPTOMS

- **Profuse catarrhal discharges of old standing, of all kinds, especially if they are offensive, tenacious and difficult to detach**
- Excellent for cancerous and other grave diseases of the liver accompanied by jaundice
- General muscular lameness and soreness; aching in limbs; staggering gait
- Headache; dull heavy ache in temples and forehead on waking in the morning
- Tenacious, thick, nauseous mucous from mouth and throat. Taste bitter and nauseous, with offensive breath
- **Strong desire for acids, but loathing for food**
- Liver disorder – aching pain in liver, fullness, drowsiness with persistent sleeplessness and a dull, heavy headache
- Itching of jaundice; urticaria associated with liver affections
- Nasal obstruction or post-nasal catarrh often accompany jaundice or a disordered liver
- Abundant, offensive secretion of tenacious mucous in the throat which is difficult to detach
- Throat constricted with a rough feeling and a constant desire to swallow stringy mucous
- **Sharp pains around the heart with increased, audible pulsations, but slow pulse**
- Thick, yellow, acrid, foetid leucorrhoea
- **Sensation as of insects under the skin, especially on face**
- Disturbed, unrefreshing sleep with frequent wakings and bad dreams

CLINICAL

- Cancer
- Parotiditis
- Stomatitis
- Jaundice
- Intestinal catarrh
- Post-nasal catarrh
- Pharyngeal ailments
- Sore throat
- Bronchorrhoea
- Leucorrhoea
- Urticaria
- Insomnia

MODALITIES

- **Aggravation:** Warmth of bed, after sleep, after breakfast, in the morning, from motion
- **Amelioration:** In open air, eating, breakfast

REMEDY RELATIONSHIP

- **Compare:** Ptel., Corn., Chel., Lept., Fago., Kali-bi., Hydr., Dig.
- **Antidote:** Dig. in jaundice

MYRISTICA SEBIFERA

INTRODUCTION
- **Common name:** Brazilian cuba
- **Family:** *Myristicaceae*
- **Source:** Vegetable kingdom
- **Part used:** Red, acrid, poisonous gum obtained by incising the bark
- **Prover:** Mure

SPHERE OF ACTION
- Ears
- Gastrointestinal system
- Injuries
- Musculoskeletal system
- Cellular tissues
- Periosteum
- Skin

CONSTITUTION
- Indicated in inflammations of the skin, periosteum and cellular tissues where it hastens suppuration and shortens its duration
- **Temperament:** Nervous, scrofulous
- **Thermal:** Ambithermal
- **Miasm:** Sycosis

MIND
- Concentration impossible
- Dreams – of buildings, beginning at upper part, of business, of disputes
- Heedless, careless
- Vexed by a song which keeps running in the head
- Indifference, apathy regarding business
- Stupefaction, as if intoxicated

KEYNOTE SYMPTOMS
- It is a remedy of great antiseptic powers
- For inflammation of skin, cellular tissues and periosteum; also traumatic infections; hastens suppuration and shortens its duration
- Indicated in phlegmonous inflammation
- **Its use often does away with use of the knife; acts more powerfully often than *Hepar sulphuris* or *Silicea terra***
- Coppery taste which excites spitting of blood; burning in the throat
- **Tongue cracked and white; entire mouth, tonsils and pharynx painful and sensitive to contact**
- Fistula-in-ano; stool mixed with yellow mucous
- Inflammation of middle ear, tympanitis. Suppuration of middle ear, otitis media
- Very effective in suppurative processes affecting the joints
- Hands are stiff, as if from squeezing something for a long time; pain in hands worse when they touch each other
- Specific action in panaritium. Pain in the fingernails with swelling of the phalanges
- Fistulae, carbuncles, abscesses, malignant pustule; for inflammation of the skin

CLINICAL
- Suppurations
- Traumatic infections
- Homoeopathic antiseptic
- Parotiditis
- Stomatitis
- Fistula-in-ano
- Otitis media
- Scrofulous osteitis
- Panaritium
- Cellulitis
- Phlegmonous erysipelas
- Carbuncles
- Boils
- Abcesses
- Ulcers
- Eczema
- Fistulae
- Whitlow

MODALITIES
- **Aggravation:** Touch, contact
- **Amelioration:** In open air

REMEDY RELATIONSHIP
- **Compare:** Nux-m., Sil., Calc-s., Sulph., Pyrog.

NAJA TRIPUDIANS

SPHERE OF ACTION

- Mind
- Heart
- Nervous system
- Medulla oblongata
- Cerebellum
- Respiratory system
- Female genital system

INTRODUCTION

- **Common name:** Cobra venom
- **Family:** *Elapidae*
- **Source:** Animal kingdom
- **Part used:** Venom obtained by compressing the gland
- **Prover:** Russell and Stokes

CONSTITUTION

- Suits conditions depending upon degeneration of motor cells
- Depression of both mental and physical powers. **All complaints have a tendency to settle around the heart**
- Tendency to collapse and swooning fits
- **Temperament:** Nervous
- **Miasm:** Syphilis, Sycosis
- **Thermal:** Chilly

MIND

- Suicidal insanity, loathing of life
- **Broods constantly over imaginary troubles and misfortunes**
- Fear of death, disease, rain, misfortune
- Dreads to be left alone
- Forgetful, absentminded; wondering of mind, irresolution
- Nervous, excited, tremulous
- Depressed, melancholic, as if everything was done wrong and cannot be rectified
- Anxiety from pain in region of heart
- Aversion to talking
- Ailments from grief, sorrow, anticipation

KEYNOTE SYMPTOMS

- Acts primarily upon the nervous system, particularly upon the pneumogastric, glossopharyngeal and respiratory nerves
- Produces a typical case of bulbar paralysis with no haemorrhage but only oedema
- Left side principally affected; inability to lie on the left side
- **Sensation of a hot iron running throughout the system**
- Chronic, nervous palpitation, especially after public speaking
- Organs seems to be drawn together, especially heart and ovary
- All complaints have a tendency to settle around the heart, hypertrophy and valvular lesions
- Very susceptible to cold
- Marked surging of blood upwards
- Control of sphincters lost; loss of power of limbs
- **All complaints aggravate after sleep**
- Severe headache with intense depression; sensation of a blow from behind on head and neck
- Grasping at the throat with sensation of choking. Constriction of chest and throat
- Respiration slow, shallow, laboured, difficult; asthmatic constriction of chest, cannot expand lungs
- Oppressive weight on chest, as if a hot iron has been run in; dull, heavy pain in chest; sharp pain, worse on deep inspiration
- Acute and chronic septic endocarditis; heart affections after infectious diseases
- Low blood pressure
- **Pulse irregular in force but regular in rhythm**
- Marked dyspnoea and prostration due to a weak heart
- **Aching in left ovary with pain in the heart**
- With heart symptoms, pain in forehead and temples concomitant

CLINICAL

- Suicidal insanity
- Bulbar paralysis
- Spinal irritation
- Headache
- Migraine
- Ptosis
- Spasmodic stricture of oesophagus
- Otalgia
- Otitis media
- Hay fever
- Sore throat
- Dyspnoea
- Asthma
- Angina pectoris
- Chronic hypertrophy of heart
- Valvular diseases of heart
- Cardiac asthma
- Endocarditis
- Rheumatic carditis
- Pericarditis
- Myelitis
- Leucorrhoea
- Ovarian affections

MODALITIES

- **Aggravation:** At night, walking, left side, touch, riding in a carriage, after menses, from stimulants, cold air
- **Amelioration:** Lying on right side, walking, riding in open air, sneezing

REMEDY RELATIONSHIP

- **Compare:** Serpent poisons generally. Bung-f., Lach., Crot-h., Spig., Spong., Ars., Cact., Mygal., Dig., Carb-v., Camph., Gels., Caust., Agar., Aur.
- **Antidoted by:** Ammonia, tobacco

NAPHTHALINUM

INTRODUCTION
- **Common name:** Tar camphor, Naphthalene
- **Group:** Chemical compound
- **Source:** Mineral kingdom
- **Formula:** $C_{10}H_8$
- **Prover:** Lippincott

SPHERE OF ACTION
- Eyes
- Gastrointestinal system
- Respiratory system
- Urinary system
- Skin

MIND
- Mania, delirium, intoxication, loss of consciousness
- Restlessness
- Anxiety
- Lying as if stupefied by a narcotic

MODALITIES
- **Aggravation:** During night, while urinating
- **Amelioration:** Open air, from loosening clothes

KEYNOTE SYMPTOMS
- Sudden onset of symptoms – fever, headache, loss of appetite, allergies
- General muscular twitching; staggering, drunken gait
- Marked affinity for the eyes – **it produces detachment of the retina; papillo-retinal infiltration; deposits in patches upon the retina; soft cataract; corneal opacity**
- It is given in material doses **for the expulsion of worms, especially threadworms**
- Allergy, especially hay fever – acute coryza with fluent, excoriating discharge and much sneezing
- Paroxysms of cough, following each other in rapid succession that the patient cannot breathe – whooping cough, asthma. Cough with a blue or purple face
- Dyspnoea with sighing inspiration. Emphysema of aged with asthma
- Breathing irregular, laboured, asthmatic. Expectoration tenacious
- Soreness in the chest
- Irritation of the periphery of the urinary apparatus. Sudden, violent desire to urinate; meatus red, swollen. Pain in bladder, urine black; incontinence

CONSTITUTION
- Marked affinity for eyes. Face pale with a yellowish hue, stupefied
- **Temperament:** Nervous
- **Thermal:** Chilly
- **Miasm:** Syphilis

CLINICAL
- Corneal opacity
- Amblyopia
- Retinal detachment
- Cataract
- Worms
- Pinworms
- Catarrh
- Coryza
- Hay fever
- Whooping cough
- Bronchitis
- Phthisis pulmonalis
- Emphysema
- Asthma
- Dyspnoea
- Cystitis
- Black urine
- Pyelonephritis
- Urethral caruncle
- Balanitis
- Gleet
- Gonorrhoea
- Skin diseases
- Dermatitis
- Psoriasis
- Eczema
- Typhoid

REMEDY RELATIONSHIP
- **Compare:** Dros., Cor-r., Coc-c. Terp-h., Salol., Carb-ac, Arn., Bell., Ip., Thuj., Petros., Cina, Teucr., Ars., All-c., Sabad.

NATRIUM CARBONICUM

SPHERE OF ACTION
- Mind
- Gastrointestinal system
- Respiratory system
- Mucous membranes
- Urinary system
- Female genital system
- Skin

INTRODUCTION
- **Common name:** Sodium carbonate
- **Group:** Salt
- **Source:** Mineral kingdom
- **Formula:** $Na_2CO_3.10H_2O$
- **Prover:** Hahnemann

CONSTITUTION
- Suits light haired people of leucophlegmatic, temperament with an aversion to physical or mental exercise and open air
- Suits gentle, sacrificing people with a pale face and blue rings, around the eyes
- **Temperament:** Nervous, leucophlegmatic, hydrogenoid
- **Thermal:** Chilly
- **Miasm:** Psora

MIND
- Sad, depressed and melancholic
- Difficulty in comprehension
- Inability to think or perform any mental labour
- Confused, forgetful
- Dreams anxious, frightful; of journey, thunder, floods, death, quarrels, thieves
- Anxious and restless during thunderstorm
- Cheerful and jocular, even though sad within
- Mental fatigue
- Sadness and weeping from music; music causes tendency to suicide
- Inability to assimilate ideas when reading or writing
- Cross, irritable, especially during fever; disposition to be angry
- Aversion to society or the presence of certain people

KEYNOTE SYMPTOMS
- Great debility and worse from slightest mental or physical exertion
- Emaciation, anaemia and bloating; exhaustion
- It stimulates cellular activity and increases oxidation and metabolism
- Has an irritating action upon the skin – chapped hands and face, rough dry skin, herpes, warts, eczema, ulcers, vesicular eruptions and scrofulous skin conditions
- Irritating effects also seen on mucous membranes – from the mouth to the anus, eyes, nose, vaginal tract, respiratory tract, etc.
- Swelling and induration of glands
- Discharges are thick, yellow and offensive
- Congestion and catarrhal condition of head
- **Chronic effects of sunstroke; debility from heat of summers**
- Headache from sun or working under strong light; in hot weather; alternates with digestive problems
- **Oversensitive to, or ailments due to errors in diet**
- Indigestion, flatulence and bloating; weak digestion; sour eructations
- **Children cannot tolerate milk, diarrhoea from starch, milk**
- **Yellow substance like pulp of orange in stool; sudden call for stool**
- Nasal catarrh, bad smell of nasal secretion. Post-nasal catarrh, hawking of mucous from the throat
- Bearing down sensation; heaviness in the pelvic region, worse sitting, better moving
- Cervix is indurated or has a congenital defective growth on the anterior vaginal wall
- Leucorrhoea – thick, yellow, ropy, offensive and irritating
- Sterility due to lack of retention of semen due to excessive discharge of mucous from the vagina after coitus
- Weak ankles, they turn easily; twitching in muscles and limbs
- Freckles, yellow spots or blotches and pimples on skin

CLINICAL
- Tumours
- Necrosis
- Sunstroke
- Headache
- Photophobia
- Malassimilation
- Food allergies
- Milk allergy
- Belching
- Dyspepsia
- Flatulence
- Gastritis
- Peptic ulcer
- Irritable bowel syndrome
- Throat affections
- Lung affections
- Cystitis
- Enuresis
- Infertility
- Leucorrhoea
- Urethritis
- Spermatorrhoea
- Gonorrhoea
- Rheumatism
- Gout
- Weak ankles
- Eczema
- Herpes
- Freckles
- Pimples
- Chapped hands
- Warts
- Ichthyosis

MODALITIES
- **Aggravation:** From music, in the sun, excessive summer heat, mental exertion, a thunderstorm, noise, milk, dietic errors, physical exertion, drafts, getting wet, damp weather
- **Amelioration:** Eating, sweating, motion, pressure, rubbing, boring finger in ear or nose

REMEDY RELATIONSHIP
- **Compare:** Sodii bicarbonas, Nat-s., Calc., Sep., Nat-m., Caust., Lyc., Ant-c., Lil-t.
- **Antidoted by:** Ars., Camph.
- **Follows well:** After, Sep. in bearing down, Kalium salts
- **Compatible:** Sep., Puls., Calc., Nux-v., Sulph.

SPHERE OF ACTION

- Mind
- Eyes
- Gastrointestinal system
- Respiratory system
- Blood
- Lymphatic system
- Musculoskeletal system
- Genital system
- Skin

INTRODUCTION

- **Common name:** Sodium chloride
- **Group:** Salt
- **Source:** Mineral kingdom
- **Formula:** NaCl
- **Prover:** Hahnemann

CONSTITUTION

- Suits anaemic, chlorotic individuals with tendency to catarrh
- Emaciated, thin people, most notable around the neck; cachectic people
- Suits people who are oversensitive to all influences and have an oily, waxy look
- **Temperament:** Nervous, tuberculous, scrofulous
- **Thermal:** Chilly
- **Miasm:** Psora, Syphilis, Sycosis

NATRIUM MURIATICUM

MIND

- Acute and chronic grief
- **Reserved and introverted; emotionally shut down. Sighing, sulking**
- Severe depression with feeling of isolation; sad before menses
- Hypochondriacal, tired of life
- Psychic causes of disease; ill-effects of grief, fright, anger.
- **Consolation aggravates; detests consolation**
- **Appears to bid for sympathy yet angry when consoled**
- Irritable, gets into a passion about trifles
- Hates people who have offended them
- Aversion to the presence of strangers while urinating
- Aversion to men in women
- Dwells on past unpleasant memories. Holds grudges for years
- Prefers to be alone, to cry
- Makes mistakes in speaking; speaks what he does not intend to; awkward, hasty speech
- Young girls fall in love with married men

KEYNOTE SYMPTOMS

- Marked emaciation and poorly nourished on account of digestive problems
- Marked emaciation during summer complaints, from malaria, anaemia; most observable in the neck
- Great weakness and weariness, felt in the morning in bed
- Coldness – cold limbs, cold sensation along the spine
- Dry skin and mucous membranes – of mouth, throat, rectum, vagina, etc., or thick, white or clean, watery, albuminous and acrid discharges
- **Headache – migrainous, blinding, with photophobia, from sunrise to sunset; from grief. Anaemic headache of school girls**
- **Crack down the middle of lower lip**
- **Intense craving for salt. Excess salt in body leads to salty taste and corrosive skin**
- **Mapped tongue with red insular patches; numbness and tingling of tongue**
- Great liability to take cold; hay fever; coryza
- Tears stream down face on coughing
- Leucorrhoea acrid, watery, debilitating
- Menses suppressed from grief; low sex drive since grief
- Sterility with too early and too profuse menses
- Seminal emission soon after cotion with increased desire; weakness of organ with retarded emission
- Numbness of one side or parts lain on with paralysis
- Fingers or parts seem too short; constrictive sensation throughout
- Spinal irritation and paralysis after sexual excesses, grief, anger
- Spine oversensitive to pressure, touch
- Crusty eruptions in bends of limbs, behind ears, margin of scalp. Greasy skin
- Periodic, intermittent fevers with predominant chill. Chill from 10 to 11 am with thirst

CLINICAL

- Depression
- Stomatitis
- Anaemia
- Chlorosis
- Debility
- Malignancy
- Multiple sclerosis
- Goitre
- Headache
- Migraine
- Seborrhoea
- Photophobia
- Eye strain
- Stomatitis
- Gastritis
- Peptic ulcer
- Enlarged spleen
- Irritable bowel syndrome
- Constipation
- Catarrh
- Sinusitis
- Hay fever
- Heart affections
- Arrhythmia
- Hypertension
- Premenstrual syndrome
- Dysparunia
- Leucorrhoea
- Menstrual problems
- Sterility
- Spermatorrhoea
- Sciatica
- Gout
- Eczema
- Psoriasis
- Suicidal state
- Tinea
- Herpes
- Urticaria
- Erysipelas
- Malaria
- Fever blisters
- Insomnia

MODALITIES

- **Aggravation:** At 10 or 11 am, at the seashore or from sea air, heat of sun or stove, summers, strong emotions, consolation, sex, bread, fat, mental exertion, talking, writing, reading, lying down.
- **Amelioration:** In open air, cool bathing, going without regular meals; lying on right side sitting up, talking long, rest, rubbing, sweating, tight clothing

REMEDY RELATIONSHIP

- **Complementary:** Apis, Sep., Ign.
- **Compare:** Bry., Apis., Nat-c., Nat-i., Borx., Puls., Nat-s, Calc., Ign., Sep., Thuj., Graph., Alum.
- **Nat-m. is the chronic of Ign., which is its vegetable analogue.**
- **Followed by:** Sep. and Thuj.
- **Antidotes:** Arg-n., Quinine
- **Antidoted by:** Smelling Nit-s-d., Phos.

NATRIUM PHOSPHORICUM

SPHERE OF ACTION
- Mind
- Nervous system
- Gastrointestinal system
- Respiratory system
- Musculoskeletal system

INTRODUCTION
- **Common name:** Phosphate of soda, Disodium hydrogen phosphate
- **Group:** Salt
- **Source:** Mineral kingdom
- **Formula:** $NaPO_3$
- **Prover:** Farrington

CONSTITUTION
- Suits ailments with excess of acidity
- For marasmus of bottle fed babies
- Face is pale or red on alternate sides, body smells sour and glands are swollen
- **Temperament:** Nervous
- **Thermal:** Chilly
- **Miasm:** Psoric, Tubercular

MIND
- Fear, worse at night, that something will happen
- Imagines that pieces of furniture are persons, that he hears footsteps in the next room
- Mind dull, confused, worse mental exertion
- Irritable before breakfast
- Indifferent to loved ones, everything
- Easily offended, sensitive
- Sad, melancholic, especially after emissions, masturbation, from music

KEYNOTE SYMPTOMS
- Suits ailments caused by excess of lactic acid. Acid diathesis; ailments with excess of acidity
- **Discharges golden yellow, acidic, acrid, excoriating, sour**
- **Desires strong tasting things, eggs, beer, which ameliorate; aversion to bread and butter.** Worse acids, citrus fruits, alcohol, milk, sugar, fatty food and bitter foods
- Sourness – sour belching, sour vomiting. Heartburn, acidity and waterbrash. Peptic ulcer and attacks of gastralgia. Jaundice.
- Empty feeling in the stomach
- Constipation alternates with diarrhoea; anus excoriated, cutting pain in anus during stool, greenish jelly-like diarrhoea; desire for stool after coition
- One ear red hot, frequently itchy with acidity
- Inflammatory condition of the throat with sensation of a lump. **Golden yellow, creamy coating at the back of the roof of the mouth and tongue**
- Urine acidic; burning during urination; frequent urging to urinate
- Menses too early, pale, thin, watery; sterility from acid, sour secretions from the vagina; leucorrhoea – creamy or honey coloured or acrid and watery
- Skin yellow, itching, especially of ankles; eczema with honey coloured secretion; crusta lactea with golden yellow scabs

CLINICAL
- Leucocytosis
- Aphthae
- Dyspepsia
- Heartburn
- Acidity
- Peptic ulcer
- Jaundice
- Worms
- Threadworms
- Diarrhoea
- Post-nasal catarrh
- Tuberculosis
- Diabetes
- Vaginitis
- Leucorrhoea
- Gout
- Hives
- Boils
- Blisters

MODALITIES
- **Aggravation:** Sugar, milk, thunderstorm, mental exertion, walking upstairs, bitter foods, fatty foods
- **Amelioration:** Cold

REMEDY RELATIONSHIP
- **Compare:** Nat-lac., Nat-ns., Nat-sil-f., Nat-sel., Nat-sulo., Nat-s-c., Nat-tel., Calc., Rob., Phos.

SPHERE OF ACTION

- Mind
- Meninges
- Head
- Gastrointestinal system
- Liver
- Respiratory system
- Skeletal system
- Genital system
- Skin

INTRODUCTION

- **Common name:** Glauber's salt, Sodium sulphate
- **Group:** Salt
- **Source:** Mineral kingdom
- **Formula:** $Na_2SO_4.10H_2O$
- **Prover:** Schreter and Nenning

CONSTITUTION

- Hydrogenoid constitution leading to complaints due to living in damp houses, basements or cellars
- **Temperament:** Bilious, hydrogenoid
- **Thermal:** Chilly
- **Miasm:** Sycosis

NATRIUM SULPHURICUM

MIND

- Sad, gloomy, inclined to weep
- Inability to think; mental exertion aggravates
- **Music unbearable, causes depression**
- Wants to commit suicide by shooting or hanging; suicidal impulses; has to use a lot of self control to prevent oneself from doing so
- Fear of crowd, evil
- Aversion to be spoken to
- Aversion to life
- Dreams of fighting, running water
- Very irritable and ill-humoured in the morning
- Melancholic with periodical attacks of mania
- Cheerful after stools
- Mental ailments after a fall, blow or injury to the head

KEYNOTE SYMPTOMS

- **Marked periodicity of complaints** is a keynote
- Ill-effects of falls, blows, concussions or injuries to head. Headache, blindness or other physical and mental complaints since head injury
- Discharges are thick, yellow and greenish
- Conjunctiva yellow; conjunctivitis with granular lids; intense photophobia; sensitive to sunlight. Scrofulous ophthalmia
- **Toothache better by holding cold water in the mouth; gums burn like fire**
- **Tongue dirty greenish-gray or greenish-brown coat, especially at the root**
- **Want of appetite; repugnance to food**
- **Burning thirst for very cold drinks, especially in the evening**
- Sour vomiting, bilious vomiting, acid dyspepsia with heartburn, flatulence and duodenal catarrh. Burning in abdomen and anus
- Liver ailments – sore, enlarged, congested with sharp stitching pains, cannot bear clothes around abdomen. Gall stone colic
- Stools – involuntary, while passing flatus; loose morning stools; great size of faecal mass
- Nose bleed during menses; nasal catarrh with thick, yellow discharge
- Cough with thick, ropy, greenish, copious expectoration; must hold chest while coughing
- Asthma, specially of malarial districts; humid asthma of children; occurs early in the morning; every fresh cold brings on the attack
- **Lower lobe of left lung is affected.** Empty, all gone feeling in chest; pain through left lower chest; stitches on left side of chest
- Gonorrhoea – thick, yellowish-green discharge. Yellowish-green leucorrhoea in women after gonorrhoea
- **Every spring skin complaints reappear. Tendency to warts**
- Soft fleshy excrescences or condylomata on male genital organs

CLINICAL

- Debility
- Head injuries
- Convulsions
- Concussions
- Opisthotonos
- Myelitis
- Spinal meningitis
- Epilepsy
- Headache
- Migraine
- Photophobia
- Toothache
- Biliousness
- Flatulence
- Liver affections
- Jaundice
- Hepatitis
- Diarrhoea
- Epistaxis
- Hoarseness
- Cough
- Dyspnoea
- Asthma
- Pneumonia
- Diabetes
- Leucorrhoea
- Herpetic vulvitis
- Gonorrhoea
- Rheumatism
- Sciatica
- Blisters
- Herpes

MODALITIES

- **Aggravation:** Damp basements or dwellings, damp weather, lying in one position, water in any form, head injury, early morning
- **Amelioration:** Dry weather, pressure, sitting up (cough), changing position, open air, warm dry air

REMEDY RELATIONSHIP

- **Compare:** Nat-suc., Nat-ch., Fel, Mom-b., Pulm-v., Bold., Nat-i., Nat-hsulo., Sulph., Thuj., Merc., Still., Nat-m. and Sulph.
- **Complementary:** Ars., Thuj.

NITRICUM ACIDUM

INTRODUCTION

- **Common name:** Nitric acid, Aqua fortis
- **Group:** Acid
- **Source:** Mineral kingdom
- **Fromula:** HNO_3
- **Prover:** Hahnemann

SPHERE OF ACTION

- Mind
- Eyes
- Gastrointestinal tract
- Respiratory system
- Mucous membranes
- Urinary system
- Genital system
- Skin

CONSTITUTION

- Suits old people with marked weakness
- Hydrogenoid constitution
- For lean persons with rigid fibre, dark complexion, hair and eyes, suffering from chronic diseases and have a tendency to diarrhoea
- **Temperament:** Nervous
- **Thermal:** Chilly
- **Miasm:** Psora, Syphilis, Sycosis

MIND

- Sensitive to noise, pain, touch, jar
- Constantly thinks about past troubles
- Hateful, vindictive, self-willed, headstrong, hates people who have offended them
- Irritable. Violent anger, fits of rage and cursing
- Fear of death, morbid fear of cholera
- Dependency. Hopeless despair. Indifference. Pessimism.
- Anxiety regarding health; from loss of sleep
- Sadness before menses
- No disposition to work; thoughts vanish after mental exertion

KEYNOTE SYMPTOMS

- **Tendency to haemorrhages – from nose, uterus, haemorrhoids, ulcers, bladder**
- **Ulcers – in mouth, throat, tonsils, skin, cervix, etc., which bleed easily; are sensitive and have splinter-like pains**
- Muco-cutaneous junctions most affected, particularly of the mouth, throat and arms. All orifices are swollen, red and fissured
- Cachexia, due to syphilis; intermittent fevers, anaemia, etc.
- Bones painfully sore; decay and exostosis of bones
- **Splinter-like, shooting pains in affected parts; pain appears and disappears suddenly**
- Sensation of a band around affected parts like head, bone, etc.
- **Discharges are very offensive, especially urine, perspiration, faeces and leucorrhoea. Discharges are also acrid, thin and dirty brown**
- Ulcers in soft palate; bleeding gums, bloody saliva, putrid breath. **Tongue – clean, red, wet with a furrow in the center**
- Discharge of a foetid, watery substance from the anus that keeps it constantly moist
- Diarrhoea and dysentery – watery and blood streaked, with pieces of membrane like scrapings of intestines and tenesmus
- Constipated with fissures in rectum. Great straining but little passes. Violent cutting pains after stools, lasting for hours. After stools, irritable and exhausted. Haemorrhoids bleed easily and come out with each stool
- **Urine is scanty, dark, offensive – smells like horse's urine; feels cold on passing**
- Uterine haemorrhage after childbirth or curetting. Hair from genitals fall off
- Large, jagged warts – bleed on washing; exuberant granulations

CLINICAL

- Haemorrhages
- Actinomycosis
- Caries of mastoid
- Mastoiditis
- Syphilitic iritis
- Fissures
- Fistulae
- Haemorrhoids
- Constipation
- Dysentery
- Cholera
- Proctitis
- Tinnitus
- Ozaena
- Epistaxis
- Polyps
- Asthma
- Involuntary micturition
- Metrorrhagia
- Superficial erosion of cervix
- Ulcers
- Herpes
- Warts
- Condylomata
- Corns

MODALITIES

- **Aggravation:** Evening and at night, after midnight, contact, change of temperature of weather, while sweating, on walking, cold air, jar, motion.
- **Amelioration:** While riding in a carriage, steady pressure, mild weather

REMEDY RELATIONSHIP

- **Complementary:** Ars. Calad., Lac-c., Sep.
- **Inimical to:** Lach.
- **Follows well:** Calc., Hep., Merc., Nat-c., Puls., Thuj.; but is most effective after Kali-c.
- **Compare:** Merc., Kali-c., Thuj., Hep., Calc.
- **Antidotes:** Merc.

NUPHAR LUTEUM

INTRODUCTION
- **Common name:** Yellow pond lily
- **Family:** *Nymphaeaceae*
- **Source:** Vegetable kingdom
- **Part used:** Rhizome
- **Prover:** Pitet

SPHERE OF ACTION
- Gastrointestinal system
- Musculoskeletal system
- Urinary system
- Male genital system
- Skin

MIND
- Impatient to slightest contradiction
- Sympathetic, compassionate towards animals, suffering; feels great pain on seeing the suffering of animals
- Excessive moral sensibility

MODALITIES
- **Aggravation:** After least excess of any kind, the day after sex, diarrhoea worse early morning, itching worse in the evening
- **Amelioration:** Pressure

CONSTITUTION
- Prescribed for cases with marked depression of the male generative system, generally associated with headache
- **Temperament:** Nervous, impatient, sympathetic
- **Thermal:** Chilly
- **Miasm:** Syphilis

KEYNOTE SYMPTOMS
- Produces nervous weakness, with marked symptoms in the sexual sphere; for severe depression of male generative sphere
- Weakness after coition; from diarrhoea
- Sore, bruised pains in head, thorax, posterior part of thighs; worse jar, walking
- Pityriasis capitis with marked itching and falling out of hair
- Brilliant sparks before the eyes when coughing
- Acute or chronic enterocolitis; slow digestion
- **Early morning, yellow diarrhoea with severe exhaustion is a keynote**
- **Urine has copious, reddish sand which adheres to the vessel**
- Complete absence of sexual desire and erection. Impotency; involuntary emissions during stool or when urinating; spermatorrhoea
- Pain in testicles and penis

CLINICAL
- Weakness
- Headache
- Pityriasis capitis
- Enterocolitis
- Colitis
- Morning diarrhoea
- Diarrhoea
- Sexual weakness
- Impotency
- Spermatorrhoea
- Involuntary emission
- Enlarged testicles
- Enlarged penis
- Prostatic cancer
- Backache
- Itching
- Typhoid

REMEDY RELATIONSHIP
- **Compare:** In sexual weakness- Agn., Kali-br., Lyc., Sel., Yohim; in diarrhoea – Chel., Gamb., Sulph., Nymph.

NUX MOSCHATA

SPHERE OF ACTION

- Mind
- Nervous system
- Gastrointestinal system
- Respiratory system
- Musculoskeletal system
- Female genital system
- Sleep

INTRODUCTION

- **Common name:** Nutmeg
- **Family:** *Myristicaceae*
- **Source:** Vegetable kingdom
- **Part used:** Seeds
- **Prover:** Helbig

CONSTITUTION

- For women and children with dry skin, who rarely perspire; have stiff, straight hair; have a delicate constitution
- For weakness and dyspepsia of old age
- **Temperament:** Nervous, hydrogenoid
- **Thermal:** Chilly
- **Miasm:** Syphilis

MIND

- Very forgetful, absence of mind, indifference; loss of memory
- Vanishing of thoughts while reading, talking, writing; weak memory with headache
- Does not recognize well known streets; complete loss of memory of past life
- Senile dementia; Alzheimer's diseases
- Does her household duties automatically, but if interrupted, does not recollect what she has done
- Confusion, especially during pregnancy
- Feels as if in a dream, spaced out feeling; bewildered
- Changeable mood – laughing and crying
- Clairvoyant; sense of impending dissolution
- Hysteria and mania; loss of emotional control; makes ridiculous gestures
- Sense of duality – thinks she has two heads, seems to be two persons
- Irresistible drowsiness
- Ailments from overtaxing mental powers, grief, disappointed love

KEYNOTE SYMPTOMS

- **Dryness of mucous membranes** – of mouth, tongue, skin, eyes, etc. **with thirstlessness and want of perspiration**
- Drowsiness and sleepiness accompany all complaints, along with chillness, coldness and thirstlessness
- Giddiness, a cheerful, lazy feeling, staggering, as if drunk
- Tendency to fainting spells, at stools, menses, from standing long, sight of blood, pain, heart failure
- Eyes feel very dry, too dry to close the lids
- Mouth is so dry that **saliva seems like cotton; tongue adheres to the roof of the mouth**
- Toothache during pregnancy
- Flatulent dyspepsia, hiccough and craving for highly seasoned food. Excessive bloating of the abdomen
- Rectum inactive; stool is soft; yet is unable to expel it. Faintness during or after stool
- Cough is loose after eating, dry after drinking and worse from the warmth of the bed
- Menses – variable and irregular. Uterine haemorrhage
- Threatened abortion in hysterical women, disposed to fainting

CLINICAL

- Hysteria
- Dryness
- Apoplexy
- Narcolepsy
- Alzheimer's disease
- Epilepsy
- Vertigo
- Syncope
- Headache
- Toothache
- Hiccups
- Dyspepsia
- Flatulence
- Colic
- Constipation
- Haemorrhoids
- Aphonia
- Hoarseness
- Hysterical cough
- Asthma
- Palpitation
- Incontinence of urine
- Menstrual irregularities
- Uterine haemorrhage
- Uterine prolapse
- Leucorrhoea
- Gout
- Rheumatism
- Chilblains
- Drowsiness
- Sleepiness

MODALITIES

- **Aggravation:** Cold, wet windy weather, weather changes, cold food, water and cold washing, menses, mental exertion, excitement, shock, emotions, pregnancy, jar, motion, lying in painful side
- **Amelioration:** In dry warm weather, warm room, wrapping up warmly, moist heat.

REMEDY RELATIONSHIP

- **Compare:** Nux-v., Puls., Rhus-t., Ign., Asaf., Orni., Myris.
- **Antidoted by:** Camph., Gels., Valer., Zinc., Op., Nux-v.
- Nux-m. antidotes mercurial inhalation, lead colic, oil of turpentine, spirituous liquors, and especially the effects of bad beer
- **Antidotes:** Ars., Laur., Rhod.
- **Compatible:** Nux-v., Puls., Ant-t., Rhus-t., Lyc.

NUX VOMICA

INTRODUCTION

- **Common name:** Poison nut, Kuchla
- **Family:** *Loganiaceae*
- **Source:** Vegetable kingdom
- **Part used:** Seeds
- **Prover:** Hahnemann

SPHERE OF ACTION

- Mind
- Sensory and motor centers
- Spinal cord
- Nervous system
- Gastrointestinal system
- Respiratory system
- Cardiovascular system

CONSTITUTION

- Suits conditions incident to a modern life style; leading a sedentary life with much mental exertion
- Debauched, thin, irritable, over zealous people inclined to get angry very fast
- Thin spare, nervous, quick, active people with dark hair and complexion
- **Temperament:** Bilious, zealous
- **Thermal:** Chilly
- **Miasm:** Sycosis

MIND

- Very irritable, head strong, self-willed, overzealous and fiery temperament.
- Angry and impatient. Easily offended, quarrelsome
- Fault finding; can't bear contradiction; gets angry and violent without provocation
- Sensitive to all impressions. Can't bear light, noises, odours. Does not want to be touched
- Workaholic, ambitious and competitive; very fastidious
- Time passes too slowly
- The least ailment affects them; hypochondriacal
- Melancholic, desire for solitude and tranquility
- Anxiety and restlessness in the evening

KEYNOTE SYMPTOMS

- Pre-eminently a male remedy – for businessmen who suffer from its cares and worries
- **For ailments incident to a modern and sedentary lifestyle,** found in long office hours, over studies
- Useful for ailments from the ill-effects of wine, women, rich food, tobacco and sedative drugs; indulgent people
- **One of the best remedies to commence treatment of cases that have been drugged by strong allopathic treatment**
- Affects nervous system, produces excessive sensitiveness. Twitching and jerkings; spasms, convulsions, tetanic seizures with consciousness, worse slightest touch, better by being grasped tightly
- Neuralgia – violent, lightening-like pains, twisting, jerking
- Sensation in vertex as if a nail were driven in
- Vertigo with momentary fainting. Feeling of intoxication; hangover, headache with irritability
- Sour taste, nausea and vomiting in the morning; with much retching; indigestion from alcohol
- Hiccups from over eating; stomach region very sensitive to pressure
- Dyspepsia from drinking strong coffee; craves stimulants, alcohol, bitter and pungent things; loves fats
- Bruised soreness of abdominal walls; gastric headache; umbilical and inguinal hernia, especially in infants
- Weak liver from a bad diet, alcohol, drugs, fats and spices
- Constipation with constant, **ineffectual urging for stool;** as if part remained unexpelled; blind heamorrhoids,
- Epistaxis in the morning. Cold; nose stuffed up at night and outdoors
- Asthma with fulness of stomach; shallow and oppressed breathing
- Angina from excess of coffee, tobacco or alcohol
- Metrorrhagia, dysmenorrhoea with a constant urging to stool

CLINICAL

- Behavioural disorders
- Alcoholism
- Delirium tremens
- Hangover
- Drug addiction
- Tobacco habit
- Neuralgia
- Motion sickness
- Multiple sclerosis
- Tetanus
- Convulsions
- Opisthotonos
- Myelitis
- Indigestion
- Nausea
- Colic
- Bilious attacks
- Liver affections
- Hernia
- Inflammatory bowel disease
- Irritable bowel syndrome
- Peptic ulcer
- Ulcerative colitis
- Crohn's disease
- Constipation
- Haemorrhoids
- Rectal fissure
- Influenza
- Colds
- Asthma
- Hypertension
- Angina pectoris
- Arrhythmia
- Pyelonephritis
- Renal calculi
- Prostatitis
- Premenstrual syndrome
- Hydrocoele
- Impotence
- Lumbago
- Arthritis
- Sciatica
- Insomnia

MODALITIES

- **Aggravation:** Early morning, waking at 4 a.m., mental exertion, after over eating, touch, noise, anger, spices, narcotics, dry weather, in cold air, liquor, stimulants, drugs, tabocco, uncovering, disturbed sleep
- **Amelioration:** In the evening, while at rest, lying down after a nap, in damp wet weather, strong pressure, from free discharges, hot drink, hot milk

REMEDY RELATIONSHIP

- **Complementary:** Sulph., Sep.
- **Inimical:** Zinc.; must not be used before or after.
- **Follows well:** Ars., Ip., Phos., Sep., Sulph., Carb-v.
- **Followed:** Bry., Puls., Sulph.
- Nux-v. should be given on retiring or several hours before going to bed; it acts best during repose of mind and body.
- **Compare:** Stry., Kali-c., Hydr., Bry., Lyc., Graph., Ign., Nux-m., Carb-v., Calc., Cic., Bell., Acon., Ars., Puls.
- **Antidotes:** Coff., Ign., Cocc.

OENANTHE CROCATA

INTRODUCTION
- **Common name:** Water dropwart
- **Family:** *Umbelliferae*
- **Source:** Vegetable kingdom
- **Part used:** Root
- **Prover:** Ray

SPHERE OF ACTION
- Mind
- Nervous system
- Gastrointestinal system
- Respiratory system
- Musculoskeletal system
- Skin

MIND
- Tendency to cry over small things
- Furious delirium; insanity, hallucinations; behaves as if drunk
- Grasps at imaginary objects
- Does not like being questioned
- Delirium tremens
- Coma after convulsions
- Restless when delirious. Moves constantly from place to place; talks continuously, without knowing what is being said

MODALITIES
- **Aggravation:** During menses, during pregnancy, from sexual disturbances, water, injury
- **Amelioration:** Rest, pressure ameliorates deep pain in thorax

KEYNOTE SYMPTOMS
- **Very effective for the purpose of checking epileptiform convulsions of childhood and pregnancy**
- Sudden, violent and severe epileptic convulsions; followed by complete unconsciousness
- **Convulsive twitching of facial muscles**
- Convulsions with a swollen, livid face, foaming at the mouth, feeble pulse and prostration
- Convulsions, epilepsy, worse menses, pregnancy, childbirth, abortion, menopause; epilepsy since birth control pills
- Patient is cold, as if dead during convulsions
- **Offensive, profuse sweat**
- Complete loss of appetite with debility; craves cold drinks
- Spasms of the diaphragm – distressing hiccups
- Burning in throat and stomach with a disturbed intellect; nausea and vomiting
- **For obstinate vomiting which continues for days and is not relieved by anything**
- Numbness and feebleness of limbs from disorders of the sexual sphere
- Skin affections – leprosy and ichthyosis. Rosy red blotches on face, arms, chest and abdomen
- Yawns a lot; drowsy, is roused with difficulty. Snores loudly during deep sleep

CONSTITUTION
- Indicated in cases of status epilepticus, worse during menses and pregnancy with a livid countenance and red spots on the face
- **Temperament:** Nervous
- **Thermal:** Chilly
- **Miasm:** Syphilis

CLINICAL
- Delirium tremens
- Hystero-epilepsy
- Epilepsy
- Convulsions
- Tetanus
- Opisthotonos
- Lock jaw
- Trismus
- Pupils dilated
- Nausea
- Vomiting
- Oesophagitis
- Pharyngitis
- Puerperal eclampsia
- Menstrual convulsions
- Sciatica
- Leprosy
- Ichthyosis

REMEDY RELATIONSHIP
- **Compare:** Cic., Kali-br., Con., Pic-ac.

Oenanthe crocata

OLEANDER

SPHERE OF ACTION
- Eyes
- Nervous system
- Gastrointestinal system
- Heart
- Musculoskeletal system
- Skin

INTRODUCTION
- **Common name:** Rose laurel, Nerium oleander
- **Family:** *Apocynaceae*
- **Source:** Vegetable kingdom
- **Part used:** Leaves
- **Prover:** Hahnemann

CONSTITUTION
- Face pale, sunken with blue rings around the eyes and burning, very sensitive skin
- **Temperament:** Nervous
- **Thermal:** Chilly
- **Miasm:** Syphilis

MIND
- Dullness, sluggishness, difficulty of thinking and comprehending; dullness of intellect
- Memory weak, slow perception
- Confusion while reading, especially a long sentence
- Cannot bear contradiction
- Violent anger followed by speedy repentance
- Melancholy with obstinate constipation
- Sadness and lack of confidence and power
- Morose, peevish, ill-humoured

KEYNOTE SYMPTOMS
- Feeling of cramp-like tension throughout the body, as if the bones were broken
- Sensations of vibrations; buzzing and humming sensation in body
- **Involuntary discharges. Involuntary urination. Stool passes when emitting flatus.**
- Corrosive itching on the forehead and edge of hair. Eruptions on scalp and humid, foetid areas behind the ears and occiput
- Violent itching on scalp; after scratching, smarting sensation, as if raw
- Sensation as if eyes were drawn backwards, into the head
- **Can see objects only when looking at them sideways; diplopia**
- **Canine hunger with hurried eating but no appetite**
- Emptiness in stomach and chest after eating, better by brandy. Borborygmus with profuse flatus
- Lienteric stools in the morning
- Unable to speak, or speaks with difficulty; difficulty in articulation
- Palpitations with weakness and an empty feeling in the chest, better brandy
- Weakness and trembling in nursing women; can hardly walk across the room
- **Paralytic condition and cramp-like contractions of upper limbs; weakness of lower limbs. Constant cold feel**
- Skin is very sensitive, least friction causes soreness and chapping. Violent itching eruptions, that bleed and ooze. Nocturnal burning.
- Numbness of skin or itching; want of sensation in the whole body

CLINICAL
- Paralysis
- Hemiplegia
- Oedema
- Vertigo
- Meningitis
- Eruptions on scalp
- Diplopia
- Strabismus
- Vomiting
- Diarrhoea
- Dyspnoea
- Palpitations
- Chapping
- Pimples
- Eczema
- Herpes
- Pruritus

MODALITIES
- **Aggravation:** Open air, undressing, rest, friction of clothes, scratching, rubbing
- **Amelioration:** Looking sideways, having brandy

REMEDY RELATIONSHIP
- **Compare:** Con., Nat-m., Rhus-t., Caust., Lath., Hyos., Nux-v., Staph., Chin., Arg-n., Phos., Ph-ac.
- **Antidotes:** Camph., Sulph.
- **Compatible:** Con., Lyc., Puls., Spig., Sep., Rhus-t., Nat-m.

OLEUM ANIMALE

SPHERE OF ACTION
- Mind
- Nervous system
- Gastrointestinal system
- Musculoskeletal system
- Urinary system
- Genital system

INTRODUCTION
- **Common name:** Dippel's animal oil, Bone oil
- **Source:** Animal kingdom
- **Part used:** Obtained in the preparation of animal charcoal and is then purified
- **Prover:** Nenning, Hartlaub and Trinks

CONSTITUTION
- Affinity for the nervous system, especially the pneumogastric nerve
- **Temperament:** Nervous
- **Thermal:** Chilly
- **Miasm:** Syphilis

MIND
- Sad, introverted, absorbed in self
- Distracted and absentminded
- Vanishing of thoughts
- Nervous irritability
- Ill-tempered
- Indolent, taciturn, thoughtful

KEYNOTE SYMPTOMS
- Left side predominantly affected
- It affects the nerves especially pneumogastric nerve
- Useful in neuralgias and migraine. Cramp-like pain in different parts
- Sensation of chilliness, worse in a warm room, better in open air
- Stitching, burning pains, as if being pierced with hot needles
- Affected parts feel sore; flesh feels torn from the bones
- 'Pulled upward' and 'from behind forward' pains in malar bones, testicles, mammae; symptoms appear here and there or in single parts
- **Toothache, better by pressing teeth together and sensation of coldness in tips of teeth**
- **Sensation as if stomach was full of water swashing back and forth**
- Chest feels constricted; stitches in the breast from behind forward
- **Polyuria; greenish urine; frequent and urgent desire to micturate with tenesmus and scanty discharge**
- Polyuria of perfectly clear urine; especially with migraine or any nervous disorder; or profuse, pale urine of fish brine odour, worse migraine or hysteria
- Breast cancer with burning, sticking pains, radiating in all directions
- Long standing neuralgia of spermatic cord – excruciating attacks; sensation as if testicles were seized and pulled forcibly upwards
- Rheumatic pain, tremulous weakness of hands, knees, feet, etc.; shuffling gait

CLINICAL
- Neurasthenia
- Cancer
- Headache
- Migraine
- Amblyopia
- Cataract
- Myopia
- Facial paralysis
- Toothache
- Waterbrash
- Flatulence
- Diarrhoea
- Constipation
- Bronchitis
- Asthma
- Polyuria
- Breast cancer
- Retraction of testes
- Neuralgia of spermatic cord
- Prostatic hypertrophy
- Rheumatism

MODALITIES
- **Aggravation:** From cold, suppressions, noises, before, during and commencement of menses, warm room, hot drinks
- **Amelioration:** Rubbing, pressure, stretching, changing position, open air

REMEDY RELATIONSHIP
- **Compare:** Puls., Ars., Sil., Sep., Ign., Gels., Agar., Phos., Carb-v.
- **Antidoted by:** Camph., Op., Nux-v.
- **Followed well:** Bry.
- **Followed well by:** Sep.

SPHERE OF ACTION

- Pancreas
- Liver
- Respiratory system
- Heart
- Musculoskeletal system
- Female genital system
- Skin

INTRODUCTION

- **Common Name:** Cod-liver oil
- **Family:** *Gadide*
- **Source:** Animal kingdom
- **Part used:** Oil is obtained from the livers of Gadus morrhua and some allied fishes
- **Proper:** Neidhard

CONSTITUTION

- Suits emaciated, dwarfish, chilly babies and children who cannot tolerate milk
- A nutrient used for emaciation; atrophy of infants
- **Temperament:** Nervous, scrofulous
- **Thermal:** Chilly
- **Miasm:** Syphilis, Tubercular

OLEUM JECORIS ASELLI

MIND

- Insanity, madness, feeling of
- Sensation as if out of her mind
- Feels miserable all over, with great nervous irritation
- Sadness, depression
- Restlessness, anxiety

KEYNOTE SYMPTOMS

- Cod liver oil is a nutrient and affects the chest, liver, pancreas and tendons
- Atrophy of infants; emaciation, with a hot head and hands; restless and feverish at nights with a tendency to catarrh; **sweats mostly on the head, neck and hands; cannot tolerate milk**
- Indicated in emaciation, lassitude, phthisis and scrofulous diseases; also rheumatic affections
- **Yellowness, yellow discharges** – expectoration, leucorrhoea, etc. Yellowness of skin
- Soreness, sore pain – in liver, chest, throat, abdomen, ovaries, kidneys, points, back, etc.
- Pains in liver and liver region, with marked soreness and heaviness
- Hoarseness; sharp, stitching pains, burning spots. Dry, hacking, tickling cough, especially at night
- Tuberculosis in beginning stage; haemoptysis
- Palpitation of heart present as a concomitant to other symptoms
- Re-establishes or increases menstrual flow
- Aching in elbows, knees, sacrum; rigid muscles and tendons; burning in palms
- Marked fever symptoms; constantly chilly towards the evening; hectic fever and night sweats

CLINICAL

- Dwarfishness
- Emaciation
- Malnutrition
- Anaemia
- Lassitude
- Night sweats
- Goitre
- Alopecia
- Milk crusts
- Liver ailments
- Diarrhoea
- Dysentery
- Constipation
- Haemoptysis
- Whooping cough
- Tuberculosis
- Palpitations
- Leucorrhoea
- Arthritis
- Rheumatism
- Eczema
- Ringworm
- Hectic fever

MODALITIES

- **Aggravation:** From milk, exposure to cold air, living in cold, damp areas, touch, motion, stooping, riding, walking
- **Amelioration:** Rest

REMEDY RELATIONSHIP

- **Compare:** Chol., Tub., Phos., Iod., Gad., Fel., Phos., Bac.

ONOSMODIUM VIRGINIANUM

INTRODUCTION

- **Common name:** False gromwell
- **Family:** *Boraginaceae*
- **Source:** Vegetable kingdom
- **Part used:** Whole plant
- **Prover:** Green

SPHERE OF ACTION

- Head
- Eyes
- Heart
- Urinary system
- Genital system
- Musculoskeletal system

CONSTITUTION

- For cases with want of power of concentration and coordination; who cannot concentrate their thoughts, focus eyes, coordinate muscles or have a disturbed sense of proportion
- **Temperament:** Nervous
- **Thermal:** Chilly
- **Miasm:** Syphilis

MIND

- Irresolute, confused, forgetful, slow thinking
- Weakness of memory for what was about to done, what had just been done, for what has been read, for what he is about to say
- **Fear of falling while going up or down the stairs**
- Want of power of concentration and co-ordination
- Disturbance in sense of proportion; minutes seem like hours
- Depressed, listless

KEYNOTE SYMPTOMS

- Prostration, weariness feeling as if born tired
- Neurasthenia – muscles, sore aching in breast
- **Severe dryness, especially of nose, mouth and throat**
- Migraine from eyestrain
- Ocular muscles tense; paralysis of internal eye muscles; optic disc hyperaemic, retinal vessels engorged. Pain in eyeballs, between orbit and ball
- Eyes – aching, stiff, tired from over straining, but without redness
- **Craving for ice water and cold drinks which ameliorate**
- Abdomen feels bloated; griping and grumbling
- Discharge from posterior nares or a stuffed up feeling
- Pain in the heart; pulse rapid, irregular
- Sexual neuraesthenia, loss of sexual desire in both sexes; depressed or lost sexual life in women
- Leucorrhoea yellowish, acrid, profuse, offensive
- **Great muscular prostration; staggering, sensation as if walking on cotton.** Numbness and tingling in legs, feet
- **Menses too early and prolonged. Constantly feels as if menses would appear.** Soreness in uterine region.

CLINICAL

- Memory loss
- Prostration
- Muscular prostration
- Weariness
- Neurasthenia
- Staggering gait
- Locomotor ataxia
- Vertigo
- Headache
- Migraine
- Eye affections
- Vision blurred
- Diplopia
- Colour blindness
- Eyestrain
- Amblyopia
- Asthenopia
- Meniere's disease
- Sexual neurasthenia
- Mastitis
- Psychological impotence

MODALITIES

- **Aggravation:** From eyestrain, sprains, jar, motion, sexual excesses, warm humid air
- **Amelioration:** Cold drinks, undressing, eating, rest, sleep, lying on the back

REMEDY RELATIONSHIP

- **Compare:** Nat-m., Lil-t., Gels., Ruta, Myos., Helio., Symph., Sep., Pic-ac.

Onosmodium virginianum

SPHERE OF ACTION

- Mind
- Nervous system
- Gastrointestinal system
- Musculoskeletal system
- Genitourinary system
- Skin

INTRODUCTION

- **Common name:** Papaver somniferum, Poppy, Afeem
- **Family:** *Papaveraceae*
- **Source:** Vegetable kingdom
- **Part used:** Gummy juice
- **Prover:** Hahnemann

CONSTITUTION

- Their face is red, bloated, swollen, dark and appears intoxicated
- Especially adapted to children and old people with light hair, lax muscle and want of physical irritability
- **Temperament:** Nervous
- **Thermal:** Ambithermal, hot
- **Miasm:** Sycosis

OPIUM

MIND

- Stupor and coma. Coma from injury, fright, drug overdose, sunstroke; apoplexy
- Fears; after fright; which remains, that is the image recurs
- **Complaints in children from fright of the mother during pregnancy**
- Liars; tendency to lie. Blunted morals. No conscience.
- Blissful, peaceful, sensous, dreamy, sluggish, dull. Sensation of happiness, carefulness. Mental exhaltation and vivid imaginations; simulates imagination
- Thinks he is not at home
- Indifferent to pain or pleasure
- Tendency to start
- Dreams of cats, dogs and black forms
- Unable to understand or appreciate his sufferings
- Delirious, talking with eyes wide open; deceptive vision, taste; perversion of all senses
- Patient wants nothing

KEYNOTE SYMPTOMS

- Ailments of drunkards and drug addicts; ailments that originate from fright, anger, shame or excessive joy
- Lack of vital reaction with insensibility of the nervous system and general sluggishness
- Increased sensitiveness and activity of the muscles subject to will that is, involuntary muscles and diminution of it in involuntary muscles
- Lessens voluntary movements, contracts eyes, depresses higher intellectual faculties, lessens self control, especially of sphincters
- Tremors, twitching, jerking during sleep. Epilepsy while sleeping
- All complaints are accompanied by sopor, painlessness, a heavy, stupid, comatose sleep and stertorous breathing
- **Marasmus; child looks like a wrinkled, dried, old man.** Veins of face distended. Face – besotted, dusky and mottled.
- Pupils fixed, staring, glassy, dilated, non-reactive to light
- Hard, bloated, tympanitic abdomen; faecal vomiting; incarcerated hernia
- **Severe constipation, painless, impacted stools especially in babies; no desire for stool; stools like round, hard, black balls which look like sheep dung**
- Stools may also be involuntary, black, offensive and frothy
- Retained or involuntary urination after fright. Loss of power or sensibility of bladder
- Suppression of menses or threatened abortion, or suppression of lochia after fright with sopor
- Checks all secretions, except of the skin. Sweaty skin
- **Hot perspiration all over the body except lower limbs**
- **Heavy, stupid, comatose sleep. Breathing stops on sleeping. Also the contrary condition – very sleepy but cannot sleep, distant noises keep patient awake**

CLINICAL

- Hystero-epilepsy
- Chronic fatigue syndrome
- Sepsis
- Cerebral accident
- Concussion
- Meningitis
- Seizures
- Paralysis
- Epilepsy
- Convulsions
- Opisthotonos
- Apoplexy
- Coma
- Delirium tremens
- Vertigo
- Lead colic
- Intestinal obstruction
- Hernia
- Constipation
- Puerperal convulsions
- Snoring
- Insomnia
- Sleep apnoea

MODALITIES

- **Aggravation:** During and after sleep, while perspiring, from warmth, stimulants, sunstroke, alcohol, suppressed discharges, fear, emotions
- **Amelioration:** From cold things, constant walking, uncovering

REMEDY RELATIONSHIP

- **Compare:** Apis, Bell., Gels., Nux-m., Morph., Cod., Chel., Sang., Psor., Thuj., Sulph.
- **Antidotes:** Acute Opium poisoning: Atropinum and black coffee. Chronic Opium poisoning: Ip., Nux-v., Passi., Berb. is useful to counteract the Opium habit.
- **Followed well by:** Acon., Bry., Hyos., Bell., Ant-t., Nux-m., Nux-v.

SPHERE OF ACTION

- Mind
- Eyes
- Gastrointestinal system
- Heart
- Musculoskeletal system
- Urinary system

INTRODUCTION

- **Common name:** Oxalic acid, Sorrel acid
- **Group:** Salt
- **Source:** Mineral kingdom
- **Formula:** $(CO_2H)_2 \cdot 2H_2O$
- **Prover:** Kock, Neidhard, Dubbs and Smith

CONSTITUTION

- Corresponds to neurasthenic cases which suffer from intense neuralgias
- For cardiac troubles in extremely nervous people
- **Temperament:** Nervous, haemorrhagic, rheumatic
- **Thermal:** Chilly
- **Miasm:** Psora, Syphilis

OXALICUM ACIDUM

MIND

- Very cheerful; very exhilarated, thoughts and action
- All complaints are aggravated by thinking about the condition; will bring on the pains when they are not actually present
- Aversion to talk
- Mania

KEYNOTE SYMPTOMS

- Predominantly, a left sided remedy – left sided rheumatism, left sided paralysis, etc.
- Neurasthenia; weak, cold, livid and numb all over
- Muscular prostration, numbness and tingling
- **Excruciating pains; lightening-like; terrible neuralgic pains; violent pain in spots;** worse thinking about pain
- Hyperaesthesia of retina. Severe pain in eyes; eyes feel expanded
- **Cannot eat strawberries; violent pain in epigastrium, better by discharge of flatus**
- Gastroenteritis; colic, burning in small spots in the abdomen
- Hoarseness, burning sensation from throat down. Left lung painful; paralysis of the tensors of vocal cord. Dyspnoea; short, jerking inspirations; nervous aphonia
- **Angina pectoris – sharp, lancinating pain in the left lung coming on suddenly, depriving of breath.** Heart symptoms alternate with aphonia
- Frequent and copious urine. Burning in the urethra. Urine contains oxalates.
- Wrist painful, as if sprained; weak, trembling hands and feet

CLINICAL

- Confusion
- Collapse
- Neuralgia
- Multiple sclerosis
- Motor paralysis
- Convulsions
- Tetanus
- Myelitis
- Meningitis
- Headache
- Retinal hyperaesthesia
- Gastralgia
- Gastroenteritis
- Colic
- Constipation
- Aphonia
- Altered voice
- Hoarseness
- Dyspnoea
- Tuberculosis
- Angina pectoris
- Aortic insufficiency
- Renal calculi
- Oxaluria
- Urethritis
- Spermatic cord neuralgia
- Seminal vesiculitis
- Testicle induration
- Rheumatism
- Lumbago
- Backache
- Urticaria

MODALITIES

- **Aggravation:** Thinking of symptoms, mental exertion, strawberries, motion, left side, evening, night, early morning, light
- **Amelioration:** After stools

REMEDY RELATIONSHIP

- **Compare:** Ars., Colch., Arg-met., Pic-ac., Cice., Scol., Casein., Kali-ox., Ip., Verat., Ph-ac., Puls.
- Lime water is an antidote to Ox-ac. poisoning

OXYTROPIS LAMBERTI

INTRODUCTION
- **Common name:** Locoweed, Crazyweed
- **Family:** *Papilionaceae*
- **Source:** Vegetable kingdom
- **Part used:** Whole plant excluding root
- **Prover:** W.S. Gee

SPHERE OF ACTION
- Mind
- Nervous system
- Eyes
- Gastrointestinal system
- Respiratory system
- Musculoskeletal system
- Genitourinary system

MIND
- Indifferent to all influences and interests
- Stimulation of mind – pleasant intoxicated feeling
- Desires to be alone, aggravation from company
- Disinclined to work, or talk, or study
- Severe mental depression
- Worse, thinking of symptoms
- Monomania
- Dreams of quarreling or of pleasant, lascivious nature
- Restless sleep
- Can't think; cannot concentrate thoughts; forgets familiar words or names

MODALITIES
- **Aggravation:** Thinking of symptoms, immediately after eating, every other day
- **Amelioration:** After sleep, on side lain on

KEYNOTE SYMPTOMS
- It has a marked action upon the nervous system, producing uncertain, staggering or backward gait. There is trembling and a sense of emptiness. All reflexes are lost; paralysis
- Loss of power to control movement of body or limbs. Tendon reflexes lost
- Pains come and go quickly, but muscles remain sore and stiff
- Pain and stiffness in muscles of back and neck
- Paralysis of nerves and muscles of eyes
- **Thirstlessness, though there is great dryness of mouth in the morning on waking. Metallic taste.**
- Belching as after taking an aerated drink with colicky pains
- **Anal sphincter seems relaxed; stools slip from the anus like lumps of jelly**
- Urging to micturate when thinking of it. Pain in kidneys with some tenderness
- Pain in testicles and along the spermatic cord, down the thighs

CONSTITUTION
- Suits cases with marked symptoms of the nervous system like uncertain, staggering gait, loss reflexes, etc. and a pleasant intoxicated feeling
- **Temperament:** Pleasant or depressed
- **Thermal:** Chilly
- **Miasm:** Syphilis

CLINICAL
- Depression
- Locomotor ataxia
- Reflexes lost
- Staggering gait
- Vertigo
- Amblyopia
- Paralysis of eye muscles
- Sphincters relaxed
- Cystitis
- Ovarian pain
- Testicular pain
- Impotence
- Orchitis

REMEDY RELATIONSHIP
- **Compare:** Astra-m., Lath., Ox-ac., Bar-c. (Loco plant is rich in Bar-c.), Lol., Phys., Lyc.

PAEONIA OFFICINALIS

INTRODUCTION
- **Common name:** Paeony
- **Family:** *Ranunculaceae*
- **Source:** Vegetale kingdom
- **Part used:** Root
- **Prover:** Praktichen and Helbig

SPHERE OF ACTION
- Gastrointestinal system
- Respiratory system
- Musculoskeletal system
- Skin

MIND
- Afraid to talk to someone
- Senses – dull, blunted; entering a warm room after a walk
- Very affected by bad news
- Anxiety, with apprehension in the evening
- Ill-humoured, depressed
- Dreams – terrifying nightmares of death of relatives

MODALITIES
- **Aggravation:** Touch, pressure, night, motion, walking, during stool, coming into a warm room
- **Amelioration:** Drinking water helps nausea with vertigo

KEYNOTE SYMPTOMS
- Chronic, painful **ulcers, oozing an offensive moisture;** ulcers **especially upon lower parts of body** like leg, foot, toes; also breast, rectum
- **Shooting or splinter like pains; rolls on floor from pain**
- Haemorrhoids, large and ulcerated, with fissures; intolerable pain during and after stools; anal fistulae
- Painful, sensitive ulcers and fissures in rectum
- **Biting, itching in anus; orfice swollen; burning in the anus after stool followed by internal chilliness**
- Sticking pain in left chest, heat in chest
- Ulceration of perineum and anus, purple in colour, covered with crust. Oozing an offensive moisture
- Pain in wrists and fingers, knees and toes; weakness of legs preventing walking
- Ulcers form from pressure, as in case of shoe bites or bedsores
- Skin is sensitive, painful, itching, burning, as from nettle rash
- Pain in corns
- Sleep is restless, unrefreshing and disturbed by many dreams. Has terrifying dreams and nightmares

CONSTITUTION
- For rectal and anal symptoms
- For chronic ulcers on lower parts of the body
- **Temperament:** Nervous, haemorrhagic
- **Thermal:** Chilly
- **Miasm:** Psora, Sycosis

CLINICAL
- Nightmares
- Vertigo
- Rectal tenesmus
- Diarrhoea
- Constipation
- Fissures
- Fistula-in-ano
- Haemorrhoids
- Threadworms
- Breast ulcers
- Perineal ulcer
- Arthritis
- Rheumatism
- Bedsores
- Ulcers
- Abscesses
- Varicose veins
- Shoe bites

REMEDY RELATIONSHIP
- **Complementary:** Plat.
- **Compare:** Arg-met., Helon., Lil-t., Apis., Glech., Ham., Sil., Aesc., Rat., Nit-ac.
- **Antidoted by:** Aloe., Rat.

PALLADIUM METALLICUM

INTRODUCTION

- **Common name:** Palladium
- **Group:** Metal
- **Source:** Mineral kingdom
- **Formula:** Pd
- **Prover:** Hering

SPHERE OF ACTION

- Mind
- Gastrointestinal system
- Respiratory system
- Heart
- Musculoskeletal system
- Urinary system
- Female genital system
- Skin

MIND

- **Delusion that he is neglected, that he is not appreciated**
- Haughty; wounded pride wants to be flattered in company. Longs for the good opinion of others
- **Love of approbation – gives too much importance to others judgement**
- Inclined to use violent language and expressions
- Keeps up brightly when in company, much exhausted afterwards
- Excitement in company
- Weeping mood with prolapsus uteri
- Lachrymose mood
- Impatient
- Time passes too slowly

MODALITIES

- **Aggravation:** Emotions, chagrin, standing after social functions, exertion
- **Amelioration:** Touch, pressure, diversion, rubbing, after sleep, after stools, rest, in company

KEYNOTE SYMPTOMS

- It affects the ovaries especially right, uterus and mind
- Motor weakness, aversion to exercise
- Sensation as if head was swung backwards and forwards
- Pain which travels in a band across the top of the head, from ear to ear
- Bruised soreness of abdomen. Sensation as if intestines being bitten; intestines feel strangulated
- Glairy mucous from throat, frequent hawking of small solid lumps
- Painful gynaecological conditions of nervous women who appear hale and hearty in public or social functions, but collapse afterwards
- Uterine prolapse, retroversion and protrusion. Subacute pelvic peritonitis. Shooting and burning pain in the pelvis.
- **Menstrual discharge while nursing**
- Pain and swelling in right ovarian region
- **Glairy, yellow leucorrhoea before and after menses**
- Stitching pain in right breast, near the nipple
- Fleeting, neuralgic pain in extremities limbs feel tired and heavy. Pruritus of limbs
- Tired feeling in the lumbosacral region. **Rheumatic pain in right shoulder**
- **Itching all over after undressing. Warts on knuckles**

CONSTITUTION

- For individuals with 'love of approbation', which easily gives way to 'wounded pride and fancied neglect'. Such patients are better in society and aggravated after the party
- For ovarian and uterine complaints associated with the above mental condition
- **Temperament:** Sanguine, irritable, haughty
- **Thermal:** Chilly
- **Miasm:** Psora

CLINICAL

- Headache
- Flatulence
- Subpelvic peritonitis
- Diarrhoea
- Constipation
- Ovarian pain
- Ovarian cyst
- Ovarian tumour
- Menorrhagia
- Retroversion
- Uterine prolapse
- Leucorrhoea
- Arthritis
- Rheumatism
- Sciatica
- Pruritus
- Warts

REMEDY RELATIONSHIP

- **Antidoted by:** Chin., Glon., Bell.
- **Compare:** Irid., Osm., Plat. Apis, Graph., Podo., Arg-met., Lach., Lil-t., Cimic., Sulph., Helon., Tarent., Hep., Cean.

PAREIRA BRAVA

INTRODUCTION
- **Common name:** Virgin Vine, Velvet leaf
- **Family:** *Menispermaceae*
- **Source:** Vegetable kingdom
- **Part used:** Root
- **Prover:** Fox

SPHERE OF ACTION
- Urinary system
- Genital system
- Musculoskeletal system

MIND
- Restlessness
- Anxiety
- Melancholy

MODALITIES
- **Aggravation:** 3 to 6 a.m.
- **Amelioration:** Through the day

CONSTITUTION
- Suits old people with urinary complaints
- **Temperament:** Bilious
- **Thermal:** Chilly
- **Miasm:** Sycosis

KEYNOTE SYMPTOMS
- Cartilaginous induration of the mucous membrane of urethra and bladder
- **Severe pain in left lumbar region from the left kidney following the course of the ureter**
- Renal colic. Prostatic affections and inflammation of the bladder
- Bladder constantly feels distended, with pain
- Inflammation of urethra; itching along the urethra
- **Constant urging to urinate, with great straining; pain from penis down the thighs, while making an effort to urinate**
- **Pains and strangury compel the patient to go down on his knees and hands with head firmly pressed against the floor;** patient remains in this position for 10 to 20 minutes; **thereafter he starts perspiring and finally urine passes without interruption,** accompanied by tearing and burning pains
- **Black, bloody, foaming urine, depositing a brick dust sediment**
- **Urine** contains large amounts of viscid, thick, white mucous and **smells strongly of ammonia**
- Enlarged prostate with retention of urine
- Violent pain in glans penis, especially when urinating, with discharge of mucous
- Dribbling after micturition

CLINICAL
- Genitourinary obstruction
- Renal colic
- Dysuria
- Cystitis
- Urethritis
- Leucorrhoea
- Gonorrhoea
- Prostatic enlargement
- Arthritis
- Rheumatism

REMEDY RELATIONSHIP
- **Compare:** Pariet., Chim., Fab., Pichi, Uva, Hydrang., Berb., Oci., Hedeo., Sabal.

SPHERE OF ACTION

- Mind
- Head
- Eyes
- Cerebrospinal system
- Gastrointestinal system
- Respiratory system
- Musculoskeletal system

INTRODUCTION

- **Common name:** One berry, Herb Paris
- **Family:** *Liliaceae*
- **Source:** Vegetable kingdom
- **Part used:** Whole plant
- **Prover:** Stapf

CONSTITUTION

- For cases presenting with garrulity, vivacity and love for prattling with affections of the head, eyes or spinal cord
- **Temperament:** Nervous, loquacious
- **Thermal:** Chilly
- **Miasm:** Sycosis

MIND

- Loquacious mania, gossiping. Garrulous, prattling
- Foolish talk and silly actions
- Inclination to treat others with contempt and rudeness
- Imaginary foul smells – bread and milk smell like putrid meat
- Utters absurdities

PARIS QUADRIFOLIA

CLINICAL

- Neuralgia
- Headache
- Trigeminal neuralgia
- Exophthalmos
- Ciliary paralysis
- Ciliary neuralgia
- Hiccups
- Hoarseness
- Laryngitis
- Tracheitis
- Cough
- Cervical spondylosis
- Frozen shoulder
- Arthritis
- Rheumatism
- Backache

KEYNOTE SYMPTOMS

- Generally a left sided remedy
- **Coldness of right side of the body, left hot**
- Objects seem rough to touch; disorder of sense of touch
- Sensation of heaviness, numbness; parts feel too big or drawn together
- Sensation of expansion and consequent tension in the head. The head feels too large and the scalp too tight.
- Eye feel too big and heavy for the sockets. Affections of eyebrows
- **Sensation of a string pulling the eyeballs to the occiput**
- **Tongue dry on waking up, without thirst**
- Sinking feeling and hunger soon after a meal
- Catarrhal complaints; stuffed feeling at root of nose. Painless hoarseness
- Whole body painful, especially when touched; joints feel broken
- Sense of weight and weariness in the nape of the neck and across the shoulders. Fingers numb, numbness of upper limbs

MODALITIES

- **Aggravation:** Touch, mental exertion, thinking, eyestrain, after eating, animation, smoking
- **Amelioration:** Pressure, rest, belching

REMEDY RELATIONSHIP

- **Compare:** Past,. Sil., Calc., Nux-v., Rhus-t., Bell., Crot-t., Lach., Meph., Stram., Cimic., Agar.
- **Incompatible:** Ferr-p.
- **Antidoted:** Coff.
- **Compatible:** Led., Calc., Lyc., Phos., Nux-v., Sep., Rhus-t., Sulph.

PASSIFLORA INCARNATA

INTRODUCTION
- **Common name:** Passion flower, Maypop
- **Family:** *Passifloraceae*
- **Source:** Vegetable kingdom
- **Part used:** Leaves
- **Prover:** Hale

SPHERE OF ACTION
- Mind
- Nervous system
- Gastrointestinal system
- Respiratory system
- Musculoskeletal system
- Skin

MIND
- Insomnia of infants and aged, and the mentally worried and overworked
- Sleeplessness, with restlessness and a suicidal tendency
- Excitable, nervous, restless
- Hysteria, acute mania
- Neurosis of children
- Alcoholism, delirium tremens
- Drug addiction – breaks off habit

MODALITIES
- **Aggravation:** Mental worries, exhaustion, mental excitement, night, nervousness
- **Amelioration:** Remaining quiet

KEYNOTE SYMPTOMS
- Quieting effect on nervous system, thus acts as an antispasmodic in conditions like asthma, whooping cough, spasms, convulsions, puerperal convulsions, etc.
- Tetanus of new born, convulsions in children with neuralgia or during teething
- **Tetanus, mostly affecting the trunk with marked opisthotonos**
- Restless and wakeful sleep in infants and aged who are mentally worried with a tendency to convulsions
- Neuroses of children, worm fever, dentition, spasms
- Painful diarrhoea and irritable haemorrhoids
- Tedious labour pains making the patient nervous and excitable
- Sleeplessness of alcoholics and drug addicts

CONSTITUTION
- For a quietening effect on the nervous system. Thus, used as an antispasmodic and an efficient nervine
- **Temperament:** Nervous
- **Thermal:** Chilly
- **Miasm:** Psora, Syphilis

CLINICAL
- Nervousness
- Hysteria
- Mania
- Delirium tremens
- Morphine habit
- Neuralgia
- Spasms
- Convulsions
- Tetanus
- Epilepsy
- Opisthotonos
- Trismus
- Diarrhoea
- Constipation
- Worm fever
- Haemorrhoids
- Whooping cough
- Asthma
- Puerperal convulsions
- Chancre
- Sciatica
- Erysipelas
- Insomnia

REMEDY RELATIONSHIP
- **Compare:** Cean., Nux-v., Ph-ac., Chin.
- **Antidotes:** Quinine

PETROLEUM

SPHERE OF ACTION

- Mind
- Gastrointestinal system
- Respiratory system
- Musculoskeletal system
- Genitourinary system
- Skin

INTRODUCTION

- **Common name:** Crude rock oil, Coal oil
- **Group:** Hydrocarbon
- **Source:** Mineral kingdom
- **Prover:** Hahnemann

CONSTITUTION

- Suits slender people with light hair and skin, with a tendency to skin diseases in winter
- Suits long lasting, deep seated, wasting diseases
- **Temperament:** Nervous, haemorrhagic
- **Thermal:** Chilly
- **Miasm:** Psora, Syphilis

MIND

- Mental weakness and forgetfulness. Loss of memory
- Mental confusion in open air
- Worries, but don't know why
- Aggravation from mental emotions
- Sadness during menses
- Low spirited with dimness of sight
- **During sleep or delirium, imagines that one leg is double or that another person lies alongside him in the same bed, that there are two babies in the bed, etc.**
- Feels that death is near and must hurry to settle affairs
- Irritable, quarrelsome nature; easily offended, vexed at everything
- Presence of strangers aggravates

KEYNOTE SYMPTOMS

- **Diarrhoea after cabbage, only during daytime; stool watery and gushing with itching of anus**
- Coldness in spots in abdomen, heart and after scratching
- Leucorrhoea, profuse, albuminous. Genitals in women sore, moist; aversion to sex
- Herpetic eruptions on the perineum, prostate inflamed and swollen; sweaty genitals
- Chlorosis in girls, with or without ulceration of the stomach
- **Emaciation, especially of the chest**
- Fingertips rough, cracked and fissured, especially in winters; fingertips never look clean; can't wash hands as it causes them to chap
- Fissures and cracks, especially in skin folds, nipples; cracks bleed easily, worse winters
- **Skin dry, rough, parchment-like, thick; worse in folds. Thick, greenish crusts, burning and itching.**
- Chilblains moist, itch and burn, become purple. Psoriasis of hands.
- Very sensitive skin; slightest scratch makes skin suppurate
- Ailments from riding in cars, ships, aircraft; motion sickness
- **Nausea with accumulation of water in the mouth; vomits a bitter green substance**
- Nostrils ulcerated and cracked, burn. Itching at the tip of the nose
- Light red haemorrhages, worse lifting or riding

CLINICAL

- Anaemia
- Sprains
- Motion sickness
- Vertigo
- Occipital headache
- Blepharitis
- Hypermetropia
- Halitosis
- Dyspepsia
- Heartburn
- Gastralgia
- Diarrhoea
- Constipation
- Haemorrhoids
- Nostrils ulcerated
- Diphtheria
- Cystitis
- Urethritis
- Bed wetting
- Cracks
- Fissures
- Herpetic eruptions
- Psoriasis
- Eczema
- Rhagades
- Bedsores
- Chilblains

MODALITIES

- **Aggravation:** Motion, during a thunderstorm, in winters, from dampness, vexation
- **Amelioration;** Dry weather, warm air, lying with head high

REMEDY RELATIONSHIP

- **Compare:** Carb-v., Graph., Sulph., Phos.
- **Antidoted by:** Nux-v., Cocc.
- **Antidotes:** Nit-ac., Lead poisoning
- **Compatible:** Bry., Calc., Lyc., Sep., Sil., Nit-ac., Sulph., Puls., Nux-v.

PHELLANDRIUM AQUATICUM

SPHERE OF ACTION

- Eyes
- Gastrointestinal system
- Respiratory system
- Breasts
- Female genital system

INTRODUCTION

- **Common name:** Water dropwort
- **Family:** *Umbelliferae*
- **Source:** Vegetable kingdom
- **Part used:** Fruit and seeds
- **Prover:** Nenning and Richter

CONSTITUTION

- Suits feeble, irritable people with weak and deficient nutrition
- **Temperament:** Nervous, lymphatic
- **Thermal:** Chilly
- **Miasm:** Psora, Syphilis

MIND

- Sad, anxious, profoundly meditative
- Occasional extravagant merriment
- Dreams of lightening with fright or of a robbery in which he received many blows
- Peevish arrogance

KEYNOTE SYMPTOMS

- Clang-like striking on metal in brain wakes patient up
- Tired feeling when walking
- Headache involves nerves to the eyes. Sensation of weight in vertex, aching and burning in temples above eyes
- **Craves sour things, beer and milk. Aversion to cold water**
- **Everything tastes sweet**
- Cough with profuse and foetid expectoration; cough compels patient to sit up
- **Tuberculosis, generally affecting the middle lobe; right side more affected than left;** offensive, profuse expectoration and cough in phthisis, emphysema and bronchitis
- Intolerable pains in lactiferous tubes between the acts of nursing. Sticking pain in the right breast, near the sternum. Pain in nipples each time child is put to breast.
- Hectic fever with profuse, debilitating perspiration, intermittent, with pain in arms

CLINICAL

- Vertigo
- Headache
- Ciliary neuralgia
- Lachrymation
- Photophobia
- Diarrhoea
- Hoarseness
- Coryza
- Cough
- Dyspnoea
- Haemoptysis
- Bronchitis
- Emphysema
- Phthisis
- Breast affections
- Mastitis
- Intermittent fever

MODALITIES

- **Aggravation:** Open, cold air, using eyes, after dinner, on appearance of menses, after alcohol
- **Amelioration:** While nursing

REMEDY RELATIONSHIP

- **Compare:** Con., Phyt., Sil., Ant-i., Myos-a.
- **Antidoted by:** Rheum

Phellandrium aquaticum

239

PHOSPHORICUM ACIDUM

SPHERE OF ACTION

- Mind
- Nervous system
- Gastrointestinal system
- Respiratory system
- Musculoskeletal system
- Genitourinary system

INTRODUCTION

- **Common name:** Phosphoric acid, Orthophosphoric acid
- **Group:** Acid
- **Source:** Mineral kingdom
- **Formula:** H_3PO_4
- **Prover:** Hahnemann

CONSTITUTION

- Suits originally strong constitutions weakened by loss of fluids, excesses and violent and acute diseases
- Suits children and young people who have grown too rapidly, are tall, slender and slim, and are mentally any physically overtaxed
- Mild, yielding disposition
- **Temperament:** Nervous, scrofulous, haemorrhagic
- **Thermal:** Chilly
- **Miasm:** Sycosis, Syphilis

MIND

- Dizziness of mind; when reading, many other thoughts come to patient's mind, confusing him
- Listless, apathetic and greatly indifferent. Dull; answers slowly and incorrectly
- Brain fag; cannot collect thoughts or find the right word. Difficult comprehension
- Mental debility followed by physical debility
- Effects and prostrated from grief, mental shock or disappointed love
- **Aversion to talking, wants to be alone. Wants nothing and cares for nothing**
- Homesickness with a tendency to cry, weight loss, insomnia and pining. **Pining with emaciation**
- Hysteria during menopause
- Delirium with marked stupefaction
- Becomes unconscious after strong emotions
- Dread regarding future; hopelessness

KEYNOTE SYMPTOMS

- For complaints from a weak immunity caused by violent acute diseases, grief, loss of vital fluids and excesses
- Marked debility producing nervous exhaustion, weakness is better by a short nap. **It is a convalescent remedy**
- Haemorrhages of dark blood
- Tendency to decay, external parts become black, senile, gangrenous
- Bruised soreness, like growing pains
- Neurosis of stump after amputation
- **Copious discharge of urine and sweat**
- Weakened sphincters – faeces and urine pass involuntarily
- Pressure in eyes, naval, on top of head. School girls headache
- Pain as if eyeballs forcibly pressed together in the head
- Meteoric distention and **passage of large quantities of offensive, garlicky smelling flatus; pain in umbilical region**
- Persistent, painless, profuse, watery or lienteric diarrhoea, with little debility, especially in children with rickets
- Weak feeling in chest from talking or coughing; dry cough from a ticking sensation, as from a feather in the chest. Salty expectoration
- **White milky urine – becomes milky on standing.** Polyuria, diabetes
- Child passes a great quantity of urine during enuresis
- Uterus bloated, as if filled with wind
- Deficient sexual power in men; weakness from excessive masturbation or sexual activity

CLINICAL

- Mental weakness
- Brain fag
- Anxiety
- Homesickness
- Emaciation
- Neurasthenia
- Fatigue
- Debility
- Anaemia
- Growing pains
- Cancer pains
- Purpurea
- Formication
- Vertigo
- Headache
- Hairfall
- Amblyopia
- Heartburn
- Flatulence
- Diarrhoea
- Lienteria
- Bronchitis
- Enuresis
- Diabetes
- Phosphaturia
- Sexual weakness
- Self-abuse
- Physometra
- Impotence
- Spermatorrhoea
- Masturbation
- Periosteal inflammation
- Rachitis

MODALITIES

- **Aggravation:** From mental affections, loss of vital fluids, especially seminal, self abuse, sexual excesses, talking causes weakness in chest, emotions, grief, chagrin, cold draft, music
- **Amelioration:** Warmth, after a short sleep, after stools

REMEDY RELATIONSHIP

- **Compare:** Carc., Chin., Nux-v., Pic-ac., Mur-ac., Phos., Lac-ac., Oeno., Nect., Puls., Sil.
- **Antidoted by:** Camph., Coff., Staph.
- **Followed well by:** Ferr-p. Ars., Bell., Sulph., Sep., Nux-v., Puls., Lyc., Caust.

PHOSPHORUS

INTRODUCTION

- **Common name:** Phosphorus
- **Group:** Element
- **Source:** Mineral kingdom
- **Formula:** P
- **Prover:** Hahnemann

SPHERE OF ACTION

- Mind
- Eyes
- Mucous and serous membranes
- Cerebrospinal system
- Gastrointestinal system
- Respiratory system
- Heart
- Musculoskeletal system
- Genitourinary system
- Skin

CONSTITUTION

- Suits young people who grow too rapidly
- People with waxy, translucent skin
- Suits tall, slender, narrow chested people with fine features and long fingers, inclined to stoop. Pale, sickly complexion
- **Temperament:** Sanguine, nervous, haemorrhagic
- **Thermal:** Chilly
- **Miasm:** Psora, Tubercular, Syphilis

MIND

- Melancholic, wants sympathy and consolation; with violent crying or interrupted by fits of involuntary laughter
- Mental prostration from trifles, weary of life; repugnance to labour
- Laughs on serious matters or when sad
- Anxious, restless, fidgety, **worse lying on left side or during a thunderstorm**
- Emotionally oversensitive; over-sensitive to external impressions; tendency to start from noises
- Great apathy, sluggishness; amativeness, shamelessness; approaching insanity
- Anger, passion and violence
- Desires to be magnetized
- Clairvoyant, ecstasy, great flow of ill-assorted ideas of insanity
- Fear of dark, of thunderstorms, of future or that something bad will happen
- Sympathetic and sensitive to the pains and sufferings of others

KEYNOTE SYMPTOMS

- Left sidedness of all complaints
- Insidious onset, gradually increasing debility ending in a severe or rapid disease
- Suddenness of symptoms – sudden prostration, fainting, sweating, pains, etc.
- Swelling of both eyelids
- Haemorrhages – recurrent, vicarious, small wounds bleed much; blood streaked discharges
- Tendency to disorganize blood and cause fatty degeneration of blood vessels, tissues and organs. Thus, it produces a picture of destructive metabolism
- Irritates, inflames and degenerates mucous and serous membranes, spinal cord and nerves
- **Burning anywhere and everywhere over the body**
- It destroys bone tissue, especially **of the spine, lower jaw and tibia**
- Oversensitive to external impressions like odours, touch, light, sound and electrical changes like thunderstorms
- Green halo around candle light, letters appear red; atrophy of optic nerve
- Tremendous **thirst for cold, iced drinks, ice creams, refreshing things**
- **Desires salt, chocolate, acids and spicy foods.** Aversion to warm drinks and food. Bad effects of eating too much salt.
- Throws up ingesta by the mouthful. **Water is vomited as soon as it gets warm in the stomach**
- Weak, empty, all gone sensation in the abdomen
- Post-operative vomiting
- Painless, copious, exhausting diarrhoea
- **Extremely foetid stool, flatus; long, narrow, hard stool like dogs stool, difficult to expel**
- Tightness in chest; oppression as of a great weight on chest. Breathing is quickened. Dry cough, worse talking and cold air.
- Joints stiff, easily dislocated, weak, worse exertion

CLINICAL

- Nervous debility
- Haemorrhages
- Emaciation
- Haemophilia
- Blood extravasations
- Purpura haemorrhagica
- Polycythaemia
- Neuritis
- Locomotor ataxia
- Epilepsy
- Cancer
- Lipoma
- Polyps
- Osteomyelitis
- Bone fragility
- Mastoiditis
- Vertigo
- Headache
- Retinal bleeding
- Glaucoma
- Cataract
- Optic nerve atrophy
- Vitreous opacities
- Scurvy
- Hoarseness
- Chilblains
- Decayed teeth
- Toothache
- Gastritis
- Atrophy of liver
- Hepatitis
- Cirrhosis
- Pancreatic disease
- Diarrhoea
- Epistaxis
- Coryza
- Aphonia
- Cough
- Haemoptysis
- Pneumonia
- Tuberculosis
- Asthma
- Pulmonary oedema
- Endocarditis
- Myocarditis
- Nephritis
- Bright's disease
- Haematuria
- Diabetes
- Syphilis
- Breast affections
- Metritis
- Nymphomania

MODALITIES

- **Aggravation:** Evening, before midnight, twilight, lying on left or painful side, during a thunderstorm, weather changes, warm food and drink, odours, noise, emotions, mental exertion. Cold air relieves the head and face symptoms but aggravates those of chest, throat and neck
- **Amelioration:** In the dark, lying on right side, from being rubbed or mesmerized, from cold food, cold water, until it gets warm, sitting

REMEDY RELATIONSHIP

- **Complementary:** Ars., All-c., Lyc., Sil., Nux-v., Sanguiso., Phos-pchl.
- **Incompatible:** Caust.
- **Compare:** Tub. follows Phos. well and compliments its action. Phos-h., Amph., Thymol., Calc., Chin., Ant-t., Sep., Lyc., Sulph.
- **Follows well:** After, Calc. or Chin.

PHYSOSTIGMA VENENOSUM

INTRODUCTION
- **Common name:** Calabar bean
- **Family:** *Leguminosae*
- **Source:** Vegetable kingdom
- **Part used:** Seeds
- **Prover:** Christison

SPHERE OF ACTION
- Eyes
- Heart
- Nervous system
- Gastrointestinal system
- Respiratory system
- Musculoskeletal system

CONSTITUTION
- For paralysis, tremors, trismus tetanus and chorea; paralytic state of mind and body
- **Temperament:** Nervous
- **Thermal:** Chilly
- **Miasm:** Psora, Syphilis

MIND
- Uncommon mental activity, **cannot stop thinking; mind active even during sleep**
- Nervous, irritable
- Nothing seems right
- Too many things in the room, continually counting them
- Paralytic state of mind and body from grief
- Mentally exhausted – cannot concentrate, cannot remember anything
- Exhilarated in the morning, gloomy towards noon

KEYNOTE SYMPTOMS
- Depressed motor and reflex activity of the cord causing loss of sensibility to pain and muscular weakness followed by complete paralysis
- Spinal irritation, loss of motility
- **Muscles refuse to obey** will; fluttering tremors in muscles, they are drawn into knots
- Darting pains here and there
- **Flushes of heat, especially in palms. Offensive odour from hands**
- Horror of cold water, drinks or bathing; cold water feels too cold. Slightest draught of air renews the shuddering
- Severe headache, cannot bear to raise the eyelids
- Paralysis of accommodation; astigmatism, increasing myopia, profuse lachrymation
- Twitching of ocular muscles or that of the nose
- Contraction of pupil and ciliary muscles
- Spasm of ciliary muscles. Irritability after using eyes
- Irregular menstruation, with palpitation
- Locomotor ataxia; numbness in paralysed parts, crampy pain in limbs; pain in right popliteal space.

CLINICAL
- Ataxia
- Chorea
- Poliomyelitis
- Spinal irritation
- Tetanus
- Paralysis
- Trismus
- Glaucoma
- Myopia
- Mydriasis
- Twitching of eyelids
- Partial blindness
- Photophobia
- Night blindness
- Muscae volitantes
- Astigmatism
- Blepharospasm
- Globus hystericus
- Gastralgia
- Constipation
- Coryza
- Post-diphtheritic paralysis
- Fatty degeneration of heart
- Arthritis
- Hemiplegia
- Paraplegia
- Blisters

MODALITIES
- **Aggravation:** Lying on left side, in church, on waking, motion, jar, descending, stepping, pressure, bathing
- **Amelioration:** Cool open air, closing eyes, sleep, lying on right side or abdomen, exerting will, keeping feet warm

REMEDY RELATIONSHIP
- **Compare:** Bell., Con., Cur., Gels., Hyper., Stry., Esin., Esin-sal., Muscin., Thebin., Pipe.
- **Antidote:** Atropia

PHYTOLACCA DECANDRA

INTRODUCTION

- **Common name:** Poke-root, American nightshade
- **Family:** *Phytolaccaceae*
- **Source:** Vegetable kingdom
- **Part used:** Roots
- **Prover:** Hahnemann

SPHERE OF ACTION

- Mind
- Glands
- Gastrointestinal system
- Respiratory system
- Breasts
- Musculoskeletal system
- Urinary system

CONSTITUTION

- Cancerous constitution
- Suits glandular and syphilitic affections, sensitive to cold weather
- **Temperament:** Nervous, glandular, rheumatic
- **Thermal:** Chilly
- **Miasm:** Syphilis

MIND

- Loss of personal delicacy; complete shamelessness and indifference to exposure of her person
- Melancholy, gloom, indifference to life, is sure she will die; predicts death
- Desires death in the morning on waking
- Disgust for business
- Irritability, nervousness and restlessness
- Disinclined towards mental exertion
- Indifference towards life

KEYNOTE SYMPTOMS

- **Glandular remedy. Glands hardened like stone.** There is glandular swelling with heat and inflammation. Particularly affects breasts and tonsils
- Affinity for fibrous and osseous tissues, fascias and sheathes of muscles
- General muscular soreness, patient moans and groans
- **Pains flying like electric shocks, rapidly shifting, shooting, lancinating.** Pains come and go suddenly, change place
- Discharges are shreddy, stringy
- Tendency to boils; papular and pustular lesions, squamous eruptions
- Cannot tolerate pain, oversensitive to pain; becomes unconscious from pain
- Dentitional ailments in children with an **irresistable desire to bite teeth together. Tongue has a fiery, red tip**
- **Throat sore, better swallowing cold drinks, worse warm drinks;** feels rough, narrow and hot; throat red or bluish-red in colour
- Tonsillitis with swollen fauces. **Pain shoots into ears on swallowing**
- Suppressed, scanty urine with pain in kidney region
- Affinity for mammary glands – enlarged, heavy, hard, stony and swollen with tenderness. Hard and painful nodosities
- Cracks and small ulcers around nipples
- **Pain radiates from nipple all over the body when child nurses**
- Breasts very sensitive; pressure with hand ameliorates pain
- Rheumatism, after tonsillitis, accompanied by lassitude, patient wants to lie down all the time; wandering pains. Syphilitic bone pains
- Hip joint disease, sciatica – pain shoots from sacrum down the outer aspect of thighs, to knees and toes
- Tendency to hasten suppuration. Pus is ichorous, foetid and watery

MODALITIES

- **Aggravation:** When it rains, exposure to damp cold weather, movement, changes of weather, during menses, right side, swallowing especially hot drinks
- **Amelioration:** Warmth, dry weather, lying on abdomen, left side

CLINICAL

- Glands enlarged
- Cancer
- Tumours
- Vertigo
- Iritis
- Retarded dentition
- Glossitis
- Mumps
- Ozaena
- Diphtheria
- Pharyngitis
- Tonsillitis
- Dyspnoea
- Nephritis
- Breast abscess
- Fibrocystic breast disease
- Mastitis
- Breast tumour
- Syphilis
- Venereal buboes
- Orchitis
- Bone affections
- Arthritis
- Rheumatism
- Bursitis
- Tendonitis
- Gout
- Sciatica
- Plantar fasciitis
- Boils

REMEDY RELATIONSHIP

- **Compare:** Kali-i., its analogue. Tincture of Phyt-b., Bry., Rhus-t., Merc., Sang., Arum-t.
- **Inimical:** Merc.
- **Antidotes:** Milk and salt, Bell., Mez.

PICRICUM ACIDUM

INTRODUCTION

- **Common name:** Picric acid, Trini-trophenolum
- **Group:** Acid
- **Source:** Mineral kingdom
- **Formula:** $C_6H_2OH(NO_2)_3$
- **Prover:** Parisel

SPHERE OF ACTION

- Head
- Eyes
- Ears
- Cerebrospinal system
- Gastrointestinal system
- Genitourinary system
- Musculoskeletal system

CONSTITUTION

- Suits physically and mentally worn out people of dark complexion and dirty appearance
- Suits anaemic and cachectic people
- **Temperament:** Nervous, anaemic, cachectic
- **Thermal:** Chilly
- **Miasm:** Psora, Sycosis, Syphilis

MIND

- Dull and unable to concentrate or read more than a few minutes at a time; cannot collect thoughts
- Brain fag
- Mental weakness and confusion, unable to take on projects; mental exertion aggravates
- Sexual desire and lascivious thoughts in presence of any woman; lewd
- Lack of will power
- Dementia with prostration; sits still, listless
- Anxiety, fear of failure in an exam

KEYNOTE SYMPTOMS

- Neurasthenia. Myelitis with spasms and prostration
- Tired heavy feeling all over the body, especially the limbs, worse exertion, great weakness
- **Headaches** especially, occipital headaches, **relieved by bandaging tightly; worse mental exertion and sexual excitement**
- Chronic catarrhal conjunctivitis with copious, thick, yellow discharge
- **Bitter taste with unquenchable thirst. Aversion to food at noon.**
- Uraemia with complete anuria
- Inflammation of kidneys with profound weakness and dark, bloody, scanty urine; dribbling urine
- **Pain in the left ovary and leucorrhoea before menstruation**
- Extreme prostration from frequent seminal emissions
- Priapism, hard erection, with pain in testicles up the spermatic cord. Prostatic enlargement. Impotency with tendency to boils.
- Degeneration of the spinal cord with paralysis
- Acute ascending paralysis, feet cold, cannot get warm
- Burning along the spine, in legs
- Weakness and pain in back. Pins and needles sensation in extremities

CLINICAL

- Weak memory
- Brain fag
- Cerebral softening
- Neurasthenia
- Debility
- Muscular debility
- Pernicious anaemia
- Spinal cord degeneration
- Acute ascending paralysis
- Locomotor ataxia
- Myelitis
- Hemiplegia
- Headache
- Styes
- Conjuctivitis
- Vomiting
- Boils in ear
- Diabetes
- Haemoglobinuria
- Uraemia
- Anuria
- Nephritis
- Sexual excitement
- Ovaritis
- Impotency
- Priapism
- Prostatic hypertrophy
- Writer's palsy
- Lumbago
- Burns
- Boils
- Carbuncles

MODALITIES

- **Aggravation:** Least mental or physical exertion, motion, study, wet weather, mental shock, fatigue
- **Amelioration:** From cold and cold water, tight pressure, bandaging, rest

REMEDY RELATIONSHIP

- **Compare:** Ox-ac., Gels., Phos., Sil., Arg-n., Zinc-pic., Ferr-pic., Calc-pic., Kali-p., Ph-ac., Petr.

PINUS SYLVESTRIS

INTRODUCTION
- **Common name:** Scotch pine, Scotch fir
- **Family:** *Pinaceae*
- **Source:** Vegetable kingdom
- **Part used:** Young shoot
- **Prover:** Domeures

SPHERE OF ACTION
- Gastrointestinal system
- Musculoskeletal system
- Skin

MIND
- Hurried, hasty, occupation in; desires to do several things at once, but cannot finish any
- Undertakes many things but perseveres with nothing
- Anxious, despondent
- Dullness of mind, unable to think; caused by any exertion
- Sudden vanishing of thoughts

MODALITIES
- **Aggravation:** Walking, exertion, touch, morning, evening
- **Amelioration:** Rest, open air

KEYNOTE SYMPTOMS
- Chilliness alternately with flushing of face
- Scalp sensitive to touch; sensation of fullness, dullness and heaviness of head
- Face alternately red and pale
- Glandular swellings; liver and spleen enlarged and painful
- **Itching of anus; discharge of threadworms**
- Nose itches. Severe epistaxis, several days in succession
- The chest seems thin, as if it would give way to pressure
- Increased bronchial mucous
- Severe boring, burning pain in kidney region. **Burning on urination, increased flow of strong smelling urine.** Spasm of bladder.
- **Emaciation of lower limbs and weak ankles in children.** Cramp in calves. Late walking in rickety and scrofulous children.
- Stiffness; gouty and paralytic pain in limbs, bones and joints, especially finger joints
- Nettle rash, itching all over, in general, especially around joints and abdomen

CONSTITUTION
- For weak ankles with tardiness in walking in rachitic children and emaciation of lower limbs
- **Temperament:** Nervous, gouty, rheumatic, scrofulous
- **Thermal:** Chilly
- **Miasm:** Psora, Sycosis, Syphilis

CLINICAL
- Emaciation
- Headache
- Squint
- Diarrhoea
- Constipation
- Haemorrhoids
- Epistaxis
- Amenorrhoea
- Dysmenorrhoea
- Stiff joints
- Arthritis
- Rheumatism
- Gout
- Weak ankles
- Cramps in calves
- Urticaria
- Nettle rash

REMEDY RELATIONSHIP
- **Compare:** Pin-l, Abies-c., Abies-n., Ter., Sabin., Juni., Thuj., Aloe, Benz-ac., Sulph.

Pinus sylvestris

PIPER METHYSTICUM

SPHERE OF ACTION
- Mind
- Gastrointestinal system
- Musculoskeletal system
- Urinary system
- Skin

INTRODUCTION
- **Common name:** Kava-kava, Kavae rhizoma
- **Family:** *Piperaceae*
- **Source:** Vegetable kingdom
- **Part used:** Rhizome

CONSTITUTION
- For cases with silent and drowsy intoxication with incoherent dreams and loss of muscular power
- Cases with a highly strung nervous system
- **Temperament:** Nervous, bilious
- **Thermal:** Ambithermal
- **Miasm:** Psora, Sycosis, Syphilis

MIND
- Lively and inclined to work
- Dreams – curious, non-sensical, amorous, wild, of journeys, alternating with half conscious waking
- Restlessness, wants to change position all the time
- Mentally exhalted
- Want of vigour
- Timid, apprehensive

KEYNOTE SYMPTOMS
- **All symptoms, especially pains are temporarily better by diverting the mind or changing the topic**
- Tense as if every nerve was strung up to the highest pitch; trembling
- Emaciation and decrepitude
- Weakness in the morning, better on rising and moving around. Want of tone and life in all functions towards night
- **Frontal brain – 'solid with pain', moves down to the base of the brain and cervical spine**
- Persistent sensation of enlargement of head
- Vertigo and dizziness, better on closure of eyes
- **Velvety fur coating on tongue at night**
- Constipation – hard, large, light coloured. Burning in rectum
- Increased micturation, burning during micturition in urethra; gonorrhoea and gleet; cystitis
- Hands feel paralyzed; pain in the thumb joint; pain in right arm; numbness of right elbow
- Lower limbs numb and weak, is unable to stand
- Skin dry, where it is thick as on hands and feet, with scales, cracks and ulcers. Fall of scales leaves white spots which generally ulcerate

CLINICAL
- Vertigo
- Dizziness
- Flatulent colic
- Constipation
- Burning micturation
- Cystitis
- Dysuria
- Gonorrhoea
- Chordee
- Orchitis
- Arthritis deformans
- Rheumatism
- Ulcers
- Eczema
- Ichthyosis
- Leprosy

MODALITIES
- **Aggravation:** Thinking, reading, walking, going downstairs
- **Amelioration:** Open air, moving, turning mind to another topic, changing position

REMEDY RELATIONSHIP
- **Compare:** Chaul., Cub., Pip-n., Mati., Rhus-t., Ox-ac., Coff., Pic-ac., Aven., Arg-n., Acon., Cham.
- **Antidoted by:** Rhus-t., Puls.

PIX LIQUIDA

SPHERE OF ACTION
- Mucous membranes
- Gastrointestinal system
- Respiratory system
- Blood
- Skin

MIND
- Irritability, worse contradiction
- Restlessness
- Anxiety

MODALITIES
- **Aggravation:** Night
- **Amelioration:** Rest

INTRODUCTION
- **Common name:** Pine tar
- **Family:** *Coniferae*
- **Source:** Vegetable kingdom
- **Part used:** A product of dry distillation of various coniferous woods
- **Prover:** Jeanes

KEYNOTE SYMPTOMS
- Great exhaustion
- Action on various mucous membranes
- Constant vomiting of black vomit, with pain in the stomach
- Dark coloured stool and urine
- A drug to be considered when the patient has bronchial irritation after influenza and other infectious diseases with profuse muco-purulent sputum which has an offensive taste and odour
- A remedy for chronic bronchitis, bronchiectasis and tuberculosis
- **Pain at third left costal cartilage, where it joins the rib**
- Suppuration of left lung with pain at third rib; rales
- **Eruptions, especially on back of hands, itching intolerably at night, bleed on scratching**
- Desquamation of skin, skin cracked

CONSTITUTION
- **A 'stimulant expectorant' in chronic bronchitis and tuberculosis, and a 'stimulant' for skin ailments like psoriasis and scaly eczema**
- **Temperament:** Anxious
- **Thermal:** Ambithermal
- **Miasm:** Sycosis

CLINICAL
- Alopecia
- Vomiting
- Stomach pain
- Influenza
- Post-influenza
- Cough
- Bronchitis
- Bronchiectasis
- Tuberculosis
- Chest pain
- Itching
- Pruritus
- Acne
- Scaly eczema
- Psoriasis

REMEDY RELATIONSHIP
- **Compare:** Kreos., Petr., Pin-s., Eupi., Ter., Carb-ac., Ther.

PLATINUM METALLICUM

INTRODUCTION

- **Common name:** Platina
- **Group:** Metal
- **Source:** Mineral kingdom
- **Formula:** Pt
- **Prover:** Stapf

SPHERE OF ACTION

- Mind
- Gastointestinal system
- Musculoskeletal system
- Genital system

CONSTITUTION

- Predominantly a women's remedy with too frequent and too profuse menses; sexual organs very sensitive
- Suits thin, hysterical women with dark hair
- **Temperament:** Bilious, sanguine
- **Thermal:** Chilly
- **Miasm:** Psora, Syphilis

MIND

- Mental and physical symptoms alternate
- Changeable moods – weeps and laughs alternately
- Unkind, quarrelsome and rude. Contempt for others; fault finding
- Feels she does not belong to her own family or has no place in the world. Feels everything is changed or different
- Irresistible impulse to kill her own husband or children
- Religious mania alternating with sexual excitement
- Hysteria, before menses. Perverted social desire – nymphomania, worse during menses
- Oversensitive mind, emotions and nerves
- Disordered sense of proportion – objects seem smaller or strange
- Feels all people are physically and mentally inferior to her. Superiority complex of royal blood of the highest degree
- **Proud and over-estimation of one's self; looks down upon others.** Arrogant, haughty. Wounded pride.

KEYNOTE SYMPTOMS

- Mental symptoms alternate with sexual symptoms
- Several symptoms are a reflex from the ovaries, uterus and sexual organs
- Marked tendency to anaesthesia, paralysis, localised numbness and coldness
- Pains increase and decrease gradually
- **Sensation of band about the part affected or as if bandaged**
- Constriction around forehead; cramp-like, squeezing pain. Numbness with headache
- **Sensation of coldness, creeping and numbness on entire right side of face.** Prosopalgia with numbness of malar bones
- Sense of constriction in stomach
- **Ravenous hunger with continuous nausea with anxiety,** trembling and lassitude
- Painter's colic; pressing and bearing down pains in the abdomen, extending into the pelvis; pinching around the umbilical region
- **Constipation, stools retarded, black, passed in small quantities after a lot of straining**
- Constipation in travellers who are constantly changing food and water. Stool as if burnt, **adheres to the rectum like soft clay**
- Constipation in travellers who are constantly changing food and water. Stool as if burnt, adheres to the rectum like soft clay
- Excessive sexual desire, leading to masturbation, nymphomania
- Ovaritis with sterility; vaginismus, sex is impossible. Sleeps with legs far apart. Amenorrhoea in emigrants.
- Menses too early, too profuse; metrorrhagia – dark, clotted with spasms and painful, bearing down pains; dysmenorrhoea
- Unnaturally increased sexual desire in men with voluptuous tickling and itching

CLINICAL

- Depression
- Hysteria
- Neurasthenia
- Numbness
- Spasms
- Cramps
- Epilepsy
- Neuralgia
- Malignancy
- Obesity
- Headache
- Prosopalgia
- Bell's palsy
- Bulimia
- Nausea
- Colic
- Painter's colic
- Diarrhoea
- Constipation
- Haemorrhoids
- Sexual disorders
- Sexual mania
- Nymphomania
- Suppressed menses
- Amenorrhoea
- Dysmenorrhoea
- Metrorrhagia
- Ovaritis
- Ovarian cyst
- Pruritus vulvae
- Sterility
- Vaginismus
- Arthritis
- Rheumatism
- Herpes

MODALITIES

- **Aggravation:** Emotions, chagrin, sex, during menses, touch, pressure, sitting, standing, bending backwards, evening, night
- **Amelioration:** Sunshine, walking in open air, stretching, motion

REMEDY RELATIONSHIP

- **Compare:** Rhod., Stann., Valer., Sep., Plat-m., Sed-ac., Plat-m-n., Aur., Croc., Ign., Kali-p., Puls.
- **Antidote:** Puls., Plat. antidotes the bad effects of lead
- **Compatible:** Lyc., Bell., Puls., Ign., Rhus-t., Verat., Sep.

PLUMBUM METALLICUM

INTRODUCTION

- **Common name:** Lead
- **Group:** Metal
- **Source:** Mineral kingdom
- **Formula:** Pb
- **Prover:** Hartlaub, Trinks, Hering and Nenning

SPHERE OF ACTION

- Mind
- Eyes
- Cerebrospinal system
- Gastrointestinal system
- Circulatory system
- Musculoskeletal system
- Genitourinary system

CONSTITUTION

- Suits men, more than women, especially of a dry, bilious constitution who are hypochondriacal or disposed to religious monomania
- Marasmus in infants, with large and hard abdomen, pale, emaciated face, and extreme constipation
- **Temperament:** Anxious, bilious
- **Thermal:** Hot
- **Miasm:** Sycosis, Syphilis

MIND

- Intellectual apathy; increasing slowness, slow perception. Deficiency of ideas
- Timidity about appearing in public; restless, anxiety and yawning; sighing
- Mentally exhausted from physical labour
- **Fear of being assassinated; thinks everyone is going to murder her**
- Feigns sickness or exaggerates her condition; inclined to deceive
- Cursing, wild delirium with a distorted face; imbecility, mania
- Memory poor, especially for words. Struggle to find the right word to express himself. Slow perception, weakness or loss of memory
- Mental depression, quiet, melancholic, no enjoyment in ordinary things

KEYNOTE SYMPTOMS

- Excessive and rapid emaciation
- General sclerotic conditions, especially affects the blood, alimentary and nervous system
- **Blue line along margin of gums; gums swollen; tremors of naso-labial muscles**
- Violent colic with sensation as if abdominal wall is drawn by a string to the spine. Intense colic, radiating to all parts of the body. Obstructed flatus. Abdomen retracted.
- **Constipation; hard, lumpy, black stools like sheep dung.** Neuralgia of rectum; anus drawn up
- Cardiac weakness; pulse soft, small, dicrotic
- Chronic interstitial nephritis with severe pain in abdomen. Kidney irritation; urine scanty, albuminous, of low specific gravity
- Loss of sexual power; testicles drawn up, feels constricted
- **Progressive muscular atrophy;** infantile paralysis. **Paralysis of lower limbs, of single muscles, wrist drop**
- Pain in atrophied limbs. Loss of patellar reflex. Cramps in calves
- Pain in right big toe at night
- Stinging and tearing pain in limbs; also twitching, tingling and numbness
- Lead paralysis is chiefly of extensors, of forearms or upper limbs, from centre to periphery, with partial anaesthesia or excessive hyperaesthesia, preceded by pain
- Takes strange attitudes and positions in bed during sleep. Jerks during sleep

CLINICAL

- Dementia
- Neuro degenerative disorders
- Cerebral accident
- Multiple sclerosis
- Parkinson's disease
- Neuritis
- Paralysis
- Stroke
- Progressive muscular atrophy
- Spasms
- Paraplegia
- Tremors
- Marasmus in infants
- Anaemia
- Amaurosis
- Glaucoma
- Gastralgia
- Lead poisoning
- Painter's colic
- Strangulated hernia
- Intussusception
- Constipation
- Haemorrhoids
- Tinnitus
- Claudication
- Contractures
- Arteriosclerosis
- Angina pectoris
- Aneurysm
- Interstitial nephritis
- Bright's disease
- Vaginismus
- Menorrhagia
- Induration of breasts
- Wrist drop
- Gout
- Anidrosis

MODALITIES

- **Aggravation:** At night, from motion, touch, open air, clear weather, foggy weather
- **Amelioration:** Rubbing, hard pressure, stretching limbs, rest, lying down, bending double ameliorates colic

REMEDY RELATIONSHIP

- **Compare:** Plb-act., Plb-i., Alum., Plat., Op., Podo., Merc., Thal., Plect., Plb-chr., Plb-p., Nux-v.
- **Antidotes:** Plat., Alum., Petr., Sul-ac., Zinc., Plat.

PODOPHYLLUM PELTATUM

SPHERE OF ACTION

- Mind
- Mucous membranes
- Gastrointestinal system
- Female genital system

INTRODUCTION

- **Common name:** May apple
- **Family:** *Berberidaceae*
- **Source:** Vegetable kingdom
- **Part used:** Rhizome
- **Prover:** Williamson

CONSTITUTION

- For complaints of pregnant and parturient women, with sensation as if intestines were falling down
- Bilious attacks in people who suffer from gastrointestinal derangement with profuseness of discharges.
- **Temperament:** Nervous, bilious
- **Thermal:** Chilly
- **Miasm:** Psora

MIND

- Mental fatigue from business
- Ailments from emotional excitement
- Anxious in the twilight, with anxiety felt more in the abdomen after stool; anxiety as if he would be ill
- Loquacity with delirium, from eating acidic fruits; changes topics of conversation; quickly from one subject to another
- Fear of impending disease, that he would be very ill, when waking up in the morning
- Depression of spirits, disgust of life
- Restless and fidgety

KEYNOTE SYMPTOMS

- Right sided remedy – throat, ovary, hypochondrium
- **Headache alternating with diarrhoea; headache in winters and diarrhoea in summers**
- Hydrocephalus; rolling of head from side to side with moaning and vomiting
- Great desire to press gums together
- **Tongue – broad, large, moist with a burning sensation and imprint of teeth**
- Difficult dentition in children with grinding of teeth at night; head hot, rolling from side to side; hot, glowing cheeks; and diarrhoea
- Viscid mucous in mouth, coating teeth
- Thirst for large quantities of cold water
- Abdomen distended with sensation of weakness and sinking. Can lie comfortably only on the stomach
- Constantly shaking and rubbing the liver region with hands
- Torpidity of liver, portal engorgement, haemorrhoids, hypogastric pains, fullness of superficial veins and jaundice. Liver region painful
- Pendulous abdomen after confinement
- **Stools – watery, profuse, painless, putrid, prostrating, gushing, with jelly-like mucous and prolapse of rectum**
- Diarrhoea early in the morning, in hot weather, after acid fruits
- Diarrhoea in children while being bathed or washed
- Weakness of muscles and ligaments causing prolapse of rectum and uterus on passing stools or over straining
- Marked loquacity during chill and heat stage of fever
- Right ovarian neuralgia. Uterine prolapse from over lifting or straining, especially during pregnancy, post-parturition; with haemorrhoids
- Moaning during sleep, with eyes half closed

CLINICAL

- Brainfag
- Alcoholism
- Fidgety
- Neuralgia
- Debility
- Brain affections
- Spinal meningitis
- Convulsions
- Hydrocephalus
- Headache
- Vertigo
- Photophobia
- Dentitional complaints
- Vomiting
- Gastralgia
- Gastroenteritis
- Diarrhoea
- Dysentery
- Cholera morbus
- Cholera infantum
- Constipation
- Worms
- Prolapsed rectum
- Prolapsed uterus
- Suppressed eruptions
- Chillblains

MODALITIES

- **Aggravation:** Early morning, in hot weather; during dentition, motion, during and after stools, milk, acid fruits
- **Amelioration:** Pressure, rubbing the liver region, lying on abdomen

REMEDY RELATIONSHIP

- **Compare:** Aloe, Chel., Coll., Lil-t., Merc., Nux-v., Sulph., Mand., Prune. (colitis)
- It antidotes the bad effects of Mercury.
- **After:** Ip., Nux-v., in gastric affections; after Calc. and Sulph. in liver diseases

POLYGONUM HYDROPIPEROIDES

INTRODUCTION

- **Common name:** Mild water pepper, smartweed
- **Family:** *Polygonaceae*
- **Source:** Vegetable kingdom
- **Part used:** Whole plant
- **Prover:** Dr W.E. Payne

SPHERE OF ACTION

- Gastrointestinal system
- Respiratory system
- Musculoskeletal system
- Genitourinary system
- Skin

MIND

- Gloomy views of life, dislike of change and excessive dread of death
- Great depression followed by excessive irritability
- Anxiety, restlessness, melancholy
- Hopeless foreboding, worse after sleep
- Epilepsy and hysteria
- Sleep full of dreams

MODALITIES

- **Aggravation:** Cold, damp, pressure of clothes, rising
- **Amelioration:** Warmth

KEYNOTE SYMPTOMS

- Cutting pains or pulsating, flashing, wandering pains, especially in extremities
- **Sensation of coldness alternated or coincided with heat in same or other parts.** For example, **coldness of right side of face, when pain in left side** was most severe; **burning in chest with cold feeling in pit of stomach;** feet burning then suddenly cold
- **Voracious appetite. Thirst for cold water, yet drinking causes nausea**
- Painful engorged veins. Varicosis, haemorrhoids and rectal pockets
- Interior of anus studded with itching eminences
- Inflammation of kidneys from cold. Cutting pains along ureters to bladder. Strangury, pains in bladder
- Aching in hips, in loins in women; sensation as if hips were being drawn together; sensation of weight and tension in pelvis
- Metrorrhagia, and also amenorrhoea in young girls
- Acrid, excoriating leucorrhoea
- Pain and soreness in testicles, spermatic cord and neck of bladder when urinating. Itching and stinging of prepuce
- Pulsating, flashing, wandering pains in prostate
- Superficial ulcers and sores on lower extremities, especially in women during climacteric

CONSTITUTION

- For young girls suffering from amenorrhea, having an aversion to sex
- Tendency to varicose veins
- **Temperament:** Nervous, bilious
- **Thermal:** Chilly
- **Miasm:** Psora, Sycosis, Syphilis

CLINICAL

- Flatulent colic
- Gastritis
- Diarrhoea
- Constipation
- Haemorrhoids
- Laryngitis
- Cough
- Nephritic colic
- Nephritis
- Amenorrhoea
- Metrorrhagia
- Prostatitis
- Orchitis
- Arthritis
- Rheumatism
- Sciatica
- Varicose veins
- Dry skin
- Eczema
- Ulcers
- Chronic erysipelas

REMEDY RELATIONSHIP

- **Compare:** Card-m. in ulcers; Ham., Senec., Polyg-pe., Polyg-s., Polyg-a.

Polygonum hydropiperoides

PRIMULA OBCONICA

SPHERE OF ACTION
- Gastrointestinal system
- Respiratory system
- Musculoskeletal system
- Skin

MIND
- Anguish before stools
- Disposition to contradict
- Irritability, worse contradiction
- Restlessness
- Anxiety
- Oversensitivity

MODALITIES
- **Aggravation:** Physical exertion, pain in abdomen worse by bending from side to side
- **Amelioration:** Rest

INTRODUCTION
- **Common name:** Primrose
- **Family:** *Primulaceae*
- **Source:** Vegetable kingdom
- **Part used:** Whole plant
- **Prover:** Rev. F.H. Brett

KEYNOTE SYMPTOMS
- **Right sided** complaints
- **Intermittence of symptoms**
- Deep infiltration and tension of tissues; blisters, especially on fingers
- Paralysed sensation. Weakness, burning irritation and discolouration of skin
- **Diminished facial irritation, alternates with pharyngeal soreness**
- Papular eruptions on the chin, burning at night
- Skin complaints with febrile symptoms
- Urticaria-like eruptions. Erysipelas with severe itching, worse at night, red and swollen
- **Purple blotches on the back of hands,** palmar surface is stiff
- Small papules on a raised base
- Eczema – papular and excoriated. Eruptions between fingers

CONSTITUTION
- For moist eczema, papular eruptions on the chin and swollen eyelids in sensitive patients
- For deep infilteration and tension of tissues
- **Temperament:** Nervous, haemorrhagic
- **Thermal:** Chilly
- **Miasm:** Psora, Syphilis

CLINICAL
- Weakness
- Blepharitis
- Splenitis
- Hepatitis
- Constipation
- Pharyngitis
- Arthritis
- Rheumatism
- Eruptions
- Blisters
- Erysipelas
- Papules
- Eczema
- Burns
- Erythema multiforma

REMEDY RELATIONSHIP
- **Compare:** Chen-v., (weakness in the lumbar and lower dorsal region); Rhus-t., Fago., Verat.

PRUNUS SPINOSA

SPHERE OF ACTION
- Eyes
- Gastrointestinal system
- Heart
- Urinary system
- Skin

INTRODUCTION
- **Common name:** Black thorn
- **Family:** *Rosaceae*
- **Source:** Vegetable kingdom
- **Part used:** Flower bud used, just before flowering
- **Prover:** Wahle

CONSTITUTION
- For old people with dark complexion, ciliary neuralgia and oedema
- **Temperament:** Nervous, haemorrhagic
- **Thermal:** Chilly
- **Miasm:** Psora, Syphilis

MIND
- **Restlessness which does not allow one to remain in one place, walks about constantly with dyspnoea and short breathing**
- Sighing, as if climbing a high and steep mountain
- Complaining; morning in bed, weeping tearful mood
- Dreams – of furuncles, of salty things
- Anxiety with difficulty in breathing
- Hurried, hasty while walking
- Morose, cross, irritable, fretful, ill-humoured, peevish
- Aversion to walk from sadness

KEYNOTE SYMPTOMS
- Pre-eminently a right sided remedy
- **Pressive pains** – out pressive and out **shooting; shooting from within out;** felt in the skull, eyes, root of nose and ears
- Sensation as if air inhaled does not reach the pit of the stomach
- Shooting pains, like lightening
- Ciliary neuralgia; bursting pain in the right eyeball
- Sudden pain in the right eye as if it would burst
- Toothache – as if teeth were pulled out
- Flatulence presses on bladder resulting in cramps in the bladder, forcing the patient to double up
- Hard nodular stool with rectal pain, as if an angular body was present, with slimy diarrhoea
- Cramp-like pain in the bladder region
- Oppression of chest; anxious, short respiration
- Spasmodic tenesmus of bladder and rectum at close of urination; strangury
- Sensation as if urine passes upto the glans and then returns causing pain in urethra
- Tenesmus of bladder, must hurry, impelled to micturate.
- Ankle and foot feel sprained

CLINICAL
- Anasarca
- Dropsy
- Oedema
- Neuralgia
- Ciliary neuralgia
- Vitreous opacity
- Glaucoma
- Choroido-retinitis
- Irido-cyclitis
- Toothache
- Ascites
- Diarrhoea
- Dysentery
- Constipation
- Angina pectoris
- Tenesmus of bladder
- Dysuria
- Strangury
- Pedal oedema
- Finger frozen
- Herpes zoster

MODALITIES
- **Aggravation:** Stooping, ascending, motion, jar, pressure, night
- **Amelioration:** Rest, bending double

REMEDY RELATIONSHIP
- **Compare:** Laur., Prun-p., Prun-v., Pyrus.

Prunus spinosa

PSORINUM

SPHERE OF ACTION
- Mind
- Gastrointestinal system
- Respiratory system
- Heart
- Musculoskeletal system
- Urinary system
- Skin

INTRODUCTION
- **Common name:** Scabies vesicle
- **Group:** Nosode
- **Source:** Animal kingdom
- **Part used:** Serous fluid of a scabies vesicle
- **Prover:** Hahnemann (proved seropurulent matter of scabies vesicle) Gross (proved product of 'psora sica') or Hering (proved the salt from a product of psora)

CONSTITUTION
- Pale, sick, delicate people who do not sleep day or night, they fret, worry and cry. Child good, plays all day, troublesome and screams all night
- Peevish, unhealthy looking children
- Pale, delicate, sallow, greasy face with humid eruptions on the face, especially chin and neck with swelling of the upper lip, subject to diseases of glands and skin or suppressed eruptions
- **Temperament:** Nervous, bilious, scrofulous
- **Thermal:** Chilly
- **Miasm:** Psora, Sycosis

MIND
- Nervous, restless people who are easily startled
- Hopeless. Despair of recovery when sick
- Makes own and others life miserable
- Sensitiveness
- Fears – he will die, his business will fail, of fire, of being alone, of going mad, of future, of poverty, of health, of cancer
- Poverty consciousness
- Lack of vitality
- Deep anxiety states, with restlessness and anxiety; especially when riding in a carriage
- Suicidal thoughts. Great despondency. Pessimistic. Sentimental.

KEYNOTE SYMPTOMS
- For complaints of psoric origin
- In chronic cases when well selected remedies fail to act
- Lack of vitality or reaction after severe acute diseases. Marked debility from loss of vital fluids, after acute diseases independant of organic disease
- Chilly remedy, wants warm clothing even in summer. Sensitive to every change in weather
- **Patients – adults and children appear dirty and unhealthy with a disagreeable odour about them which no amount of washing can remove**
- Profuse perspiration on least exertion, after acute diseases – with relief of all suffering
- **All secretions** – diarrhoea, menses, leucorrhoea, perspiration, saliva, nasal mucous – **have a filthy, carrion-like odour**
- Feels unexplicably well the day before about to get ill
- Hair dry, lusterless, tangles easily, glues together
- Headache preceded by flickering before eyes, by dimness of vision or blindness; hungry during attacks
- Tongue, gums – ulcerated; **tough mucous of foul taste adheres to the soft palate**
- Profuse, offensive saliva; tough mucous in the throat, recurring, quinsy – eradicates it's tendency. **Expectoration of cheesy, pea-like balls of disgusting taste**
- **Eructations taste like bad eggs.** Very hungry all the time; must eat something in the middle of the night
- Horrible, offensive, almost involuntary, dark, watery, thin, dirty greenish stools – at night and towards morning
- Obstinate constipation from inactivity of rectum; with severe pains. Burning haemorrhoids
- Dry coryza with stoppage of nose; post-nasal discharge
- Hay fever appearing regularly every year with an asthmatic, eczematous or psoric history
- Tonsil swollen; rough; dysphagia with pain in ears
- Asthma worse sitting up, better lying down. Cough returns every winter
- Provides immunity from catching colds
- Dry, scaly eruptions – in bends of elbows and knees – disappear in summer, reappear in winter
- Intolerable itching, worse warmth of bed or by scratching
- Increased secretion from sebaceous glands – oily skin

CLINICAL
- Depression
- Phobic disorders
- Anxiety
- Debility
- Plica polonica
- Crusta lactea
- Headache
- Blepharitis
- Chronic ophthalmia
- Nausea
- Diarrhoea
- Constipation
- Haemorrhoids
- Colds
- Ozaena
- Hay fever
- Chronic otorrhoea
- Otitis media
- Quinsy
- Tonsillitis
- Adenoids
- Pharyngitis
- Bronchitis
- Asthma
- Cardiac weakness
- Arthritis
- Backache
- Sciatica
- Dermatitis
- Psoriasis
- Acne
- Boils
- Abscesses
- Ulcers
- Scabies
- Eczema
- Urticaria
- Herpes zoster
- Insomnia

MODALITIES
- **Aggravation:** Coffee – *Psorinum* patient does not improve while using coffee, changes of weather, in hot sunshine, from cold, dread of the least cold air or draft, suppressions
- **Amelioration:** Heat, warm clothing even in summer, when quiet, lying with head low

REMEDY RELATIONSHIP
- **Compare:** Ped. in lack of reaction; Calc., Nat-ars., Gaert.
- **Complementary:** Sulph. and Tub.
- **Followed well:** Bry., Alum., Borx., Hep., Sulph., Tub.
- **After:** Lac-ac., in vomiting of pregnancy; Arn. in traumatic affections of ovaries; Sulph. follows Psor. well in mammary cancer. "Whether derived from purest gold or purest filth, our gratitude for its excellent service forbids us to inquire or care.— P.B. Bell.

PTELEA TRIFOLIATA

INTRODUCTION

- **Common name:** Water ash, Hoptree
- **Family:** *Rutaceae*
- **Source:** Vegetable kingdom
- **Part used:** Bark of root
- **Prover:** Hale

SPHERE OF ACTION

- Head
- Gastrointestinal system
- Liver
- Respiratory system
- Musculoskeletal system
- Skin

CONSTITUTION

- Adapted to young people with an atonic state of stomach and liver affections
- **Temperament:** Nervous, bilious
- **Thermal:** Chilly
- **Miasm:** Psora, Syphilis

MIND

- Liveliness after eating, followed by depression an hour later
- **Unusual energy and tendency to hurry; always in a haste with lassitude and weariness**
- Thoughts chase each other through the mind, impossible to fix attention
- Sad, depressed, dejected, melancholic; tendency to worry in the morning after waking
- Dull, stupid, dazed, confused with a riddled feeling in the head
- Memory weak – for things and names. Makes mistakes while writing and spelling; unable to read
- Irritable, nervous, starts from sudden noises

KEYNOTE SYMPTOMS

- Headache, better after breakfast. Dull frontal headache, as if a sharp corner was pressing against the top of the head; as if the skull would be pressed outwards by a sharp plug
- **Tongue – rough, swollen, coated; papillae red and prominent**
- All symptoms disappear suddenly after eating something
- Atonic state or stomach. Liver affections
- Eructations, nausea, vomiting. Feeling of corrosion, heat and burning in the stomach. Stomach feels empty after eating
- **Liver and stomach symptoms are aggravated by lying on the left side and better by lying on the right side**
- Heaviness in region of liver. Liver sore, swollen and sensitive to pressure
- **Copious expulsion of ascarides**
- Stool followed by tenesmus and succeeded by itching and smarting at the anus
- Stool – hard, difficult with much straining and smarting
- Sensation of pressure on the lung and of suffocation when lying on the back
- Asthma, dyspnoea; cramp-like pains in the cardiac region

CLINICAL

- Headache
- Glossitis
- Nausea
- Vomiting
- Dyspepsia
- Atonic gastroenteritis
- Hepatomegaly
- Jaundice
- Hepatitis
- Colic
- Diarrhoea
- Dysentery
- Constipation
- Worms
- Dyspnoea
- Bronchitis
- Asthma
- Nightmares
- Insomnia

MODALITIES

- **Aggravation:** Lying especially on the left side, early morning, on waking, mental exertion, hot room, moving eyes
- **Amelioration:** Eating sour and acidic things, cold air, morning, evening

REMEDY RELATIONSHIP

- **Compare:** Merc., Mag-m., Nux-v., Chel.

SPHERE OF ACTION

- Gastrointestinal system
- Respiratory system
- Urinary system
- Female genital system

INTRODUCTION

- **Common name:** Common flea, Human flea
- **Family:** *Pulicidae*
- **Source:** Animal kingdom
- **Part used:** Whole animal

CONSTITUTION

- Suits people who are old looking and have a wrinkled face with marked urinary symptoms
- **Temperament:** Nervous, haemorrhagic
- **Thermal:** Chilly patient
- **Miasm:** Psora, Syphilis

MIND

- Very impatient, cross, does not want to be looked at or spoken to
- Irritable
- Anxious
- Melancholic
- Memory confused; cannot think
- Restlessness

PULEX IRRITANS

CLINICAL

- Faintness
- Headache
- Loss of appetite
- Nausea
- Vomiting
- Diarrhoea
- Constipation
- Varicose veins
- Asthma
- Cystitis
- Urethritis
- Involuntary micturation
- Amenorrhoea
- Menses delayed
- Leucorrhoea
- Gonorrhoea
- Orchitis
- Acute prostatitis
- Lumbago
- Fever
- Urticaria
- Measles
- Acne
- Insomnia

KEYNOTE SYMPTOMS

- Chilly while sitting besides the fire
- Sensation of a glow all over the body
- Frontal headache with an enlarged feeling of the eyes
- Foulness of breath, taste, stool, urine, skin odour
- **Thirsty, especially during headache. Metallic taste**
- Abdomen bloated; stools very offensive
- Capricious hoarseness. Expectoration black
- Involuntary micturation; urine scanty with frequent urging, pressure on the bladder and burning in the urethra
- Cannot retain urine, must attend to the call immediately
- Irritable bladder during menses. Increased salivation during menses
- **Cotton ball sensation inside vagina;** amenorrhoea
- Stains of menses and leucorrhoea are very hard to wash out. Menses late, scanty, thick

MODALITIES

- **Aggravation:** Left side, moving about
- **Amelioration:** Sitting or lying down

REMEDY RELATIONSHIP

- **Compare:** Ox. acidum, Lyco., Staph., Nux-v., Carbo. veg.
- **Antidoted by:** Nux-v., Camph.

PULSATILLA NIGRICANS

SPHERE OF ACTION

- Mind
- Ears
- Eyes
- Gastrointestinal system
- Respiratory system
- Veins
- Female genital system

INTRODUCTION

- **Common name:** Wind flower
- **Family:** *Ranunculaceae*
- **Source:** Vegetable kingdom
- **Part used:** Whole plant
- **Prover:** Hahnemann

CONSTITUTION

- For beautiful people with fair, fine hair, blue eyes and soft lax muscles, who are anaemic and chlorotic
- Women inclined to be fleshy, with scanty, and protracted menses
- **Temperament:** Nervous, phlegmatic
- **Thermal:** Chilly
- **Miasm:** Psora, Syphilis, Sycosis

MIND

- Hypochondriacal moroseness
- Morbid fear of opposite sex
- Fastidious, very emotional
- Forsaken feeling in the evening; history of abandonment, grief
- Dreams – frightful
- Religious melancholy
- Easily discouraged
- **Mild, gentle, yielding disposition**
- **Timid; weeps easily, almost impossible to detail her ailments without weeping;** weeps easily before menses
- Changeability of mental condition
- Great sensitiveness. Likes sympathy, better by consolation, on being held or hugged
- Full of cares for domestic affairs
- Child wants to be carried slowly and caressed

KEYNOTE SYMPTOMS

- **Changeability of symptoms** – no two stools are alike, no two chills are alike, erratic temperatures in fever, well one hour, miserable the next, etc.
- **Contradictory symptoms like** – patient is chilly but has an aversion to heat, mouth dry but patient is thirstless, etc.
- Patient though chilly, seeks open air; does not want to be covered
- Never well since puberty
- **All discharges from mucous membranes are thick, bland, greenish-yellow, but vaginal discharges are acrid**
- Wandering pains – drawing, tearing, erratic, shifting rapidly from one part to another; with constant chillness
- Headache from overloaded stomach or rich fatty foods like pastries, ice cream, etc.
- **Thirstlessness with all complaints. Dry mouth without thirst**
- **Yellow or white coated tongue.** Greasy taste. Food, especially bread tastes bitter. Altered taste. Aversion to fatty foods, warm foods and drinks
- All gone sensation in stomach, especially in tea drinkers
- Indigestion, abdominal colic from rich, greasy, fatty food
- Diarrhoea, only at night, watery, greenish-yellow; no two stools alike; after eating fruits
- Blind haemorrhoids with itching and sticking pains, weight as of a stone
- Dry cough in evening and at night; loose cough in the morning. Pressure on chest with soreness
- Menses too late, scanty, thick, clotted, changeable and intermittent. Flow intermits. Creamy, acrid, excoriating leucorrhoea.
- Wide awake in the evening; irresistible sleepiness in the afternoon. Feels uncomfortable with one pillow. Lies with hands above the head.

CLINICAL

- Dementia
- Melancholy
- Anxiety
- Depression
- Anaemia
- Varicose veins
- Alopecia
- Vertigo
- Migraine
- Styes
- Conjunctivitis
- Toothache
- Mumps
- Heartburn
- Waterbrash
- Dyspepsia
- Flatulence
- Vomiting
- Gastritis
- Piles
- Diarrhoea
- Dysentery
- Otalgia
- Otitis media
- Anosmia
- Sinusitis
- Cough
- Bronchitis
- Asthma
- Cystitis
- Urethritis
- Ovarian cyst
- Menorrhagia
- Dysmenorrhoea
- Amenorrhoea
- Leucorrhoea
- Uterine prolapse
- Sterility
- Arthritis
- Rheumatism
- Intermittent fever
- Eczema
- Chickenpox
- Measles
- Urticaria
- Sleeplessness

MODALITIES

- **Aggravation:** In a warm closed room, evening, twilight, on beginning to move, lying on the left, or on the painless side, very rich, fat, indigestible food, the diseased side, warm applications, heat
- **Amelioration:** Open air, lying on painful side, cold air or cool room, eating or drinking cold things, cold applications, consolation

REMEDY RELATIONSHIP

- **Compare:** Cycl., Kali-bi., Kali-s., Sulph., Pent. often indicated after Puls. in later colds; Joan., Atri., Puls-n. identical effects
- **Antidotes:** Coff., Cham., Nux-v.
- **Complementary:** Kali-m., Lyc., Sul-ac.; Kali-m. its chemical analogue. Sil. is the chronic of Puls. in nearly all ailments.
- **Follows well:** Kali-bi., Lyc., Sep., Sil., Sulph.

PYROGENIUM

INTRODUCTION

- **Common name:** Pyrogen, Pyrexin, Sepsin
- **Group:** Nosode
- **Source:** Animal kingdom
- **Part used:** A product of decomposed lean beef in water, allowed to stand in the sun for 2-3 weeks
- **Prover:** John Drysdale

SPHERE OF ACTION

- Mind
- Gastrointestinal system
- Respiratory system
- Heart
- Genitourinary system
- Skin

CONSTITUTION

- For septic states, when the best selected remedy fails to relieve or permanently improve, with marked restlessness
- For latent pyogenic infections, where symptoms keep relapsing after the apparent simillimum
- **Temperament:** Nervous, bilious
- **Thermal:** Chilly
- **Miasm:** Psora, Sycosis, Syphilis

MIND

- Useful in all septic states with intense restlessness
- Restlessness and delirium during fever
- Frightful restlessness, better when first beginning to move; constant motion
- Activity of the brain – making speeches and writing articles at night
- Loquacity, thinking and speaking faster than ever before, especially during delirious fever
- Whispering or muttering to herself
- Full of anxiety and insane notions
- Excited, anxious and sensitive
- Confused. Sense of duality. Irritable.
- Hallucinations, that he is very wealthy; sees phantoms, images
- Bed feels too hard, tosses about
- Desire to be rocked

KEYNOTE SYMPTOMS

- Infection, suppuration, sepsis; conditions that begin from acute infections
- Chronic ailments dating back to septic conditions
- Marked restlessness, constantly on the move to relieve soreness
- **Discharges are horribly offensive** – breath, mucous, diarrhoea, vomit, leucorrhoea, menses, lochia, etc.
- Delirium with much activity of the brain and restlessness. Painless throbbing in the head
- Aching in all limbs; sore, bruised; bed feels too hard. Prostrate, yet restless
- Throbbing of neck muscles, seen as waves, running up from the clavicles
- **Taste sweetish, pus-like, foetid**
- **Tongue is large, flabby, clean, dry, smooth, as if varnished**
- Coffee ground vomiting
- **Constipation from complete inertia;** obstinate stools – large, black, or like small black balls
- Diarrhoea, offensive, brownish-black, painless, involuntary
- Severe tenesmus of bladder and rectum
- Fan-like motion of alae nasi
- Threatening heart failure, especially in zymotic and septic fevers; palpitations; conscious of the heart
- **Septicaemia following miscarriage; septic puerperal infection;** uterine haemorrhages
- Foetus or secundines retained for days with horribly offensive discharge
- Septic fever; chills begin in the back, between scapulae; coldness and chilliness with palpitations
- Sudden rise of fever or temperature. **High grade with pulse absolutely out of proportion to the temperature;** cold clammy sweat, which is horribly offensive and profuse but sweating does not cause a fall in temperature
- Hallucinations persistent even after the fever comes down

CLINICAL

- Sepsis
- Numbness
- Cellulitis
- Lymphangitis
- Soreness
- Headache
- Glossitis
- Nausea
- Haematemesis
- Food poisoning
- Peritonitis
- Diarrhoea
- Constipation
- Influenza
- Diphtheria
- Endometritis
- Retained placenta
- Metrorrhagia
- Amenorrhoea
- Pelvic inflammatory disease
- Puerperal peritonitis
- Malaria
- Septic fever
- Puerperal fever
- Typhoid
- Abscesses
- Pigmentation
- Ulcers
- Bed sores
- Wounds
- Insomnia

MODALITIES

- **Aggravation:** Cold, damp, sitting
- **Amelioration:** From motion, heat, hot bathing, hot drinks, pressure, changing position

REMEDY RELATIONSHIP

- **Compare:** Strept., Staph., Pyrog., Echi., Carb-v., Ars., Lach., Rhus-t., Bapt., Carb-ac., Op., Psor., Sec., Verat.
- **Complementary:** Bry.

RADIUM BROMATUM

INTRODUCTION

- **Common name:** Radium bromide
- **Group:** Salt
- **Source:** Mineral kingdom
- **Formula:** $RaBr_2$
- **Prover:** Diffenbach

SPHERE OF ACTION

- Gastrointestinal system
- Respiratory system
- Musculoskeletal system
- Urinary system
- Female genital system
- Skin

CONSTITUTION

- For restless people with chronic rheumatism and great weakness
- **Temperament:** Nervous, bilious
- **Thermal:** Chilly
- **Miasm:** Psora, Sycosis, Syphilis

MIND

- Apprehensive, depressed
- Fear of being alone, of the dark, wants someone near
- Great desire to be with people
- Tired and irritable
- **Dreams of passing urine, of fire, of commiting suicide, great desire to be with people**
- Anxiety as if something was going to happen
- Unable to think clearly, with dull frontal headache all the time
- Easily vexed

KEYNOTE SYMPTOMS

- Severe aching pains all over; with restlessness; better moving; deep pain in joints
- Electric shocks through the body, especially during sleep
- **Metallic taste in mouth with increased salivation. Pricking sensation at end of tongue**
- **Craving for pork. Aversion to sweets, ice creams, meat of which she is very fond.**
- Long standing ulcers. Nausea, sinking sensation, belching of gas, empty feeling
- **Colic in abdomen, better bending double and passing stools**
- Pain over McBurney's point and at the location of sigmoid flexure. Full of gas – extremely flatulent.
- Dry, spasmodic cough; persistent with tickling in the suprasternal fossa
- Irritation of kidney with brick red sediment, albuminuria and hyaline casts. Nephritis with rheumatic symptoms
- Haemorrhages from uterus. Retained placenta. Delayed and irregular menses with backache.
- Rheumatoid arthritis, osteoarthritis, spondylosis, cracking in shoulder
- Arms feel heavy. Legs, arms and neck feel hard and brittle
- Lumbosacral backache, relieved by continuous motion
- Dermatitis of finger. Trophic changes in finger nails
- Itching all over with burning as if on fire. Necrosis and ulceration

CLINICAL

- Cancer
- Vertigo
- Trigeminal neuralgia
- Nausea
- Appendicitis
- Diarrhoea
- Constipation
- Piles
- Pruritus ani
- Hypotension
- Nephritis
- Enuresis
- Albuminuria
- Dysmenorrhoea
- Pruritus vulvae
- Arthritis
- Rheumatism
- Cervical spondylosis
- Lumbago
- Gout
- Fever
- Itching
- Rodent ulcer
- Ulcers
- Burns
- Radiation burns
- Necrosis
- Epithelioma
- Moles
- Naevi
- Dermatitis
- Acne rosacea
- Pimples

MODALITIES

- **Aggravation:** On getting up, warmth of bed, smoking
- **Amelioration:** Open air, continuous motion, hot bath, lying down, pressure

REMEDY RELATIONSHIP

- **Compare:** Anac., X-ray, Rhus-t., Sep., Uran-n., Ars., Puls., Caust.
- **Antidotes:** Rhus-v., Tell.

RANUNCULUS BULBOSUS

INTRODUCTION

- **Common name:** Buttercup
- **Family:** *Ranunculaceae*
- **Source:** Vegetable kingdom
- **Part used:** Whole plant
- **Prover:** Franz

SPHERE OF ACTION

- Mind
- Gastrointestinal system
- Respiratory system
- Heart
- Musculoskeletal system
- Urinary system
- Skin

CONSTITUTION

- For bad effects of alcoholic beverages, especially mental effects
- Vesicular eruptions, on the face in clusters with bright red cheeks
- **Temperament:** Nervous
- **Thermal:** Chilly
- **Miasm:** Psora, Syphilis

MIND

- Fear of ghosts in the evening; does not want to be alone
- Hasty, irritable and quarrelsome, especially in the morning
- Oppression with weeping
- Loss of ideas; vanishing of thoughts on reflection
- Obtuseness of intellect
- Bad mental effects of alcohol; delirium tremens
- Depression of spirits with a desire to die

KEYNOTE SYMPTOMS

- For all bad effects of alcohol like hiccup, delirium tremens, epilepsy, weakness, fainting, etc.
- Pains – lancinating, sticking, jerking, out pressing, stitching, as if bruised with external sensitivity
- Sensitiveness to touch, sore bruised sensation. Soreness of affected parts
- Pains appear in paroxysms, excited or precipitated by atmospheric changes, inflammatory, neuralgic or myalgic
- Smarting in eyes, nose and fauces. **Eyes smart as if from smoke**
- Painful indigestion; accumulation of saliva in the mouth; hot, putrid eructations with pressure on sternum and laboured breathing. Burning at cardiac end of stomach
- **Removes bad effects of alcoholic drinks**
- Frequent expulsion of very foetid flatus
- Chilliness in chest when walking in open air; stitches in chest
- Intercostal neuralgia; intercostal rheumatism worse inspiration, motion or lying on the painful side; as if sternum, ribs and intercostal spaces are bruised
- Muscular pain along margins of shoulder blades in women with small burning spots from sedentary employment
- Burning and severe itching; herpetic eruptions. Itching in palms; blister-like eruptions on palms
- **Herpes – blue vesicles and horny scabs with intolerable burning, itching; especially on chest and back**

CLINICAL

- Alcoholism
- Delirium tremens
- Pains
- Neuralgia
- Photophobia
- Day blindness
- Glaucoma
- Indigestion
- Hiccough
- Gastritis
- Hay fever
- Bronchitis
- Pneumonia
- Pleurodynia
- Pleurisy
- Pleuritic
- adhesions
- Intercostal pain
- Ovarian neuralgia
- Arthritis
- Rheumatism
- Sciatica
- Lumbago
- Fibrositis
- Callosities
- Herpes zoster
- Chilblains
- Blisters
- Corns
- Vesicular eruptions
- Eczema

MODALITIES

- **Aggravation:** Contact, motion, atmospheric changes, especially, wet stormy weather, open air, cold air brings on all sorts of ailments
- **Amelioration:** Standing, sitting bent forward

REMEDY RELATIONSHIP

- **Compare:** Ran-a., Ran-fl., Ran-g., Ran-r., Bry., Crot-t., Mez., Euph., Acon., Arn., Clem.
- **Incompatible:** Sulph., Staph.
- **Antidotes:** Bry., Camph., Rhus-t.

RAPHANUS SATIVUS

INTRODUCTION
- **Common name:** Black garden radish
- **Family:** *Cruciferae*
- **Source:** Vegetable kingdom
- **Part used:** Fresh root
- **Prover:** Nusser

SPHERE OF ACTION
- Head
- Eyes
- Throat
- Gastrointestinal system
- Respiratory system
- Female genital system
- Skin

CONSTITUTION
- Suits hysterical, mental and nervous system
- Seborrhoea with greasy skin and distended abdomen; oedema of lower eyelids
- **Temperament:** Hysterical
- **Thermal:** Ambithermal
- **Miasm:** Sycosis

MIND
- Nymphomania
- Great dislike for her own sex
- Sadness alternating with hopefulness
- Aversion to children, especially girls
- Mental and physical fatigue
- Irritable
- Neglected feeling
- Sense of intoxication on getting up in the morning, excitement of brain
- Melancholic, fearful
- Want of spirit
- Marked anguish with fear of death; patient wants religious consolation
- Forgetful during menses

KEYNOTE SYMPTOMS
- Headache; brain feels tender and sore. Oedema of lower eyelids
- **Teeth feel as if made of papermache**
- Sensation as if a hot foreign body like a ball going up from the uterus to the throat. Burning in the epigastrium followed by hot, putrid eructations and headaches; sensation as if a number of balls rising from the abdomen to the throat
- **Appetite without hunger at 4 am, in bed. Constant violent thirst; drinks more than micturates**
- One of the most flatulent remedies. Great accumulation and incarceration of flatus – almost stops breathing. Hard abdomen, no flatus emitted upwards or downwards.
- Increases biliary and salivary secretion, with pain and stitches in the liver and spleen regions
- Intestines prominent; pad-like swelling of intestines. Diarrhoea; stools liquid, frothy, profuse, brown and accompanied with colic
- Post-operative gas pains
- **Urine turbid with yeast-like sediment, produces thick urine like milk**
- Menses profuse and long lasting
- Nervous irritation of genitals, titilation of parts
- Numbness, heaviness and paralytic pain in hands, soles, buttocks; numbness in parts near painful bones. Sensation of swelling of bones

CLINICAL
- Hysteria
- Headache
- Toothache of pregnancy
- Nausea
- Vomiting
- Globus hystericus
- Flatulence
- Flatulent colic
- Incarcerated flatus
- Diarrhoea
- Constipation
- Laryngitis
- Pharyngitis
- Sexual insomnia
- Nymphomania
- Seborrhoea
- Pemphigus

MODALITIES
- **Aggravation:** At night, in morning on waking, eating, drinking, jar, touch
- **Amelioration:** Walking in open air

REMEDY RELATIONSHIP
- **Compare:** Mom-b., (worse, near splenic flexure); Carb-v., Anac., Arg-n., Brassi.
- **Follows well:** Lyc., Coch., Cheir., Brass., Thlasp.

RATANHIA PERUVIANA

INTRODUCTION

- **Common name:** Krameria mapato, Rhatany root
- **Family:** *Leguminosae*
- **Source:** Vegetable kingdom
- **Part used:** Root
- **Prover:** Hartlaub and Trinks

SPHERE OF ACTION

- Teeth
- Nipples of breast
- Respiratory system
- Heart
- Female genital system
- Rectum

CONSTITUTION

- Suits thin, emaciated, greatly anxious people with sunken eyes. Passive, delicate haemorrhages make patient pale and exhausted
- For nervous women to prevent miscarriage
- **Temperament:** Nervous, bilious
- **Thermal:** Chilly
- **Miasm:** Psora, Sycosis, Syphilis

MIND

- Anxious
- Athenic
- Irritable
- Efficiency to perform work
- Restless, quarrelsome
- Peevish
- Exhausted due to haemorrhages of the passive type
- Tired, overworked, prostrated
- Restless due to bowel complaints
- Apprehensive depression when alone, wants company

KEYNOTE SYMPTOMS

- Bursting in head after stools
- **Twitching in upper eyelids; eyes feel constricted, as if compressed by a vice**
- White spots before eyes, obstructing sight
- **Terrible toothache in early months of pregnancy; teeth feel elongated, especially after lying down**
- Molars feel elongated, sensation as if
- Violent hiccough causing pain in stomach, after dinner
- **Burning sensation on the tip of the tongue**
- Stool has to be forced out with a great effort
- Hard, dry stools with much straining. Haemorrhoids protrude during stool followed by long lasting aching and burning in the anus. Excruciating pains after stools
- Fissures of anus with great constriction, burning like fire, temporarily relieved by cold water. Sensitiveness of rectum
- **Sensation as if a splinter of glass were sticking in the anus and rectum, burning for hours after stool; relieved by hot water application**
- Pinworms, itching of anus
- Fissures of nipples in nursing women

CLINICAL

- Pterygium
- Hiccough
- Flatulence
- Colic
- Diarrhoea
- Constipation
- Fistula-in-ano
- Anal fissures
- Haemorrhoids
- Pinworms
- Rectal neuralgia
- Cracked nipples
- Arthritis
- Housemaid's knee
- Backache

MODALITIES

- **Aggravation:** Anxiety, exertion, touch, eating, at night
- **Amelioration:** Hot water application, walking in open air, emission of flatus

REMEDY RELATIONSHIP

- **Compare:** Canth., Carb-ac., Iris, Sulph., Thuj., Paeon., Crot-t., Sang-n., Dol., Slag.
- **Analogue:** Lyc.

RHAMNUS CALIFORNICA

SPHERE OF ACTION
- Head
- Eyes
- Heart
- Gastrointestinal system
- Genitourinary system

INTRODUCTION
- **Common name:** California coffee tree
- **Family:** *Rhamnaceae*
- **Source:** Vegetable kingdom
- **Part used:** Bark collected in spring and kept for atleast one year before using

CONSTITUTION
- For a flushed, hot, glowing face, in mentally dull and dazed individuals
- **Temperament:** Nervous, haemorrhagic
- **Thermal:** Chilly
- **Miasm:** Psora, Syphilis

MIND
- Nervous
- Restless and irritable
- Concentration is difficult, especially for studies
- Dull and dazed
- Aversion to work
- Lassitude
- Melancholic
- Anxiety

KEYNOTE SYMPTOMS
- **Muscular pains and soreness**
- Soreness of parts – head, throat, chest, extremities. Tenderness in right intercostal muscle
- Soreness, especially in occiput and vertex, worse bending
- Deep **right sided headache.** Bursting feeling in head with every step. Dizzy feeling. Twitching of eyelids.
- Constipation, tenesmus and dry stool. Flatulent diarrhoea.
- Dullness of hearing. Soreness deep of the ear, while swallowing
- Variation of pulse, slow pulse
- Increased urination. Tickling in anterior urethra. Small morning drop.
- Sexual desire increased
- Unable to control muscular action. **Legs sore, walks like a drunken man**
- Inflammatory rheumatism; joints are swollen and painful

CLINICAL
- Headache
- Gastralgia
- Constipation
- Deafness
- Pleurodynia
- Rheumatic heart
- Tachycardia
- Cystitis
- Increased micturition
- Increased sexual desire
- Gonorrhoea
- Dysmenorrhoea
- Arthritis
- Rheumatism
- Backache
- Lumbago

MODALITIES
- **Aggravation:** In the evening

REMEDY RELATIONSHIP
- **Compare:** Rham-cath. or Rham-f. (a rheumatic remedy); Cas-s.

RHEUM PALMATUM

SPHERE OF ACTION
- Mind
- Hair
- Teeth
- Mucous membranes
- Gastrointestinal system
- Respiratory system
- Skin

INTRODUCTION
- **Common name:** Rhubarb
- **Family:** *Polygonaceae*
- **Source:** Vegetable kingdom
- **Part used:** Rhizome
- **Prover:** Hahnemann

CONSTITUTION
- For children, especially during dentition.
- For impatient children with cold sweat on the face; smell sour, even after bathing
- For pregnant and nursing women. For urinary complaints after an abortion
- **Temperament:** Anxious, nervous
- **Thermal:** Chilly
- **Miasm:** Psora

MIND
- Children cry, scream and toss about all night, impatient; desires many things, cry, dislike even favourite things
- Restlessness
- Irritability
- Nocturnal sleeplessness
- Finds temporary satisfaction after their whims are gratified. Impossible to satisfy
- Ugly, unpleasant
- Obstinate, forgetful

KEYNOTE SYMPTOMS
- **Sourness of all discharges;** breath smells sour, stools are sour, whole body smells sour. No amount of washing will remove the sourness
- **Sweat on scalp, constant and profuse, asleep or awake,** hair always wet. **Cold sweat on face, especially around the mouth and nose**
- Twitching of eyelids and corner of mouth giving the appearance of frowning
- Dentitional disorders including – wind colic; sour smell of body which remains even after washing. Children during dentitional diarrhoea; child irritable, restless; cries and tosses about whole night. Halitosis.
- Desires many kinds of food but cannot eat them; becomes repugnant
- Sour, flat, slimy taste. **Food tastes bitter. Profuse and offensive saliva.**
- **Stools – pappy, slimy, whitish, turn green on the diaper, sour, with shivering and colic which is severe – must bend double, worst just before stool.** Colicky, even ineffectual urging to evacuate, altered faecal stool. Diarrhoea with colic.
- Weak bladder – urine cannot be discharged without an effort

CLINICAL
- Blepharitis
- Dentitional disorders
- Twitching of lips
- Halitosis
- Wind colic
- Diarrhoea
- Constipation
- Cough
- Asthma
- Distension of bladder

REMEDY RELATIONSHIP
- **Compare:** Mag-p., Hep., Podo., Cham., Ip., Coloc., Mag-c., Staph., Sulph.
- **Antidotes:** Camph., Cham.
- **Complementary:** Mag-c. when milk disagrees and child has a sour odor. May be given after abuse of Magnesia, with or without rhubarb, if stools are sour

MODALITIES
- **Aggravation:** Uncovering, after eating, moving about, nursing a child
- **Amelioration:** Warmth, wrapping up, lying bent

RHODODENDRON CHRYSANTHUM

INTRODUCTION

- **Common name:** Snow-rose, Golden flowered rhododendron
- **Family:** *Ericaceae*
- **Source:** Vegetable kingdom
- **Part used:** Flower buds (when well developed but not opened) and leaves
- **Prover:** Seidel

SPHERE OF ACTION

- Mind
- Ears
- Eyes
- Gastrointestinal system
- Respiratory system
- Musculoskeletal system
- Male genital system

MIND

- Confused and stupid. Confusion in the morning and after coition
- Forgets what he is talking about; leaves out whole words while writing
- Fear of thunder in nervous persons
- Dread of storms
- Aversion to business
- Easily affected by wines
- Delirium – staggers; falls asleep on knees
- Starts and appears terrified in sleep but wakes up cheerful
- Mental derangement
- Excessive indifference, with dread of all kinds of labour
- Frightful visions. Morose humour
- Brain, as if in a fog

MODALITIES

- **Aggravation:** Stormy, windy weather, electrical changes in the atmosphere, on approach of thunderstorm, at night, towards morning.
- **Amelioration:** From wrapping the head warmly, dry heat, exercise after the storm breaks, eating.

KEYNOTE SYMPTOMS

- **Nervous people who dread a storm and are particularly afraid of thunder; better warmth, wrapping the head**
- Ciliary neuralgia, darting like arrows through the eyes. Sensation of dryness and burning in the eyes. Contraction of one pupil while the other is dilated.
- **Swollen gums, toothache in damp weather and before a storm. Stumps of teeth loosened**
- Difficulty in hearing with whizzing and ringing in ears. Hearing better in the morning
- Violent pleuritic pains causing breathlessness and speechlessness
- Hydrocoele in boys from birth
- Orchitis, sensation in glands as if they were being crushed
- Testicles, especially left, swollen, painful, drawn up. Induration and swelling of testes after gonorrhoea
- Stiffness in the neck. **Pains in the bones in spots, reappearing with change of weather**
- Pain in the shoulders, arms and wrists
- Gouty inflammation of great toe. Rheumatic drawing, tearing pains in limbs, worse rest and stormy weather. Joints swollen.
- Cannot get sleep or remain asleep unless legs are crossed at the ankles

CONSTITUTION

- Tendency to faint in young girls of phthisical tendency who grow too rapidly and are upset by thunderstorms
- Gouty and rheumatic subjects, who are worse before a storm
- **Temperament:** Nervous
- **Thermal:** Chilly
- **Miasm:** Psora, Syphilis

CLINICAL

- Neuralgia
- Cramps
- Headache
- Ciliary neuralgia
- Prosopalgia
- Toothache
- Tinnitus
- Pleuritic pains
- Renal dropsy
- Gonorrhoea
- Hydrocoele
- Epididymitis
- Orchitis
- Arthritis
- Rheumatism
- Gout
- Bursitis
- Injury to tendons

REMEDY RELATIONSHIP

- **Compare:** Ampe-qu. (hydrocoele and renal dropsy); Dulc., Rhus-t., Nat-s., Bry., Con., Calc., Led., Lyc. and Sep.

RHUS GLABRA

INTRODUCTION

- **Common name:** Smooth upland sumach
- **Family:** *Anacardiaceae*
- **Source:** Vegetable kingdom
- **Part used:** Leaves and bark
- **Prover:** A.V. Marshall

SPHERE OF ACTION

- Mind
- Hair
- Teeth
- Mucous membranes
- Gastrointestinal system
- Respiratory system
- Skin

MIND

- Distaste for society
- Dull; forgetful
- Indifferent to surrounding objects
- Delusion that he is incorporeal; delusions of floating in air
- Dreams of flying
- Irritability
- Anxiety, weakness
- Gloomy, tired
- Stupid

MODALITIES

- **Aggravation:** After sleep
- **Amelioration:** Movement

KEYNOTE SYMPTOMS

- Exhaustion and painful fatigue
- Great debility. Profuse perspiration arising from debility
- Tendency to ulceration and putrefaction
- **Dull, heavy headache on walking, ameliorated by exercise**
- Dull, heavy pain in front and top of the head
- **Tongue is furred white**
- Soft, spongy gums; bleeding from the mouth
- Several, small, sensitive ulcers on the oral mucous membrane, opposite the bicuspids
- Disinfects bowels so that the flatus and stools are free from odour

CONSTITUTION

- Suits pale, nervous, anaemic patients who are excessively weak
- **Temperament:** Nervous
- **Thermal:** Chilly
- **Miasm:** Psora, Syphilis

CLINICAL

- Fatigue
- Exhaustion
- Prostration
- Weakness
- Headache
- Stomatitis
- Glossitis
- Gingivitis
- Scurvy
- Flatulence
- Gastritis
- Diarrhoea
- Constipation
- Pharyngitis

REMEDY RELATIONSHIP

- Said to be antidotal to the action of Mercury and has been employed in the treatment of secondary syphilis after mercurialization
- **Compare:** Rhus-t., Anac.

RHUS TOXICODENDRON

INTRODUCTION

Common name: Poison ivy, Poison ash
Family: *Anacardiaceae*
Source: Vegetable kingdom
Part used: Leaf
Prover: Hahnemann

SPHERE OF ACTION

- Mind
- Eyes
- Mucous membranes
- Gastrointestinal system
- Respiratory system
- Heart
- Musculoskeletal system
- Urinary system
- Skin

CONSTITUTION

- Suits patients with a rheumatic diathesis, who are very listless because of the pains which are better by moving about
- **Temperament:** Nervous, bilious
- **Thermal:** Chilly
- **Miasm:** Psora, Sycosis, Syphilis

MIND

- Extreme restlessness, with a desire for continuous change in position
- Impatient and hurried
- Delirium with fear and suspicion of being poisoned
- Dreams of exertion
- Sad, patient begins to weep without knowing why, worse in the evening
- Anxiety, sadness, helplessness and profound despondency
- Anxiety for own children
- Causeless weeping. Irritability
- Answers correctly, but slowly, or hastily, or reluctantly
- Great apprehension; listless
- Sensorium cloudy

KEYNOTE SYMPTOMS

- **One of the trios of restlessness, cannot stay in one place**
- Sensitive to open air–exposing the hand from under the bed cover produces cough
- **Ailments from getting wet, especially after being over heated**
- Ailments from spraining or straining a muscle, tendon or part
- Swollen eyes, oedematous old injuries of the eyes, ulceration of cornea. Lids inflamed, agglutinated, swollen
- Jaws crack when chewing. Swollen face. Pain in maxillary joint.
- Fever blisters around the mouth and on the chin; corners of mouth ulcerated
- Headache in the occiput
- **Marked thirst, with dryness of mouth and tongue. Desires cold drinks, though it aggravates cough, chill; worse after ice cold water**
- **Dry, sore, red, cracked tongue with a red triangular tip**
- Diarrhoea in typhoid fever, worse during night, better during the day
- Tearing pains down the thighs in dysentery
- Tonsillitis, after riding in cold wind; swollen glands; stitching pain on swallowing
- Dry cough during chill stage of fever
- Prolapse of uterus from over-stretching or straining
- Swelling and intense itching of vulva
- Lochia thin, protracted, offensive, diminished with shooting pains, extending upward in the vagina
- Affects fibrous tissues, joints, tendons, sheaths, aponeurosis causing pain and stiffness
- Pain, stiffness, lameness on first moving after rest or on getting up in the morning; better by walking or continued motion; motion limbers up the patient, thus feels the need for change of position regularly
- Hot, painful swelling of joints, sensitive to touch. Tearing pains in tendons, ligaments and fasciae. Limbs stiff, paralysed, sensitive to cold air.
- Cracking in joints, especially on stretching
- Erysipelas; red, swollen, itching intensely

MODALITIES

- **The great characteristic of Rhus-t. is that with few exceptions the pains occur and are worse during repose and are ameliorated by motion**
- **Aggravation:** Before a storm, cold, wet rainy weather, night, midnight, getting wet while perspiring; rest, lying on the back or on the right side
- **Amelioration:** Warm, dry weather, wrapping up; warm or hot things, motion, change of position, moving affected parts

CLINICAL

- Cellulitis
- Septicaemia
- Paralysis
- Hemiplegia
- Neuralgia
- Beri beri
- Crusta lactea
- Orbital cellulitis
- Suppurative iritis
- Photophobia
- Parotiditis
- Influenza
- Bronchitis
- Asthma
- Angina pectoris
- Enuresis
- Menstrual disorders
- Abortion
- Menorrhagia
- Metrorrhagia
- Arthritis
- Rheumatism
- Gout
- Sciatica
- Cervical spondylosis
- Fibrositis
- Tendonitis
- Typhoid
- Eczema
- Chilblains
- Vesicles
- Erysipelas
- Herpes zoster
- Impetigo
- Urticaria

REMEDY RELATIONSHIP

- **Complementary:** Bry., Calc-f., Phyt. In urticaria follow with Bov. Bry.
- **Inimical:** Apis. must not be used before or after.
- **Antidotes:** Bathing with milk and Grin. lotion is very effective. Plb., Anac., Crot-t., Grin., Mez., Cypr., Graph.
- **Compare:** Rhus-r., Rhus-d., Arn., Bapt., Lach., Ars., Hyos., Op. Bry., Rhod., Nat-s., Sulph.
- Sepia, often quickly > itching and burning of Rhus-t., the vesicles drying up in a few days

Rhus toxicodendron

RHUS VENENATA

INTRODUCTION
- **Common name:** Poison elder
- **Family:** *Anacardiaceae*
- **Source:** Vegetable kingdom
- **Part used:** Stem and leaves
- **Prover:** Bute

SPHERE OF ACTION
- Mind
- Mucous membranes
- Gastrointestinal system
- Respiratory system
- Musculoskeletal system
- Skin

CONSTITUTION
- Adapted to a rheumatic diathesis; affected part becomes red
- Patient has a swollen face, especially under the right eye
- **Temperament:** Nervous
- **Thermal:** Chilly
- **Miasm:** Psora, Syphilis

MIND
- Great sadness, no desire to live, loathing of life
- Everything seems gloomy, sad
- Concentration difficult
- Restlessness, nervousness
- Thoughts disconnected
- Dreams of death, murder
- Thoughts of suicide
- Weeps with great despondency
- Apprehension
- Delirium ends in stupor
- Irritability, worse contradiction

KEYNOTE SYMPTOMS
- Great lassitude. Swelling of whole body with intolerable irritation. Marked restlessness.
- Sensation as if hot blood rushing along the blood vessels
- Dizzy when first getting out of bed
- Heavy frontal headache, worse stooping
- **Eyes almost closed due to swelling of lids; sensation of sand in them**
- Sensation as if tongue, was scalded; sensation extends to the mouth and throat during dinner
- **Tongue–red tip with fissure in the middle; vesicles on the under surface**
- Burning and itching in rectum; haemorrhoids; discharge of blood after stool
- Pharynx and oesophagus irritable. Swallowing painful and difficult, food seems to stop midway to stomach. Pain half way down the oesophagus.
- **Sensation of a hair in the throat way back**
- Dry, teasing, fatiguing cough, tonsils red and congested. Frequent desire to swallow but swallowing is difficult.
- Pains come and go suddenly, wander about; upward and downward along the periosteum
- Bruised feeling in all limbs; all muscles are stiff. Affects parts where bones are directly covered by skin like – forehead, knuckles, etc.
- Rheumatism before a storm
- Skin dark red; erysipelas; vesicles
- Menses with large clots and soreness of vagina

CLINICAL
- Septicaemia
- Cellulitis
- Vertigo
- Ptosis
- Corneal ulcer
- Conjunctivitis
- Nausea
- Vomiting
- Diarrhoea
- Constipation
- Bronchitis
- Pneumonia
- Asthma
- Dysuria
- Dysmenorrhoea
- Prostatitis
- Arthritis
- Rheumatism
- Typhoid fever
- Tinea cruris
- Phlegmonous erysipelas
- Urticaria
- Scab formation
- Eczema
- Injuries

MODALITIES
- **Aggravation:** Hot weather, damp days, before stools, touch, pressure, rest
- **Amelioration:** Open air, moderate exercise

REMEDY RELATIONSHIP
- **Antidote:** Clem., Rhus-d. is identical to it. It antidotes Rad-br. and follows it well.
- **Compare:** Anac.

ROBINIA PSEUDOCACIA

INTRODUCTION

- **Common name:** Yellow locust, False acacia
- **Family:** *Leguminosae*
- **Source:** Vegetable kingdom
- **Part used:** Bark of root and stem
- **Prover:** Burt

SPHERE OF ACTION

- Mind
- Nervous system
- Gastrointestinal system
- Respiratory system
- Musculoskeletal system
- Male sexual system

CONSTITUTION

- Body smells sour, with indigestion, dyspepsia. Acidity, especially at night
- **Temperament:** Nervous
- **Thermal:** Chilly
- **Miasm:** Psora, Syphilis

MIND

- Irritability due to indigestion
- Sadness, despondency, mental depression; desires death
- Fear of disgrace
- Anguish, as from tickling soles
- Anguish from pain in stomach
- Can hardly tell what she is doing
- Memory weak for what he had just thought
- Weeping, tearful mood
- Nymphomania, erotic madness
- Nervousness
- Anxiety
- Timidity
- Afraid of crowds
- Very low spirited

MODALITIES

- **Aggravation:** At night, from motion, lying down aggravates acidity
- **Amelioration:** Rest

KEYNOTE SYMPTOMS

- **Chief keynote is acidity, especially if there is nocturnal aggravation**
- Sourness of all discharges – sour eructations, vomiting, stool, sweat etc.
- Smell of the body sour, sour sweat
- Vertigo and dullness of head in whatever position it is placed
- **Sensation as if brain is revolving, worse lying on right side**
- Gastric headache with acid vomiting due to a sour stomach, from fats, meat, cabbage, turnips, gravies, flatulent foods
- Steady headache with sensation as if head is full of boiling water
- Facial neuralgia spreading to the eyes, forehead and teeth with contraction or spasmodic pain in the jaws, as if they were disarticulated
- **White coating on tongue with a red tip**
- Dyspepsia, flatulence, especially at night on lying down, patients smell sour
- Regurgitation of acid and bitter substances; everything turns to acid
- Sour eructations and profuse, intensely sour vomiting which sets the teeth on edge
- Neuralgia or severe, sharp pains in stomach associated with acidity
- **Acrid, yellowish leucorrhoea having an extremely foetid smell**

CLINICAL

- Headache
- Migraine
- Eructations
- Hyperacidity
- Reflux oesophagitis
- Heartburn
- Dyspepsia
- Gastralgia
- Gastritis
- Nausea
- Vomiting
- Flatulence
- Neuralgia of stomach
- Peptic ulcer
- Hiatus hernia
- Morning diarrhoea
- Diarrhoea
- Constipation
- Cough
- Urticaria
- Eczema
- Psoriasis
- Rash

REMEDY RELATIONSHIP

- **Compare:** Mag-p., Arg-n., Orex-tann., (hyperchlorhydria; deficient acid and slow digestion; 14 hourly doses); Cyt-l., Rheum., Calc., Aeth., Mag-c., Puls. (in acidity); Chin., Carb-v., Lyc., (in flatulence); Nux-v.

RUMEX CRISPUS

INTRODUCTION

- **Common name:** Yellow dock
- **Family:** *Polygonaceae*
- **Source:** Vegetable kingdom
- **Part used:** Rhizome
- **Prover:** Houghton

SPHERE OF ACTION

- Mind
- Mucous membrane
- Gastrointestinal system
- Respiratory system
- Heart
- Musculoskeletal system
- Urinary system
- Skin

CONSTITUTION

- For those with a nervous and tubercular diathesis; patients with extremely sensitive skin and mucous membranes
- **Temperament:** Nervous, bilious
- **Thermal:** Chilly
- **Miasm:** Psora, Sycosis, Syphilis

MIND

- Suicidal mood
- Stagnation of ideas; lassitude and uneasiness
- Restlessness in the evening. Low spirited, with a serious expression on the face
- Indifferent about his surroundings
- Disinclined to mental exertion
- Irritability
- Sadness
- Anxiety

KEYNOTE SYMPTOMS

- Extremely sensitive to cold air, even open air
- Diminishes secretions of mucous membranes while exhalting sensitivity of mucous membranes in the larynx and trachea
- Lymphatics enlarged and secretions perverted
- Sharp pains, neuralgias; pains – neither fixed nor constant
- Marked flatulence and rumbling in abdomen; annoying borborygmi
- Early morning diarrhoea with gastralgia and cough, driving the patient out of bed
- Violent sneezing; irritations and itching in nostrils extending to pharynx
- Nose dry, obstructed. Profuse mucoid discharge from nose and trachea. Thin, watery, frothy expectoration by the mouthful; later stringy and tough.
- Hoarseness, voice uncertain; worse in the evening, after exposure to cold
- **Rawness of larynx and trachea when coughing; hawks up tenacious mucous**
- Dry, hacking, teasing cough, preventing sleep; aggravated by pressure, talking, inspiring cold air, at night, uncovering
- Incessant tickling in the throat pit, extends down to the bifurcation of trachea, causes cough. Touching the throat pit brings on cough; cough as if a piece of phlegm is stuck in the chest
- **Cough causes expulsion of urine; may even cause miscarriage in women in early months of pregnancy**
- Intense itching in various parts; worse exposure to cold air and when undressing

CLINICAL

- Lymphatics enlarged
- Epithelioma of face
- Nausea
- Vomiting
- Flatulence
- Gastritis
- Jaundice
- Diarrhoea
- Constipation
- Haemorrhoids
- Fissure
- Epistaxis
- Rhinitis
- Sinusitis
- Laryngitis
- Pharyngitis
- Complete aphonia
- Lump in throat
- Cough
- Bronchitis
- Urticaria
- Eczema

MODALITIES

- **Aggravation:** Cool or cold air, lying down, in the evening, left chest; uncovering, inhaling
- **Amelioration:** Warmth, keeping mouth covered to exclude cold air, wrapping up, discharge of offensive flatus

REMEDY RELATIONSHIP

- **Compare:** Caust., Sulph., Bell., Rumx., contains chrysophanic acid to which the skin symptoms correspond. Lapa., Dros., Hyos., Phos., Sang.
- **Antidoted by:** Bell., Camph., Con., Hyos., Lach., Phos.

RUTA GRAVEOLENS

INTRODUCTION

- **Common name:** Rue bitterwort
- **Family:** *Rutaceae*
- **Source:** Vegetable kingdom
- **Part used:** Whole plant
- **Prover:** Hahnemann

SPHERE OF ACTION

- Bones
- Periosteum
- Muscles
- Nerves
- Joints
- Eyes
- Urinary bladder
- Uterus
- Skin

CONSTITUTION

- Suited to robust, sanguinous persons with tendency to haemorrhages from the nose, gums and rectum
- **Temperament:** Restless, nervous
- **Thermal:** Chilly
- **Miasm:** Psora, Sycosis

MIND

- Suspicious, imagines that he is always being deceived
- Disposition to quarrel and contradict
- Anxiety as from a troubled conscience. Anxious, irritable, rigid patients
- Melancholy and moral dejection
- Remorse
- Slowness of conception
- Mental dullness and aversion to thinking
- Confusion of mind
- Starting from sleep on slightest touch
- Delusion someone is behind him
- Irritability, worse contradiction
- Anxiety, panic and fear of death during fever

KEYNOTE SYMPTOMS

- Marked lassitude, weakness and despair, with heaviness in all limbs
- **Parts upon which patient lies are painful, as if bruised.** Sore, lame, bruised feeling all over, as from blows or falls. **Coccyx feels as if injured.**
- Tendency to formation of deposits on the periosteum, tendons, joints, especially wrists
- Physical restlessness – keeps changing position frequently. Ankles feel dislocated
- **Bad effects of mechanical injuries,** dislocations, fractures, injury or affections of periosteum causing marked soreness
- Lameness remaining after sprains
- Amblyopia, asthenopia, from over straining or over exertion of eyes. Aching in eyes with blurred vision.
- **Eyes burn, feel strained, hot from sewing or reading fine print.** Disturbances of accommodation
- Constipation; difficult stools, passed after straining. Rectal prolapse every time bowels move. Rectum protrudes on stooping.
- Pressure on neck of bladder, as if full even after urinating; constant urging to micturate. Wrists feel as if sprained
- Flat, smooth warts on palms of hands

MODALITIES

- **Aggravation:** Lying down, from cold, wet weather, eyestrain, over exertion injury, lifting
- **Amelioration:** Lying on back, warmth, rubbing, motion

CLINICAL

- Scrofulous exostosis
- Sprains
- Injuries
- Amblyopia
- Asthenopia
- Strained eyes
- Conjunctivitis
- Constipation
- Rectal prolapse
- Lower bowel cancer
- Involuntary urination
- Prolapse of uterus
- Arthritis
- Rheumatism
- Sciatica
- Backache
- Dislocation
- Fracture
- Periostitis
- Warts
- Ganglion
- Erysipelas

REMEDY RELATIONSHIP

- **Compare:** Arn., Arg-n., Con., Euphr., Phyt., Rhus-t., Symph., Rat., Card-m. (rectal irritation); Jab., Sil.
- **Follows well:** Arnica, it hastens the curative process in the joints; after Symph., in injuries of bones.
- **Antidote:** Camph.
- **Complementary:** Calc-p.

Ruta graveolens

SABADILLA

INTRODUCTION
- **Common name:** Cevadilla seeds
- **Family:** *Liliaceae*
- **Source:** Vegetable kingdom
- **Part used:** Seeds
- **Prover:** Hahnemann

SPHERE OF ACTION
- Mind
- Head
- Eyes
- Mucous membranes
- Gastrointestinal system
- Respiratory system
- Female genital system

MIND
- Hysterical paroxysms caused by fright
- Delusions as to the state of his body
- Miserable; angry; erroneous, fixed personal ideas or illusions that some horrible throat disease has come on and will be fatal
- Irritable, easily startled
- Nervous symptoms–reflex from worms, alternate nervous and physical symptoms
- Nervous twitching from worms; hysteria after fright, formications
- Anxiety
- Cannot perform mental labour without headache

MODALITIES
- **Aggravation:** Cold and cold drinks, full moon, mental exertion
- **Amelioration:** Warm food and drink, being wrapped up

KEYNOTE SYMPTOMS
- **Periodicity, almost clock-like,** making it useful in intermittent fevers and neuralgias
- Sensitive to cold air; every exposure settles in the nose and throat
- Twitching, convulsive trembling or catalepsy from worms
- Violent itching of hairy scalp, itches till it bleeds; itching in vertex, as from vermin; and anus and rectum as from ascarides
- Headache from thinking too much, after every work, eating
- Headache unilateral, on alternate sides of forehead with taenia
- Sneezing, spasmodic with watery coryza, lachrymation, redness of eyes and frontal headache
- Unilateral obstruction of nose alternately. Aversion to the smell of garlic; even to the smell of flowers
- Nose itching, tingling, very dry, must rub or pick at it
- Sore throat beginning on left side, with sensation of a lump or a foreign body in the throat, constant necessity to swallow, with a great desire for warm drinks and food which relieve; with difficulty in swallowing
- **Persistent, violent, abortive chill starting in the lower extremities, goes from below upwards, lachrymation during paroxysm of fever with absence of thirst**
- Horny, deformed, thickened nails

CONSTITUTION
- For persons with light hair, fair complexion and a relaxed, weak muscular system
- Especially suited to children disposed to worms
- **Temperament:** Nervous
- **Thermal:** Chilly
- **Miasm:** Psora, Syphilis

CLINICAL
- Allergy
- Blisters
- Headache
- Flatulence
- Diarrhoea
- Constipation
- Pin worms
- Rhinitis
- Influenza
- Hay fever
- Otitis media
- Pharyngitis
- Tonsillitis
- Diphtheria
- Pleurisy
- Asthma
- Cancer

REMEDY RELATIONSHIP
- **Compare:** Coloc., Colch., Lyc., where < is from 4 to 8 pm; Puls., Sabad. > in open air. Verin., Nux-v., Arund. and Poll., Phle., Cumin. (hay fever).
- **Follows:** Bry. and Ran-b. well in pleurisy, and has cured after Acon. and Bry. failed.
- **Complementary:** Sep.
- **Antidotes:** Puls., Lyc., Con., Lach.

SABAL SERRULATA

INTRODUCTION

- **Common name:** Saw palmetto
- **Family:** *Palmaceae*
- **Source:** Vegetable kingdom
- **Part used:** Ripe fruit

SPHERE OF ACTION

- Mind
- Gastrointestinal system
- Respiratory system
- Genitourinary system

CONSTITUTION

- For pale, irritable, confused patients with apathy and indifference
- **Temperament:** Nervous
- **Thermal:** Chilly
- **Miasm:** Psora, Syphilis

MIND

- Languor, apathy, indifference
- Fear of going to sleep, starts up with fear as patient dozes off
- Anger, worse sympathy
- Restlessness
- Suspicious
- Foresaken feeling
- Neglected feeling
- Gloomy
- Anxiety
- Confused, dull
- Sad and melancholic before menses
- Broods over her symptoms

MODALITIES

- **Aggravation:** Cold damp cloudy weather, early morning, sympathy, before menses
- **Amelioration:** From milk, after sleep

KEYNOTE SYMPTOMS

- General and sexual debility. Promotes nutrition and tissue building
- Fear of going to sleep. Vertigo with headache
- Belching and acidity. Desire for milk
- Copious expectoration with catarrh of the nose
- Irritability of genitourinary organs. Organs feel relaxed and cold
- **Homoeopathic catheter, cystitis with prostatic troubles**
- Ovaries tender, enlarged; suppressed and perverted sexual inclination
- Small, underdeveloped mammae; breasts shrivel
- Prostatic trouble like prostatic enlargement, epididymitis, **difficulties in passing urine and discharge of prostatic fluid**
- Wasting of testes in men and loss of sexual power
- Prostatic enlargement and irritation of neck of bladder. Enuresis due to paralysis of sphincter vesicae

CLINICAL

- Neuralgia
- Migraine
- Iritis
- Toothache
- Rhinitis
- Sinusitis
- Otitis media
- Chronic bronchitis
- Pericarditis
- Rheumatic heart disease
- Valvular disorders
- Sexual weakness
- Pains of cancer of urinary tract
- Enuresis
- Cystitis
- Undeveloped mammae
- Ovaries enlarged
- Chronic gonorrhoea
- Benign enlargement of prostate
- Prostatic hypertrophy
- Epididymitis

REMEDY RELATIONSHIP

- **Compare:** Ph-ac., Stigm., Santal., Apis. In prostatic symptoms: Ferr-pic., Thuj., Pic-ac. (more sexual erethism); Pop. (prostatic enlargement with cystitis)

SABINA

INTRODUCTION
- **Common name:** Savine
- **Family:** *Juniperaceae*
- **Source:** Vegetable kingdom
- **Part used:** Leaf and stem
- **Prover:** Hahnemann

SPHERE OF ACTION
- Head
- Serous membranes
- Fibrous membranes
- Gastrointestinal system
- Respiratory system
- Female genital system

MIND
- Music is unbearable; it produces nervousness; goes through the bone and marrow
- Restlessness, nervousness and hysteria
- Melancholy, does not like making a conversation
- Sadness, dejection, discouraged
- Anxiety with fear and apprehension
- Gloomy, morose, listless
- Weakness of memory
- Weeps aloud
- Hypochondriacal

MODALITIES
- **Aggravation:** From least motion, warm air or room, heat.
- **Amelioration:** Cool open fresh air.

KEYNOTE SYMPTOMS
- Violent pulsations, wants windows open
- Vertigo with suppressed menses. Headache bursting, appears suddenly, diminishes slowly
- **Desires lemonade;** tympanitic destention of abdomen
- **Drawing pains in small of back from sacrum to pubis** in nearly all diseases. Labour-like pains
- Pain from sacrum to pubis, from below upwards, shooting up the vagina
- Haemorrhage from the uterus, flow partly red, partly clotted; worse least motion, better by walking
- Menorrhagia in women who abort readily. Inflammation of uterus and ovaries after abortion
- Menses – profuse, bright, early, discharge of blood between periods with sexual excitement
- **Profuse, milky, starchy, ropy leucorrhoea**
- **Promotes expulsion of moles or foreign bodies from the uterus**
- Retained placenta from atony of uterus; intense after pains
- Persons with arthritic pain. Rheumatic affections of the heel

CONSTITUTION
- For women who menstruate very early in life, chlorotic women having tendency to miscarriage; particularly in the third month
- Gouty or rheumatic diathesis
- **Temperament:** Nervous
- **Thermal:** Chilly
- **Miasm:** Psora, Syphilis

CLINICAL
- Granulation
- Diarrhoea
- Constipation
- Epistaxis
- Cystitis
- Nymphomania
- Gonorrhoea
- Abortion
- Retained placenta
- Uterine haemorrhages
- Premature labour
- Metrorrhagia
- Dysmenorrhoea
- Menorrhagia
- Leucorrhoea
- Arthritis
- Rheumatism
- Gout
- Adenomyosis
- Condylomata
- Warts
- Figwarts

REMEDY RELATIONSHIP
- **Complementary:** Thuj.
- **Compare:** Sang., Rosm., Croc., Calc., Tril-p., Ip., Mill., Erig., Sec.
- **Antidote:** Puls.
- **Follows:** Thuj. in condyloma and sycotic affections.

SALIX NIGRA

INTRODUCTION
- **Common name:** Black willow
- **Family:** *Salicaceae*
- **Source:** Vegetable kingdom
- **Part used:** Bark
- **Prover:** Wright

SPHERE OF ACTION
- Gastrointestinal system
- Respiratory system
- Male genital system
- Female genital system
- Musculoskeletal system

CONSTITUTION
- Suits those with a red, swollen face; hysteria and nervousness; affects the sexual organs
- **Temperament:** Nervous, haemorrhagic
- **Thermal:** Chilly
- **Miasm:** Psora, Syphilis

MIND
- Hysteria and nervousness
- Restlessness and nervousness before menses
- Sexual thoughts, lascivious dreams
- Lasciviousness, lustfulness
- Erotic insanity
- Nymphomania
- Anxiety
- Melancholy

KEYNOTE SYMPTOMS
- Congestion, redness, especially of face, nose; eyes blood-shot
- **Painful roots of hair**
- Tired sleepy state. Disposition to lie down and sleep
- Haemorrhages from nose, uterine fibroids
- Nervousness and restlessness before and during menses
- Ovarian congestion, neuralgia
- Moderates sexual passion, sexual dreams
- Seminal emissions in presence of women, or while talking to them
- Painful movement of the testicles
- Soreness of muscles
- **Coldness of hands and feet, even in summers**
- Pain across sacral region

CLINICAL
- Hysteria
- Nervousness
- Alopecia
- Diarrhoea
- Constipation
- Epistaxis
- Nymphomania
- Menorrhagia
- Ovarian neuralgia
- Acute gonorrhoea
- Orchitis
- Masturbation
- Spermatorrhoea
- Arthritis
- Rheumatism
- Backache

MODALITIES
- **Aggravation:** Mental stress, before and during menses, touch
- **Amelioration:** Rest

REMEDY RELATIONSHIP
- **Compare:** Yohim., Canth., Con., Agn., Pic-ac., Dam., Aven., Sabal.

SAMBUCUS NIGRA

SPHERE OF ACTION
- Mucous membranes
- Gastrointestinal system
- Respiratory system
- Genitourinary system

INTRODUCTION
- **Common name:** Elder
- **Family:** *Caprifoliaceae*
- **Source:** Vegetable kingdom
- **Part used:** Leaves and flowers
- **Prover:** Hahnemann

CONSTITUTION
- Suits scrofulous, robust people who have suddenly become emaciated; also cyanosis of face and red burning spots on cheeks
- For scrofulous children with a tendency for respiratory diseases
- **Temperament:** Nervous, bilious
- **Thermal:** Chilly
- **Miasm:** Psora, Sycosis, Syphilis

MIND
- Changeable, variable mood. Restless, nervous, fretful and ill-humoured during sweat stage
- Easily startles from sleep. Delusions of ghosts, phantoms, frightful images on closing eyes
- Easily frightened – fear of impending danger, of suffocation, at night after waking

KEYNOTE SYMPTOMS
- Colic with nausea and flalutence
- Spasmodic affections of the larynx, chest and nasal passages
- Obstructions and snuffles of infants or new borns with dry coryza preventing breathing and nursing
- **Child awakens suddenly, nearly suffocated, blue in face, must sit up; gasps for breath, then goes to sleep and the attack repeats again**
- Sudden suffocation or strangling cough waking patient after mid-night, with violent sweat
- Attacks of suffocation as in the last stage, as if he would die
- **Inspiration normal but expiration difficult during dyspnoea**
- Dry, deep cough preceeds paroxysm of fever
- Acute nephritis with dropsy and vomiting
- Oedema, dropsical swellings of various parts of the body especially legs, instep and feet
- Skin bloated, swollen; general dropsy. Heat and perspiration on face
- Sweats or gets short of breath with many symptom
- Dry heat during sleep; marked perspiration during the day or upon waking. Dreads uncovering

CLINICAL
- Dropsy
- Oedema
- Cyanosis
- Flatulence
- Rhinitis
- Snuffles
- Laryngitis
- Spasm of glottis
- Laryngospasm
- Croup
- Pertussis
- Bronchitis
- Asthma
- Dyspnoea
- Nephritis
- Arthritis
- Rheumatism
- Eczema
- Fever paroxysm

MODALITIES
- **Aggravation:** During rest, sleep, after eating fruit
- **Amelioration:** Sitting up in bed, motion, most of the pain occurs during rest and disappears during motion

REMEDY RELATIONSHIP
- **Compare:** Chin., Chlor., Ip., Meph., Sulph, Op. and Samb-c.
- **Follows well:** After Op. in bad effects of fright.
- **Antidotes:** Ars., Camph., relieves ailments from abuse of Ars.

SANGUINARIA CANADENSIS

SPHERE OF ACTION

- Mind
- Mucous membranes
- Gastrointestinal system
- Respiratory system
- Female genital system

INTRODUCTION

- **Common name:** Blood root
- **Family:** *Papaveraceae*
- **Source:** Vegetable kingdom
- **Part used:** Rhizome
- **Prover:** Bute and Dovoney

CONSTITUTION

- For affections of mucous membranes especially that of respiratory tract; vasomotor disturbances causing congestion, circumscribed redness of cheeks, burning in palms and soles, flushes of heat, etc.
- **Temperament:** Nervous, haemorrhagic
- **Thermal:** Chilly
- **Miasm:** Psora, Syphilis

MIND

- Great torpidity and aversion to mental work in wet weather
- Irritability, worse contradiction
- Feeling of helplessness because of a sensation of being paralysed
- Confusion of mind
- Melancholy, sadness
- Delusion that she is in a car or a train and begs others to hold her
- Anxiety, wants to be held
- Day dreaming, she lies with her eyes wide open, one thought chasing another
- Painfully sensitive to noise with irritability

KEYNOTE SYMPTOMS

- Burning in various parts like, eyes, chest, throat, nose, palms and soles
- Gastric origin of headaches; symptoms ascend from stomach to head, ending in bilious vomiting. **Periodical sick headache; pain begins in occiput, spreads upwards and settles over eyes, especially right eye; sensation as if head would burst; relieved by sleep**
- Cancer of rectum
- Rush of blood to head and chest with circumscribed redness of cheeks in the afternoon with respiratory complaints
- Oedema of larynx, trachea sore
- **Cough dry, relieved by passing flatus.** Spasmodic cough after influenza and whooping cough; returns with every fresh cold
- Haemoptysis from suppressed menses. Severe dyspnoea and constriction of the chest
- Asthma with stomach disorders
- **Diarrhoea appears as coryza improves**
- Valvular disease with lung disease
- Menses offensive, profuse. Soreness of breasts. Climacteric disorders like hot flushes
- **Rheumatism of the right shoulder, left hip joint and nape of neck.** Burning in the soles and palms
- Pain in places least covered by flesh like tibia, knuckles, etc.
- Feet hot, at night puts them out of bed. Burning and ebullitions

CLINICAL

- Neuralgia
- Headache
- Migraine
- Nausea
- Diarrhoea
- Constipation
- Tinnitus
- Ozaena
- Rhinitis
- Influenza
- Hay fever
- Nasal polypi
- Laryngitis
- Pharyngitis
- Tonsillitis
- Aphonia
- Tuberculosis
- Asthma
- Dyspnoea
- Hydrothorax
- Valvular disease
- Climacteric disorders
- Galactorrhoea
- Rheumatism

MODALITIES

- **Aggravation:** Sweets, right side, motion, touch
- **Amelioration:** Acids, sleep, darkness

REMEDY RELATIONSHIP

- **Complementary:** Ant-t.
- **Compare:** Just., Dig., Bell., Iris, Meli., Lach., Ferr., Op., Sulph., in climacteric affections; Chel., Phos., Sulph., Verat-v., in chronic bronchitis or latent pneumonia
- **After:** Bell. fails in scarlatina
- As a dynamic remedy for the narcosis of Op.

SANICULA AQUA

INTRODUCTION
- **Common name:** Sanicula springs, Mineral spring water
- **Group:** Water
- **Source:** Mineral kingdom
- **Prover:** O.G. Gundlach

SPHERE OF ACTION
- Tongue
- Gastrointestinal system
- Respiratory system
- Genitourinary system

CONSTITUTION
- Suits emaciated people where skin hangs in folds
- For a debilitated constitutions who are ill-nourished and weak, with constant changes in symptoms
- **Temperament:** Nervous, bilious
- **Thermal:** Hot
- **Miasm:** Psora, Sycosis

MIND
- Headstrong, obstinate, touchy, children
- Irritable, least word offends, misconstrues everything
- Aversion to touch
- Restlessness to move from place to place
- Desire to travel. Forgetful
- Constantly changing. Cross, irritable, then quickly laughs; crossness alternates with play-fulness
- Constantly changing occupation
- Dread of darkness, dread of downward motion, constant irresistable desire to look behind
- Throws herself backward from anger

KEYNOTE SYMPTOMS
- Marasmus; progressive emaciation. Child looks old, dirty, greasy and brownish; skin around neck wrinkled and hangs in folds
- Child kicks off clothing even in coldest weather
- Head and neck sweats profusely during sleep, wetting the pillow
- **Tongue burns, must protrude it; ringworm of tongue**
- **The odour of stool is of rotten cheese which follows despite bathing**
- **Constipation – no desire for stool** till a large accumulation takes place. After marked straining, **stools partially expelled receds. Large evacuation of small, dry, grey balls which have to be removed mechanically.**
- **Diarrhoea is changeable in character and colour; like scrambled eggs, scum of frog pond, frothy**
- **Stool square, as if carved with a knife**
- Incontinence of urine and faeces – sphincter unreliable
- Vaginal discharge or leucorrhoea has smell of fish brine
- Great weakness and bearing down sensation, as if pelvic contents would escape, desire to support parts by placing hand, with leucorrhoea
- Excoriation of skin around genitals, anus and perineum
- Backache – stubborn and touchy; sensation as if back is in two pieces
- Offensive foot sweat between toes making them sore
- Fever, but no thirst

CLINICAL
- Carsickness
- Seasickness
- Scaly dandruff
- Nausea
- Vomiting
- Flatulence
- Distention
- Diarrhoea
- Constipation
- Fissure-in-anus
- Enuresis
- Leucorrhoea
- Dysmenorrhoea
- Uterine prolapse
- Rickets
- Eczema
- Boils
- Foot sweat

MODALITIES
- **Aggravation:** Moving arms backward, jar, motion, strain
- **Amelioration:** Warmth, vomiting, open air

REMEDY RELATIONSHIP
- **Compare:** Abrot., Alum., Calc., Sil., Sulph., Sanicula aqua must not be confounded with the Sanicle, also called Sanic. This is used in various nervous affections, resembling Valer.
- **Related to:** Abrot., Alum., Borx., Calc., Graph., Nat-m., Sil., and others of our great antipsorics.

SPHERE OF ACTION

- Mucous membranes
- Gastrointestinal system
- Respiratory system
- Musculoskeletal system
- Sexual system

MIND

- Anxiety from exertion
- Irritability at trifles
- Discouraged
- Sadness
- Melancholy
- Restlessness
- Gloomy

MODALITIES

- **Aggravation:** Night, motion
- **Amelioration:** Open air

INTRODUCTION

- **Common name:** L(+) Lactic acid, d-lactic acid
- **Group:** Acid
- **Source:** Mineral kingdom
- **Part used:** $CH_3CH(OH)COOH$
- **Prover:** Griggs

SARCOLACTICUM ACIDUM

KEYNOTE SYMPTOMS

- **Invaluable in spinal neurasthenia, muscular weakness,** dyspnoea, incidental to myocardial weakness
- Tired feeling with muscular prostration. Soreness all over
- Vomiting due to general toxaemia
- Influenza with violent nausea and vomiting, and marked prostration
- Constriction in the pharynx; sore throat; tickling in the throat
- Extreme weakness from climbing stairs; stiffness of thighs and calves; cramps in the calves
- Restless at night; difficulty in falling asleep

CONSTITUTION

- For epidemic influenza with great prostration and tired feeling. Feels sore all over, especially in the afternoon. Tired feeling in the morning on getting up.
- **Temperament:** Nervous
- **Thermal:** Chilly
- **Miasm:** Psora, Syphilis

CLINICAL

- Muscular prostration
- Paralytic weakness
- Spinal neurasthenia
- Myocardial weakness
- Cramps
- Stiffness
- Nausea
- Vomiting
- Diarrhoea
- Constipation
- Influenza
- Laryngitis
- Pharyngitis
- Dyspnoea
- Asthma
- Rheumatism

REMEDY RELATIONSHIP

- **Compare:** Eup-per., Arn., Bry.

Sarcolacticum acidum

SARSAPARILLA OFFICINALIS

SPHERE OF ACTION

- Mucous membranes
- Gastrointestinal system
- Respiratory system
- Genitourinary system
- Skin

INTRODUCTION

- **Common name:** Smilax, Wild liquorice
- **Family:** *Liliaceae*
- **Source:** Vegetable kingdom
- **Part used:** Rhizome and root
- **Prover:** Hahnemann

CONSTITUTION

- Suits children with faces like old people and enlarged abdomen
- Suits dark haired people of lithic or sycotic diathesis
- **Temperament:** Nervous, bilious
- **Thermal:** Chilly
- **Miasm:** Sycosis, Syphilis

MIND

- Despondent, gloomy, without cause
- Depression and anxiety from pain
- Easily offended, sensitive
- Irritability, ill-humoured
- Restlessness, anxiety
- Fickleness, changeable disposition
- Impatient

KEYNOTE SYMPTOMS

- Nausea, vomiting and headache. Apathae, salivation.
- Rumbling and fermentation in abdomen; much flatus
- Sensation of emptiness in stomach after a meal
- Colic and backache at the same time
- **Can pass urine only when standing; urine dribbles while sitting**
- **Excruciating pain from right kidney downwards.** Pain causes depression. Painful distention of bladder with tenderness
- Excruciating pain at the conclusion of urination
- **White sand in the urine; sand in urine or on diaper; child screams before and while passing it.** Renal colic and dysuria in infants
- Passage of gravel or small calculi; renal stone and colic
- Urine scanty, slimy, flaky, sandy and copious. Urine passes in a thin, feeble stream.
- Nipples – small, withered, retracted, cracked
- Bloody seminal emission. Horrible stench on genitals. Itching of scrotum and perineum.
- Suppressed gonorrhoea; discharge of white turbid urine and tenderness of bladder; cystitis
- Rheumatic pains after gonorrhoea
- Itchy, humid eruptions on forehead, before menses
- Cracks in hands and soles of feet with pain and burning. Skin hard, indurated
- Dry, emaciated, shrivelled skin, lying in folds
- Ulceration around finger tips. Cutting sensation, burning under nails
- Rash on exposure to open air, especially in spring. Herpetic eruptions

CLINICAL

- Marasmus
- Aphthae
- Dyspepsia
- Diarrhoea
- Cholera infantum
- Dysentery
- Constipation
- Emphysema
- Asthma
- Cystitis
- Retention of urine
- Suppression of urine
- Urethritis
- Bright's disease
- Pyelonephritis
- Renal calculus
- Physometra
- Nocturnal emissions
- Prostatitis
- Arthritis
- Rheumatism
- Eczema
- Herpes
- Ulcers
- Rhagades
- Onychia

MODALITIES

- **Aggravation:** Dampness, at night, after micturating, when yawning, in spring, before menses
- **Amelioration:** Warmth, uncovering neck and chest

REMEDY RELATIONSHIP

- **Complementary:** Merc., Sep., either of which follows well
- **Compare:** Berb., Lyc., Nat-m., Phos., Petr., Sass., Saur., Cuc-c.
- **Antidote:** Bell.
- Frequently called for after abuse of Mercury

SCROPHULARIA NODOSA

SPHERE OF ACTION
- Mucous membranes
- Gastrointestinal system
- Respiratory system
- Female genital system

INTRODUCTION
- **Common name:** Knotted figwort
- **Family:** *Scrophulariaceae*
- **Source:** Vegetable kingdom
- **Part used:** Whole plant
- **Prover:** Franz

CONSTITUTION
- For scrofulous conditions wherever enlarged glands are present with weakness, prostration and paleness
- **Temperament:** Nervous
- **Thermal:** Chilly
- **Miasm:** Psora, Syphilis

MIND
- Delusions; objects appear on closing eyes
- Anxiety about the future
- Despondency, depression from motion
- **Much troubled about the past and very apprehensive about the future**
- Miserable and sluggish feeling in mind when moving about
- Restlessness
- Melancholy

CLINICAL
- Cancerous glands
- Hodgkin's disease
- Nodosities
- Drowsiness
- Vertigo
- Crusta lactea
- Photophobia
- Haemorrhoids
- Otitis media
- Dyspnoea
- Bronchitis
- Asthma
- Breast tumour
- Pruritus vaginae
- Epithelioma
- Eczema

KEYNOTE SYMPTOMS
- Powerful remedy whenever enlarged glands are present
- Weakness, wants to lie down. Too weak to speak
- Dizziness, fullness and pressure in vertex. Vertigo in upright position and felt in vertex
- **Accumulation of sweetish saliva in several parts of tongue**
- Painful, bleeding, protruding piles
- Eczema around ears. Inflammation around the auricle
- Violent dyspnoea. Oppresion of chest. Pain around bifurcation of trachea.
- Nodosities in the breast
- **Pricking, itching,** all over the skin, **worse at the back of the hands and between fingers**
- Excessive drowsiness in the forenoon and afternoon, before and after meals

MODALITIES
- **Aggravation:** Lying on right side, after food, in the morning, pressure
- **Amelioration:** Warm room

REMEDY RELATIONSHIP
- **Compare:** Op., Lob-e., Ruta, Carc., Con., Aster., Dig., Grat., Euphr.
- **Followed by:** Dig.
- **Antidoted by:** Bry.

Scrophularia nodosa

SECALE CORNUTUM

SPHERE OF ACTION
- Mucous membranes
- Gastrointestinal system
- Respiratory system
- Muscular fibres
- Female genital system

INTRODUCTION
- **Common name:** Ergot of rye
- **Family:** *Hyporeaceae*
- **Source:** Vegetable kingdom
- **Part used:** Fresh dried fungus
- **Prover:** Hartlaub and Trinks

CONSTITUTION
- For old people, especially thin, scrawny, old women with sunken eyes and blue circles around them; are pale, pinched, dry and shrivelled
- Women of lax fibre, everything seems loose and open with tendency to passive haemorrhages
- **Temperament:** Nervous, haemorrhagic
- **Thermal:** Hot
- **Miasm:** Psora

MIND
- Discouragement and timidity
- Restlessness. Insanity, very suspicious because of it
- Fear of death with desire to jump into water
- Maniacal fear, or depressed by fear
- **Puerperal mania – exposes the body, tears at genitals, inserts finger into vagina and scratches until it bleeds. Idea of modesty lost**
- Laughs, claps her hands over head
- Madness, indication to bite or drown himself
- Irritable
- Sadness and melancholy
- Great anxiety, anguish

KEYNOTE SYMPTOMS
- Produces contractions of unstriped muscle fibres. Facial and abdominal muscles twitch
- General atrophy and emaciation. Rapid emaciation of paralysed parts
- Cramps commence in the face, extending over whole body. Spasmodic distortion. Lock-jaw.
- Numbness, crawling as if mice creeping all over, under the skin
- Haemorrhagic diathesis, copious flow of thin, black, watery blood; slightest wound causes bleeding for weeks
- Burning of all parts, as if sparks of fire were falling on parts, worse from heat
- **Cold to touch, yet cannot bear to be covered. Aversion to heat. All conditions are better from cold.**
- **Tongue dry, cracked, coated thick. Tingling at the tip of the tongue which is stiff**
- Unnatural, ravenous appetite and thirst unquenchable
- **Craving for acids, sours and lemonades**
- Very exhausting, painless, involuntary, profuse, watery, putrid, brown diarrhoea with icy coldness
- Collapse in cholera disease, skin cold yet cannot bear to be covered
- Epistaxis, dark, oozing; worse slight touch; with exhaustion. Epistaxis in alcoholics
- Enuresis in old people
- Brownish, offensive leucorrhoea
- Circulatory imbalances. Dark, passive, unclotted, uterine haemorrhages. Continuous oozing of watery blood till next period.
- **Threatened abortion around third month**
- Pains during labour weak, feeble, irregular – no expulsive action; followed by long, painful after-pains
- Suppression of milk in scrawny, exhausted women. Breasts do not fill properly
- Tonic spasms – especially of all extensors; convulsions, tetanus
- **Gangrene – dry, senile, cold.** Varicosities seems loose and open. Vessels flabby causing passive haemorrahages.

CLINICAL
- Anaemia
- Numbness
- Formication
- Convulsions
- Seizure disorder
- Haemorrhages
- Claudication
- Raynaud's syndrome
- Locomotor ataxia
- Hairfall
- Incipient cataract
- Diabetic retinitis
- Diarrhoea
- Cholera
- Constipation
- Epistaxis
- Enuresis
- Albuminuria
- Uterine haemorrhage
- Puerperal metritis
- Miscarriage
- Leucorrhoea
- Fibroma
- Carbuncles
- Petechiae
- Ecchymosis
- Gangrene
- Ulcerations
- Varices

MODALITIES
- **Aggravation:** Heat, warmth from covering of all affected parts, all diseases worse from heat, touch, motion, exertion
- **Amelioration:** In cold air, getting cold, uncovering affected parts, rubbing, fanning, stretching out limbs

REMEDY RELATIONSHIP
- **Compare:** Ergot., Bran-n-o., Cinnm., Colch., Ars., Aur-m. 2x; Agro. Ust., Carb-v., Pituin., Cinnm. in post-partum haemorrhage; it increases labour pains, controls profuse or dangerous flooding, is always safe, while Ergot is always dangerous
- **Antidotes:** Camph., Op
- **Similar to:** Ars., but cold and heat are opposite
- Resembles Colch. in cholera morbus

SELENIUM METALLICUM

INTRODUCTION

- **Common name:** Selenium
- **Family:** Element
- **Source:** Mineral kingdom
- **Formula:** Se
- **Prover:** Hering

SPHERE OF ACTION

- Mind
- Nervous system
- Gastrointestinal system
- Respiratory system
- Male genital system

CONSTITUTION

- Adapted to light complexioned blondes with marked emaciation of face and hands, legs or feet
- **Temperament:** Nervous
- **Thermal:** Chilly
- **Miasm:** Psora, Syphilis

MIND

- Extremely sad, despairing
- Uncompromising
- Melancholic
- Mental labour fatigues patient
- Cannot take mental exertion
- **Lascivious thoughts, with impotency**
- Forgetfulness when awake, with distinct recollection during half sleep
- Forgetfullness in business, recollects in dreams whatever he has forgotten
- Great loquacity, fond of conversing, especially in the evening
- When excited, stammers, uses syllables of words in wrong connection

KEYNOTE SYMPTOMS

- Great mental and physical debility, especially from sexual excesses and after debilitating diseases
- Great debility, easy exhaustion – mental and physical, during old age; worse heat
- Left sided affections
- Ill-effects of debauchery
- Inability to bear a draught of air – causes pain in head, limbs, etc.
- Throbbing in vessels of whole body, especially abdomen
- Emaciation of affected parts
- Hair falls off head, eyebrows, whiskers and genitals
- Headache of drunkards, after debauchery, from strong odours and tea
- **Desires – liquors, especially brandy; ill-effects from sugar, salt food, tea, lemonade**
- **Tongue thick white coated in the morning**
- Chronic liver affections; liver enlarged and painful with a fine rash over the liver region
- Constipation – large, hard stools, impacted; removed by mechanical aid
- Hoarseness, from long use of voice, in singers with discharge of clear, starchy mucous
- Weakness, debility and relaxation, especially seen in the sexual sphere
- Sexual neurasthenia. **Increased desire but decreased ability.** Impotence; **dribbling of semen during sleep.** Dribbling of prostatic fluid. **Penis relaxed.**
- Paralytic pain in lumbosacral region in the morning
- Itching around finger joints, between fingers; eruptions between fingers
- Sleepless till midnight; wakes up early

CLINICAL

- Debility
- Alcoholism
- Hairfall
- Alopecia
- Headache
- Hiccough
- Constipation
- Aphonia
- Hoarseness
- Laryngitis
- Haemoptysis
- Prostatitis
- Prostatorrhoea
- Impotency
- Hydrocoele
- Spermatorrhoea
- Psoriasis
- Eczema
- Comedones
- Seborrhoea oleosa
- Acne
- Scabies
- Insomnia

MODALITIES

- **Aggravation:** Draft of air, in the sun, from lemonade, tea or wine, after sleep, in hot weather, wine, mental exertion
- **Amelioration:** Taking cold water or cold air into the mouth, after sunset

REMEDY RELATIONSHIP

- **Compare:** Phos. in genitourinary and respiratory symptoms; Arg-met. and Stann. in laryngitis of singers or speakers; Alum., hard stool, inactive rectum. Agn., Calad., Sulph., Tell., Ph-ac.
- **Follows well:** Calad., Nat-m., Staph., Ph-ac., in sexual weakness.
- **Itch checked by mercurials or sulphur often requires Selenium.**
- **Incompatible:** Chin.
- **Antidotes:** Ign., Puls.

SENECIO AUREUS

INTRODUCTION
- **Common name:** Golden ragwort, Life root
- **Family:** *Compositae*
- **Source:** Vegetable kingdom
- **Part used:** Whole plant
- **Prover:** Small

SPHERE OF ACTION
- Mucous membranes
- Gastrointestinal system
- Respiratory system
- Musculoskeletal system
- Female genital system

CONSTITUTION
- Suits women and little girls of nervous temperament with circumscribed spots on the face and chest
- **Temperament:** Nervous, haemorrhagic
- **Thermal:** Chilly
- **Miasm:** Psora, Syphilis

MIND
- Irritable, worried, undecided
- Sadness, despondency, dejection, dullness
- Mental depression, gloom; melancholy alternating with a cheerful mood
- Hysteria at night; with sleeplessness. Inability to fix mind
- Ecstasy alternating with sadness
- Inability to fix mind on one subject for any length of time
- Aversion to thinking during menses
- Meditation during menses
- Feeling of homesickness
- Dreams of writing, of intellectual character
- Nervousness

KEYNOTE SYMPTOMS
- Lassitude during daytime – sleepless at night with vivid unpleasant dreams, wants to lie down, tired all morning
- Pains are radiating, shifting, lancinating, in head, eyes, face, abdomen, etc.
- Left side more affected as in face, head, etc.
- Wave-like dizziness from occiput to sinciput
- **Aversion to sweets; coffee**
- Dryness of fauces, throat, mouth
- Early stages of liver cirrhosis
- Stools – thin, dark, bloody, passed with tenesmus
- Fullness of nasal passages with burning, sneezing, profuse flow and a raw sensation
- Dyspnoea on ascending; dry teasing cough
- **Tendency to take cold before menses**
- Backache with congested kidneys
- Functional amenorrhoea of young girls
- Menses retarded, suppressed; alternating with epistaxis or nasal catarrh
- Before menses, inflammatory condition of throat, chest and bladder but after flow (menstrual) commences, all these symptoms improve
- Menses may be either premature and profuse or retarded or absent
- Violent anaemic dysmenorrhoea, with urinary symptoms
- Lascivious dreams with involuntary emissions

CLINICAL
- Nervousness
- Homesickness
- Tenesmus
- Cirrhosis of liver
- Diarrhoea
- Constipation
- Epistaxis
- Coryza
- Hoarseness
- Aphonia
- Laryngitis
- Pharyngitis
- Pneumonia
- Pleurisy
- Nephritis
- Irritable bladder
- Cystitis
- Amenorrhoea
- Dysmenorrhoea
- Vicarious menses
- Involuntary emissions
- Enlarged prostate
- Backache
- Sleeplessness

MODALITIES
- **Aggravation:** Cold, open air, night, afternoon, sitting, dampness
- **Amelioration:** Bending forward, onset of menses

REMEDY RELATIONSHIP
- **Compare:** Senec-j. (cerebrospinal irritation, rigid muscles, chiefly of neck and shoulders; also, in cancer), Alet., Caul., Sep., Arn., Calen., Bellis-p., Puls., Helon., in uterine complaints; Caps., and Ph-ac. in homesickness

SEPIA OFFICINALIS

INTRODUCTION

- **Common name:** Cuttle fish
- **Family:** *Sepiadae*
- **Source:** Animal kingdom
- **Part used:** Inky juice of the cuttle fish
- **Prover:** Hahnemann

SPHERE OF ACTION

- Mind
- Mucous membranes
- Gastrointestinal system
- Respiratory system
- Urinary system
- Female genital system
- Skin

CONSTITUTION

- Suits persons, especially women of dark hair, rigid fibre but mild and easy disposition who are sensitive to all impressions
- **Washer women's remedy.** Tell-tale face – yellow saddle across nose and cheeks, butterfly pigmentation on face – yellow; scrofulous and pot bellied women
- **Temperament:** Anaemic, chlorotic, sanguine
- **Thermal:** Chilly
- **Miasm:** Sycosis

MIND

- Greedy, miserly
- **Indifference, hardness, indolent**
- Aversion to family, to those loved best, to sympathy, to company, yet dreads to be alone
- Tearful, great sadness and weeping
- Any demand by family is viewed as a further burden and met with anger
- Excitable, affectionate, oversensitive, introverted, loves dancing
- Shrieking at children, cannot control her anger
- Nobody knows what she will do next
- Anxiety, fear over trifles
- Fear of ghosts, poverty
- Stasis, sluggishness, indifference, detached, disconnectedness
- Sad, morose
- Irritability, depression, desperation
- Dread of being alone, of men
- Very sensitive; must not be found fault with

KEYNOTE SYMPTOMS

- Flushes of heat, especially during climacteric; asscends from pelvic organs; with anxiety and faintness, followed by perspiration
- Sensation of a lump or ball internally; sensation of a lump in the rectum, prostate, uterus, anus, throat, etc.
- **Faints easily, especially while kneeling at church, after getting wet, extremes of heat or cold. Faints after slightest exertions**
- Sensitive to cold air; chills easily
- Stasis, laxness, prolapse, varicosities of viscera. Weariness and misery
- Coldness in vertex with headache; at menstrual nisus, with scanty flow. Hairfall after chronic headache or during climacteric
- The sight or thought of food sickens; morning sickness of pregnancy
- Empty feeling in stomach; all gone feeling, not better by eating. **Tongue foul but becomes clear at each menstrual period**
- **Craving for vinegar, acids and pickle; aversion to fats. Always worse after taking milk**
- Constipation during pregnancy, confinement; stools hard, knotty, in balls; sense of weight or ball in anus
- **Infantile diarrhoea; worse from boiled milk**
- Thick, greenish discharge from nose; chronic nasal catarrh with marked post-nasal droppings
- **Prolapse of uterus and vagina; bearing down, must cross limbs to prevent it**
- Menses irregular; either late and scanty, or early and profuse
- Profuse sweat on genitals, especially scrotum
- Pains extend from other parts on to the back, with shuddering
- Itching; not ameliorated by scratching; especially in bends of elbows and knees
- Herpes circinatus in isolated spots

CLINICAL

- Depression
- Chronic fatigue syndrome
- Anaemia
- Gastritis
- Peptic ulcer
- Infantile diarrhoea
- Constipation
- Haemorrhoids
- Rectal fissure
- Pruritus ani
- Ozaena
- Sinusitis
- Cough
- Stress incontinence
- Enuresis
- Cystitis
- Sexual dysfunction
- Dysparunia
- Amenorrhoea
- Menorrhagia
- Uterine prolapse
- Vaginitis
- Endometriosis
- Leucorrhoea
- Menopause
- Nausea of pregnancy
- Pelvic inflammatory disease
- Premenstrual syndrome
- Miscarriage
- Arthritis
- Rheumatism
- Sciatica
- Lumbago
- Varices
- Hirsutism
- Cholasma
- Ringworm
- Urticaria
- Condyloma
- Prostatitis
- Psoriasis
- Herpes
- Warts

MODALITIES

- **Aggravation:** In afternoon or evening; from cold air or dry east wind, sexual excesses, at rest, sultry, moist weather, before a thunderstorm (Psor.), washing, laundry, after sweat
- **Amelioration:** Warmth of bed, hot applications; violent exercise, pressure, after sleep

REMEDY RELATIONSHIP

- **Complementary:** Nat-m., Phos. Nux-v. intensifies action. Guaj. often beneficial after Sep.
- **Inimical:** Lach., Puls.
- **Compare:** Lil-t., Murx., Sil., Sulph., Asper., Orig-d., Lapo.
- **Similar:** Lach., Sang., Ust., in climacteric irregularities of circulation
- Frequently indicated after Sil., Sulph.
- A single dose often acts curatively for many weeks

SERUM ANGUILLAE

INTRODUCTION
- **Common name:** Eel serum
- **Family:** *Anguillidae*
- **Source:** Animal kingdom
- **Part used:** The serum

SPHERE OF ACTION
- Gastrointestinal system
- Liver
- Respiratory system
- Heart
- Kidneys
- Muscular system

MIND
- Irritable disposition
- Cross
- Dissatisfied
- Anxiety, restlessness, gloomy, melancholic

MODALITIES
- **Aggravation:** Deep inspiration, swallowing, noise, odour
- **Amelioration:** Rest

KEYNOTE SYMPTOMS
- Toxic action on the blood destroying its globules
- **Hypertension and oliguria without oedema**
- Mitral insufficiency, asystole with or without oedema, dyspnoea and difficult urinary secretion
- Heart disease with anuria
- In cardiac uraemia, it ends renal obstruction and produces abundant diuresis
- Kidneys affected either from cold, infection or intoxication where the attack is characterised by oliguria, anuria and albuminuria; **this remedy re-establishes diuresis and rapidly arrests albuminuria**
- Renal obstruction, acute nephritis with uraemia, oliguria and arterial hypertension
- Acute nephritis with threatening uraemia

CONSTITUTION
- For cases with hypertension and oliguria, but no oedema
- For cases with presence of albumin and renal elements in urine, haemoglobinuria and prolonged anuria
- **Temperament:** Nervous, haemorrhagic
- **Thermal:** Chilly
- **Miasm:** Psora, Syphilis

CLINICAL
- Hypertension
- Oedema
- Diarrhoea
- Constipation
- Mitral insufficiency
- Cardiac uraemia
- Nephritis
- Diuresis
- Anuria
- Uraemia
- Oliguria
- Albuminuria
- Renal obstruction diuresis
- Haematuria

REMEDY RELATIONSHIP
- Great analogy exists between Eel serum and the venom of Vipera
- **Compare:** Vip., Lach.

SILICEA TERRA

INTRODUCTION

- **Common name:** Pure silica, Pure flint, Silicon dioxide
- **Group:** Element
- **Source:** Mineral kingdom
- **Formula:** SiO_2
- **Prover:** Hahnemann

SPHERE OF ACTION

- Mind
- Mucous membranes
- Glands
- Gastrointestinal system
- Respiratory system
- Musculoskeletal system
- Skin

CONSTITUTION

- **Suited to stone cutters ailments**
- Constitutions suffering from deficient nutrition due to defective assimilation
- Scrofulous, rachitic children with a large head, open fontanelles and sutures, pot bellied abdomen, who are slow in learning to walk and sweat much about the head
- Suited to nervous, weak, irritable people with fine skin, pale, light complexion and lax muscles
- **Temperament:** Anxious
- **Thermal:** Chilly
- **Miasm:** Psora, Sycosis

MIND

- Apathy, indifference
- Lack of stamina, want of grit, mental labour difficult
- Afraid of failure
- Very sensitive – physically and mentally to all external impressions
- **Averse to and aggravation from mother's milk, vomits it**
- Sensitive, delicate, well behaved
- Fixed ideas; children have fits of obstinacy, sometimes because of fixed opinions; head strong
- Mentally weak, feeble, faint-hearted
- Timid, answers only to the mother. Irritable when aroused
- **Pin mania – thinks only of pins, fears them, looks for them, collects them**
- Ill-humour on least provocation, from excessive nervous debility
- Patient likes to be magnetized which ameliorates
- Night walking

KEYNOTE SYMPTOMS

- Induration and suppuration of glands – cervical, parotid, axillary, mammary inguinal, sebaceous, etc.; generally without pain
- **Promotes expulsion of foreign bodies from tissues** like, fish bones, needles, bone splinters, etc.
- Highly chilly, lacks vital heat; hugs the fire, suffering parts feel cold
- Diseases of bones, caries and necrosis; fistulous burrowings. **Soft spongy bones.**
- Defective nutrition. Lack of stamina. Debility. **Children late learning to walk.**
- **Full moon, new moon aggravation**
- Convulsions start from solar plexus
- Ailments accompanied by pus formation; suppurative processes. Controls suppurative processes of soft tissues, bones, periosteum – maturing abscesses or reducing excessive suppuration when desired.
- Discharges – acrid and corrosive
- Ill-effects of vaccination; suppressed foot sweat; intolerant to alcoholic stimulants
- Ailments from taking cold in the feet
- **Offensive, profuse sweat on head and neck – wetting the pillow**
- **Hair-like sensation on tongue**
- Offensive, painless diarrhoea with cadaverous odour
- Chronic diarrhoea in soldiers due to sleeping on damp grounds
- Constipation which is offensive, from inactivity of rectum; always before and during menses; stools recede again when partly expelled
- **Pricking as of a pin in tonsil.** All colds settle in throat. Violent cough on lying down with thick, yellow, lumpy expectoration
- Profuse, acrid, corroding, milky leucorrhoea gushing with itching of pudenda
- Profuse menses with icy coldness all over the body
- Discharge of blood from vagina when child takes the breast
- Nipples sore have fistulous ulcers, drawn in
- **Carrion-like offensive odour of feet, with excoriation between toes.** Icy cold, sweaty feet
- Every injury suppurates. Hurts fester. Affections of nails – crippled

MODALITIES

- **Aggravation:** Cold, during menses, during new moon, uncovering, especially the head, lying down, light, noise, from washing, vaccination
- **Amelioration:** Warmth, especially from wrapping up the head, all the symptoms except gastric are ameliorated by cold food (Lyc.), in summers, wet humid weather

CLINICAL

- Injuries
- Strains
- Foreign bodies, splinters
- Paralysis
- Convulsions
- Epilepsy
- Headache
- Corneal ulcers
- Iritis
- Choroiditis
- Cataract
- Trachoma
- Keratitis
- Photophobia
- Pyorrhoea
- Fistula-in-ano
- Haemorrhoids
- Painless diarrhoea
- Constipation
- Rectal fissure
- Otorrhoea
- Quinsy
- Ozaena
- Vaginal cyst
- Leucorrhoea
- Arthritis
- Rheumatism
- Caries
- Necrosis of bones
- Unhealthy skin
- Vesicles
- Erysipelas
- Pustules
- Corns
- Panaritium
- Bunions
- Ingrowing toe nails
- Keloid
- Abcesses

REMEDY RELATIONSHIP

- **Complementary:** Thuj., Sanic., Puls., Fl-ac., Merc. and Sil. do not follow each other well
- **Compare:** Hep., Kali-p., Pic-ac., Calc., Phos., Nat-sil., Ferr-cy., Sil-mar., Vitrum—Crown glass. Arund-d., Get., Ruta, Sanic.
- **Follows well:** Calc., Graph., Hep., Nit-ac., Phos.
- **Is followed well by:** Hep., Fl-ac., Lyc., Sep.
- **Sil. is the chronic of Puls.**

Silicea terra

SPHERE OF ACTION

- Mucous membranes
- Ears
- Nose
- Gastrointestinal system
- Respiratory system
- Female genital system

INTRODUCTION

- **Common name:** Black mustard
- **Family:** *Cruciferae*
- **Source:** Vegetable kingdom
- **Part used:** Seeds
- **Prover:** Cattell and Butler

CONSTITUTION

- Suits women who are anxious and of irritable disposition, scalp is hot and itchy
- **Temperament:** Nervous
- **Thermal:** Chilly
- **Miasm:** Sycosis

MIND

- Irritable disposition
- Cross, dissatisfied without cause, must guard herself constantly or be uncivil and pettish
- Dreams vivid or lascivious
- Answers abruptly
- Restlessness
- Difficulty in thinking, studying

SINAPIS NIGRA

CLINICAL

- Hiccough
- Heartburn
- Belching
- Diarrhoea
- Constipation
- Painful conditions of nose
- Coryza
- Rhinitis
- Middle ear disease
- Otitis media
- Hay fever
- Cough
- Tonsillitis
- Pharyngitis
- Hoarseness
- Asthma
- Arthritis
- Rheumatism
- Blisters
- Insomnia

KEYNOTE SYMPTOMS

- Catarrh of bladder, stomach, air passages but mucous membranes, dry and hot; no discharge
- Scalp hot and itchy. Dull feeling in vertex, as if empty
- **Offensive breath, smelling like onions**
- **Sweat on upper lip and forehead. Sweat better when nausea comes on**
- Colic pains come on while bent forward, better sitting up straight
- Secretions from the nose are thick, lumpy, acrid, scanty and burning
- **Stoppage of left nostril all day, or in the afternoon and evening**
- Mucous from posterior nares feels cold. Scanty, acrid discharge. Nostrils alternately stopped. Dryness of anterior nares.
- **Loud coughing spells;** hacking cough, **relieved by lying down; barking expiration**
- Rheumatic pain in the intercostal and lumbar muscles

MODALITIES

- **Aggravation:** Touch, pressure, motion, evening, stooping, thinking of symptoms
- **Amelioration:** Mental diversion, sitting erect, eating a hearty meal

REMEDY RELATIONSHIP

- **Compare:** Sulph., Caps., Coloc., Sin-a., Thios., Coch., Sang. (scalded sensation on tongue)
- Mustard oil by inhalation act on the sensory nerve endings of trigeminal nerve

SOLIDAGO VIRGAUREA

INTRODUCTION

- **Common name:** Golden rod
- **Family:** *Compositae*
- **Source:** Vegetable kingdom
- **Part used:** Whole plant except root
- **Prover:** Rademacher and Guliken

SPHERE OF ACTION

- Mucous membranes
- Respiratory system
- Urinary system
- Female genital system

CONSTITUTION

- Suits scrofulous subjects
- Suits cases arising from or complicated by the defective action of kidneys
- **Temperament:** Bilious
- **Thermal:** Chilly
- **Miasm:** Sycosis

MIND

- Irritable disposition
- Cross
- Gloomy
- Melancholic
- Frustrated
- Neglected feeling

MODALITIES

- **Aggravation:** Pressure, at night
- **Amelioration:** Profuse urination

KEYNOTE SYMPTOMS

- Marked sensation of weakness
- **Diseases arising from, or complicated with defective function of kidney are very likely to be benefitted by this remedy**
- Paroxysms of sneezing
- Abundant mucous secretion or expectoration on coughing; chronic catarrh of lungs; allergies
- Asthma with noctornal dysuria; bronchitis with profuse, purulent expectoration
- Kidneys are sensitive to pressure
- Sometimes makes use of the catheter unnecessary
- Backache due to renal congestion
- Difficulty in urinating due to mechanical pressure on the bladder as by a fibroid of the uterus or an enlarged prostate
- Pain in kidneys extending forward to the abdomen
- **Urine – dark, reddish-brown, with thick sediment; with epithelial cells and mucous; scanty, voided with difficulty**
- Clear, offensive, stinking urine
- **Rheumatic pain in the legs. Legs can be moved horizontally, but when moved perpendicularly, they feel lame**
- Blotches on skin, especially hands and feet, itching intolerably dropsy and threatened gangrene

CLINICAL

- Tumours
- Dropsy
- Ophthalmia
- Constipation
- Dyspnoea
- Tuberculosis
- Bronchitis
- Asthma
- Bright's disease
- Haematuria
- Albuminuria
- Dysuria
- Renal calculus
- Fibroids
- Lumbago
- Backache
- Gangrene
- Exanthema

REMEDY RELATIONSHIP

- **Antidote:** Iodof. 2x antidotes poison of Golden rod.
- **Compare:** Ars., Hydrang., Sabal., Santa., Tritic.

SPIGELIA ANTHELMIA

INTRODUCTION

- **Common name:** Pink root, Animal worm grass
- **Family:** *Loganiaceae*
- **Source:** Vegetable kingdom
- **Part used:** Whole plant – dried
- **Prover:** Hahnemann

SPHERE OF ACTION

- Mind
- Eyes
- Nervous system
- Gastrointestinal system
- Respiratory system
- Cardiovascular system
- Sexual system

CONSTITUTION

- Suits anaemic, debilitated subjects of rheumatic diathesis
- For scrofulous children suffering from ascaris lumbricoides
- For people with light hair, who are pale, thin, weak and bloated, having wrinkled yellow skin
- **Temperament:** Nervous, bilious
- **Thermal:** Chilly
- **Miasm:** Psora, Sycosis, Syphilis

MIND

- **Afraid of sharp, pointed things likes pins and needles; delusion about pins**
- Anxiety with palpitation and deep constriction of the chest; regarding the future; regarding his family; conscience
- Full of worries and cares, especially about relatives
- Sad, depressed, to the extent of suicidal mania, especially in the evening
- Weak memory; absence of ideas
- Unfit for intellectual labour

KEYNOTE SYMPTOMS

- **Pains and neuralgia – violent, burning like hot wires, stitching and jerking**
- Pains press outwards from within, from below upwards, especially in the eyeballs
- **It is a sun remedy – headache begins at sunrise, it is at the height at noon and subsides by sunset**
- **Neuralgias generally left sided,** of head, eyes, face, teeth, heart; **especially of fifth cranial nerve**
- Body is painfully sensitive to touch; the part touched feels chilly
- Sharp, stabbing, sticking pain through the eyeballs back into the head; from cold, damp, rainy weather
- Prosopalgia, involving the eye, malar bone, teeth; left sided; from morning to sunset; worse cold, rainy weather
- Foetid breath and foetid flatus marked symptoms, especially with helminthiasis
- **Toothache, better while eating or lying down; worse tobacco, cold drinks; with shivering, palpitation and agitation**
- Stammering with worm affections, repeats first syllable 3 or 4 times
- Child refers to the naval as the most painful part
- Chronic catarrh with postnasal dropping of bland mucous, choking at night
- **Dyspnoea, must lie on the right side with head high**
- Angina pectoris; neuralgia extending to one or both arms; aggravation from movement
- Pulse weak, irregular; pericarditis with sticking pains, palpitation and dyspnoea

CLINICAL

- Neuralgia
- Hyperthyroidism
- Headache
- Migraine
- Glaucoma
- Iritis
- Prosopalgia
- Toothache
- Halitosis
- Worms
- Diarrhoea
- Constipation
- Otitis media
- Sinusitis
- Dyspnoea
- Angina pectoris
- Arrhythmia
- Pericarditis
- Rheumatic heart disease
- Aneurysm
- Weak pulse
- Rheumatic carditis
- Valvular disorders

MODALITIES

- **Aggravation:** From motion, noise, light, touch, turning the eyes, from every shaking, commotion, or concussion, washing, in the sun, rising
- **Amelioration:** Lying on right side with the head high, inspirations, rest, warmth, steady firm pressure

REMEDY RELATIONSHIP

- **Compare:** Acon., Ars., Cact., Dig., Kali-c., Kalm., Naja, Spong. in heart affections. Spig-m., Cimic., Arn. (Spig. is the chronic of Arn.); Cinnb. (supraorbital pain); Naja, Sabad., Teucr., Cina.
- **Antidote:** Puls., Cocc., Aur., Camph.
- **Antidotes:** Merc., Colch.

SPONGIA TOSTA

SPHERE OF ACTION
- Mind
- Mucous membranes
- Gastrointestinal system
- Respiratory system
- Genitourinary system

INTRODUCTION
Common name: Roasted sponge
Family: *Porifera*
Source: Animal kingdom
Part used: Whole animal
Prover: Hahnemann

CONSTITUTION
- Especially adapted to diseases of children and women with light hair, lax fibre, fair complexion, swollen glands, and who have a larynx which is sensitive to touch
- **Temperament:** Tubercular
- **Thermal:** Chilly
- **Miasm:** Psora

MIND
- **Irresistible desire to sing; with excessive mirth; followed by sadness**
- Fear of future; tired of life
- Anxiety; fear and terror of approaching death with suffocation due to choking; of fatal termination of disease
- Timidity; incessantly tormented by a frightening scene from the past
- Weeps with dreams, with whooping cough, with heat, with sweat
- Despondent about loss of sexual power
- Obstinate and improper behaviour
- Every excitement increases the cough
- Mental obtuseness with complete disinclination for mental labour
- Quarrelsome; tired of life

KEYNOTE SYMPTOMS
- Worse after sleep or sleeps into aggravation
- **Swelling and induration of glands** like thyroid gland, cervical glands, etc.
- Dryness of mucous membranes of air passages. **Cough – dry, barking, croupy; worse sweets, cold drinks, lying with head low, cold winds and better eating or drinking warm things**
- Hoarse, voice – cracked and feels faint. Chest weak, can scarcely talk
- Larynx dry, burns and feels constricted; sensitive to touch; sensation of a plug in the larynx
- Croup, worse during inspiration and before midnight
- Dry, chronic sympathetic cough of organic heart disease
- **Sensation as if breathing through a sponge**
- Suffocation causes anxiety. Inflammation of the larynx, trachea and bronchi. Feeling of stoppage of wind pipe
- Sore throat, worse after eating sweets
- Respiration, wheezing, whistling, short and difficult; cold clammy sweat all over
- Surging of blood to chest, as if it would force out upwards
- Thyroid gland swollen, suffocative paroxysms especially at night
- Angina pectoris with rapid and violent palpitations. Awakened suddenly after midnight with pain and suffocation; is hot, flushed and frightened to death; valvular insufficiency
- **Amenorrhoea with asthma;** during menses wakes with suffocative spells
- Spermatic cord and testicles swollen, tender, painful, bruised. Maltreated orchitis

CLINICAL
- Goitre
- Adenitis
- Laryngeal phthisis
- Sinusitis
- Laryngitis
- Pharyngitis
- Diphtheria
- Cough
- Bronchitis
- Wheezing
- Croup
- Asthma
- Tuberculosis
- Angina pectoris
- Valvular insufficiency
- Endocarditis
- Aneurysm of descending aorta
- Arthritis
- Rheumatism
- Orchitis
- Epididymitis

MODALITIES
- **Aggravation:** Dry cold wind, ascending, motion, walking, touch, pressure, before midnight
- **Amelioration:** Descending, lying with head low, eating and drinking warm things

REMEDY RELATIONSHIP
- **Compare:** Acon., Hep., Brom., Lach., Merc-i-f. (goitre), Arn., Caust., Iod., Nux-m., sputa loosened but must be swallowed again
- **Follows well:** Acon., Hep., in cough and croup when dryness prevails; after, Spong., Hep., when mucous commences to rattle

SQUILLA MARITIMA

INTRODUCTION
- **Common name:** Sea onion, Squill
- **Family:** *Liliaceae*
- **Source:** Vegetable kingdom
- **Part used:** Bulb
- **Prover:** Hahnemann

SPHERE OF ACTION
- Mucous membranes
- Gastrointestinal system
- Respiratory system
- Musculoskeletal system
- Urinary system

CONSTITUTION
- For cases where hands and feet are icy cold while the rest of the body is warm
- **Temperament:** Nervous, bilious
- **Thermal:** Chilly, ambithermal
- **Miasm:** Psora, Sycotic, Syphilis

MIND
- Indolent
- Haughty
- Malicious
- Easily angered
- Aversion to mental or physical labour
- Irritability, worse contradiction

KEYNOTE SYMPTOMS
- Slowly developing complaints
- Useful in dropsical conditions with great weakness and weariness of body
- Acts upon mucous membranes of respiratory, digestive and urinary systems; for ailments requiring several days to reach their maximum intensity
- Increased lachrymation; eyes feel irritated. Child bores into eyes with fists
- Pressure like a stone on the stomach
- Pains or disorders of spleen with stitches under the left free ribs
- **Child rubs the face with fists during coughing**
- Cough with sneezing; cough of measles
- Fluent coryza, margins of nostril feel sore. Sneezing
- **Change of weather from warm to cold and cold drinks provoke cough. Inability to sit during cough.**
- Becomes tired and eventually lies down after cough although there is inclination to cough. Violent, furious, exhausting cough with profuse, salty, slimy expectoration.
- Dyspnoea, with stitches in the chest
- **For chronic bronchitis of old people with dyspnoea, mucous rales and scanty urine**
- Profuse urination. Involuntary spurting of urine while coughing. Frequent calls to micturate at night, passing large quantities
- Tender feet – feet get sore from standing, as in shop girls

CLINICAL
- Involuntary stools
- Coryza
- Sneezing
- Cough
- Bronchitis
- Dyspnoea
- Pneumonia
- Asthma
- Broncho-pneumonia
- Arteriosclerosis
- Involuntary urination
- Measles

MODALITIES
- **Aggravation:** Motion, exertion, early morning, ascending, uncovering
- **Amelioration:** Rest, lying down, wrapping warmly

REMEDY RELATIONSHIP
- **Compare:** Dig., Stroph-h., Apoc-h., Bry., Kali-c., Squil.
- **Follows well:** Dig., if it fails to relieve water logged cases
- **Antidoted by:** Camph.

STANNUM METALLICUM

SPHERE OF ACTION
- Nervous system
- Gastrointestinal system
- Respiratory system
- Female genital system

INTRODUCTION
- **Common name:** Tin
- **Group:** Element
- **Source:** Mineral kingdom
- **Formula:** Sn
- **Prover:** Hahnemann

CONSTITUTION
- Suits a pale, sunken, sickly countenance with dark rings around the eyes
- Profound debility with profuse muco-purulent discharges on a tubercular base. Even talking causes severe weakness
- **Temperament:** Nervous, tubercular
- **Thermal:** Chilly
- **Miasm:** Psora, Tubercular

MIND
- Very sad and despondent. Melancholic
- Disinclination to talk, extreme exhaustion of mind
- Anxious, weak and irritable
- Disposition to weep. She feels like crying all the time; can cry at any time but crying makes her worse
- Restlessness with anxiety; mental symptoms ameliorated as soon as menses start
- Hopelessness, discouraged
- Ill-humour with taciturnity. Sudden fits of passion
- Dread of seing people

KEYNOTE SYMPTOMS
- Great debility and profound weakness is a keynote
- Feels weak, dizzy and faints, especially when going downstairs
- Pains appear and disappear gradually
- Aching in temples, forehead. Headache, increasing and decreasing gradually. Drawing pain in malar bones and orbits
- **Nausea and vomiting from the odour of cooked food**
- Empty, sinking, all gone sensation in chest and stomach
- Abdominal colic – cramp-like; relieved by hard pressure or by pressing the abdomen against a knee or shoulder
- Passes worms, lumbrici with stools
- Obstinate acute coryza, influenza with cough
- Dry, deep, husky, hollow voice, relieved by expectoration
- **Chest feels sore, weak; can hardly talk**
- Deep, hollow, cough – in paroxysms of three with empty sensation in chest
- **Sweetish and salty expectoration; copious, yellow-green pus**
- **Respiration short, oppressive; stitches on the left side while breathing**
- Bearing down sensation – uterine prolapse with a weak sinking feeling in stomach. Menses early and profuse
- Leucorrhoea with considerable prostration of strength
- Paralytic weakness; drops things. Limbs suddenly give out on attempting to sit
- Bitter taste, heat in evening during fever with exhausting night sweats
- **Sweat – on forehead and nape of neck, debilitating, especially towards morning; with mouldy, musty odour**

CLINICAL
- Anaemia
- Debility
- Paralysis
- Spasms
- Convulsions
- Epilepsy
- Neuritis
- Typewriter's paralysis
- Neuralgia
- Headache
- Nausea
- Vomiting
- Abdominal disorders
- Gastralgia
- Worms
- Colic
- Hoarseness
- Expectoration
- Cough
- Chest affections
- Bronchitis
- Asthma
- Uterine prolapse
- Leucorrhoea
- Ulceration
- Hectic fever
- Insomnia

MODALITIES
- **Aggravation:** Laughing, singing, talking, lying on right side, warm drinking, gentle motion, touch, lying down
- **Amelioration:** Coughing or expectorating relieves hoarseness, hard pressure, bending double, rapid motion

REMEDY RELATIONSHIP
- **Compare:** Stann-i., Caust., Calc., Sil., Tub., Bac., Helon. Myrt-ch.
- **Complementary:** Puls.
- **Follows well:** Caust.
- **Followed by:** Calc., Phos., Sil., Sulph., Tub.

STAPHYSAGRIA

INTRODUCTION

- **Common name:** Stavesacre, Louse seeds
- **Family:** *Ranunculaceae*
- **Source:** Vegetable kingdom
- **Part used:** Seeds
- **Prover:** Hahnemann

SPHERE OF ACTION

- Mind
- Eyes
- Teeth
- Gastrointestinal system
- Throat
- Respiratory system
- Genitourinary organs
- Skin

CONSTITUTION

- For nervous affections with marked irritability and diseases of the genitourinary tract
- Person was insulted but being too dignified to fight, subdued his wrath becoming sick, exhausted and trembling
- **Temperament:** Nervous
- **Thermal:** Chilly
- **Miasm:** Psora, Syphilis

MIND

- **Ill-effects of anger and insults; envy and chagrin; thwarted pride**
- Sensitive to slightest mental impressions and least action or harmless word offends
- Great indignation about things done by himself
- Very apathetic and indifferent, low spirited and has weak memory
- Children cry for things which when given are pushed and thrown away
- Dwells on sexual subjects, sexual sins and excesses
- **Very sensitive about what others say regarding them**
- Hypochondriacal
- Prefer solitude
- Violent outbursts of anger
- Indolent

KEYNOTE SYMPTOMS

- Suppression of emotions and anger, suppressed sexuality leading to masturbation
- Mechanical injuries from sharp instruments; post-surgical pain
- Styes, tumours or chalazae on eyelids, in succession, leaving hard nodosities behind
- **Intense craving for tobacco**
- Toothache during menses, in sound and decayed teeth, worse cold air, cold drinks or from touch of food. **Teeth turn black and crumble, decay on edges.** Salivation, spongy gums. Bleed easily.
- Stomach–flabby, weak, feels relaxed. Desire for stimulants. Nausea after abdominal surgery.
- Colic with pelvic tenesmus after anger, following abdominal surgery. Incarcerated flatus
- Cough only in daytime excited by cleaning the teeth, from anger and indignation, and by tobacco smoke
- **Intolerable urging to urinate, still patient has to wait for a long time**
- Irritable bladder of married women – honeymoon cystitis; sensation as if a drop of urine was rolling down the urethra
- Pain after lithotomy. Burning in urethra when micturating and when not micturating
- Dyspnoea after coitus
- **Parts sensitive in women; vulva so sensitive, can barely wear a napkin**
- Prostatic problems, frequent micturation. Spermatorrhoea, especially after self-abuse
- Crural neuralgia; dull aching pains extending to hip joint
- Inflammation of phalanges with sweating and suppuration. Arthritic nodes
- Backache, worse in morning before rising
- Eczema – oozes acrid moisture from under the crusts; scratching changes location of itching. Night sweats
- Sleepy all day, awake all night, bodyache all over

CLINICAL

- Depression
- Nymphomania
- Neuralgia
- Post-surgical pain
- Cerebral accidents
- Chorea
- Chalazae
- Styes
- Blepharitis
- Iritis
- Strabismus
- Pyorrhoea
- Peptic ulcer
- Diarrhoea
- Constipation
- Dyspnoea
- Cystitis
- Enuresis
- Honeymoon cystitis
- Urethritis
- Uterine prolapse
- Masturbation
- Spermatorrhoea
- Post-surgical orchitis
- Prostatitis
- Arthritis
- Rheumatism
- Figwarts
- Psoriasis
- Eczema
- Insomnia

MODALITIES

- **Aggravation:** Mental affections, from anger, indignation, grief, mortification, loss of fluids, tobacco, onanism; sexual excesses; from touch on affected parts
- **Amelioration:** At night, rest, warmth, after breakfast

REMEDY RELATIONSHIP

- **Compare:** Caust., Coloc., Ign., Lyc., Puls., and Staph. act well after each other
- **Inimical:** Ran-b., either before or after
- **Complementary:** Caust., Coloc.
- **Antidote:** Camph.

STELLARIA MEDIA

SPHERE OF ACTION
- Eyes
- Musculoskeletal system
- Liver
- Skin

INTRODUCTION
- **Common name:** Chickwood
- **Family:** *Caryophyllaceae*
- **Source:** Vegetable kingdom
- **Part used:** Whole plant when flowering

CONSTITUTION
- For a condition of stasis, congestion and sluggishness of all functions
- **Temperament:** Nervous
- **Thermal:** Chilly
- **Miasm:** Sycosis

MIND
- Great irritability
- Lassitude
- Indisposed to work
- Dull
- Anxious
- Restless
- Gloomy

CLINICAL
- Headache
- Blepharitis
- Corneal ulcer
- Hepatomegaly
- Jaundice
- Diarrhoea
- Constipation
- Arthritis
- Rheumatism
- Gout
- Synovitis
- Cervical spondylosis
- Psoriasis
- Insomnia

KEYNOTE SYMPTOMS
- Liver enlarged, swollen, with stitching pains; sensitive to pressure. Clay-coloured stools
- Constipation or alternate constipation and diarrhoea
- Rheumatic pains – sharp, sudden, shifting, darting, wandering. Stiffness of joints, parts sore to touch, bruised feeling
- Chronic rheumatism; **rheumatic pain in calves of legs, in different parts of the body**
- Enlarged, inflamed gouty finger joints. Pain in shoulders and arms
- **Rheumatic pains shifting in nature** – now in the ankle, now in the knee, now in the shoulder
- Neck muscles stiff and sore

MODALITIES
- **Aggravation:** In the morning, from warmth, tobacco
- **Amelioration:** In the evening, from cold air, motion

REMEDY RELATIONSHIP
- **Compare:** Puls. (similar is rheumatism, pains shifting, worse rest, warmth; better cold air)

Stellaria media

STICTA PULMONARIA

SPHERE OF ACTION
- Head
- Eyes
- Gastrointestinal system
- Respiratory system
- Joints
- Musculoskeletal system
- Genitourinary system

INTRODUCTION
- **Common name:** Lungwort
- **Family:** *Stictaceae*
- **Source:** Vegetable kingdom
- **Part used:** Whole plant
- **Prover:** S.P. Burdick

CONSTITUTION
- Suited to neuralgic, rheumatic, gouty individuals
- Broken down, nervous and rheumatic ailments
- **Temperament:** Nervous
- **Thermal:** Chilly
- **Miasm:** Sycosis, Syphilis

MIND
- **Great desire to talk about anything or everything. Can't keep her tongue still; does not care whether anyone listens**
- Confusion of ideas, cannot concentrate on them
- Gloomy, melancholic, sad
- Feels as if floating in air

KEYNOTE SYMPTOMS
- Burning in eyelids and eyes; soreness of eyeballs
- Diarrhoea; stool profuse, frothy
- Severe coryza with violent sneezing; intense headache and conjunctivitis which is preceded or followed by rheumatism and swelling of small joints
- **Nose blocked with a constant need to blow the nose; discharge absent or dries quickly forming crusts. Dry scabs.**
- Dryness of nasal membrane. Dull, heavy pressure at the root of the nose with catarrh and headache
- Severe harassing cough – dry, incessant and hacking, at night preventing sleep; can neither sleep nor lie down, must sit up; worse inspiration
- **Cough, after sunset, till vomiting occured; cures cough often left by measles, whooping cough, influenza; follows colds**
- In phthisis or haemoptysis, symptoms of cough with sudden pain from sternum to spine, constant, worse movement with oppression of chest
- Inflammatory condition of the joints with redness. Rheumatic pains precede catarrhal symptoms. Swelling and stiffness of hands and feet.

CLINICAL
- Haemorrhage
- Falls
- Paralysis
- Chorea
- Headache
- Photophobia
- Conjunctivitis
- Blepharitis
- Diarrhoea
- Rhinitis
- Influenza
- Tracheitis
- Whooping cough
- Bronchorrhoea
- Tuberculosis
- Angina pectoris
- Arthritis
- Rheumatism
- Sciatica
- Cervical spondylosis
- Bursitis
- Housemaids knee
- Agalactia
- Measles

MODALITIES
- **Aggravation:** As the day advances, lying down, at night, motion
- **Aggravation:** Pressure, open air, free discharges

REMEDY RELATIONSHIP
- **Compare:** Dat-a., Bougmanica, Cetr., Ery-a., Dros., Still., Rumx., Samb.

SPHERE OF ACTION

- Mind
- Mucous membranes
- Gastrointestinal system
- Respiratory system
- Heart
- Genitourinary system
- Skin

INTRODUCTION

- **Common name:** Indian corn, Corn-silk, Maize, Zea maydis
- **Family:** *Graminae*
- **Source:** Vegetable kingdom
- **Part used:** Corn silk

CONSTITUTION

- Adapted to a uric acid and phosphatic diathesis
- Generally found useful in chronic cases only
- **Temperament:** Nervous, bilious
- **Thermal:** Chilly
- **Miasm:** Psora, Sycosis, Syphilis

STIGMATA MAYDIS

MIND

- Gloomy
- Tired
- Restless
- Anxious
- Apprehensive

KEYNOTE SYMPTOMS

- Vomiting sour with pain in gastric region
- **Heart and urinary conditions combined**
- Has marked urinary symptoms and has been used with success in **organic heart disease with much oedema of lower extremities and scanty urination**
- Pain during micturation, nephritic colic. Chronic pyelitis with catarrh
- Tenesmus after urinating
- Supression and retention of urine. Discharge of small calculi, red sand and blood in urine
- Cystitis, retention, dysuria
- Enlarged prostate, with retention of urine
- Remedy for chronic malaria, chronic gonorrhoea

CLINICAL

- Dyspepsia
- Constipation
- Arteriosclerosis
- Cystitis
- Dysuria
- Retention of urine
- Urinary incontinence
- Renal calculi
- Chronic pyelitis
- Gonorrhoea
- Enlarged prostate
- Malaria

MODALITIES

Aggravation: After urination

REMEDY RELATIONSHIP

- **Compare:** Shucks; Tritic. Sabal in bladder affections; Dig., Stroph-h., in heart affections

STRAMONIUM

SPHERE OF ACTION

- Mind
- Cerebrospinal system
- Mucous membranes
- Genitourinary system
- Skin

INTRODUCTION

- **Common name:** Thorn apple
- **Family:** *Solanaceae*
- **Source:** Vegetable kingdom
- **Part used:** Fresh plant when in flower and fruit
- **Prover:** Dr Hahnemann

CONSTITUTION

- Suited in ailments like delirium, fever, mania, chorea of young plethoric people, especially children
- Cases present with heat of face with cold hands and feet; circumscribed redness of cheeks
- **Temperament:** Bilious
- **Thermal:** Chilly
- **Miasm:** Psora

MIND

- Complaints after fright
- Ailments from suppressed anger
- **Trio of delirium with a desire to escape**
- **Fear of being injured.** Delusions, about his own identity.
- Strong fears at night, of darkness. Wakes with terror.
- Cannot bear solitude or darkness, must have light and company
- Horror of shining objects, mirror, hearing running water
- Hallucinations terrify the patient; a remedy of terrors – sees ghosts, hideous animals; anxiety when going through a tunnel; hears voices, talks with spirits
- Violence and fear of violence
- Great loquacity; ceaseless talking
- Raving mania. Religious insanity
- Emotional vulnerability, paranoia schizophrenia
- Weeping in dreams
- Claustrophobia, hydrophobia

KEYNOTE SYMPTOMS

- Ailments from fright, suppressed anger, head injury, vaccination, fever, cerebral accident, shock
- Secretions and excretions are suppressed; ailments due to suppressed secretion; like menses, sweat, lochia, etc.
- Painlessness is very characteristic; with most of the complaints
- **Restlessness and nervousness – marked**
- Entire body sensitive to touch; spine sensitive – slightest pressure on spine produces out cries and ravings
- Involuntary movements, spasms, convulsions, chorea, tics, jerks; hurried movements
- Twitching of single muscles; squint
- Convulsions with consciousness; from bright light or brilliant objects
- Tonic and clonic spasms alternate
- Paralysis of one side and convulsions of the other side of the body
- Head continuously jerks from the pillow, is bent back; boing of head in to the pillow
- **Sight of water, bright light, mirror or anything glittering brings on spasms**
- Grinding of teeth
- **Difficulty in swallowing with intense thirst is a marked symptom**
- Dark, putrid, painless, involuntary, offensive diarrhoea
- **Vomiting as soon as head is raised from the pillow**
- Stammering, has to exert himself a long time before he can utter a word, makes great effort to speak
- Increased sexual desire in both sexes; lasciviousness priapism and onanism in males; nymphomania, catemania in women
- Neck stiff, cannot bend head back, opisthotonus

CLINICAL

- Behavioural disorders
- Fears
- Temper problems
- Delirium
- Mania
- Manic depression
- Phobic disorders
- Schizophrenia
- Hyperactive children
- Seizure disorder
- Chorea
- Convulsions
- Cerebral accidents
- Head injury
- Meningitis
- Delirium tremens
- Risus sardonicus
- Strabismus
- Stammering
- Diarrhoea
- Enuresis
- Sexual disorders
- Metrorrhagia
- Febrile convulsions
- Acne
- Burns
- Hirsutism
- Nightmares

MODALITIES

- **Aggravation:** Shining objects, surface of water, fright, after sleep, dark cloudy days, swallowing, suppressions, touch, at night, looking into light
- **Amelioration:** Bright light, lemon juice, company, warmth

REMEDY RELATIONSHIP

- **Compare:** Hyos., Bell., Pyrog., Lach., Agar., Cupr., Zinc., Rhus-t., Op.
- **Antidotes:** Bell, Tab, Nux-v.
- **Complementary:** Sulph.
- **Follow well:** Cupr, Bell.
- **Incompatible:** Coff.
- **Antidoted by:** Lemon juice, vinegar

STRONTIUM CARBONICUM

INTRODUCTION

- **Common name:** Carbonate of strontia, Strontium carbonate
- **Group:** Metal
- **Source:** Mineral kingdom
- **Formula:** $SrCO_3$
- **Prover:** Nenning, Schreter, Seidel, Trinks and Woost

SPHERE OF ACTION

- Mind
- Gastrointestinal system
- Respiratory system
- Musculoskeletal system
- Skin

MIND

- Delusion that he is a criminal
- **Destructiveness,** suddenly angry, beats anything that comes in his way. Delirium tremens
- **Discontented, displeased, dissatisfied**
- Dullness, sluggishness
- Shrieking, shouting during sleep
- Peevishness, with tendency to fly into a rage
- Cannot bear solitude
- Excessive forgetfulness
- Restlessness at night with sensation of smothering
- Confusion of mind from spirituous liquors; loquacious
- Anguish

MODALITIES

- **Aggravation:** Change of weather, from being quiet, when beginning to move, cold, drafts, walking
- **Amelioration:** Immersing in hot water, light, heat, sun, warm store, wrapping

KEYNOTE SYMPTOMS

- Bad effects of haemorrhages during and after surgical shock with profuse oozing of blood, coldness and prostration
- **For bad effects of x-rays, radium, nuclear exposure**
- Shock after surgeries
- Headache – boring, pressive and tensive
- Vertigo with headache and nausea
- Flushing of the face, violent pulsations of the arteries; congestion of the heart, lungs and head
- **Diarrhoea, worse at night and is very urgent – continuous urging; scarcely leaves the vessel before having to return; better after am**
- Sticking pain in the abdominal ring. Diarrhoea with burning in anus which lasts a long time after stool
- Bloody crusts in the nose; itching redness, burning of nose
- High blood pressure with a flushed face, pulsating arteries and threatened apoplexy
- Sprains and bone affections, especially the femur
- Rheumatic pains, especially of joints; cramps in calves and soles
- Pains are so severe, she thought she would faint
- **Sciatica with oedema of ankle**
- Chronic spasm of the ankle joint. Oedematous swelling. Icy cold feet.
- Venous tension of the arms; veins of hands engorged
- Violent perspiration at night

CONSTITUTION

- Suits those with a hot, red face and circumscribed redness of cheeks; blood rushes to face, pale face
- **Temperament:** Anxious
- **Thermal:** Chilly
- **Miasm:** Sycosis

CLINICAL

- Collapse
- Prostration
- Apoplexy
- Oedema
- Neuritis
- Vertigo
- Headache
- Asthenopia
- Hiccough
- Cardialgia
- Flatulence
- Diarrhoea
- Varicose veins
- Hypertension
- Arteriosclerosis
- Nephritis
- Phlebitis
- Cramps
- Sciatica
- Scrofulous bones
- Varicosities
- Sprains

REMEDY RELATIONSHIP

- **Compare:** Arn., Ruta, Sil., Bar-c., Carb-v., Stront-i. (arteriosclerosis), Stront-br. Stront-n.
- **Antidoted by:** Camph.

STROPHANTHUS HISPIDUS

INTRODUCTION

- **Common name:** Kombe seed
- **Family:** *Apocycaneae*
- **Source:** Vegetable kingdom
- **Part used:** Ripe seeds

SPHERE OF ACTION

- Heart
- Gastrointestinal system
- Respiratory system
- Muscular system
- Female genital system

CONSTITUTION

- For corpulent people with anaemia, palpitations and breathlessness
- Suits children suffering from chlorosis, anaemia and irritability of the heart
- **Temperament:** Nervous
- **Thermal:** Chilly
- **Miasm:** Sycosis

MIND

- Anxiety, especially from anticipation with palpitation of heart and tendency to breath deeply
- **Fear of ordeals**
- Floating sensation, of being lifted up during sleep
- Mentally, these patients are irritable
- Precocious loquacity in children
- Irritability, worse contradiction

KEYNOTE SYMPTOMS

- **Removes alcohol habit. Causes an aversion to it without the withdrawal symptoms**
- Temporal pain with diplopia, impaired vision; senile vertigo from cerebral anaemia
- Functional disturbances of the heart from long use of alcohol, tobacco and tea
- **Tones the heart and removes dropsical accumulations**
- Acts on the heart – increasing systole and reducing the rapidity
- Arteriosclerosis – rigid arteries of aged, mitral regurgitation with oedema and dropsy
- **Irritable heart. Pulse quickened, heart's action is weak,** rapid, irregular – due to cardiac insufficiency or muscular debility. Restores tone to brittle tissues, especially of heart muscles and valves
- Alternations – rapid pulse alternates with slow pulse. Exophthalmic goitre
- Weak, irregular pulse, fluttering sensation in cardiac region, palpitation during sleep
- Useful during climacteric period, there are aching pains through the hips and extensors of the thighs. Menorrhagia; uterine haemorrhage
- Extremites – swollen, dropsical; anasarca

CLINICAL

- Alcoholism
- Tobacco smoker
- Dipsomania
- Anaemia
- Chlorosis
- Anasarca
- Oedema
- Exophthalmic goitre
- Diplopia
- Bronchial asthma
- Pneumonia
- Angina pectoris
- Myocarditis
- Cardiac insufficiency
- Arteriosclerosis
- Cardiac asthma
- Mitral regurgitation
- Menorrhagia
- Urticaria
- Dyspnoea

MODALITIES

- **Amelioration:** Exertion, tea, tobacco, emotions
- **Aggravation:** Rest

REMEDY RELATIONSHIP

- **Compare:** Dig. (but is slower than Stroph-h. in its action), Ph-ac. (weak heart, irregular pulse, fluttering sensation in the cardiac region, palpitations during sleep, fainting) Apoc., Crat., Cact., Acon., Aven., Chin. and Nux-v. in alcoholism

SULPHUR

INTRODUCTION

- **Common name:** Brimstone
- **Family:** Element
- **Source:** Flowers of sulphur
- **Part used:** Trituration of flowers of sulphur
- **Prover:** Hahnemann

SPHERE OF ACTION

- Mind
- Nervous system
- Mucous membranes
- Gastrointestinal system
- Respiratory system
- Portal system
- Skin

CONSTITUTION

- For scrofulous people subject to venous congestions. Are quick motioned, quick tempered and plethoric
- For lean, stoop-shouldered people who walk and sit stooping
- Dirty filthy people prone to skin affections
- For hot, emaciated, by bellied children who cannot bear to be washed
- **Temperament:** Nervous, lymphatic
- **Thermal:** Hot
- **Miasm:** Psora

MIND

- Worried by trifles
- Indifference to domestic duties, too unhappy to live
- Sensitive to everything
- Hurried, impatient, sad
- Absentminded while reading, very forgetful
- Doubtful and anxious
- Unsteadiness of ideas
- Apathy and inaptitude for business aversion to buisness
- Dread of exertion, very lazy
- Religious melancholy
- **Ragged philosophers – dirty looking poeple, always speculating on religious and philosophical subjects**
- **Happy dreams, wakes up singing**
- **Delusion – everything the patient takes a fancy to, looks pretty – even rags look beautiful**
- Lachrimose; frequent weeping
- Very irritable selfish – no regard for others

KEYNOTE SYMPTOMS

- Indicated in patients with a history of suppression of skin disease by external applications
- For complaints that are continuously relapsing; disease returns again and again, especially acute diseases
- **Standing is the most uncomfortable position**
- **Burning anywhere and everywhere in the body**
- **A weak, empty, all gone sensation in the stomach, especially around 11 am – must have something to eat. Milk disagrees**
- Congestion in single parts eyes, nose, lips, anus, etc. Irregular circulation – causes local burning, throbbing, congestion, flushes of heat, etc.
- All the discharges like leucorrhoea, nasal discharge are acrid and offensive
- **Hot patient yet persistently refuses to take a bath;** bathing and heat aggravate
- It facilitates absorption of serous or inflammatory exudates in pleura, joints, etc.
- Chronicity. Burning. Congestion. Redness
- Ascending effects
- Early morning diarrhoea, driving patient out of bed; painless
- Dry, unhealthy hair and skin; every little injury suppurates
- Soles burn, must uncover them
- Redness of orifices and parts near orifices like lips, anus, vulva, nostrils, etc.; they are also sore and hypersensitive
- Dyspnoea; difficult respiration, must open windows. Rattling of mucous

CLINICAL

- Vertigo
- Headache
- Meningitis
- Eye affections
- Keratitis
- Stomatitis
- Parotid hypertrophy
- Nausea
- Liver derangement
- Diarrhoea
- Constipation
- Haemorrhoids
- Worms
- Ear affections
- Deafness
- Epistaxis
- Influenza
- Laryngitis
- Adenoids
- Tonsillitis
- Lung affections
- Asthma
- Pneumonia
- Tenesmus
- Leucorrhoea
- Arthritis
- Rheumatism
- Eruptions
- Acne
- Barber's itch
- Boils
- Lichen planus
- Weeping eczema
- Herpes
- Polypus
- Freckles
- Ringworm
- Measles
- Varices
- Catnap sleep
- Sleep disorders

MODALITIES

- **Aggravation:** Standing, rest, stooping, bathing, washing, 11 am, at night, milk, suppressions, warmth, heat
- **Amelioration:** Open air, motion, sweating, walking, drawing up affected limbs

REMEDY RELATIONSHIP

- **Compare:** Acon., Ars., Merc., Calc., Lyc., Sep., Sars., Puls., Apis., Bry., Psor., Lach., Sul-ac.
- **Complementary:** Aloe, Psor., Acon., Ars., Lyc., Sep., Puls., Thuj.
- **Antidoted by:** Acon., Camph., Cham., Chin., Merc., Puls., Sep., Rhus-t., Thuj.

SPHERE OF ACTION

- Mind
- Gastrointestinal system
- Respiratory system
- Female genital system

INTRODUCTION

- **Common name:** Snowberry
- **Family:** *Caprifoliaceae*
- **Source:** Vegetable kingdom
- **Part used:** Berry
- **Prover:** Burdick

CONSTITUTION

- Suits women during pregnancy and menstruation
- **Temperament:** Nervous
- **Thermal:** Ambithermal
- **Miasm:** Psora

MIND

- Irritable
- Nervous, restless
- Depressed
- Likes to stay alone
- Gloomy, melancholic

SYMPHORICARPUS RACEMOSUS

CLINICAL

- Gastric disturbances
- Nausea
- Vomiting of pregnancy
- Dyspepsia
- Flatulence
- Abdominal distention
- Gastralgia
- Gastric ulcer
- Duodenal ulcer
- Diarrhoea
- Constipation

KEYNOTE SYMPTOMS

- Aversion to all food. Smell and thought of food is repugnant
- Bad taste in the mouth
- Gastric disturbances, fickle appetite, nausea, waterbrash and bitter taste
- **Deathly nausea, worse any motion, worse during menses and better lying on the back**
- Persistent vomiting of pregnancy with violent retching, better lying on the back
- Pain in the abdomen

MODALITIES

- **Aggravation:** Smell or thought of food, motion

REMEDY RELATIONSHIP

- **Compare:** Colch., Sep.

SYMPHYTUM OFFICINALE

INTRODUCTION
- **Common name:** Comfrey, Knitbone
- **Family:** *Boraginaceae*
- **Source:** Vegetable kingdom
- **Part used:** Root
- **Prover:** Croserio

SPHERE OF ACTION
- Eyes
- Bones
- Cartilage
- Periosteum
- Musculoskeletal system

MIND
- Anxiety
- Restlessness
- Irritability due to pain

MODALITIES
- **Aggravation:** Touch, motion, pressure, injuries, sprains, sexual excesses
- **Amelioration:** Warmth

KEYNOTE SYMPTOMS
- Injuries to bones, cartilages, periosteum with excessive pain
- Injuries, especially fractures
- Excessively painful old injuries to the periosteum or cartilage
- Blows from blunt instruments
- Trauma to the eyes and orbit; **pain in eye after a blow from an obtuse object**
- Toothache after injury; jaw swollen and painful after dental work
- **Pricking, stitching pains with soreness of periosteum.** Pains, especially periosteal remaining after wounds have healed
- **Non-union of bones; defective, deficient callus formation.** Comminuted fractures.
- Irritable stump after operations. Phantom limb pain after amputation
- Arthralgia, especially of the knee
- Backache from excessive sexual indulgence
- Caries of vertebrae
- Coldness of the skin

CONSTITUTION
- For traumatic injuries of bones or periosteum and for non-union of fractures
- **Temperament:** Nervous
- **Thermal:** Chilly
- **Miasm:** Psora

CLINICAL
- Pain
- Injuries to bones, cartilages, periosteum
- Old injuries
- Fractures
- Sprains
- Non-union of bones
- Blunt injuries to eyes
- Periodontal diseases
- Flatulence
- Gastralgia
- Dyspepsia
- Abdominal distention
- Dysentery
- Haemorrhoids
- Pott's disease
- Psoas abscess

REMEDY RELATIONSHIP
- **Compare:** Arn., Calc-p., Calc-f., Bry., Calen., Fl-ac., Hep., Sil., Staph., Led., Rhus-t., Hyper.

SYPHILINUM

INTRODUCTION
- **Common name:** Leusinum, Leuticum
- **Source:** Nosode
- **Part used:** The syphilitic virus
- **Prover:** Swan

SPHERE OF ACTION
- Mind
- Eyes
- Ears
- Gastrointestinal system
- Respiratory system
- Female sexual system
- Bones
- Skin

MIND
- Forgetfulness, does not remember faces, names, events, places, but remembers things previous to his illness
- Has a faraway feeling that he is not himself
- Apathy and indifference towards the future
- **Compulsive neurosis. Impulse to wash hands. Profound aversion to dirt or to touching dirty things. Compulsive checking.**
- Very nervous, laughs or weeps without cause; does not wish to be soothed
- Aversion to company. Sad and lamenting
- Despair of recovery
- Insanity. Senile dementia
- Extreme dread of night, gets worse as night approaches

MODALITIES
- **Aggravation:** At night, sundown to sunrise, seashore, in summers, protruding tongue
- **Amelioration:** Inland, at high altitudes, applied heat, daytime, slow or continued motion

KEYNOTE SYMPTOMS
- Utter prostration and debility in the morning. Impaired nutrition causing severe emaciation
- Affections of all the glands of the body
- Foetidity of all discharges and secretions – stool, urine, sweat, and all other secretions from the nose, vulva, etc.
- **Nocturnal aggravation with mental and physical breakdown**
- Destructiveness, erosion; ulceration – of mouth, nose, genitals, skin, etc.; stubborn ulceration
- Pains increase and decrease gradually, violent or linear
- **Hereditary tendency to alcoholism**
- Facial neuralgia; paralysis of one side with difficult speech; advancing hemiplegia
- Obstinate constipation for years; rectum as if tied up in strictures
- **Bones, especially those of tibia and head affected.** Bone pains or destruction; **knots in muscles**
- Bones – sore, decay; curvature of bones; exostosis
- Constant eruptions, pustular boils and abscesses in endless succession; with foul green pus

CONSTITUTION
- Especially useful when there is a hereditary tendency to alcoholism or syphilitic miasm
- Dwarfed, shrivelled, old looking babies and children with a bald head and big belly
- **Temperament:** Nervous
- **Thermal:** Chilly
- **Miasm:** Syphilis

CLINICAL
- Debility
- Alcoholism
- Compulsive disorder
- Anxiety
- Neuralgia
- Malignancy
- Hairfall
- Alopecia
- Ophthalmia
- Aphthae
- Teeth decay
- Diarrhoea
- Constipation
- Ozaena
- Otorrhoea
- Asthma
- Aneurysm
- Syphilis
- Leucorrhoea
- Chancres
- Bone disorders
- Abscesses
- Acne
- Bone pains
- Insomnia
- Psoriasis
- Scoliosis
- Night sweats

REMEDY RELATIONSHIP
- **Compare:** Merc., Kali-i., Nit-ac., Aur., Alum., Asaf., Phyt., in bone diseases and syphilitic affections

SYZYGIUM JAMBOLANUM

SPHERE OF ACTION
- Metabolism
- Endocrine system
- Urinary system
- Skin

INTRODUCTION
- **Common name:** Jambol seeds, Jamun
- **Family:** *Myrtaceae*
- **Source:** Vegetable kingdom
- **Part used:** Seed
- **Prover:** Dudgeon

CONSTITUTION
- Suits lean, thin, persons with progressive emaciation and suffering from diabetes mellitus
- **Temperament:** Nervous
- **Thermal:** Chilly
- **Miasm:** Psora, Syphilis

MIND
- Irritable
- Sad, depressed
- Anxious
- Restless
- Gloomy
- Desires company
- Tired
- Melancholic

KEYNOTE SYMPTOMS
- Fatigue, prostration, anxiety, apprehension with marked weakness and emaciation
- **Great thirst, mouth very dry**
- **Very useful in diabetes mellitus.** Causes marked reduction and disappearance of sugar in urine
- Very large amount of urine of high specific gravity passed
- Old ulcers of skin associated with diabetes mellitus
- Prickly heat in upper part of body; small red pimples that itch violently

CLINICAL
- Weakness
- Prostration
- Emaciation
- Diarrhoea
- Constipation
- Asthma
- Glycosuria
- Diabetes mellitus
- Rheumatism
- Diabetic ulcers
- Prickly heat
- Acne
- Eczema

MODALITIES
- **Aggravation:** Exertion, profuse sweating, mental stress and strain
- **Amelioration:** Rest, open air

REMEDY RELATIONSHIP
- **Compare:** Ins.—an aqueous solution of the active principle from the pancreas which affects sugar metabolism. If administered at suitable intervals in diabetes mellitus, the blood sugar is maintained at a normal level and the urine remains free of sugar. Over dosage is followed by weakness, fatigue, tremulousness and profuse sweating.

TABACUM

INTRODUCTION

- **Common name:** Tobacco
- **Family:** *Solanaceae*
- **Source:** Vegetable kingdom
- **Part used:** Leaves
- **Prover:** Hartlaub and Trinks

SPHERE OF ACTION

- Mind
- Head
- Mucous membranes
- Gastrointestinal system
- Respiratory system
- Cardiovascular system

CONSTITUTION

- For complete prostration of the entire muscular system with collapse; death-like pallor, icy coldness and sweat
- **Temperament:** Nervous, bilious
- **Thermal:** Chilly
- **Miasm:** Psora, Sycosis, Syphilis

MIND

- Forgetful, discontended
- Gloomy, melancholic; inclination to weep – weeping ameliorates
- Very despondent
- Sense of excessive wretchedness during menopause and menses
- Anxiety better by weeping. Sudden anxiety at night. Anxiety from thinking about it
- Indifference
- Does not recognize relatives
- **Unconsciousness; as if in a trance; ameliorates when cold water is poured over the head**
- Suicidal disposition, but lacks courage
- Restless, continuously changing place
- Mental faculties impaired, cannot read or study
- Feels as if someone was coming to arrest him or murder him

MODALITIES

- **Aggravation:** Motion of boat, pressure, opening eyes, evening, extremes of heat and cold
- **Amelioration:** Open fresh cold air, uncovering, abdomen, cold applications

KEYNOTE SYMPTOMS

- **Icy coldness of the surface, covered with cold sweat**
- Complete prostration and relaxation of entire muscular system
- Constriction of muscles of hollow organs like throat, chest, bladder and rectum
- **Symptoms occur in paroxysms** – asthma, vertigo, sick headache, sneezing, etc.
- Excessive vertigo on opening the eyes, on rising and looking backwards, worse indoors, better in open air
- Periodical sick headache with deathly nausea
- **Dim vision, as if sees through a veil**
- Incessant nausea with violent vomiting, on least motion, better in open air. Vomiting with faintness, cold sweat, during pregnancy with much spitting
- Terrible sinking feeling at the pit of the stomach; sense of relaxation
- Nausea, giddiness, death-like pallor, vomiting, icy coldness, sweat and intermittent pulse are characteristic
- Collapse; patient is cold but wants abdomen uncovered – it reduces the nausea and vomiting
- Diarrhoea – sudden, watery, with nausea and vomiting, prostration, cold sweat. Vigorous peristaltic activity
- Constipation – inactive bowel, rectum paralyzed
- Hemming and hoarseness of public speakers
- For high tension and arteriosclerosis of coronary arteries leading to angina
- **Palpitations, when lying on left side; subside on turning to the right side**
- Icy cold extremites with trembling

CLINICAL

- Brain fag
- Collapse
- Paroxysms
- Craving for tobacco
- Disgust for tobacco
- Seasickness
- Occipital headache
- Vertigo
- Amaurosis
- Strabismus
- Nausea
- Vomiting
- Gastraglia
- Incarcerated hernia
- Diarrhoea
- Cholera infantum
- Constipation
- Laryngitis
- Nasopharyngitis
- Tracheitis
- Intermittent pulse
- Arteriosclerosis
- Hypertension
- Angina pectoris
- Tachycardia
- Bradycardia
- Arthritis
- Rheumatism
- Pruritus
- Freckles

REMEDY RELATIONSHIP

- **Compare:** Hydrobr-ac., Camph., Verat., Ars. Nicot.
- **Antidote:** Vinegar, sour apples. Camph. is the physiological antagonist

TARAXACUM OFFICINALE

INTRODUCTION
- **Common name:** Dandelion
- **Family:** *Compositae*
- **Source:** Vegetable kingdom
- **Part used:** Whole plant
- **Prover:** Hahnemann

SPHERE OF ACTION
- Mind
- Mucous membranes
- Gastrointestinal system
- Respiratory system

MIND
- Weak memory
- Loquacity, especially during perspiration; Inclined to talk, laugh and be merry.
- Impatient and irritable
- Depressed, morose, apathetic
- **Dislikes labour but after starting, works well**

MODALITIES
- **Aggravation:** Lying down; resting, at night, fatty foods
- **Amelioration:** Touch, moving, open air

KEYNOTE SYMPTOMS
- **Great tiredness, 'lead-like heaviness', inclined to sit or lie down,** involuntary closure of eyes. Tingling, formication and numbness
- **Mapped tongue** – tongue is coated with a white film which clears off in patches leaving dark red, sensitive spots
- Debility, loss of appetite; bitter taste and eructations
- Gastric and bilious attacks, especially gastric headache
- **Hysterical tympanites;** flatulence; **sharp stitches on the left side; as if bubbles were forming and bursting in the abdomen**
- Jaundice with an enlarged and indurated liver, and mapped tongue hysterical tympanites
- Painless and frequent urging to urinate with copious discharge of urine
- **Cold finger tips; sweat between toes**
- **Profuse night sweats**

CONSTITUTION
- For liver affections with gastric complaints, debility and a mapped tongue, especially in old people
- **Temperament:** Nervous, bilious
- **Thermal:** Chilly
- **Miasm:** Psora, Sycosis, Syphilis

CLINICAL
- Debility
- Sick headache
- Mapped tongue
- Glossitis
- Biliousness
- Gastritis
- Tympanites
- Cholecystitis
- Jaundice
- Gall stones
- Constipation
- Asthma of children
- Headache

REMEDY RELATIONSHIP
- **Compare:** Bry., Chel., Hydr., Nux-v., in gastric and bilious affections; Ars., Nat-m., Merc., Ran-s., in mapped tongue

TARENTULA CUBENSIS

INTRODUCTION

- **Common name:** Cuban spider
- **Family:** *Araneideae*
- **Source:** Animal kingdom
- **Part used:** The entire living spider
- **Prover:** Monge

SPHERE OF ACTION

- Mind
- Gastrointestinal system
- Female genital system
- Skin

MIND

- Marked nervousness and associated restlessness
- Anxiety; keeps hands busy, picks fingers
- Excessive hyperaesthesia
- **Useful in hysteria where patient lacks emotional control**
- Agony due to pain; delirium due to pain

MODALITIES

- **Aggravation:** Exertion, at night, cold drinks
- **Amelioration:** Smoking, tobacco

KEYNOTE SYMPTOMS

- A toxaemic remedy acting on blood; useful in septic conditions
- Early and persistent prostration
- Septic conditions accompanied by marked burning and sharp stinging pains. Affected part is hard and covered with copious sweat
- **Loss of appetite, except for breakfast**
- Pruritus, especially around the genitals
- Restlessness of feet
- Intermittent fever with aggravation in the evening
- Abscesses where pain and inflammation predominate
- **Purplish-bluish hue of affected part, with atrocious burning pain;** gangrene, carbuncle buboes, fawns, anthrax
- Carbuncles, especially in the sloughing stage, with marked prostration and diarrhoea

CONSTITUTION

- Suits thin, emaciated, people suffering from septic conditions where incubation period is slow but further progress is rapid accompanied by marked prostration
- **Temperament:** Nervous, bilious
- **Thermal:** Chilly
- **Miasm:** Psora, Sycosis, Syphilis

CLINICAL

- Delirium
- Prostration
- Chorea
- Convulsions
- Diarrhoea
- Pruritus vulva
- Intermittent fever
- Bubonic plaque
- Itching
- Abscesses
- Carbuncles
- Senile ulcers
- Gangrene
- Insect bites

REMEDY RELATIONSHIP

- **Compare:** Agar., Ars., Bell., Cupr., Hyos., Lach., Lil-t., Med., Nux-v., Stram., Sul-ac., Tub.

TARENTULA HISPANICA

SPHERE OF ACTION

- Mind
- Nervous system
- Respiratory system
- Heart
- Female genital system

INTRODUCTION

- **Common name:** Spanish spider
- **Family:** *Araneidea*
- **Source:** Animal kingdom
- **Part used:** Entire spider
- **Prover:** Numez

CONSTITUTION

- Suits nervous, hysterical people subject to choreic affections
- Emaciation – flesh falls off the patient and eyes looks like that of a fox – cunning with a mischevious and destructive tendency
- **Thermal:** Hot
- **Temperament:** Nervous
- **Miasm:** Sycosis, Syphilis

MIND

- Paroxysms of insanity – pulls hair, has threatening manners and speech
- Fear of impending calamity
- Delusions – sees faces, monsters, ghosts, animals
- Restlessness, can't bear to see others suffering
- Must keep herself fruitlessly busy or takes a walk
- Child requires constant monitoring; disobedient
- Is foxy, sly, cunning, crafty
- Enjoys giving pain to others; kills animals for pleasure
- Kleptomania
- **Revengeful, destructive, mischevious**
- **Likes and enjoys dancing; jumps on music; sings till hoarse, likes tricks**
- Child has attention seeking syndrome
- Joking and profound melancholy; discontented
- Conceited and deceptive behaviour
- **Fakes fainting; if no one observes, there are no symptoms**

KEYNOTE SYMPTOMS

- Symptom appear periodically, return annually
- **Better by music – it first excites and then subsequently relieves**
- Agony of pains compels patient to walk the floor for nights. Great relief from rubbing the parts
- **Restlessness, cannot stay in any position; especially seen in lower limbs; must keep in motion, though walking aggravates all symptoms**
- Constant movement of legs, arms, trunk with inability to do anything; keeps tossing in bed from restlessness
- Twitching and jerking of muscles. Spinal irritability
- Hysterical hyperaesthesia
- Neuralgias, especially of the head, of great intensity, as if thousands of needles were pricking into the brain. Better by rubbing the head against the pillow
- Red, green, yellow, black colours produce a heavy mist before the eye
- **Desires raw food**
- **Cough, ameliorated by smoking, insult**
- Slight touch along spine provokes spasmodic pain in chest
- Increased desire in both sexes till the point of mania. Coitus aggravates the suffering in both
- Shameless, even after masturbation
- Intolerable pruritus vulvae in women. Spasms of uterus. Profuse menses, dysmenorrhoea with frequent erotic spasms
- In men – semen blood causing sensation of heat in its passage
- Choreic movements; weakness of legs
- Dark red and purplish colouration and swelling of skin and tissues
- Recurrent boils; malignant ulcers, carbuncles, anthrax, gangrene
- Sleepless due to nervous excitement
- Constrictive sensation – apparent imminent choking

CLINICAL

- Behavioural disorders
- Hysteria
- Multiple sclerosis
- Paralysis
- Convulsions
- Chorea
- Tumours
- Diabetes mellitus
- Headache
- Angina
- Valvular diseases
- Cardiac anxiety
- Increased libido
- Nymphomania
- Uterine fibroid
- Pruritus vulvae
- Eczema
- Boils
- Abscesses
- Carbuncles
- Gangrene
- Malignant ulcers
- Formication

MODALITIES

- **Aggravation:** Motion, contact, touch of affected parts, noise, damp cold weather, at night, in the evening, after sex
- **Amelioration:** In open air, music, rubbing affected parts, pressure, riding in a carriage, smoking

REMEDY RELATIONSHIP

- **Compare:** Ars., Pyrog., Crot-h., Echi., Anthraci., Bell., Apis., Agar., Cupr., Lach., Plat., Mygal., Naja, Ther.
- **Antidotes:** Mag-c., Puls., Cupr., Chel., Gels., Mosch., Carb-v.
- **Antidoted to:** Lach.

TEREBINTHINIAE OLEUM

INTRODUCTION
- **Common name:** Oil of turpentine
- **Family:** *Pinaceae*
- **Source:** Vegetable kingdom
- **Part used:** Oil distilled from the oleo resin obtained from various species of pinils
- **Prover:** Seidel

SPHERE OF ACTION
- Mind
- Tongue
- Mucous membranes
- Gastrointestinal system
- Respiratory system
- Urinary system
- Female genital system

MIND
- Muttering delirium
- Loathing of life, weary of life
- Suicidal disposition by hanging
- Unconsciousness after stool
- Confusion of mind ameliorated by urinating
- Intense irritability, children fly into a temper during dentition
- Fear of apoplexy, hydrophobia
- Stupefaction – inability to fix attention
- Mania; intense nervous excitement

MODALITIES
- **Aggravation:** Dampness, night, cold, lying, pressure, when urinating, sitting, touch
- **Amelioration:** Walking, stooping, motion, belching

KEYNOTE SYMPTOMS
- **Haemorrhages – passive, black, offensive,** oozing from mucous membranes; from nose, bowels, urinary tract, uterus, etc.
- **Tongue – does not clean gradually, but rapidly, in large flakes, leaving tongue smooth, glossy and red; deprived of pappillae, as if glazed**
- Tympanitis and soreness of the abdomen with diarrhoea. Enormous distention of abdomen
- Diarrhoea – watery, frequent, profuse, foetid and bloody; burning in anus and rectum
- Inflammation of kidneys with haemorrhage; nephritis after any acute disease
- **Congestion in the renal pelvis causing urine to be uniformly mixed with blood – smoky appearance of urine with coffee ground sediment or thick, yellow, slimy, muddy sediment**
- Stranguary with haematuria; constant tenesmus, spasmodic retention of urine
- **Urine is painless, cloudy, smoky, albuminous, profuse and dark in colour with the odour of violets**
- Severe burning in uterine region; with metrorrhagia
- Stands with feet apart, has no power of balancing the body. Walks bent like an old man, as if pitched forward while walking
- Unbroken chilblains with excessive itching and pulsations

CONSTITUTION
- Suits children during dentition, epistaxis and worms; nervous women
- Complaints of people with sedentary habits, especially old people
- For bleeding mucous surfaces – dark, passive, foetid. Chronic rheumatism and gouty complaints
- **Temperament:** Nervous, bilious
- **Thermal:** Chilly
- **Miasm:** Psora, Sycosis, Syphilis

CLINICAL
- Haemorrhages
- Coma
- Dropsy
- Tympanitis
- Enterocolitis
- Worms
- Ascitis
- Diarrhoea
- Diphtheria
- Violent bronchitis
- Albuminuria
- Haematuria
- Cystitis
- Bright's disease
- Nephritis
- Stranguary
- Backache
- Scarlatina
- Exanthemata
- Chilblains
- Purpurea
- Typhoid
- Malaria
- African fever

REMEDY RELATIONSHIP
- **Compare:** Alumn., Arn., Ars., Canth., Lach., Nit-ac., Sec.
- Is recommended as a prophylactic in malarial and African fevers
- **Antidote:** Phos.
- **Antidote to:** Merc., Phos.

TEUCRIUM MARUM VERUM

SPHERE OF ACTION

- Mucous membranes
- Nose
- Gastrointestinal system
- Respiratory system
- Female genital system

INTRODUCTION

- **Common name:** Cat thyme
- **Family:** *Labiatae*
- **Source:** Vegetable kingdom
- **Part used:** Whole plant
- **Prover:** Allen

CONSTITUTION

- Suits old people and children when too much medicine has produced an oversensitive condition and remedies fail to act
- **Temperament:** Nervous, bilious
- **Thermal:** Chilly, ambithermal
- **Miasm:** Psora, Sycosis, Syphilis, Tubercular

MIND

- Talking of unpleasant things by others aggravates
- Vivaciousness
- Extreme moral excitement and loquacity
- Indolence with great aversion to mental or physical exertion
- Irritable or irrascible with oversensitiveness, after eating, during heat, at puberty
- Irresistible inclination to sing, especially during fever
- Fatigue on merely hearing others converse

KEYNOTE SYMPTOMS

- Suitable after too much medicine has been taken
- Nocturnal restlessness with worms, especially ascarides
- Crawling and violent stiching pain in anus, in bed
- Itching in the anus, and constant irritation in evening in bed in the rectum – cannot sleep because of it
- Irritation and itching of nose and anus which suggests helminthiasis
- Chronic nasal catarrh with atrophy; large, offensive crusts and clinkers; loss of smell
- **Coryza with nose block on the side lain on. Mucous polyp**
- Loss of sense of smell
- Discharge of large, irregular clinkers
- Crawling in nostrils, with lachrymation or sneezing
- **Mouldy taste in throat when hawking up mucous**
- Trembling sensation in various parts with nervous excitement and marked irritability
- Numbness and tingling in limbs
- **Desire to stretch**
- Complete abscence of sweat, with very dry skin

CLINICAL

- Halitosis
- Worms
- Ascarides
- Anal itching
- Chronic nasal catarrh
- Ozaena
- Nasal polyps
- Nasal mucous polypi
- Atrophic rhinitis
- Anosmia
- Vaginal polyp

MODALITIES

- **Aggravation:** Touch, sitting, stooping, warmth
- **Amelioration:** Exercising in open air does not fatigue

REMEDY RELATIONSHIP

- **Compare:** Teucr-s. (in tuberculosis with muco-purulent expectoration; dropsy; orchitis and tuberculous epididymitis; especially in young, thin individuals with tuberculosis of the lungs, glands; bones and urogenitals, 3x), Cina, Ign., Sang., Sil.

THALLIUM METALLICUM

INTRODUCTION

- **Common name:** Thallium
- **Group:** Metal
- **Source:** Mineral kingdom
- **Formula:** Tl
- **Prover:** Lamy and Miarme

SPHERE OF ACTION

- Hair
- Nervous system
- Gastrointestinal system
- Musculoskeletal system

MIND

- Excitable state with weeping and shouting
- Hysteria with hyperaesthesia
- Weeping, tearful mood; starts crying on least provocation
- Shrieking
- Extreme irritability with violence and uneasiness
- Marked anxiety for no reason
- Apathy and depression

MODALITIES

- **Aggravation:** Pressure, touch, contact
- **Amelioration:** From walking

KEYNOTE SYMPTOMS

- Emaciation; very tired, great lassitude
- Endocrinal disorders, especially of the thyroid and adrenalin gland
- Pains neuralgic, shooting, spasmodic and lancinating like electric shocks
- Falling of hair – axillary, pubic, scalp-with great rapidity after acute and exhausting diseases
- Severe, lancinating pains in stomach and bowels, like electric shocks
- Muscular atrophy; tremors, chorea-like movements; rapid movements like convulsions
- Paralysis, trembling of lower limbs; paralytic feeling. Disorders of movement co-ordination
- Peripheral neuritis with most horrible neuralgic, spasmodic pains of tabes dorsalis or locomotor ataxia
- **Numbness and formication beginning in fingers and extending through the pelvis, perineum and inner thighs to the feet**
- Cyanosis of extremities. Dermal trophic lesions
- Great sleeper; has difficulty in falling asleep again
- Discolouration, red stripes on skin after scratching; dryness of skin
- Trophic condition of nails; deformed nails

CONSTITUTION

- For alopecia, following acute, exhausting diseases and horrible neuralgias
- For marked muscular atrophy and paraplegia
- **Temperament:** Bilious, nervous
- **Thermal:** Chilly
- **Miasm:** Syphilis, Sycosis

CLINICAL

- Alopecia
- Emaciation
- Cyanosis
- Neuritis
- Chronic myelitis
- Polyneuritis
- Paralysis
- Tremors
- Locomotor ataxia
- Baldness
- Chronic influenza
- Paraplegia
- Eczema
- Deformed nails
- Night sweats
- Insomnia

REMEDY RELATIONSHIP

- **Compare:** Lath., Caust., Arg-n., Plb., Thal-s.

THEA CHINENSIS

INTRODUCTION
- **Common name:** Tea
- **Family:** *Theaceae*
- **Source:** Vegetable kingdom
- **Part used:** Green leaves
- **Prover:** Roth

SPHERE OF ACTION
- Head
- Gastrointestinal system
- Respiratory system
- Female genital system

CONSTITUTION
- Nervous sleeplessness, heart troubles, palpitations and other complaints of old tea drinkers
- **Temperament:** Nervous, bilious
- **Thermal:** Chilly
- **Miasm:** Psora, Sycosis, Syphilis

MIND
- Nervous excitability with exaltation of intellectual faculties
- **Fear of killing her child; impulse to kill. Is suicidal and homicidal.**
- Dreams of murdering boys and girls in cold blood
- Nervous sleeplessness
- **Horrible dreams cause no horror**
- Homicidal impulses – of jumping out of a window, of putting baby in boiler
- Delirium tremens
- Delirium with ecstasy; laughs incessantly, talks in rhymes; maniacal
- Delusion – time passes too quickly
- Nervousness; want of confidence
- Temporary mental exhalation
- Ill-humoured, peevish

KEYNOTE SYMPTOMS
- Headache with a cold damp feeling at the back of the head
- Sick headaches radiating from one point
- Faint, all gone feeling, with a sinking sensation in the epigastrium; **craves acids, lemons**
- Dyspnoea, nervous sleeplessness, heart problems and dyspepsia of old tea drinkers
- Sudden production of wind in large quantities. Tendency to hernia
- Praecordial distress; palpitations. **Anxious oppression, fluttering especially on left side**
- Pulse – rapid, feeble, irregular, intermittent
- Soreness and tenderness in ovaries

CLINICAL
- Hallucinations
- Delirium
- Delirium tremens
- Neuralgia
- Headache
- Sick headaches
- Dyspepsia
- Hernia
- Diarrhoea
- Constipation
- Haemorrhoids
- Palpitations
- Nervous sleeplessness
- Insomnia

MODALITIES
- **Aggravation:** Night, open air, cold water, walking in open air, after meals
- **Amelioration:** Warm bath, warmth

REMEDY RELATIONSHIP
- **Antidote:** Kali-hp., Thuj., Ferr., Kali-i. (material doses for tea taster's cough)
- **Compare:** Sep., Sulph., Phos., Sabin., Ant-c., Hydr., Ip., Verat.
- **Antidoted by:** Beer

THERIDION CURASSAVICUM

INTRODUCTION

- **Common name:** Orange spider, Black spider of Curacoa
- **Family:** *Agelenidae*
- **Source:** Animal kingdom
- **Part used:** Entire spider
- **Prover:** Hering

SPHERE OF ACTION

- Nervous system
- Gastrointestinal system
- Respiratory system
- Skeletal system
- Female genital system

CONSTITUTION

- For cases of rachitis, caries, necrosis and scrofulous diseases of the bones – it goes to the root of evil and destroys the cause;
- Suits tubercular diathesis with over sensitivity, especially to noise
- **Temperament:** Nervous, bilious
- **Thermal:** Chilly
- **Miasm:** Psora, Sycosis, Syphilis

MIND

- Sensation, as if dying
- **Sounds penetrate through the whole body causing nausea and vertigo. Noises seem to strike painful spots on the body. Every shrill sound penetrates the teeth.**
- Extreme sensitiveness in general, especially to noise. Worse least noises
- Fruitless activity, finds pleasure in nothing; restless
- Confusion of mind, worse laughing
- Sluggishness
- Delusion – time passes too quickly
- Talkative after ingesting liquor or alcohol
- Inclined to be startled
- Want of self-confidence
- Audio and visual hallucinations

KEYNOTE SYMPTOMS

- Must lie down; weakness in the morning with sleepiness
- **Symptoms, especially of head and stomach, worse closing eyes** like vertigo, nausea, vomiting, seasickness, of preganancy, etc.
- Headache – severe, affects the eye, particularly the left one. Sick headache
- Vertigo on closing the eyes, from least noise, with nausea and vomiting
- **Craves bananas and oranges.** Violent burning in liver region with vomiting; abscess of liver.
- Violent stitches high in chest, beneath left shoulder, especially in phthisis
- Hysterical anxiety felt in the region of the heart with pain especially at puberty
- Extreme nervous sensitiveness of puberty, during menses and climacteric
- Spinal irritation; diseases of the spine and other bones. Caries, necrosis and scrofulous diseases of bones have benefitted from this drug
- **Pains in bones all over, as if broken**
- Sensitiveness between vertebrae – sits sideways, avoiding pressure on spine

CLINICAL

- Anxiety
- Panic disorders
- Seasickness
- Neuralgia
- Tetanus
- Vertigo
- Headache
- Toothache
- Liver abscess
- Chronic nasal catarrh
- Ozaena
- Allergy
- Phithisis florida
- Arrhythmia
- Nocturnal emissions
- Insomnia

MODALITIES

- **Aggravation:** Touch, pressure, on shipboard, riding in a carriage, closing the eyes, jar, noise, coitus, left side
- **Amelioration:** Warmth, from rest in horizontal position

REMEDY RELATIONSHIP

- **Follows well:** After, Calc., Lyc., Sulph.
- **Antidoted by:** Acon., mosch., Graph.
- **Compare:** Ars., Cocc., Sep., Nux-v., Iod., Con., Asar., Coff.

THLASPI BURSA PASTORIS

SPHERE OF ACTION
- Mind
- Mucous membranes
- Gastrointestinal system
- Respiratory system
- Urinary system
- Female genital system

INTRODUCTION
- **Common name:** Shepherd's purse
- **Family:** *Cruciferae*
- **Source:** Vegetable kingdom
- **Part used:** Whole plant
- **Prover:** Macfarlan and McGeorge

CONSTITUTION
- Suits gouty and haemorrhagic symptoms in women during menopause
- For effects of suppressed uterine diseases
- **Temperament:** Nervous, bilious
- **Thermal:** Chilly, ambithermal
- **Miasm:** Psora, Sycosis, Syphilis

MIND
- Impulse to walk far
- Nervous restlessness, drives her from place to place
- Causeless weeping, tearful mood with disgust for everything
- Dull and stupefied, as if haven't slept enough

KEYNOTE SYMPTOMS
- **Tendency to haemorrhages – profuse, passive, dark and clotted, from every outlet of the body**
- Craves buttermilk
- **Taste in mouth like bad eggs or bitter, slimy taste with dryness of the mouth**
- In chronic diarrhoea, when there is purely primary affection of bowel
- Abundant muco-purulent discharge from bowels after all faeces have passed
- Bleeding after nasal operations
- Often replaces the use of a catheter
- Urine – burning, passed frequently, has a strong odour. Dysuria and spasmodic retention
- **Brick dust sediment in urine, accumulation of gravel. Urine heavy, phosphatic**
- Albuminuria during pregnancy
- Metrorrhagia with severe colic, with expulsion of clots. Too frequent and copious menses. Scarcely recovers from one period before another begins
- Every alternate menstrual period. Profuse bleeding during menses.
- Leucorrhoea before and after menses; bloody, dark, offensive; stains indelibly, excites itching
- Menses and leucorrhoea leave a fast stain.
- Haemorrhages after miscarriage, abortion or labour; from uterine fibroids
- Sore pain in womb on rising

CLINICAL
- Haemorrhage
- Toothache
- Diarrhoea
- Dysentery
- Epistaxis
- Laryngitis
- Pharyngitis
- Cough
- Tuberculosis
- Chronic cystitis
- Dysuria
- Renal colic
- Renal calculus
- Stranguary
- Haematuria
- Metrorrhagia
- Menorrhagia
- Leucorrhoea
- Uterine fibroids
- Backache

MODALITIES
- **Aggravation:** Towards night, every other month, suppression of vaginal discharges or haemorrhages
- **Amelioration:** Cold bathing, dampness, rapid motion, open air, bending over

REMEDY RELATIONSHIP
- **Compare:** Sin-n., Vib., Ust., Urt-u., Croc., Tril-p., Mill.

THUJA OCCIDENTALIS

INTRODUCTION

- **Common name:** Arbor vitae
- **Family:** *Coniferae*
- **Source:** Vegetable kingdom
- **Part used:** Leaves and twigs
- **Prover:** Hahnemann

SPHERE OF ACTION

- Mind
- Mucous and cutaneous membranes
- Nervous system
- Gastrointestinal system
- Genitourinary system
- Skin

CONSTITUTION

- Hydrogenoid constitution
- For oily, greasy, unhealthy skin, dark complexion and dark hair, fleshy people
- **Temperament:** Bilious
- **Thermal:** Chilly
- **Miasm:** Sycosis

MIND

- **Fixed ideas like, a strange person is by his side, as if something was alive in the abdomen, soul and body are separate**
- He is under the control of a supernatural being
- Music is unbearable, causes weeping and trembling
- Forgetful, loss of memory
- Slowness and sluggishness. Lack of self-esteem and confidence, feelings of worthlessness
- Feels unattractive. Depression. Hiding, secretiveness, deceptiveness, lies
- Fixed ideas, delusions
- Oversensitiveness, especially emotional
- Dreams of falling

KEYNOTE SYMPTOMS

- Left sided remedy
- **Rapid exhaustion and emaciation**
- **For bad effects of vaccinations and suppressed or maltreated gonorrhoea or warts**
- **Periodicity annually or at 3 am and 3 pm**
- Flesh feels as if beaten from the bones
- Tendency to polypi – in nose, ear, uterus, anus, etc.
- Wart-like excrescences or condylomatas on mucous and cutaneous surfaces
- Headache; sensation as if temple was pierced by a nail
- Sensation as if a cold stream of air were flowing out through the eyes
- **Teeth decay at roots; crown remains intact**
- **Tea drinker's dyspepsia and toothache**
- Abdomen distended; gurgling sound; flatus protruding here and there
- **Early morning diarrhoea – as if water expelled from a bung hole**
- Constipation; severe pain in rectum compels patient to cease effort; stool receeds after being partly expelled
- Sensation as if urine trickling in urethra after micturating; violent cutting pain at close of micturation
- Haemorrhoids, cancer of rectum; piles worse when sitting
- Fistula-in-ano, fissure – painful to touch, surrounded by flat warts or moist, mucous condylomata
- Distressing, burning pain in left ovarian region, worse during menses. Coition prevented due to vaginal sensitivity
- **Sensation as if limbs made of glass or wood and would easily break**
- Dirty brown spots on skin; warts large, pedunculated. Eruptions only on covered parts – burn after scratching. Nails brittle and deformed
- **Sweat only on uncovered parts except in head; sweats when asleep only**
- Sweat – oily staining linen yellow, profuse, sour smelling and foetid. **Perspiration smells like honey or sweetish on the genitals**
- Discharges are mucopurulent, copious, foul smelling, acrid and of rancid or sweetish odour

CLINICAL

- Polypi
- Fleshy tumours
- Sarcoma
- Myxoedema
- Headache
- Keratitis
- Styes
- Syphilis iritis
- Ophthalmia
- Tarsal tumours
- Ciliary neuralgia
- Ranula
- Pyorrhoea
- Flatulence
- Hernia
- Diarrhoea
- Constipation
- Piles
- Fissure
- Fistula-in-ano
- Chronic catarrh
- Ozaena
- Asthma
- Pneumonia
- Urethritis
- Suppressed gonorrhoea
- Incontinence of urine
- Arthritis
- Rheumatism
- Warts
- Figwarts
- Condylomata
- Herpes
- Ingrowing toe nails
- Corns
- Cysts
- Eruptions
- Intermittent fever

MODALITIES

- **Aggravation:** At night, from heat of bed, at 3 am and 3 pm, from cold, damp air; narcotics, after gonorrhoea, after vaccinations, after suppressed warts
- **Amelioration:** Motion, pressure, rubbing, warmth, wrapping up, left side, drawing up limbs

REMEDY RELATIONSHIP

- **Compare:** (Hydrogenoid constitution: Calc., Sil., Nat-s., Aran., Apis, Puls.). Cupre-au., Cupre-l., Sil., Maland., Med., Merc., Cinnab., Ter., Juniperus, Sabin., Sil., Canth., Cann-s., Nit-ac., Puls., Cop., Staph., Ant-t.
- **Antidotes:** Merc., Camph., Sabin.
- **Complementary:** Sabin., Ars., Nat-s., Sil., Med., Sab.
- **Follows well:** Med., Merc., Nit-ac.

THYROIDINUM

INTRODUCTION

- **Common name:** Dried thyroid gland of the sheep
- **Group:** Sarcode
- **Source:** Animal kingdom
- **Part used:** Thyroid gland
- **Prover:** Murray

SPHERE OF ACTION

- Metabolism
- Nutrition
- Endocrine system
- Central nervous system
- Eyes
- Heart
- Genitourinary system
- Bones
- Skin

CONSTITUTION

- Suits obese, puffy people with defective metabolism; suffering from myxoedema, cretinism, cachectic debility, anaemia, asthma, goitre, etc.
- **Temperament:** Nervous, bilious
- **Thermal:** Chilly
- **Miasm:** Psora, Sycosis, Syphilis

MIND

- Irritable, sad, depressed
- Homicidal
- Fearful dreams, nightmares
- Dementia, delusions of persecution and suspicion
- Insanity and mania
- Restlessness
- Stupor alternating with restless melancholy
- Worse least opposition. Goes into a rage over trifles
- Fretfulness and moroseness
- Excited state followed by depression

KEYNOTE SYMPTOMS

- Action over the mechanism of the organs of nutrition, growth and development
- Irregular fat deposition, a state of obesity and puffiness is present. Muscular weakness and a flushed face
- Swelling of glands with stony hardness
- Prominent eyeballs – exophthalmos
- **Thick coated tongue. Bad taste in mouth**
- **Desires sweet, salt and cold drinks**
- Dry, painful cough with haemoptysis and scanty, difficult expectoration
- Weak frequent pulse with an inability to lie down – tachycardia. Severe heart pain, palpitations on least excertion. Action of heart weak with numbness of fingers
- Enuresis in weak children who are nervous and irritable. **Urine smells of violets; burning in the urethra, increased uric acid in urine**
- It has increased the flow of milk in nursing women when the flow has been deficient
- Undescended testicles in boys
- Rheumatic arthritis with tendency to obesity, coldness and cramps in extremities. Oedema of legs, cold extremities, trembling of limbs
- Delayed union of fractures or cases where nutrition of bones is affected
- Effective in a great variety of skin cases like psoriasis and eczema. Skin is dry

CLINICAL

- Anaemia
- Emaciation
- Infantile wasting
- Cachexia
- Malaise
- Unconciousness
- Fainting
- Myxoedema
- Goitre
- Cretinism
- Epileptic fits
- Chronic hydrocephalus
- Hairfall
- Prominent eyeballs
- Amblyopia
- Otitis media
- Breathlessness
- Tachycardia
- Enuresis
- Albuminuria
- Premature labour
- Amenorrhoea
- Uterine fibroid
- Deficient milk
- Rickets
- Muscular spasms
- Incomplete paraplegia
- Rheumatoid arthritis
- Psoriasis
- Pityriasis rubra
- Syphilitic eruptions
- Leprosy
- Eczema

MODALITIES

- **Aggravation:** Least exertion, stooping, cold before and during menses
- **Amelioration:** In the evening, rest, lying on abdomen

REMEDY RELATIONSHIP

- **Compare:** Spong., Calc., Fuc., Lycps-v., Thym-gl. extract
- High potencies very efficient in exophthalmic goitre

TRIFOLIUM PRATENSE

INTRODUCTION
- **Common name:** Red clover
- **Family:** *Leguminosae*
- **Source:** Vegetable kingdom
- **Part used:** Flower heads
- **Prover:** Duncan

SPHERE OF ACTION
- Gastrointestinal system
- Respiratory system
- Salivary glands

MIND
- Confused ideas in the morning
- Loss of memory, mental failure
- Stupid, dull feeling in general

MODALITIES
- **Aggravation:** At night, in open air, on waking up, after sleep
- **Amelioration:** Heat, rubbing

KEYNOTE SYMPTOMS
- Congestion – head and lungs feel full of blood. Fullness and congestion of salivary glands. Ptyalism
- Increased salivation, sensation as if mumps were coming on. Mumps with profuse salivation
- **Marked constipation; each stool followed by several drops of black blood attended by a bearing down sensation, as if bowels would collapse**
- Sensation as if were breathing in hot air, or air is full of impurities
- Hoarse and choking; chills with cough at night. Much mucous in throat, constantly trying to clear it
- Cough followed by hiccough; dry, tickling cough, especially on coming out into open air
- Whooping cough with hoarseness and choking
- Stiff neck, cramps in sternocleidomastoid muscles, relieved by heat and rubbing

CONSTITUTION
- Suits a cancerous diathesis
- **Temperament:** Nervous
- **Thermal:** Chilly, ambithermal
- **Miasm:** Psora, Sycosis, Syphilis

CLINICAL
- Cancerous tumours
- Tumour
- Cramps
- Ulceration
- Crusta lactea
- Ptyalism
- Hiccough
- Mumps
- Hoarseness
- Hay fever
- Whooping cough
- Stiff neck
- Tibial ulcers

REMEDY RELATIONSHIP
- **Compare:** Trif-r.
- **Complementary:** Calc-p.

TRILLIUM PENDULUM

INTRODUCTION

- **Common name:** Wake-robin, Birthroot
- **Family:** *Liliaceae*
- **Source:** Vegetable kingdom
- **Part used:** Subterranean part of the plant

SPHERE OF ACTION

- Blood vessels
- Mucous membranes
- Gastrointestinal system
- Respiratory system
- Female genital system

CONSTITUTION

- A haemorrhagic medicine with faintness and dizziness
- **Temperament:** Nervous, bilious
- **Thermal:** Chilly, ambithermal
- **Miasm:** Psora, Sycosis, Syphilis

MIND

- Anxiety during menses or menopause
- Aversion to conversation
- Agitated, keeps tossing about, impossible to keep still
- Mental confusion with sense of duality
- Sad, melancholic

CLINICAL

- Haemorrhage
- Toothache
- Scurvy
- Haematemesis
- Diarrhoea
- Dysentery
- Epistaxis
- Laryngitis
- Pharyngitis
- Cough
- Tuberculosis
- Haemoptysis
- Haematuria
- Uterine fibroids
- Menorrhagia
- Metrorrhagia
- Leucorrhoea
- Backache

KEYNOTE SYMPTOMS

- Haemorrhagic tendency with great faintness and dizziness. **Haemorrhage – active and passive, generally bright red.**
- Haemorrhagic medicine for bleeding from relaxed organs and blood vessels
- Tendency to putrescence of fluids; lochia suddenly becomes sanguinous
- Haemorrhage from gums and after tooth extraction
- **Desire for water or disgust for everything except cold water**
- Haemorrhage due to uterine fibroids, displacements or during pregnancy – ante or post-partum or climateric relaxation of pelvic region
- Phthisis – advanced stage with copious, purulent expectoration and haemoptysis
- **Uterine haemorrhage sensation as though hips and back were falling to pieces,** as if bones of hips, back and thighs were forced apart. **Better by tight bandaging.**
- Menses every 2 weeks, lasting a week and very profuse; flooding with fainting, dim sight, palpitations, noises in the ears, cold extremities and thirst

MODALITIES

- **Aggravation:** Climaxis, over exertion, too long a ride, every two weeks, after eating, motion aggravates haemorrhage
- **Amelioration:** Motion, tight bandage, exertion in open air, sitting erect, bending forward

REMEDY RELATIONSHIP

- **Compare:** Chin., Bell., Kali-c., Mill., Lach., Sep., Sulph., Thlas., Ust. Tril-c., Fic-r.; Sanguis., Ip., Sabin., Ham.
- **Complementary:** Calc-p., in menstrual and haemorrhagic affections

TRITICUM REPENS

SPHERE OF ACTION
- Mind
- Mucous membranes
- Urinary system
- Male genital system

INTRODUCTION
- **Common name:** Couch grass
- **Family:** *Gramineae*
- **Source:** Vegetable kingdom
- **Part used:** Rhizome
- **Prover:** Burnett

CONSTITUTION
- For irritability of the urinary bladder
- **Temperament:** Nervous
- **Thermal:** Chilly
- **Miasm:** Psora, Sycosis, Syphilis

MIND
- Dullness
- Sluggishness
- Forgetful
- Irritability, worse contradiction
- Restless
- Fearful

KEYNOTE SYMPTOMS
- Dysuria, when the ailment is mainly in the urethra
- **Frequent, difficult and painful urination.** Dense urine, causing irritation of mucous surfaces. **Gravelly urine.**
- Urinary infection, incontinence of urine. Irritability of the urinary bladder
- Catarrhal or purulent discharge from the urinary tract

CLINICAL
- Urinary infection
- Cystitis
- Dysuria
- Incontinence of urine
- Strangury
- Pyelitis
- Gonorrhoea
- Enlarged prostate

MODALITIES
- **Aggravation:** Night
- **Amelioration:** Warm bath

REMEDY RELATIONSHIP
- **Compare:** Trad. (haemorrhage from ear and upper air passages; dysuria, urethral discharge; scrotum inflamed); Chim., Senec., Pop., Baros., Uva, Polytr. (dysuria in old people; dropsy, urinary obstruction and suppression)

TROMBIDIUM MUSCAE DOMESTICAE

SPHERE OF ACTION

- Mind
- Mucous membranes
- Teeth
- Gastrointestinal system
- Respiratory system

INTRODUCTION

- **Common name:** Red acarus of the fly
- **Family:** *Acarudea*
- **Source:** Animal kingdom
- **Part used:** Red acarus found under the wing
- **Prover:** Harvey, Head, JFR and Bancroft

CONSTITUTION

- For cases of dysentery, worse by food and drink
- **Temperament:** Nervous, bilious
- **Thermal:** Chilly
- **Miasm:** Psora, Sycosis

MIND

- Disposition to contradict. Inclined to do things by contraries
- Delusion that people are enlarged, especially during vertigo
- Restlessness, must move constantly
- Loquacious, inability to keep quiet
- Inability to collect ideas and co-ordinate them
- Loss of memory
- Disposition to gape

KEYNOTE SYMPTOMS

- **Complaints aggravated by eating or drinking anything, especially symptoms of teeth, nose and tonsils**
- **Toothache – worse in the evening, from reading aloud preventing sleep**
- Griping in the hypochondrium, congestion of liver with urgent stool on rising from bed
- During stool, pain, grippe – most pronounced on the left side of the abdomen, shooting downwards
- Tenesmus with brown, thin, bloody stools
- **Much pain before and after stools. Stools only after eating** – this is characteristic of diarrhoea and dysentery
- Perspiration before stools; prostration, tenesmus, burning in anus after stools
- Cramps in calves and legs after stool
- Profuse watery nasal discharge, worse during dinner
- Skin of scalp and whiskers itchy

CLINICAL

- Dandruff
- Toothache
- Liver congestion
- Hepatitis
- Rectal tenesmus
- Diarrhoea
- Dysentery
- Haemorrhoids
- Anal prolapse
- Coryza
- Sinusitis
- Rheumatism
- Eczema

MODALITIES

- **Aggravation:** Any food or drink, after stools, touch, pressure, movement
- **Amelioration:** Warm drinks improve toothache, open air improves coryza

REMEDY RELATIONSHIP

- **Compare:** Led., Sulph., Culc., Thuj., Nit-ac., Sul-ac., Ign., Podo.
- **Antidoted by:** Staph., Merc-c.

TUBERCULINUM BOVINUM KENT

SPHERE OF ACTION

- Mind
- Mucous membranes
- Gastrointestinal system
- Respiratory system
- Female genital system
- Genitourinary system

INTRODUCTION

- **Common name:** Tuberculosis nosode
- **Group:** Nosode
- **Source:** Animal kingdom
- **Part used:** From tubercular abscess or from a glycerine extract of pure cultivation of human tubercular bacillus
- **Prover:** Nebel

CONSTITUTION

- Suits tubercular people of light complexion, blue eyes, who are blonde, tall, slim, narrow chested, with fine, long eyelashes. They take cold easily
- **Temperament:** Tubercular, scrofulous
- **Thermal:** Chilly
- **Miasm:** Tubercular

MIND

- Discontented, disobedient, destructive, obstinate, restless
- **Romantic, longs for nature, longs to find inner contentment**
- Hyperactivity; has an impulse to run; reckless
- **Desire for a change and to travel**
- Depressed, melancholic, hopeless
- Despondent and morose
- Mania alternating with melancholia
- Insomnia alternating with sopor
- **Fear of animals especially, dogs and cats**
- Disposition to use foul, filthy language; to curse and swear
- Sensitive to music
- Confusion, contradictory behaviour, changeable mood
- Precocious children; whine and complain when spoken to
- Ritualistic, superstitious

KEYNOTE SYMPTOMS

- History of tubercular affections. Takes cold easily, even on the slightest exposure to cold air; susceptible to changes in weather
- Scrofulous diathesis; enlarged glands, adenoids etc.
- Very sensitive, mentally and physically
- **Rapid and profound emaciation while eating well.** Patient is always tired; movement causes intense fatigue.
- **Great weakness with profuse night sweats**
- Symptoms are constantly changing
- **Longs for open air, wants doors and windows open,** or to ride in strong wind; sensation of suffocation, even with plenty of fresh air
- Chronic or recurrent illnesses like diarrhoea, epilepsy, arthritis, boils. Recurring infectious illnesses in childhood.
- Crops of small boils with green, foetid pus
- **Marked craving for smoked meat and fats, cold milk**
- Early morning diarrhoea, especially in children
- Enlarged tonsils and adenoids; tendency to cold which generally ends in diarrhoea
- **Tuberculosis begins in apex of lungs, especially left lung**

CLINICAL

- Autism
- Behavioural disorders
- Compulsive behaviour
- Hyperactivity
- Malignancy
- Lymphoma
- Hodgkin's disease
- Adenopathy
- Paralysis
- Plica polonica
- Alopecia
- Meningitis
- Diarrhoea
- Otorrhoea
- Perforated eardrum
- Colds
- Cough
- Croup
- Pneumonia
- Asthma
- Bronchitis
- Tuberculosis
- Tonsillitis
- Enuresis
- Amenorrhoea
- Dysmenorrhoea
- Arthritis
- Rheumatism
- Eczema
- Ringworm
- Erysipelas
- Erythema
- Acne
- Remittent fever
- Night sweats
- Nightmares

MODALITIES

- **Aggravation:** In a closed room, before a storm, cold damp winds, on waking, early morning, motion, exertion, 10 am to 3 pm, noise
- **Amelioration:** Open air, cool wind, dry mountain air especially pine forests

REMEDY RELATIONSHIP

- **Compare:** Phos., Sep., Sulph., Psor., Lach., Bac., Sil.
- **Complementary:** Bac., Phos., Calc., Chin., Kali-s., Bry.

URANIUM NITRICUM

INTRODUCTION
- **Common name:** Nitrate of uranium, Uranium nitrate
- **Group:** Metal
- **Source:** Mineral kingdom
- **Formula:** $UO_2(NO_3)_2 \cdot 6H_2O$
- **Prover:** Blake

SPHERE OF ACTION
- Mind
- Head
- Mucous membranes
- Gastrointestinal system
- Respiratory system
- Genitourinary system

CONSTITUTION
- For glycosuria, diabetes, with emaciation, debility, flatulence and general dropsy
- **Temperament:** Nervous, bilious
- **Thermal:** Chilly
- **Miasm:** Psora, Sycosis, Syphilis

MIND
- Ailments from grief, sorrow, care
- Anger, irritability
- Ill humour, not feeling well all day
- Sadness, despondency
- Dejection, mental
- Depression, gloom
- Melancholy

KEYNOTE SYMPTOMS
- Great emaciation, debility and tendency to ascites and general dropsy
- Dryness of mucous membranes and skin
- Eyelids agglutinated and inflamed
- **Ravenous appetite.** Boring pain in pyloric region. Gastric and duodenal ulcers, burning pains.
- **Duodenal ulcer better by eating.** Burning, lancinating pains in epigastrium.
- Distension of abdomen; abdomen bloated, after eating, marked flatulence
- Bronchitis with copious mucoid discharge and emaciation; chronic colds
- Causes glycosuria and increased frequency for urination
- Copious urination, diuresis. **Burning in urethra with acidic urine, unable to retain urine without pain.** Incontinence of urine.
- Males completely impotent with nocturnal emissions. Organs cold, relaxed, sweaty

CLINICAL
- Emaciation
- Dropsy
- Styes
- Blepharitis
- Flatulence
- Gastric ulcer
- Duodenal ulcer
- Liver degeneration
- Ascites
- Chronic cold
- Bronchitis
- Hypertension
- Diuresis
- Nephritis
- Enuresis
- Glycosuria
- Diabetes insipidus
- Diabetes mellitus

MODALITIES
- **Aggravation:** Night
- **Amelioration:** Deep breathing

REMEDY RELATIONSHIP
- **Compare:** Syzy., Ph-ac., Phos., Lac-ac., Arg-n., Kali-bi., Ars., Phlor., Thyr.

URTICA URENS

INTRODUCTION
- **Common name:** Stinging nettle
- **Family:** *Urticaceae*
- **Source:** Vegetable kingdom
- **Formula:** Whole plant
- **Prover:** Fiard

SPHERE OF ACTION
- Mucous membranes
- Spleen
- Gastrointestinal system
- Respiratory system
- Sexual system
- Skin

MIND
- Dullness, sluggishness
- Difficulty in thinking and comprehending
- Forgetful
- Irritability, worse contradiction
- Restless
- Fearful

MODALITIES
- **Aggravation:** Cool moist air, touch, cool bathing, annually
- **Amelioration:** On lying down

KEYNOTE SYMPTOMS
- **Symptoms return during the same season every year**
- Profuse discharge from the mucous surfaces
- Haemorrhages from various organs
- Ill-effects of suppressed nettle rash
- **Complaints from eating shellfish**
- Splenic affections. Enlargement of spleen with pain in the left hypochondrium
- Leucorrhoea extremely acrid and excoriating
- Pruritus vulvae, with stinging, itching and oedema of the parts
- Diminished secretion of milk; also to arrest the flow of milk after weaning. Excessive swelling of breasts
- **Rheumatism alternates with urticaria-like symptoms**
- **Gout with rheumatic pain in right deltoid muscle**
- Fever of gout; generally comes on at night
- Acute pain of gout in ankles and wrists
- Itching blotches, especially over fingers and hands. Heat of skin, urticaria with burning, formication and severe itching
- Burns and scalds confined to the skin only

CONSTITUTION
- For gouty and uric acid diathesis; this medicine favours elimination of uric acid
- **Temperament:** Nervous, bilious
- **Thermal:** Chilly, ambithermal
- **Miasm:** Psora, Sycosis, Syphilis

CLINICAL
- Haemorrhages
- Anaemia
- Effusion
- Angio-neurotic oedema
- Enteritis
- Peritonitis
- Splenic affections
- Ascarides
- Pin worms
- Renal colic
- Renal stone
- Calculus – prevention of
- Enuresis
- Lithiasis
- Uraemia
- Agalactia
- Pruritus vulvae
- Gout
- Rheumatism
- Deltoid rheumatism
- Urticaria
- Burns
- Chickenpox
- Bee stings
- Herpes labialis

REMEDY RELATIONSHIP
- **Compare:** Medus., Nat-m., Lac-c., Ric., Bomb-pr., Rhus-t., Apis; Chlol., Astac., Puls., Bol-lu., Anac., Lyc., Hedeo., Form.
- **Antidotal to:** Apis., Mushroom poisoning, serpent and scorpion bites

USTILAGO MAYDIS

INTRODUCTION

- **Common name:** Corn smut
- **Family:** *Ustilaginaceae*
- **Source:** Fungi
- **Part used:** Fungal galls
- **Prover:** Burt

SPHERE OF ACTION

- Mind
- Head
- Mucous membranes
- Musculoskeletal system
- Female genital system
- Male genital system

CONSTITUTION

- For congestion of various parts, in thin, tall women during climacteric with a flabby uterus
- For nervous, old men who have an irresistible tendency for masturbation
- **Temperament:** Nervous, bilious
- **Thermal:** Chilly
- **Miasm:** Psora, Sycosis, Syphilis

MIND

- Amorous disposition
- Irresistable tendency to masturbation; prostrated from sexual abuse and loss of semen
- Likes to remain alone. Seeks solitude; does not want to see or talk to anyone
- Irritability, worse contradiction, on being asked a question or to repeat something
- Fearful
- Very depressed, especially in the afternoon; sad and cries frequently
- Nervousness

KEYNOTE SYMPTOMS

- Haemorrhages; slow, passive or in clots, blood dark but watery; occasionally it forms long, dark, stringy clots
- Malaise, as if has a cold with watery discharge from the nose and eyes
- Languor and faint feeling at 11 am in a warm room
- **Muscular debility – sensation as if boiling water running along the back**
- **Sensation of a knot in the uterus, bowels, throat, etc.**
- Nervous headache from menstrual irregularities
- Loss of hair all over, especially from the head; loss of nails
- Sticky secretions matting the hair – crusta lactea
- Flabby uterus; hypertrophied, prolapsed, subinvolution. Uterine fibroids with haemorrhage
- Profuse menses, especially after a miscarriage; discharge of blood on least provocation; intermenstrual bleeding at menopause; blood bright red, clotted. Menorrhagia during menopause
- Ovaries are swollen, congested, painful, enlarged and have a burning sensation
- Left ovarian or pelvic pains radiates to the legs
- Vicarious menses from lungs and bowels
- Sensitive, spongy cervix, bleeds easily
- Profuse lochia, partly fluid, partly clotted
- Addictive tendency to masturbation in men. Spermatorrhoea with erotic fancies and lascivious dreams; also dull pain in lumbar region
- Tendency to small boils; dry skin

CLINICAL

- Haemorrhagic tendency
- Headache
- Miscarriages
- Bulky uterus
- Uterine fibroids
- Uterine haemorrhage
- Dysmenorrhoea
- Menorrhagia
- Metrorrhagia
- Vicarious menstruation
- Leucorrhoea
- Post-partum haemorrhage
- Cervical erosion
- Ovaritis
- Spermatorrhoea
- Masturbation
- Arthritis
- Lumbago
- Urticaria
- Eczema

MODALITIES

- **Aggravation:** Climacteric, motion, touch, riding aggravates backache
- **Amelioration:** Bandaging, colicky pain in abdomen better by constipation

REMEDY RELATIONSHIP

- **Compare:** Sec., Sabin., Zea-i., Sep., Thlas.

UVA URSI

SPHERE OF ACTION
- Mucous membranes
- Respiratory system
- Urinary system
- Skin

INTRODUCTION
- **Common name:** Bearberry
- **Family:** *Ericaceae*
- **Source:** Vegetable kingdom
- **Part used:** Fresh leaves gathered in autumn
- **Prover:** Noack and Trinks

CONSTITUTION
- For excessive mucous secretion from urinary and bronchial affections
- Suits old people with cystitis
- **Temperament:** Nervous, bilious
- **Thermal:** Chilly
- **Miasm:** Psora, Sycosis, Syphilis

MIND
- Desires death
- Dullness, sluggishness
- Difficulty in thinking and comprehending
- Forgetful
- Irritability, worse contradiction
- Restlessness
- Fearfulness

KEYNOTE SYMPTOMS
- Checks excessive mucous secretion in bronchial and urinary affections
- Hoarseness; tickling in the throat making patient want to cough all the time
- Constant urging and straining to micturate
- Cystitis with bloody urine; slimy, purulent urine; green urine
- Painful micturition with a burning sensation
- **Burning after discharge of slimy urine;** slime passes with blood
- Urine frequent and bloody with much tenacious mucous which can be rolled out of the vessel in large masses
- Chronic vesical irritation with pain, tenderness and catarrhal discharge; with dyspnoea, nausea and vomiting
- **Atony of the uterus causing prolonged labour**
- Uterine haemorrhage
- Urticaria without itching

CLINICAL
- Cyanosis
- Hoarseness
- Cough
- Urinary infection
- Strangury
- Cystitis
- Pyelitis
- Incontinence
- Urinary calculus
- Diabetes
- Uterine haemorrhage
- Menorrhagia
- Metrorrhagia
- Vesicles
- Pustules
- Eczema
- Urticaria

MODALITIES
- **Aggravation:** Open air, cold air
- **Amelioration:** Lying on the back ameliorate bladder symptoms

REMEDY RELATIONSHIP
- **Compare:** Arbutinum, Arctosphylos manzanita, Vaccinum myrtillus – Huckleberries

VACCININUM

INTRODUCTION
- **Common name:** Cowpox vaccine, Vaccinotoxinum
- **Group:** Nosode
- **Source:** Animal kingdom
- **Part used:** Lymph from cowpox vaccination pustule

SPHERE OF ACTION
- Mind
- Mucous membranes
- Eyes
- Gastrointestinal system
- Respiratory system
- Skin

MIND
- Crying, ill-humour, with restless sleep
- Nervous, impatient, irritable, restless
- Child wants to be carried
- Disposition to be troubled by things
- Morbid fear of getting smallpox
- **Confusion, does not remember things at the time they are needed**

MODALITIES
- **Aggravation:** After vaccination, at night
- **Amelioration:** Rest, backache relieved by lying down

KEYNOTE SYMPTOMS
- Ill-effects after vaccination
- Patient is tired and weak with indigestion and flatulence
- **Neuralgias, inveterate skin eruptions, chilliness, whooping cough, indigestion with marked flatulent distention are leading features**
- Neuralgic pain in head; frontal headache; **sensation as if forehead would split into two symmetrical parts**
- Keratitis after vaccinating
- Mouth and tongue dry
- Eruptions like variola. Small red pimples; pustular eruptions all over the body with confusion of mind. Blotches on skin.
- Skin hot and dry

CONSTITUTION
- For a morbid state of extreme chronicity with symptoms like those of sycosis
- **Temperament:** Nervous, bilious
- **Thermal:** Chilly
- **Miasm:** Sycosis

CLINICAL
- Vaccinosis
- Neuralgias
- Alopecia
- Dandruff
- Keratitis
- Indigestion
- Flatulence
- Distension
- Whooping cough
- Skin eruptions
- Acne
- Pimples
- Pustules
- Vesicles
- Leprosy

REMEDY RELATIONSHIP
- **Compare:** Vario., Maland., Thuj., Apis., Sulph., Sil., Ant-t., Dros., Cor-r.

VALERIANA OFFICINALIS

INTRODUCTION

- **Common name:** Valerian
- **Family:** *Valerianaceae*
- **Source:** Vegetable kingdom
- **Part used:** Rhizome-fresh or dried
- **Prover:** Hahnemann

SPHERE OF ACTION

- Mind
- Mucous membranes
- Gastrointestinal system
- Urinary system

MIND

- Hysterical, sensitive, sad, irritable. Persons in whom intellectual faculties predominate
- Oversensitive to all impressions
- Mental and physical dispositions change suddenly. Impulse to move. Restlessness.
- Very mobile ideas, going from one extreme to another
- Hallucinations at night
- **Feels light, as if floating in air**
- **Sudden changeability of symptoms like from highest joy to deepest sorrow**
- Anxious, hypochondriacal feeling as if objects around had been taken away, room appears desolate

MODALITIES

- **Aggravation:** From rest, standing, touch, excitement, fasting, open air, draft
- **Amelioration:** After a meal especially breakfast, after sleep, walking about, changing position, rubbing eases the cramps

KEYNOTE SYMPTOMS

- Nervous, excitable, weak; wriggles or squirms about, inclined to faint
- Red parts become white
- Pain – darting, tearing, come and go, appears suddenly, also jerking and cramping pains
- Pains manifest themselves after resting a long time in one position; better changing position, movement
- Sensation of great coldness in the head
- **Vomiting of coagulated or curdled milk in large lumps, by infants immediately after it was nursed by an irritable mother**
- Hysterical flatulence; hysterical cramps in the abdomen. Greenish, thin, watery, bloody diarrhoea
- **Sensation as if a thread is hanging down the throat**
- Sciatica – worse when standing or letting foot rest on floor; better walking
- Has affinity for tendo-achilles; pain in heels when sitting
- Sleeplessness or disturbed sleep, especially before midnight

CONSTITUTION

- Suits nervous, hysterical, irritable peoples especially women whose intellectual faculties predominate
- Nervous affections in excitable temperaments
- **Temperament:** Nervous, hysterical
- **Thermal:** Chilly
- **Miasm:** Psora, Sycosis, Syphilis

CLINICAL

- Nervousness
- Neuralgia
- Nausea
- Vomiting
- Dyspepsia
- Colic
- Diarrhoea
- Constipation
- Coryza
- Sinusitis
- Rhinitis
- Asthma
- Scanty menses
- Jerking
- Cervical spondylosis
- Cramps
- Sciatica
- Insomnia

REMEDY RELATIONSHIP

- **Compare:** Asaf., Croc., Ign., Lac-c., Spig., Sulph., Castm., Am-val., Zinc-vat.
- For the abuse of Chamomile tea
- **For pains in heels:** Agar., Caust., Cycl., Led., Mang., Phyt.
- **Antidoted by:** Bell., Camph., Coff., Puls., Cina
- **Antidotal to:** Merc.

SPHERE OF ACTION

- Mind
- Gastrointestinal tract
- Liver
- Respiratory system
- Cardiovascular system

INTRODUCTION

Common name: Vanadium
Group: Metal
Source: Mineral kingdom
Formula: V

CONSTITUTION

- For wasting diseases as it is an oxygen carrier and catalyzer
- Acts as a tonic for the digestive system after acute gastroenteric inflammation
- **Temperament:** Nervous
- **Thermal:** Chilly
- **Miasm:** Psora, Sycosis

VANADIUM METALLICUM

MIND

- Depressed; maniacal depression
- Irritability
- Sadness; alternating moods
- Feels guilty for not achieving success; fear of failure
- Excited when successful, depressed by failure
- Hysteria and melancholia
- **Dreams of being late, of futile efforts, of paralysis**

KEYNOTE SYMPTOMS

- It acts as an oxygen carrier and catalyzer. Increases the amount of haemoglobin
- Increases and stimulates phagocytes
- Weakness after exhausting diseases; profound weakness and emaciation
- Wasting diseases. Degenerative conditions of brain, liver and arteries
- Acts as a tonic for digestive functions and in the early stages of tuberculosis; good for nutritional problems and degenerative liver affections
- Disturbed fat and glucose metabolism
- Desire sweets, though digestion is weak
- Deeply pigmented patches on forehead in liver affections
- Dry, irritating, paroxysmal or convulsive cough; occasionally with haemoptysis
- Fatty degeneration of heart and liver
- Arteriosclerosis, hypertension; sensation as if heart was compressed, as if blood had no room in aorta
- Atheroma of arteries of the brain and liver
- Albumin, casts and blood in urine

CLINICAL

- Hysteria
- Debility
- Anaemia
- Raynaud's disease
- Chronic thalassemias
- Tremors
- Malnutrition
- Emaciation
- Cachexia
- Brain softening
- Vertigo
- Eye disorders
- Neuro-retinitis
- Blindness
- Anorexia
- Indigestion
- Liver affections
- Tuberculosis
- Atheroma
- Atherosclerosis
- Hypertension
- Cardiac hypertrophy
- Fatty degeneration
- Rheumatism

MODALITIES

- **Aggravation:** 7 am

REMEDY RELATIONSHIP

- **Compare:** Fatty degenerations, Phos., Ars. Addison's disease, Adren., Tub., Bac.

VARIOLINUM

INTRODUCTION
- **Common name:** Smallpox pustule
- **Group:** Nosode
- **Source:** Animal kingdom
- **Part used:** Prepared from the pus of a smallpox pustule

SPHERE OF ACTION
- Gastrointestinal system
- Respiratory system
- Genitourinary system
- Musculoskeletal system
- Back
- Skin

CONSTITUTION
- Used as a preventive of, or for protection against smallpox
- **Temperament:** Nervous, bilious
- **Thermal:** Chilly
- **Miasm:** Psora, Sycosis, Syphilis

MIND
- Irritability
- Sadness
- Fear of being alone, of death
- Restlessness
- Morbid fear of smallpox
- Delirium with initial fever

KEYNOTE SYMPTOMS
- For a bad effects of vaccinations
- **Acts as a preventive against smallpox.** Covers all cardinal symptoms of smallpox; it modifies and aids its course
- General aching in the muscles, tired all over with restlessness and backache and aching in legs
- Severe chilly creepings, as if cold water trickling down the back
- **Green vision on rising**
- **Tongue protrudes during sleep; thick, dirty yellow coating on tongue; breath horribly offensive**
- Dyspepsia; food seems to regurgitate, especially milk
- Every odour causes nausea, vomiting; deathly nausea, especially during headache. Frequent bilious vomiting with a bad, disgusting taste in the mouth
- Tympanitis, abdomen pouts upwards; patient looks pregnant
- **Sensation of a lump in right side of throat, as if throat is closed**
- Oppressed respiration. Cough with thick, viscid expectoration which may be occasionally bloody
- **Urine – dark coloured, like brandy; offensive; leaves rose tea coloured stains on cloth**
- Excruciating backache. Pain in back muscles as in rheumatism; pain as if back were broken. Pains from back, shift to abdomen.
- A great remedy for herpes, its eruption and pain; also cures the neuralgia left behind by herpes

CLINICAL
- Photophobia
- Gingivitis
- Dyspepsia
- Nausea
- Vomiting
- Constipation
- Deafness
- Cough
- Asthma
- Arthritis
- Rheumatism
- Backache
- Pustules
- Shingles
- Chickenpox
- Smallpox

MODALITIES
- **Aggravation:** Motion, after vaccination
- **Amelioration:** Rest, open air

REMEDY RELATIONSHIP
- **Compare:** Vac. (same action); Maland., Meg., Rhus-t., Ars.
- **Antidoted by:** Thuj., Vac., Sarr., Ant-t., Maland.

VERATRUM ALBUM

INTRODUCTION

- **Common name:** White hellebore
- **Family:** *Liliaceae*
- **Source:** Vegetable kingdom
- **Part used:** Rhizome
- **Prover:** Hahnemann

SPHERE OF ACTION

- Mind
- Blood vessels
- Gastrointestinal system
- Female genital system
- Musculoskeletal system

MIND

- Haughtiness, delirium; delusions, madness, sensitiveness; rude, critical; excessive anxiety and despair
- Cannot bear to be left alone, yet persistently refuses to talk, but uses abusive language on slightest provocation
- **Thinks she is pregnant, will soon deliver a baby. Delusions of impending misfortunes with howling and crying**
- **Delusions of religion and identity. Believes he is Christ, or a saviour, or a prophet;** religious affections. Excessive praying; despair of salvation
- Asks many questions
- Mania with a desire to cut and tear everything, especially clothes
- Livid, lewd, amorous; or lascivious talk; embraces everyone
- Feigns sickness; does not speak the truth
- Gay disposition. Fitful mood.
- **Nymphomania, kisses everybody before menses**
- Tired of life but has fear of dying
- Converses about others faults
- Strong tendency to be frightened; timid; apprehensive

MODALITIES

- **Aggravation:** After drinking, before and during menses, during or after stools; when perspiring, after fright, on exertion, touch, pressure, tobacco chewing
- **Amelioration:** Warmth, covering, hot drinks, walking, lying, children are better when being carried

KEYNOTE SYMPTOMS

- Ailments from disappointment in love, injured pride or honour, suppressed exanthema, opium, tobacco and alcohol
- Perfect picture of collapse with marked coldness, blueness, weakness and a feeble pulse. Rapid sinking of vital force
- Cold sweat on forehead concomitant to all symptoms
- **Icy coldness of various parts** – of face, tip of nose, feet, hands, legs, arms, stomach, abdomen, etc.
- **Sensation of a lump of ice on the vertex.** Neck too weak to hold up head
- Face – pale, blue, collapsed, hippocratic; sunken features
- **Voracious appetite, thirst for cold water in large quantities, but is vomited out as soon as it is swallowed**
- **Craving for acids and refreshing things**
- Copious vomiting and nausea on drinking and least motion
- Simultaneous vomiting and diarrhoea
- Diarrhoea – watery, copious, forcibly evacuated; with vomiting, cold sweat, colic and cramps commencing in hands and feet
- Constipation from inactivity of rectum, passes large, hard, black balls
- Menses too early, profuse, exhausting; dysmenorrhoea, with vomiting or diarrhoea; can barely stand after menses
- Soreness and tenderness in joints; cramps in calves

CONSTITUTION

- **Suited to extremes of life – old people and children**
- For anaemic, lean, choleric, melancholic and sanguine individuals who are habitually cold and deficent in vital reaction
- For cases with a hippocratic face, eyes surrounded by dark circles, cold sweat, pale face, rapid feeble pulse and cold perspiration
- **Temperament:** Sanguine, nervous
- **Thermal:** Chilly
- **Miasm:** Psora, Sycosis

CLINICAL

- Behavioural disorders
- Mania
- Hyperactivity
- Delirium
- Delusions
- Coprophagia
- Schizophrenia
- Restlessness
- Collapse
- Weakness
- Coldness
- Anaemia
- Neuralgia
- Surgical shock
- Seizures
- Raynaud's disease
- Nausea
- Vomiting
- Hiccough
- Gastroenteritis
- Inguinal hernia
- Diarrhoea
- Cholera
- Constipation
- Pneumonia
- Dysmenorrhoea
- Sciatica

REMEDY RELATIONSHIP

- **Compare:** Verin., Cho., Camph., Cupr., Ars., Cupr-ar., Narc-po., Trychs., Agar-em., Agar-ph.
- **After:** Ars., Arn., Chin., Cupr., Ip.; after Camph. in cholera and cholera morbus; after Am-c., Carb-v. and Bov., in dysmenorrhea with vomiting and purging
- **Often removes bad effects of excessive use of alcohol and tobacco**

VERATRUM VIRIDE

INTRODUCTION

- **Common name:** White American hellebore
- **Family:** *Liliaceae*
- **Source:** Vegetable kingdom
- **Part used:** Rhizome
- **Prover:** Burt

SPHERE OF ACTION

- Cerebrospinal system
- Pneumogastric nerve
- Gastrointestinal system
- Respiratory system
- Heart
- Skin

MIND

- Stupefaction, mental confusion
- Loquacity with exhaltation of ideas
- Quarrelsome and delirious; temporary delirium which changes to a happy delirious state
- Marked fear of death
- **Dreams about water**
- Depression

MODALITIES

- **Aggravation:** On rising from bed, going from a hot to a cold place, being uncovered, in winters; after confinement, motion
- **Amelioration:** Rubbing, lying with head low, eating, closing eyes

KEYNOTE SYMPTOMS

- Congestion, congestive states, with sensation of fullness; especially of the base of brain, chest (lungs), spine and stomach
- Suddenness of symptoms like – sudden fainting, prostration, nausea
- Cerebrospinal diseases with spasms, convulsions and cold, clammy, perspiration
- **Effects of sunstroke**
- Thirsty; nausea and vomiting – **smallest amount of food or drink is immediately rejected. Vomiting of thick, glairy, ropy mucous or bile**
- Hiccough excessive and painful with spasms of the oesophagus. Burning in stomach and oesophagus
- Pneumonia with a faint feeling in the stomach; violent congestion of lungs. Difficult breathing; sensation of a heavy load on the chest
- **Pulse soft, slow, weak, irregular and intermittent. Beating of the pulse throughout the body.**
- Urine – scanty with cloudy sediment
- Muscular and articular rheumatism; severe pain in joints
- Chorea – twitching during sleep. Constant jerking or nodding of the head; jerking and trembling threatened with convulsions
- Convulsive twitching; violent, electric shock-like pains in limbs. Constant aching in the back of the neck and shoulders
- Acute rheumatism and fever

CONSTITUTION

- For full blooded, plethoric people having a bloated, livid face
- **Temperament:** Nervous, bilious
- **Thermal:** Chilly
- **Miasm:** Sycosis, Syphilis

CLINICAL

- Furious delirium
- Puerperal basilar mania
- Congestions
- Prostration
- Sunstroke
- Meningitis
- Seizures
- Convulsions
- Chorea
- Tremors
- Apoplexy
- Sick headache
- Hiccough
- Nausea
- Vomiting
- Diaphragmitis
- Oesophagitis
- Gastralgia
- Diarrhoea
- Tenesmus
- Croup
- Pleurisy
- Asthma
- Pneumonia
- Heart affections
- Valvular disease
- Auricular fibrillation
- Membranous dysmenorrhoea
- Acute rheumatism
- Myalgia
- Chilblains
- Erysipelas
- Erythema
- Measles
- Malaria

REMEDY RELATIONSHIP

- **Compare:** Gels., Bapt., Bell., Acon., Ferr-p., Hyos., Sang.
- **Antidotes:** Stry. – fluid extract, 20-40 drops
- **Antidoted by:** Hot coffee

VERBASCUM THAPSUS

INTRODUCTION

- **Common name:** Mullein
- **Family:** *Scrophulariaceae*
- **Source:** Vegetable kingdom
- **Part used:** Whole plant
- **Prover:** Hahnemann

SPHERE OF ACTION

- Mind
- Face
- Ears
- Mucous membranes
- Gastrointestinal system
- Respiratory system
- Urinary system

CONSTITUTION

- For affections of the inferior branch of trigeminal nerve, ear, respiratory tract and bladder; quietens nervous, urinary and bronchial irritation
- **Temperament:** Nervous, bilious
- **Thermal:** Chilly, ambithermal
- **Miasm:** Psora, Sycosis, Syphilis

MIND

- Anxiety during daytime only
- Delusions; sensual imaginations
- Insanity, madness, anxiety with facial neuralgia
- Weakness of memory during vertigo
- Dreams of dead people
- Excessive gaiety with laughter or moroseness, ill-humour and irascibility
- Apathy

KEYNOTE SYMPTOMS

- Has a soothing effect on the entire nervous system; also acts as a soporific
- Cramping, squeezing, crushing, paralysing face-ache in malar bones. **Neuralgia** affecting zygoma, temporo-maxillary joint and ear, **with lachrymation; coryza and sensation as if parts were crushed with tongs**
- Pains of prosopalgia – benumbing, pinching, pressing, stitching, cramping; comes in flashes, occurring periodically and is worse by least movement
- Neuralgia especially affecting left side of face with lachrymation. Stiffness and soreness of joints, especially of lower limbs; cramp-like pains, lower limbs feel heavy
- **Copious accumulation of salt water in the mouth**
- Haemorrhoids with obstructed, hard stools. Inflamed and painful piles
- Earache – pains tearing, lancinating, with sensation of obstruction
- Deafness, especially from getting water in ears. Dry, scaly condition of meatus
- **Voice hoarse, deep, harsh, like a trumpet; cough – especially at night, when sleeping; frequent, dry, hollow, rough cough, which sounds like a trumpet – caused by tickling in the larynx and chest**
- Frequent desire to urinate; constant dribbling. Nocturnal enuresis
- Stiffness and soreness of joints; especially of lower limbs; cramp-like pains; lower limbs feel heavy

CLINICAL

- Neuralgia
- Paralysis
- Trigeminal neuralgia
- Mastoiditis
- Face-ache
- Prosopalgia
- Abdominal grippe
- Haemorrhoids
- Anal itching
- Deafness
- Otalgia
- Acute otitis media
- Cold
- Catarrh
- Hoarseness
- Spasmodic cough
- Chronic cough
- Nocturnal enuresis
- Cervical spondylosis
- Sciatica

MODALITIES

- **Aggravation:** Touch, pressure, change of temperature, cold drafts, stooping, walking, talking
- **Amelioration:** From talking, deep inspiration

REMEDY RELATIONSHIP

- **Compare:** Rhus-a., Caust., Plat., Sphing. (pain in zygoma), Stann., Spong., Sulph., Dros., Cor-r.

VESPA CRABRO

INTRODUCTION
- **Common name:** Live wasp
- **Family:** *Vesparae*
- **Source:** Animal kingdom
- **Part used:** Entire female insect
- **Prover:** Dufreshe

SPHERE OF ACTION
- Vasomotor system
- Mucous membranes
- Gastrointestinal system
- Female genital system
- Male genital system
- Skin

MIND
- Quaking
- Oversensitive to pain
- Feels as if dying or has delusions that he is about to die
- Convulsions with loss of consciousness. Does not answer when spoken to, looks into space. Has no recollection of the attack.
- Insensibility.
- Marked anxiety
- Low spirited

MODALITIES
- **Aggravation:** In a closed room, from a hot stove, after sleep, after eating, on motion
- **Amelioration:** Cold washing of hands

KEYNOTE SYMPTOMS
- Complaints occur periodically and in paroxysms
- Vasomotor symptoms of skin and mucous membranes with intense inflammation characterised by stinging, burning pain, as if pierced with red hot needles
- **Perspiration on parts laid upon, with itching**
- Axillary glands swollen with soreness of upper arms
- Erysipelas inflammation of eyelids with chemosis of conjunctiva
- Nausea and vomiting followed by creeping chills, from feet upwards
- **Left ovary markedly affected with frequent burning micturition** and pain in the sacrum extending upwards
- Menses preceded by depression, pain, pressure and constipation
- Erosion around external os
- Swelling of scrotum and penis
- **Erythema, with intense itching and burning, boils, all relieved by bathing with vinegar**

CONSTITUTION
- For vasomotor symptoms of the skin and mucous membranes, especially in women
- **Temperament:** Nervous, bilious
- **Thermal:** Chilly
- **Miasm:** Sycosis, Syphilis

CLINICAL
- Indurations
- Chemosis
- Conjunctivitis
- Nausea
- Vomiting
- Axillary lymphadenopathy
- Cystitis
- Urethritis
- Cervical erosion
- Cellulitis
- Erythema
- Boils
- Ulcers
- Wheals
- Eczema

REMEDY RELATIONSHIP
- **Compare:** Scorp. (salivation; strabismus; tetanus), Apis., Ars.
- **Antidote:** Semp., locally
- **Antidoted by:** Apis., Led., Camph., Salt water
- **Incompatible:** Arg-n.

VIBURNUM OPULUS

SPHERE OF ACTION
- Mind
- Gastrointestinal system
- Urinary system
- Female genital system

INTRODUCTION
- **Common name:** High cranberry
- **Family:** *Caprifoliaceae*
- **Source:** Vegetable kingdom
- **Part used:** Bark
- **Prover:** Allen

CONSTITUTION
- Suited to tall, slender, hysterical women who suffer from spasmodic and congestive affections of ovarian or uterine origin
- **Temperament:** Nervous, bilious
- **Thermal:** Chilly
- **Miasm:** Psora, Sycosis, Syphilis

MIND
- Confusion, inability to concentrate or perform mental labour
- Stupid feeling, does not know where he is or what to do
- Can't keep still
- Depressed, irritable, wants to be alone
- A great sick feeling all over
- Depression of spirits
- Hysterical
- Forgetful
- Sad

KEYNOTE SYMPTOMS
- Great sick feeling all over with pelvic complaints in hysterical subjects
- Tendency to cramps with all symptoms
- Sudden cramps and colic of abdomen
- **Frequent urging to urinate; passes copious, light coloured urine; cannot hold water on coughing or walking**
- Pelvic complaints, heavy aches or excruciating pains going from back, around to the abdomen, to the pelvis and down the thighs
- Spasmodic and membranous dysmenorrhoea
- Late, scanty menses, lasting only a few hours with cramps extending down the thighs and faintness on attempting to sit up
- **Thick, white, copious leucorrhoea – excoriating, causing smarting and itching of genitals**
- Ovarian region feels heavy and congested. Crampy, colicky pains in both ovarian regions
- Bearing down sensation, with feeling that body from waist downwards would collapse and excruciating pain in the lower abdomen. Super consciousness of internal sexual organs
- Prevents miscarriage when pains are spasmodic or threatening. Frequent miscarriages in the initial months, seeming like sterility
- Cramps and contraction in legs during pregnancy
- False pains preceding labour
- Violent and persistent after pains
- Sacral backache, as if the back would break. Lower limbs feel heavy and weak

CLINICAL
- Hysteria
- Cramps
- Ovaritis
- Leucorrhoea
- Spasmodic dysmenorrhoea
- Threatened abortion
- False labour pains
- Prolonged after pains
- Arthritis
- Rheumatism
- Lumbago

MODALITIES
- **Aggravation:** Lying on affected side, in a warm room, in a closed room, in the evening, at night, motion, sudden jar
- **Amelioration:** Rest, pressure, open air

REMEDY RELATIONSHIP
- **Compare:** Vib-p., Cimic., Caul., Sep., Xan., Sabin., Thlas.
- **Antidoted by:** Acon., Verat.

SPHERE OF ACTION

- Hair
- Blood vessels
- Gastrointestinal system
- Female genital system
- Skin

INTRODUCTION

- **Common name:** Lesser periwinkle
- **Family:** *Apocynaceae*
- **Source:** Vegetable kingdom
- **Part used:** Whole plant
- **Prover:** Rosenburg

CONSTITUTION

- Suits cases of tremulousness and tendency to start, especially on exciting the mind
- A remedy for skin affections, especially of the scalp
- **Temperament:** Nervous, bilious
- **Thermal:** Chilly, ambithermal
- **Miasm:** Psora, Sycosis, Syphilis

MIND

- Weakness and faintness with complaints
- Weakness, as if would die; fear of death
- Sad, lachrymose
- Peevish
- Quarrelsome, but it is soon followed by repentance
- Tendency to start, especially on exerting mentally
- Lascivious dreams

VINCA MINOR

KEYNOTE SYMPTOMS

- Extreme weakness and prostration, as if about to die; desire to stretch
- Eczema spots on scalp, oozing moisture, matting hair together. Corrosive itching of the scalp. Plica polonica; offensive smelling eruptions on the head
- **Hair falls out and is replaced by grey hair or short, wooly hair**
- **Redness of nose from slightest mental emotion**
- Distention of abdomen after stools
- Excessive, profuse, debilitating menses; continuous, like a stream
- Passive, continuous uterine haemorrhages due to fibroids, especially post-climacteric; haemorrhages are followed by great debility
- Marked sensitiveness of skin with redness and soreness, even from the slightest rubbing

CLINICAL

- Weakness
- Trembling
- Haemorrhages
- Plica polonica
- Crusta lactea
- Seborrhoea
- Dandruff
- Alopecia areata
- Vertigo
- Toothache
- Epistaxis
- Diphtheria
- Menorrhagia
- Ulcers
- Acne
- Eczema
- Vesicles

MODALITIES

- **Aggravation:** On stooping, walking, moving, reading, drinking liquids especially beer, swallowing, in open air, anger
- **Amelioration:** Toothache is relieved by warmth of bed

REMEDY RELATIONSHIP

- **Compare:** Olnd., Staph., Med., Mez., Viol-t., Jug-r., Ust., Graph.

VIOLA ODORATA

INTRODUCTION
- **Common name:** Violet
- **Family:** *Violaceae*
- **Source:** Vegetable kingdom
- **Part used:** Whole plant
- **Prover:** Hahnemann, Gross and Stapf

SPHERE OF ACTION
- Eyes
- Ears
- Gastrointestinal system
- Joints
- Urinary system
- Female genital system
- Skin

CONSTITUTION
- Suits dark complexioned people; tall, thin, nervous girls of mild disposition; tuberculous patients
- **Temperament:** Nervous, bilious, lymphatic
- **Thermal:** Chilly
- **Miasm:** Psora, Sycosis, Tubercular

MIND
- Hypochondriasis. Brain fag
- Easy comprehension and clearness of thought
- Emotions are predominated by intellect
- Increased activity of intellect
- Tension-mentally and physically
- Inclined to weep without knowing why
- Disobedient, childish behaviour; refuses to eat
- Sensitive; oversensitive to music, especially violin
- Great nervous debility

KEYNOTE SYMPTOMS
- Tension of the occiput and forehead; extends to upper half of face, upto the nose in front, and the cervical muscles at the back; muscles of the neck feel weak. Tendency to pain immediately above the eyebrows. Burning in the forehead.
- Scalp tense, extending to the face, nose and ears, must knit the brows
- Heat and burning in eyes; fiery appearances in serpentine circles in the field of vision
- **Worm infestation in children; itching in the anus every afternoon; helminthiasis**
- **Ear affections with pain around the orbits**
- Pains in ear shifting, wandering, burning and stretching
- Dyspnoea during pregnancy. Dry, short spasmodic cough with dyspnoea. Pertussis, with hoarseness.
- **Milky urine with a strong smell. Enuresis in nervous children.**
- **Rheumatism, generally right sided with a marked affection for the upper body, especially wrist**
- Pressing pain in right carpal and metacarpal joints. Rheumatism of deltoid muscle
- Yawning and stretching, without sleepiness
- **Dry skin – want of sweat, but has moist palms**

CLINICAL
- Hysteria
- Migraine
- Headache
- Vertigo
- Illusions of vision
- Choroiditis
- Myopia
- Worms
- Otorrhoea
- Deafness
- Hoarseness
- Whooping cough
- Dyspnoea
- Enuresis
- Rheumatism
- Measles

MODALITIES
- **Aggravation:** Cold air, cloudy weather, music, suppressed discharges, bending head backward and forward
- **Amelioration:** Bone pains better rising in the morning

REMEDY RELATIONSHIP
- **Compare:** Ulm., Chen-a., Aur., Puls., Sep., Ign., Cina, Caul.
- **Compatible:** Cor-r., in whooping cough; Cina., in worms
- **Antidoted by:** Camph.

VIOLA TRICOLOR

INTRODUCTION

- **Common name:** Pansy
- **Family:** *Violaceae*
- **Source:** Vegetable kingdom
- **Part used:** Whole plant
- **Prover:** Hahnemann

SPHERE OF ACTION

- Gastrointestinal system
- Respiratory system
- Joints
- Male genital system
- Skin

MIND

- Disobedience; irritability
- Ill-humoured, morosed with dislike of conversation
- Contrary, sadness regarding domestic affairs
- Indifference, apathy
- Nervous paroxysms following suppressed milk crust
- Very vivid, amorous dreams
- Anxiety about the heart on lying down

MODALITIES

- **Aggravation:** Open air, winter, 11 am, lying on non-painful side
- **Amelioration:** Open air improves headache but causes chilliness

KEYNOTE SYMPTOMS

- Nervous paroxysms following suppression of milk crusts
- Alopecia aereata; dandruff; cracked gummy crust on scalp exudating profuse, tenacious, yellow fluid matting hair together; scruf or custa lactea with unbearable burning, especially in children recently weaned
- **Pain in eyes, as if a hard body was present between the upper eyelid and eyeball**
- Face hot, sweats after eating
- Diarrhoea – stools watery, painful, irregular
- Urinary symptoms present as concomitants with skin affections; tinea capitis with frequent, involuntary micturation or eczema with urinary disturbances vis, sudden arrest of micturation or copious micturation
- Swallowing difficult, painful, causing hawking
- **Urine smells like cat's urine**
- Involuntary seminal emissions with vivid dreams; or at stool. Swelling of prepuce with itching, especially when standing; burning in glans
- Articular rheumatism with itching around joints
- **Eczema – impetigo, dry scabs all over when scratched, they exude a yellow water or pus which hardens into a gum-like substance**
- Eczema impetigoides of the face

CONSTITUTION

- Face hot, sweaty after eating
- For eczema of childhood
- **Temperament:** Nervous
- **Thermal:** Chilly
- **Miasm:** Sycosis

CLINICAL

- Milk crust
- Crusta lactea
- Conjunctivitis
- Flatulence
- Dyspnoea
- Pulmonary tuberculosis
- Infantile asthma
- Cystitis
- Urethritis
- Nocturnal emissions
- Arthritis
- Rheumatism
- Acne
- Tinea capitis
- Eczema
- Impetigo

REMEDY RELATIONSHIP

- **Compare:** Rhus-t., Calc., Sep., Viol-o., Lyc., Cham., Graph., Hep., Merc., Petr., Staph.
- **Compatible:** Puls., Rhus-t., Sep., Staph.
- **Antidoted by:** Merc., Camph., Puls., Rhus-t.

VIPERA BERUS

INTRODUCTION

- **Common name:** German viper, Common viper, European adder
- **Family:** *Ophidia*
- **Source:** Animal kingdom
- **Part used:** Venom
- **Prover:** Jahr

SPHERE OF ACTION

- Veins
- Gastrointestinal system
- Genitourinary system
- Skin

MIND

- **Suspicious**
- Jealous
- Irritability, worse contradiction
- Depressed
- Anxiety when alone

MODALITIES

- **Aggravation:** Cold touch, pressure, change of weather, letting affected parts hang down
- **Amelioration:** Elevating the affected part

KEYNOTE SYMPTOMS

- Haemorrhage; flow red, with clots, excessive; leading to prostration and faintness, especially at climacteric from the uterus
- Sensitive to change of weather, hot weather
- **Tongue dry, brown-black, swollen, protruding, with difficult speech**
- Violent pain in enlarged liver, with jaundice and fever; pain extends to shoulder, hip
- A remedy for all forms of epistaxis
- Inflammation of veins with marked swelling. **Varicose veins of legs, worse hanging legs down, feels as if they would burst with fullness, the pain is unbearable; better by elevating the feet.**
- Area around the varicose vein is inflamed and sensitive
- Severe cramps in lower extremities
- Boils, carbuncles, ulcers, gangrene, with bursting sensation; relieved by elevating parts

CONSTITUTION

- **For people who become prematurely old or for children whose development is arrested**
- For complaints of women at menopause
- **Temperament:** Nervous
- **Thermal:** Hot
- **Miasm:** Syphilis

CLINICAL

- Neurasthenia
- Polyneuritis
- Lymphangioma
- Haemorrhages
- Goitre
- Phlebitis
- Varicose veins
- Thrombosis
- Cancer
- Cramps
- Hepatomegaly
- Jaundice
- Epistaxis
- Haematuria
- Oligospermia
- Sterility
- Ulcers
- Boils
- Carbuncles

REMEDY RELATIONSHIP

- **Compare:** Sanguis. for haemorrhage of fluid blood, also Calc., Alumn., Am-c., Thuj., Sabin.

VISCUM ALBUM

INTRODUCTION

- **Common name:** Mistletoe
- **Family:** *Loranthaceae*
- **Source:** Vegetable kingdom
- **Part used:** Fresh leaves and berries
- **Prover:** Huber

SPHERE OF ACTION

- Gastrointestinal system
- Respiratory system
- Heart
- Musculoskeletal system
- Female genital system
- Skin

MIND

- Incoherent talk and spectral illusions
- Depressed mood, sadness, apathy, lack of optimism
- **Sensation of formication, as if a spider is crawling over the back of hand and foot**
- Delusion body is lighter than air; stupor, insensibility
- Feels as if in a dream
- Frightful thoughts on waking at night
- Fear of telephone, sensitive to noise
- Persistent thoughts, dwells on past disagreeable occurences
- Restless, nervous, impatient
- Cannot carry out intellectual activities

MODALITIES

- **Aggravation:** By least movement, in winters, from cold, on becoming chilled, suppression of menses
- **Amelioration:** Resting quietly, from counter pressure, walking in fresh air

KEYNOTE SYMPTOMS

- Sudden onset of complaints
- **Chilly even when near the stove**
- Vertigo – sudden onset, persistent sensation as if the whole skull were lifted up
- **Epilepsy, felt an aura – a glow that rose up from the feet to the head; patient seems to be on fire**
- Alimentary tract paralysed; feels as if someone is dragging her down from the waist, and immediately after that it feels as if the upper part of the body is floating in air
- **Feeling of suffocation when lying on the right side.** Dyspnoea, asthma connected with gout or rheumatism
- Valvular disease with affections of the sexual system
- Hypertrophy of heart with valvular insufficiency. Palpitation during coitus in males
- Uterine haemorrhage or profuse menses; blood partly bright and partly clotted and dark. Complaints during climacteric
- **Sharp pains in ovarian region, especially left side**
- Spinal irritation due to uterine disease
- General tremors, as if all the muscles are in fibrillatory contraction; jerking and twitching of muscles
- **Shooting, tearing pains in both thighs and upper extremities**
- Weakness especially of legs, dropsy of extremities; compressing pain in feet
- **General itching and tingling with no apparent cause is better by sweating**

CONSTITUTION

- For rheumatic and gouty complaints with neuralgia
- For slow, small and weak pulse with low tension and valvular insufficiency with affections of the sexual sphere
- **Temperament:** Nervous, bilious
- **Thermal:** Chilly
- **Miasm:** Psora, Sycosis, Syphilis

CLINICAL

- Chorea
- Vertigo
- Epilepsy
- Deafness
- Asthma
- Dyspnoea
- Valvular heart disease
- Hypertension
- Sensitive sexual organs
- Menorrhagia
- Metrorrhagia
- Dysmenorrhea
- Retained placenta
- Chronic endometritis
- Ovaralgia
- Rheumatism
- Sciatica
- Wounds

REMEDY RELATIONSHIP

- **Compare:** Sec., Conv., Bry., Puls., Rhod., Guips., Hed.
- **Follows well:** Acon. in rheumatism
- **Antidoted by:** Camph., Chin.

X-RAY

INTRODUCTION
- **Common name:** X-ray, Roentgen ray
- **Source:** Imponderabilia
- **Part used:** Dilutions are made from absolute alcohol irritated with x-rays through a glass bottle
- **Prover:** Fincke

SPHERE OF ACTION
- Blood
- Gastrointestinal system
- Female genital system
- Male genital system
- Musculoskeletal system
- Skin

CONSTITUTION
- **Suits weak, debilitated people who have had repeated exposures to x-rays producing skin lesions, often followed by cancer.** They suffer from distressing pains and affections of sexual glands.
- For bringing to surface suppressed symptoms
- **Temperament:** Tubercular
- **Thermal:** Chilly, ambithermal
- **Miasm:** Psora, Syphilis, Sycosis

MIND
- Irritable
- Desires to be alone, aversion to company
- Mental condition upset during profuse menstruation
- Dreams livid, lewd, especially in men
- Sexual desire lost due to anxiety
- Stimulates vitality, mentally and physically
- Gloomy, sad
- Suspicious
- Jealous
- Mental processes not clear, writes wrong words

KEYNOTE SYMPTOMS
- For ailments from repeated exposure to X-rays – either for therapeutic purpose or a history of radium therapy; changes take place in blood, lymphatics and bone marrow
- Patient is generally tired and feels sick. Feels lame and sore all over with trembling
- Organic changes leading to a stage of incurability
- Retardation of growth, both physical and mental
- Malignant and cancerous affections of the body
- **Sticking pain in different parts of the head and face. Dull pain in right upper jaw**
- **Pain in muscles of neck – gets sudden 'cricks', first on one side, then on the other, worse behind the ear**
- **Tongue dry, rough, sore and scraped**
- Complete loss of appetite. Nausea, aversion to meals
- Sensation of fullness in ear, ringing in the ears
- Pain in throat on swallowing
- Lost sexual desire in men, testes relaxed; oligospermia
- Atrophy of ovaries and testicles
- **Right sided sciatica;** rheumatoid arthritis
- For stubborn burns which refuse to heal
- Palms and sole are rough and scaly. Painful cracks, warty growths, thick nails.
- Skin is dry, wrinkled; dry itching eczema
- Sleeplessness. Drowsy while sitting all night, but the moment he lies down, drowsiness goes away and cannot sleep. Sleepy during the day

CLINICAL
- Fatigue
- Weakness
- Anaemia
- Leukaemia
- Cancer
- Alopecia
- Hairfall
- Atrophied ovaries/testicle
- Sterility
- Oligospermia
- Impotency
- Relaxed testicles
- Rheumatoid arthritis
- Psoriasis
- Eczema
- Non-healing ulcers
- Wounds
- Burns
- Fistulae
- Sinuses
- Corns
- Warty growths
- Ganglion
- Sleeplessness

MODALITIES
- **Aggravation:** In the afternoon, evening, at night, in bed, from movement
- **Amelioration:** Hot application

REMEDY RELATIONSHIP
- **Compare:** Cadm-s., Carc., Elec., M-arct., M-aust., M-ambo., Sec., Phos., Merc.

SPHERE OF ACTION

- Nervous system
- Mucous membranes
- Gastrointestinal system
- Respiratory system
- Female genital system

INTRODUCTION

- **Common name:** Prickly ash
- **Family:** *Rutaceae*
- **Source:** Vegetable kingdom
- **Part used:** Fresh bark
- **Prover:** Cullis

CONSTITUTION

- Especially for women of spare habit, nervous temperament and delicate organization
- Neurasthenic patients who are thin, emaciated, having poor assimilation of food with insomnia and occipital headache
- **Temperament:** Haemorrhagic, nervous
- **Thermal:** Ambithermal
- **Miasm:** Sycotic

XANTHOXYLUM FRAXINEUM

MIND

- Nervous, easily startled, hysterical
- Depression with a frightful feeling. Does not care if he is living or dead
- Delusion, is about to die; is going into decline
- Hysteria during amenorrhoea
- Indifference to life
- Dreams of flying

KEYNOTE SYMPTOMS

- Neurasthenic women who are thin, emaciated, have poor assimilation with insomnia and occipital headache
- Grinding, shooting, radiating, sudden pains or neuralgias – as if from electricity, all over the limbs
- Indigestion from overeating or from too much fluid. Dyspepsia, flatulence with dizziness and sick headache
- Chronic obstinate cough, coryza; cough dry – day and night
- **Menses – too early, too painful, thick, almost black;** menorrhagia
- Neuralgic dysmenorrhoea with violent, grinding, agonising pain in the back and down the legs; also neuralgic headache
- Leucorrhoea with amenorrhoea that is, **leucorrhoea at the time of menses**
- **Left ovarian neuralgia extending down the thighs, along the genito-crural nerves**
- For cancerous cysts removed surgically in women
- Affects the nervous system causing paralysing symptoms, especially hemiplegia. **Sciatica, worse hot weather**
- **Spinal disorders followed by paralysis, especially of the left side.** Numbness, left sided with impairment of motor nerves.
- Sleeplessness in neurasthenics. Sleep hard and unrefreshing

CLINICAL

- Neurasthenia
- Poor assimilation
- Haemorrhages
- Paralysis
- Hemiplegia
- Occipital headache
- Indigestion
- Tympanites
- Dysentery
- Aphonia
- Chronic obstinate cough
- Neuralgic dysmenorrhoea
- Menorrhagia
- After pains
- Leucorrhoea
- Sciatica
- Insomnia

MODALITIES

- **Aggravation:** 4 am, in the morning, from sleeping, dampness, moving head suddenly, getting feet wet
- **Amelioration:** Vomiting, drinking ice cold water, lying down, neck pain is better on pressure

REMEDY RELATIONSHIP

- **Compare:** Graph. Staph., Cimic., Mez., Pisc.

SPHERE OF ACTION

- Eyes
- Gastrointestinal system
- Musculoskeletal system
- Female genital system
- Skin

INTRODUCTION

- **Common name:** Tamalpais lily, Basket grass flower
- **Family:** *Melanthiaceae*
- **Source:** Vegetable kingdom

CONSTITUTION

- Suits dull, young girls who have difficulty concentrating on studies
- **Temperament:** Nervous
- **Thermal:** Chilly
- **Miasm:** Sycosis

MIND

- Forgetfulness, forgets names
- Misspells common words; writes last letters of word first
- Difficulty in concentrating on studies
- Dull
- Bewildered

XEROPHYLLUM TENAX

CLINICAL

- Brain fag
- Examination funk
- Headache
- Migraine
- Photophobia
- Conjunctivitis
- Ovaritis
- Vulvitis
- Menorrhagia
- Metrorrhagia
- Nymphomania
- Early typhoid state
- Eczematous condition
- Dermatitis
- Erythema
- Impotence

KEYNOTE SYMPTOMS

- Head feels stuffed up, pain across forehead and over eyes. Bewildered feeling; loss of consciousness
- Eyes feel sore and burn. Difficult to focus for close work
- In morning, rumbling of abdomen with desire for stools
- Increased sexual desire with ovarian and uterine symptoms in women
- **Back – feels hot from sacrum to scapulae**
- **Backache extending down the legs**
- Limbs feel stiff. Muscular lameness, trembling
- Erythema with vesication, intense itching, stinging and burning of skin
- Inflammation of skin resembling poison oak. Urticaria, eczematous eruption
- **Skin rough and cracked; feels like leather**

MODALITIES

- **Amelioration:** Application of cold water, afternoon, evening
- **Aggravation:** Application of hot water, moving affected part, morning

REMEDY RELATIONSHIP

- **Compare:** Rhus-t., Anac., Grind.

YOHIMBINUM

SPHERE OF ACTION
- Central nervous system
- Gastrointestinal system
- Female genital system
- Male genital system

INTRODUCTION
- **Common name:** Coryanthe yohimbe, Yohimbe
- **Family:** *Rubiaceae*
- **Source:** Vegetable kingdom
- **Part used:** Bark

CONSTITUTION
- For anaemic, thin, nervous, partly impotent men
- **Temperament:** Nervous
- **Thermal:** Ambithermal
- **Miasm:** Sycosis

MIND
- Sexual stimulant
- Irritability
- Desires company
- Insomnia due to thoughts of whole past life
- Brooding
- Sensitive
- Marked agitation with trembling

KEYNOTE SYMPTOMS
- Excites the central nervous system
- Agitation, with flying sensation of heat in face
- Contraindicated in acute and chronic conditions of inflammation of abdominal organs
- Hyperaemia of milk glands, stimulates the function of lactation
- Congestive conditions of the sexual organs. Menorrhagia – menses early, profuse, with exhaustion
- **Strong and lasting erections or neurasthenic impotence**
- **Fever – intense waves of heat with chilliness**
- **Sleeplessness, thoughts or events of whole past life keep him awake**

CLINICAL
- Neurasthenia
- Aphrodisiac
- Intestinal haemorrhage
- Bleeding piles
- Urethritis
- Improves lactation
- Metrorrhagia
- Menorrhagia
- Impotence
- Insomnia

MODALITIES
- **Aggravation:** Sexual excitement, during stool, at night
- **Amelioration:** Sleep

REMEDY RELATIONSHIP
- **Compare:** Canth., Graph., Phos., Pic-ac.

ZINCUM METALLICUM

SPHERE OF ACTION
- Mind
- Eye
- Mucous membranes
- Nervous system
- Gastrointestinal system
- Respiratory system
- Urinary system
- Sexual system

INTRODUCTION
- **Common name:** Zinc
- **Group:** Metal
- **Source:** Mineral kingdom
- **Formula:** Zn
- **Prover:** Hahnemann

CONSTITUTION
- Suits people who have nerve affections and are anaemic
- For sensitive, melancholic, lethargic, stupid people
- **Temperament:** Nervous
- **Thermal:** Chilly
- **Miasm:** Syphilis

MIND
- Very sensitive to noise
- Aversion to work and talk
- **Child repeats everything said to it**
- Melancholia; cerebral depression; sad when alone; depressed when sick
- Nervous exhaustion and defective vitality runs through; lethargic, stupid
- Slow weak tired; memory weak, comprehension slow; brain fag
- Ill effects of fright, grief, anger. Chorea from fright
- Anxiety and fear of theives
- Changeable moods. Weeps when angry
- Irritable in the evening
- Hysteria or causeless weeping before menses

KEYNOTE SYMPTOMS
- Ailments from suppressed discharges and eruptions; great relief from discharges
- Want of brain and nerve power; defective vitality; severe anaemia with marked prostration and restlessness; worse eating
- **Chronic affections with brain and spinal affections like twitching, jerking, trembling and fidgety feet**
- Convulsion, chorea, paralysis and vertigo from suppressed sweat or eruptions
- Conjunctivitis; conjunctiva, especially inner canthus red and inflamed
- Brain affections from sudden stoppage of diarrhoea
- Atonic dyspepsia, globus hystericum; least quantity of wine cannot be tolerated – causes headache
- Hasty eating and drinking or **greediness while eating or drinking**
- **Feels better after menses.** Violent pain in ovaries, uterus with excitement, hysteria and cannot keep still
- Large varicose veins on the legs; soles are sensitive
- **Spine sensitive, cannot bear to be touched, burning along the spine**
- Violent fidgety feeling in feet and lower extremities, must move them constantly. Stumbling, spastic gait
- Eruptions from fright. Itching in the hollow of knees, itching here and there
- **Cannot bear covering during sweat; sweat, offensive and sour smelling**

CLINICAL
- Alcoholism
- Brain fag
- Confusion
- Fidgety
- Brain affections
- Convulsions
- Chorea
- Epilepsy
- Nerve weakness
- Spinal irritation
- Debility
- Anaemia
- Meningitis
- Hydrocephalus
- Headache
- Hemicrania
- Squinting
- Photophobia
- Gastric disorders
- Spasm of oesophagus
- Gastralgia
- Diarrhoea
- Dysentery
- Cholera
- Hiccoughs
- Hepatomegaly
- Dry cough
- Dyspnoea
- Restless legs
- Varicose veins
- Eczema
- Suppressed eruptions
- Chilblains

MODALITIES
- **Aggravation:** Wine, milk, suppressed menses or discharges being heated, from noise
- **Amelioration:** Motion, with the menstrual flow, hard pressure, free discharges, appearance of eruptions, warmth, open air, scratching, rubbing eating while, free discharges

REMEDY RELATIONSHIP
- **Compare:** Agar., Cupr., Nux-v., Rhus-t., Stram., Ign., Sep., Kali-c., Bell., Puls., Lyc., Plb.,
- **Followed by:** Ign, Nux-v
- **Complementary:** Puls., Sulph., Calc-p.
- **Follows well:** Apis, Bell.
- **Incompatible:** Cham., Nux-v.
- **Antidoted by:** Camph., Ign., Hep.

Zincum metallicum

ZINGIBER OFFICINALE

INTRODUCTION

- **Common name:** Ginger
- **Family:** *Zingiberaceae*
- **Source:** Vegetable kingdom
- **Part used:** Dried rhizome
- **Prover:** Franz, Stapf and Bute

SPHERE OF ACTION

- Mind
- Head
- Mucous membranes
- Gastrointestinal system
- Respiratory system
- Genitourinary system

MIND

- Cheerful
- Good humoured, especially when the opposite state of mind is expected
- Irritability, especially in the evening, during menses
- **Dreams of churches**
- Excited
- Mental anxiety
- Forgetful, weak memory
- Nervous and fidgety

MODALITIES

- **Aggravation:** Touch, lying, motion, rising, laughing and talking, headache, evening and night, in cold air, cold damp air, from bread, from melons
- **Amelioration:** Sitting, standing, uncovering

KEYNOTE SYMPTOMS

- State of debility in the digestive system, sexual system and respiratory system
- **Head – sensation as if it is too large;** congestion of blood to head, especially temples
- Sensation as if contents of head passed into forehead and nose on stooping
- Hemicrania, sudden glimmering before eyes; violent, neuralgic, intermittent headache – becomes insane with pain
- **Ailments from eating melons, bread and drinking impure water; food and water poisoning**
- **Taste of food remains for long, especially of bread and toast**
- Nasal mucous membrane affected – ozaena and post-nasal discharge
- Asthma of gastric origin; breathing difficult; patient must sit up to breathe, but despite the severity of paroxysm there is anxiety. Asthma without anxiety
- Prolonged retention of urine or complete cessation of kidney function
- **Dull aching in both kidneys with frequent desire to urinate**

CONSTITUTION

- For a debilitated state of the digestive tract, sexual organs and respiratory system
- For complete cessation of function of kidneys
- Complaints from eating melons and drinking impure water
- **Temperament:** Anxious
- **Thermal:** Chilly
- **Miasm:** Psora

CLINICAL

- Headache
- Hemicrania
- Food poisoning
- Indigestion
- Flatulence
- Hepatitis
- Diarrhoea
- Dysentery
- Haemorrhoids
- Ozaena
- Post-nasal discharge
- Hoarseness
- Asthma
- Urine suppressed
- Acute renal failure
- Albuminuria
- Bright's disease
- Typhoid

REMEDY RELATIONSHIP

- **Compare:** Calad., Ars., Chin., Sulph., Nux-v.
- **Antidoted by:** Nux-v.

ORIGIN OF HOMOEOPATHY

THE FOUNDER OF HOMOEOPATHY: CHRISTIAN FREDRICH GOTTFRIED SAMUEL HAHNEMANN

10th April 1755	Birth of **Samuel Hahnemann in Meissen**, a little town in the state of Saxony in Germany. Third child of Christian Gottfried, a porcelain-painter in a porcelain factory.
20th July 1767-1770	Primary education was completed in Town school of Meissen and Prince school. He was a brilliant, hardworking student and took much interest in, Botany, Mathematics, Geometry and study of languages, had command over Greek, Latin, English, French, German, Hebrew, Spanish, Arabic, Polish, Siberian, Syriac. He had his own herbarium.
1775	*"The wonderful construction of human hand"* was a famous school leaving speech, delivered by Hahnemann. Higher education was completed in Leipsic university. In Vienna, got attached to a famous hospital of Brother of Mercy. Where he became the favourite pupil of Dr Von Quarin renowed physician of his time.
1779	24 year old Hahnemann got his M.D degree from the university of Erlangen on his thesis *"A consideration of the aetiology and therapeutics of spasmodic affection"*. He also translated few books from English to Germany.
17th November 1781	Hahnemann got married to **Johanna Leopoldine Henriette Kuechler,** step daughter of a chemist in Dessau Herr (Mr) Haesseler. He worked as a Medical officer of health at Gommern. *"The Wholesome manufacture of the chemical or the science of preparing chemical products in factories"* 2 volumes made him a famous translator.
1783	Hahnemann and Johanna Henriette Kuchler, both were proud parents of eleven children. 1st son **HENRIETTE** born in Gommern in 1783. 2nd **FRIEDRICH** born at Dresden in Nov 30, 1786. 3rd **WILHELMINE** born at Dresden in 1788. 4th **AMALIE** married to Dr Leopold Suss. 5th **CAROLINE** died unmarried. 6th &7th Twins **FREDERIKA**, married clothing Inspector Dellbruck in Stotteritz. 8th **ERNST** born at Konigslutter in 1798. 9th **ELEONORE**, married to Herrklemmen afterward to Dr Wolff. 10TH **CHARLOTTE** born at Leipsic.
1789	Hahnemann's first volume of *"Friend of Health"* was published.
1790	Hahnemann while translating *"A Treatise on materia medica"* by Dr William Cullen, came across a passage about Peruvian bark, or Cinchona where Cullen stated that quinine which is a substance purified from the bark of the cinchona tree was good for treatment of malaria. So, Hahnemann decided to investigate further.
1796	Hahnemann discovered a new system of medicine in which a drug that produces similar symptoms to a disease which cancel each other in some way, thereby restoring the patient to health. He described this phenomenon as *"SIMILIA SIMILIBUS CURENTUR"*, or *"LIKE CURES LIKE"*
1797	Law of simplex.
1805	Hahnemann's *"Medicine of Experience"* was published.
1810	Bible of homoeopathy, *"Organon of the Rational art of Healing"*.

1811-1821	Hahnemann's eight volumes of *"Materia Medica Pura"* were published.
1828	Hahnemann's *"Chronic disease"* was published.
1829	Lesser writings.
18th Jan 1835	Hahnemann got married second time to a young french lady **Madame Melanie D. Hervilly,** 45 years younger to him, and moved to Paris.
2nd July 1843	Death of Samuel Christian Gottfried Hahnemann in Paris, on his tomb words were written -----*"Non inutilis vixi"*------ it means *"I have not lived in vain"*.

PREPARATION OF HOMOEOPATHIC REMEDIES

SOURCE

1. Vegetable kingdom: e.g Aconite, Allium cepa, Nux vomica
2. Animal kingdom: e.g Cantharis, Tarentula, Naja, Sepia
3. Mineral kingdom: e.g Petroleum, Carbo veg, Argentum nitricum
4. Nosodes: Psorinum, Pyrogenum, Syphilinum, Tuberculinum
5. Sarcodes: Thyroidinum, Insulinum, Adrenalin, Cholesterinum
6. Imponderabilia: Radium, X-Ray, Electricity

PREPARATION

Homoeopathic drugs from plants and animals:

Step 1	Plant materials such as leaves, roots and flower heads, whole plants are chopped finely and dissolved in water.
Step 2	Dissolved mixture is put in a large glass vessel, to it is added 90% alcohol and 10% water.
Step 3	Mixture of chopped plant, alcohol and water is stored for several days, weeks, a month.
Step 4	Stored macerated mixture is filtered and only liquid part is extracted from it which is called 'mother tincture', it is then stored in a dark glass bottle.
Step 5	One drop of mother tincture is diluted with a mixture of water and alcohol and succussed. Most commonly used scales are decimal and centesimal. To produce 1C potency, one drop of mother tincture is added to 99 drops of alcohol and water mixture. 2C potency is prepared with one drop of 1C mixture added to 99 drops of alcohol and water mixture and succussed.
Step 6	Once the mixture reaches the required strength and potency, few drops of it is added to globules or lactose sugar or granules or powder which is dispensed to the patient in a glass vial.
Step 7	Radium brom and X-ray drugs are prepared by exposing rays of ultra sound and x-ray to a vial containing alcohol, and then potentised.

DIFFERENT METHODS OF HOMOEOPATHIC DRUG ADMINISTRATION

1	Oral methods	By mouth: 1. Syrups, 2. Elixirs, 3. Mixtures, 4. Emulsions, 5. Powders, 6. Capsules 7. Pills
2	Parenteral method	Injection: 1. Subcutaneous, 2. Intramuscular, 3. Intravenous, 4. Intrathecal, 5. Bone marrow injection, 6. Intraperitoneal
3	Mucosal absorption method	1. Rectal absorption in the form of supposition, 2. Nasal septum: Inhalation
4	Skin absorption method	1. Ointment, 2. Liniment, 3. Lotion

CLINICAL CASE HISTORY

1	Introduction of the patient	Name, Age, Sex, Address, Occupation, Income, Marital status, Phone number
2	Personal history	Appetite, Desire, Aversion, Thirst, Urine, Stool, Perspiration, Menstrual history
3	Past medical and surgical history	Hypertension, Jaundice, Epilepsy, Rheumatic fever, Tuberculosis, Diabetes mellitus, Operation major or minor
4	Drugs	Drug details, Allergy to drug
5	Smoking/alcohol consumption	Past and present history
6	Social and family history	Marital status, Social circumstances, Health of all family members, Death, Illness.
7	Vital data	Pulse, Blood pressure, Respiratory rate, Temperature
8	Systemic enquiry	Inspection, Palpation, Percussion and Auscultation of the system affected
1	CVS:	Chest pain
		Angina pectoris
		Breathlessness
		Palpitation
		Hypertension
		Ankle swelling
2	RS:	Cough
		Breathlessness
		Haemoptysis
		Night sweat
		Wheezing
		Rales, Rhonchi
3	GIT:	Weight
		Appetite
		Dysphagia
		Dyspepsia
		Abdominal pain
		Bowel habit
		Stool consistency
		Faecal incontinence
		Rectal bleeding

4	Genito-urinary system	Urinary frequency
		Dysuria
		Incontinence
		Haematuria
		Menstrual cycle
		Post menopausal bleeding
		Impotence
		Sexual orientation
5	Musculoskeletal system:	Mobility
		Arthralgia
		Joint stiffness
		Swelling
6	CNS:	Pain
		Reflexes and Tone
7	Mind:	Emotion
		Intellect
		Desires
		Aversion
		Moods and disposition
		Love, Hate, Fear, Hallucination, Delusion, Perversion, Jealousy, Suspiciousness, Mania

POTENCY SELECTION

Selection of potency in homoeopathy is a debated question, so each homoeopath has to frame some rules in his mind regarding potency selection to get good results. Higher the potency, more intense the central disturbance it can produce in a living organism. So, for best selection of potency we have to select it at the level which is just above the level of the central disturbance of the patient during his diseased state.

Potency selection is an art and each Homoeopath masters it from his own clinical experience. Some guideline points which one must keep in mind during thorough case taking for potency selection are:

SELECTION OF POTENCY

	High potency (1M, 10M, CM, etc.)	**Medium potency** (30C – 200C)	**Low potency** (30X, 12X, 6X, 3X)
Nature of the disease	Acute cases	Sub acute cases	Chronic cases
Pace of disease	Fast / rapid	Medium	Slow
Susceptibility	High susceptibility	Moderate susceptibility	Low susceptibility
Onset of disease	Sudden onset	Medium to slow	Gradual onset
Suppression of disease	Less suppression	Medium suppression	Complete suppression
Characteristic symptoms	Predominance of characteristic symptoms	Slightly matching symptoms	Pathognomic, or absence of symptoms
Mental picture	Prominent totality of mental picture	Slightly matching mental picture	Few mental symptoms available
Reaction	Good reaction	Medium reaction	Low reaction
Age of the patient	Children, young people, robust vigorous person	Middle age, sluggish, obese person	Old age, elderly people, deaf, dumb person, Mentally and physically handicapped
Vitality	Good vitality	Medium vitality	Low vitality
Miasm	Psora, Tubercular miasm	Sycotic miasm	Syphilitic miasm
Aetiological factor	Exciting cause	Maintaining cause	Maintaining cause
Pathology of symptoms	Reversible symptoms	Slightly reversible	Irreversible, advance pathology
Disease zone	Functional changes	Structural changes	Destructive changes
Constitution	Intellectual person, sedentary worker, non addicted person	Sluggish person	Hard working, labourers, addicted person
Palliation	Less palliation	Minimum palliation	Severe palliation
Pattern of disease	More clear	Clear	Less clear

	High potency (1M, 10M, CM, etc.)	Medium potency (30C – 200C)	Low potency (30X, 12X, 6X, 3X)
Drugs	Sulph., Calc., Lyco.	Thuja, Medo., Nat sulph.	Syph., Bac., Pyrog., Thyr.
Remedy	Acute remedy (Bell., Aco., Hep. sulph.)	Intercurrent remedy (Sulph., Med., Tub.)	Chronic constitutional remedy (Lach., Plat., Nat mur.)

HOMOEOPATHIC REMEDY

S. No.	Remedy	Common Name	Family
1	Abrotanum	Southernwood	Compositae
2	Aceticum acidum	Glacial acetic acid	C, H, O
3	Aconitum napellus	Monkshood	Ranunculaceae
4	Actea racemosa	Black cohosh	Ranunculaceae
5	Adrenalinum	Extract of suprarenal bodies	$C_3H_3A_2O_1$
6	Aesculus hippocastum	Horse chestnut	Sapindacea
7	Aethusa cynapium	Fool's parsley	Umbellifera
8	Agaricus muscarius	Toadstool	Fungi
9	Agnus castus	Chaste tree	Verbenacea
10	Allium cepa	Onion	Liliaceae
11	Aloe socotrina	Socotrine aloes	Liliaceae
12	Alumina	Pure clay	Al_2O_2
13	Ambra grisea	Ambergris	Nosode
14	Ammonium carbonicum	Smelling salts	$N_2H_4O_2$, CO_2
15	Ammonium muriaticum	Sal ammoniac	NHCl
16	Amylenum nitrosum	Nitrite of amyl	$C_{10}H_{11}O$, NO_3
17	Anacardium orientale	Marking nut	Anacardiaceae
18	Anthracinum	Anthrax poison	Nosode
19	Antimonium crudum	Sulphide of antimony	SbS_3
20	Antim tart	Tartar emetic	$K(Sb)C_4H_4O_6 + 1/2H_2O$
21	Apis mellifica	Poison of the honey bee	Apidae
22	Apocynum cannabinum	Indian hemp	Apocynaceae
23	Argentum metallicum	The metal	Ag
24	Argentum nitricum	Silver nitrate	$AgNO_3$
25	Arnica montana	Leopard's bane	Compositae
26	Arsenicum album	White oxide of arsenic	As_2O_3
27	Arum triphyllum	Indian turnip	Araceae
28	Asarum europeum	European snake root	Aristolochiacea

S. No.	Remedy	Common Name	Family
29	Asterias rubens	Star fish	Radiata
30	Aurum metallicum	Gold	Au
31	Baptisia tinctoria	Wild indigo	Leguminosae
32	Baryta carbonica	Barium carbonate	$BaCo_3$
33	Belladonna	Deadly nightshade	Solanaceae
34	Benzoicum acidum	Benzoic acid	$CH_6H_5CO.OH$
35	Berberis vulgaris	Barberry	Berberidaceae
36	Bismuthum	Hydrated oxide of bismuth	Bi_{12}, O_3OH_2
37	Borax	Biborate of soda	$Na_2Ba_4O_7.10H_2O$
38	Bovista	Puffball	Fungi
39	Bromium	Bromine	The element
40	Bryonia	White bryony, Wild hop	Cucurbitaceae
41	Cactus grandiflorus	Night blooming cereus	Cactacea
42	Caladium	American arum	Araceae
43	Calcarea arsenicosa	Arsenite of lime	
44	Calcarea ostrearum	Middle layer of oyster shell	$CaCO_3$
45	Calcarea phosphorica	Phosphate of lime	$Ca_3(PO_4)_2$
46	Calendula	Marigold	Compositae
47	Camphora	Camphor	Lauraceae
48	Cannabis indica	Indian hemp	Urticaceae
49	Cannabis sativa	Hemp	Urticaceae
50	Cantharides	Spanish flies	Cantharideae
51	Capsicum	Cayenne pepper	Solanaceae
52	Carbo animalis	Animal charcoal	
53	Carbo vegetabilis	Vegetable charcoal	
54	Carbolicum acidum	Glacial carbolic acid	C_6H_5OH
55	Caulophyllum	Blue cohosh	Berberidaceae
56	Causticum	Hahnmann's tinctora acris sine kali	
57	Chamomilla	Matricaria chamomilla	Compositae
58	Chelidonium majus	Celandine	Papaveraceae

S. No.	Remedy	Common Name	Family
59	Cholesterinum	Cholesterine	$C_{26}H_{44}O$
60	Cicuta virosa	Water hemlock	Umbelliferae
61	Cina	Worm seed	Compositae
62	Cinchona	Peruvian bark	Rubiaceae
63	Coca	Erythroxylon coca	Lineae
64	Cocculus	Cocculus indicus	Menispermaceae
65	Coffea cruda	Coffee	Rubiaceae
66	Colchicum autumnale	Meadow saffron	Liliaceae
67	Collinsonia canadensis	Stone root	Labiatae
68	Colocynthis	Squirting cucumber	Cucurbitaceae
69	Conium maculatum	Poison hemlock	Umbelliferae
70	Crocus sativus	Saffron	Iridaceae
71	Crotalus horridus	Poison of rattlesnake	Crotalidae
72	Croton tiglinum	Croton oil seeds	Euphorbiaceae
73	Cuprum metallicum	Copper	Cu
74	Cyclamen europaeum	Sow bread	Primulaceae
75	Digitalis purpurea	Foxglove	Scrophulariaceae
76	Dioscorea villosa	Wild yam	Dioscoreaceae
77	Diphtherinum	Homoeopathic antitoxin	A nosode
78	Drosera rotundifolia	Sundew	Droseraceae
79	Dulcamara	Bitter-sweet	Solanaceae
80	Equisetum hyemale	Scouring rush	Equisetaceae
81	Eupatorium perfoliatium	Boneset	Compositae
82	Euphrasia	Eyebright	Scrophularaceae
83	Ferrum metallicum	Iron	The element
84	Fluoricum acidum	Hydrofluoric acid	HF
85	Gelsemium	Yellow jasmine	Loganiaceae
86	Glonoinum	Nitro-glycerine	$C_3H_5(NO_2)O_3$
87	Graphites	Black lead	Amorphous carbon
88	Hamamelis virginica	Witch hazel	Hamamelaceae

S. No.	Remedy	Common Name	Family
89	Helleborus niger	Christmas rose	Ranunculaceae
90	Helonias dioica	Unicorn plant	Melanthaceae
91	Hepar sulphuris	Sulphuret of lime	CaS
92	Hydrastis canadensis	Golden seal	Ranunculaceae
93	Hyoscyamus niger	Henbane	Solanaceae
94	Hypericum perforatum	St. John's wort	Hypericaceae
95	Ignatia	St. Ignatius bean	Loganiaceae
96	Iodum	Iodine	The element
97	Ipecacuanha	Ipecac	Rubiaceae
98	Kali bichromicum	Potassium bichromate	$K_2Cr_2O_7$
99	Kali bromatum	Potassium bromide	KBr
100	Kali carbonicum	Potassium carbonate	$K_2O_2Co_2$
101	Kalmia latifolia	Mountain laurel	Ericaceae
102	Kreosotum	Kreosote	A distillation of wood tar
103	Lachesis	Surukuku snake poison	Ophidia
104	Lac caninum	Dog milk	Animal product
105	Lac defloratum	Skimmed milk	
106	Ledum palustre	Marsh tea	Ericaceae
107	Lilium tigrinum	Tiger lily	Liliaceae
108	Lobelia inflata	Indian tobacco	Lobeliaceae
109	Lycopodium clavatum	Wolf's foot; Club moss	Lycopodiaceae
110	Lyssinum	The saliva of a rabid dog	A nosode
111	Magnesium carbonicum	Carbonate of magnesia	$MgCO_3.\ 3H_2O$
112	Magnesium muriaticum	Chloride of magnesia	MgCl
113	Magnesium phosphoricum	Phosphate of magnesia	$MgHPO_4.\ H_2O$
114	Medorrhinum	The gonorrheal virus	A nosode
115	Melilotus alba	Sweet clover	Leguminosae
116	Menyanthes trifoliata	Buck bean	Gentianaceae
117	Mercurius	Quicksilver	The element
118	Mercurius corrosivus	Corrosive sublimate	$HgCl_2$

S. No.	Remedy	Common Name	Family
119	Mercurius dulcis	Calomel	Hg_2Cl_2
120	Mercurius cyanide	Cyanide of mercury	$Hg(CN)_2$
121	Mercurius proto-iodatus	Iodide of mercury	Hg_2I_2
122	Mercurius solubilis	Hahnemann's soluble mercury	Black oxide
123	Mercurius sulphuricus	Sulphate of mercury	$HgSo_4$
124	Mezereum	Daphne mezereum	Thymelaceae
125	Millefolium	Yarrow	Compositae
126	Murex purpurea	A mollusc	Muricidae
127	Muriaticum acidum	Hydrochloric acid	HCl
128	Naja tripudians	Cobra virus	Elapidae
129	Natrum carbonicum	Carbonate of soda	$Na_2CO_3.10H_2O$
130	Natrum muriaticum	Common salt	NaCl
131	Natrum sulphuricum	Sodium sulphate	$NaOSo_3.10Aq$
132	Nitricum acidum	Nitric acid	HNO_3
133	Nux moschata	Nutmeg	Myristicaceae
134	Nux vomica	Poison nut	Loganiaceae
135	Opium	Poppy	Papaveraceae
136	Petroleum	Coal or rock oil	Anthracite
137	Petroselinum	Parsley	Umbelliferae
138	Phosphoricum acidum	Glacial phosphoric acid	HPO_3
139	Phosphorus	Phosphorus	The element
140	Physostigma	Calabar bean	Leguminosae
141	Phytolacca decandra	Poke root	Phytolacaceae
142	Picricum acidum	Picric acid	$HC_6H_2(NO_2)_3O$
143	Platina	Platinum	Pt
144	Plumbum	Lead	Pb
145	Podophyllum	May apple	Berberidaceae
146	Psorinum	A product of psora	A nosode
147	Pulsatilla	Anemone	Ranunculaceae
148	Pyrogenium	A product of sepsis	A nosode

S. No.	Remedy	Common Name	Family
149	Ratanhia	Rhatany	Polygalaceae
150	Ranunculus bulbosus	Buttercup	Ranunculaceae
151	Rheum	Rhubarb	Polygonaceae
152	Rhododendron	Snowrose	Ericaceae
153	Rhus toxicodendron	Poison oak	Anacardiaceae
154	Rumex crispus	Yellow dock	Polygonaceae
155	Ruta graveolens	Rue	Rutaceae
156	Sabadilla	Cevadilla	Liliaceae
157	Sabina	Savine	Coniferae
158	Sambucus nigra	Elder	Caprifoliaceae
159	Sanguinaria	Bloodroot	Papaveraceae
160	Sanicula	Mineral spring water	Apiaceae
161	Sarsaparilla	Wild liquorice	Smilaceae
162	Secale cornutum	Spurred rye, Ergot	A fungus, A nosode
163	Selenium	Selenium	Se
164	Sepia	Cuttle fish	Mollusca
165	Silicea	Pure silica	Silicic oxide
166	Spigelia	Pinkroot	Loganiaceae
167	Spongia tosta	Roasted sponge	Spongia
168	Stannum	Tin	Sn
169	Staphysagria	Stavestcre	Ranunculaceae
170	Stramonium	Thorn Apple	Solanaceae
171	Sulphur	Brimstone, Flowers of sulphur	The element
172	Sulphuricum acidum	Sulphuric acid	H_2SO_4
173	Symphytum	Comfrey	Borraginaceae
174	Syphilinum	Syphilitic virus	A nosode
175	Tabacum	Tobacco	Solanaceae
176	Taraxacum	Dandelion	Compositae
177	Tarentula	Tarentula: Cuben and Spanish	Araneideae
178	Terebinthiniae	Oil of turpentine	A volatile oil

S. No.	Remedy	Common Name	Family
179	Theridion curassavicum	Orange spider	Araneideae
180	Thlaspi bursa pastoris	Shepherd's Purse	Cruciferae
181	Thuja occidentalis	Tree of life; White cedar	Coniferae
182	Trillium pendulum	Wake robin	Smilaceae
183	Tuberculinum-bacillinum	Pus (with Bacilli) from tubercular abscess	A nosode
184	Valeriana	Valerian	Valerianaceae
185	Variolinum	Pus from smallpox pustule	A nosode
186	Veratrun album	White hellebore	Melanthaceae
187	Veratrum viride	Green hellebore	Melanthaceae
188	Zincum metallicum	Zinc	The element

HOMOEOPATHIC PULSE

No.	REMEDY	PULSE
1.	Aceticum acidum	Full, intermittent, slow, soft
2.	Aconitum napellus	Abnormal, feeble, frequent, elevated, soft, tremulous
3.	Aesculus hippocastanum	Frequent, full, soft, weak
4.	Aethusa cynapium	Frequent, accelerated, exalted, elevated, irregular
5.	Agaricus muscarius	Small, intermittent, quick in the morning, slow, feeble, unequal
6.	Agnus castus	Abnormal, elevated, rapid, tremulous, irregular
7.	Aloe socotrina	Frequent, accelerated, elevated, full, intermittent
8.	Alumina	Febrile, frequent, accelerated, irregular, thready
9.	Ambra grisea	Abnormal, frequent, rapid, fast
10.	Ammonium carbonicum	Accelerated, elevated, rapid, hard, tense
11.	Amygdala amara	Slow, full and hard
12.	Anacardium orientale	Frequent, elevated, accelerated
13.	Antimonium crudum	Sometimes a few quick beats then three or four slow ones
14.	Antimonium tartaricum	Accelerated, full, hard, strong, aggravated by motion
15.	Apis mellifica	Strong, weak, small, soft, intermittent
16.	Arsenicum album	Suppressed even while the beats of the heart are frequent and irritated
17.	Argentum metallicum	Accelerated, elevated, fast, innumerable
18.	Argentum nitricum	Abnormal, frequent, after vexation intermittent
19.	Arnica montana	Strong, full, hard, irregular, soft, thready
20.	Arsenicum iodatum	Frequent and feeble, frequent and full or contracted and accelerated
21.	Asafoetida	Small, full, intermittent, irregular
22.	Aurum muriaticum	Fever with hard spasmodic pulse and great restlessness, pulse – 80, 90, 100 / minute
23.	Baptisia tinctoria	Weak, soft, irregular, full, frequent, fast, accelerated
24.	Baryta carbonica	Soft, small, abnormal, frequent, fast
25.	Baryta muriatica	Full and frequent
26.	Belladonna	Hard and tight, large, frequent, strong and quick, intermittent, elevated, rapid
27.	Berberis vulgaris	Weak, frequent, fast, rapid, slow and hard

No.	REMEDY	PULSE
28.	Bismuthum subnitricum	Abnormal, frequent, fast, elevated
29.	Borax veneta	Quick
30.	Bovista	Febrile, abnormal, frequent, rapid
31.	Bromium	Slow, intermittent, rapid, accelerated
32.	Bryonia alba	Weak, soft, fast, rapid, irregular
33.	Caladium seguinum	Full, hard, bounding
34.	Calcarea carbonica	Quick or slow
35.	Camphora officinalis	Small, hard, slow, full, imperceptible
36.	Cannabis indica	Rapid, intermittent, slow, irregular, soft
37.	Cannabis sativa	Abnormal, small, soft
38.	Cantharis vesicatoria	Increased, full, early in the morning, after the pains: hard and full as in febrile inflammation
39.	Capsicum annuum	Intermittent, irregular
40.	Carbo vegetabilis	Feeble and depressed, frequent, irregular
41.	Cereus bonplandii	Dicrotic and several intermissions within a minute
42.	Chamomilla	Tense, soft, small, irregular, hard, full, frequent
43.	Chenopodium	Accelerated in the evening, during frequent coryza or quick early in the morning with hot breath and dry lips
44.	Chelidonium majus	Slow, small, irregular, hard, frequent
45.	Chininum sulphuricum	Strong almost undulating frequent, quick and rather hard, accelerated
46.	China	Quick and hard, quick and irregular or slow and feeble
47.	Colchicum autumnale	Irregular, hard and full, pulse – 91, 100. Fluttering, contracted, abnormal
48.	Conium maculatum	Collapse of the pulse, large, slow pulse
49.	Crotalus horridus	Feeble and quick then feeble and slow, intermittent pulse
50.	Cuprum aceticum	Frequent, small, hard, contracted, at times regular and at other irregular
51.	Cuprum arsenicosum	Small, quick, irritated or else spasmodically contracted pulse
52.	Cuprum metallicum	Full but of ordinary quickness
53.	Digitalis purpurea	Full, irregular, very slow, weak, intermittent every fifth, seventh beat
54.	Dulcamara	Full, hard, imperceptible, jerking
55.	Euphrasia	Frequent, elevated, rapid, soft
56.	Ferrum phosphoricum	Frequent, accelerated, fast, rapid
57.	Ferrum aceticum	Scarcely perceptible or hard and full

No.	REMEDY	PULSE
58.	Gelsemium sempervirens	Irregular, soft, strong, tremulous, weak
59.	Glonoinum	Rapid, slow, irregular, weak, accelerated
60.	Helleborus niger	Pale sunken contenance, no pulse
61.	Heloderma	Pulse 56-72, full and jerky
62.	Hyoscyamus niger	Small quick intermittent pulse scarcely percetible
63.	Hypericum perforatum	Quick rather hard, accelerated pulse
64.	Indigo	Spasmodic pulse of 70 beats
65.	Iodium	Small very frequent, compressed, small, very accelerated
66.	Kalium chloricum	Pulse accelerated by 10, 15 or 20 beats
67.	Kalium hydriodium	Accelerated, frequent
68.	Kalium phosphoricum	Sluggish and below normal standard from enfeebled nervous system
69.	Kalium sulphuricum	Quick and throbbing
70.	Kreosotum	Small and subdued pulse, natural but perceptible in every part of the body as soon as she remains quite
71	Lachesis mutus	Constant, small, quick and faint
72.	Laurocerasus	Pulse of unequal strength, quick and feeble, slow, hard
73.	Lobelia inflata	More full and weaker than usual
74.	Manganum aceticum	Irregular, scarcely perceptible, now quick, now slow
75.	Menyanthes	Small, slow, intermittent, low, 52 beats/min
76.	Mercurius iodum	Over 100, small and weak
77.	Mercurius solubilis	Feeble, slow and trembling, quick and violent beating of the pulse
78.	Mercurius phosphoricus	Frequent, small, quick, feeble, tremulous
79.	Mezereum	Full, hard, tense, intermittent
80.	Morphinum	Small, irregular pulse
81.	Morphinum purum	Fever with intermittent, small and contracted pulse
82.	Natrum muriaticum	Rapid and intermittent
83.	Nitricum acidum	Feverish heat with quick pulse
84.	Nux vomica	Collapse of the pulse with full consciousness, small and quick or intermittent
85.	Opium	Strong, quick pulse which frequently becomes weak and intermittent
86.	Oxalicum acidum	More frequent and harder than usual
87.	Platinum metallicum	Abnormal, fast, innumerable, rapid, elevated

No.	REMEDY	PULSE
88.	Plumbum metallicum	Undulating pulse, slow, tense, thready, tremulus
89.	Podophylum	Abnormal, rapid, slow, weak
90.	Pulsatilla nigricans	Abnormal, frequent, rapid, slow
91.	Sepia officinalis	Intermittent, full, slow, irregular, spasmodic, tremulous weak
92.	Silicea terra	Full, hard, rapid, irregular
93.	Sulphur	Thready, full, hard, irregular, imperceptible
94.	Spongia	Rapid, intermittent, febrile
95.	Stramonium	Small, quick and scarcely perceptible
96.	Thuja occidentalis	Slow, soft, full, frequent, febrile, fast
97.	Veratrum album	Weak, small, slower than beat of the heart
98.	X-ray	Slow, weak, intermittent, with rheumatic and cancerous diathesis

HOMOEOPATHIC TONGUE

No.	REMEDY	CHARACTERISTIC SYMPTOMS
1.	Aconitum napellus	Tip of the tongue is swollen with white coating
2.	Adonis vernalis	Dirty yellow tongue, sore, feels as if scalded
3.	Aesculus hippocastanum	Metallic taste, thickly coated, feels scalded
4.	Agaricus muscarius	Taste sweet, splinter like pain in tongue, tremulous, white coated
5.	Ailanthus glandulosa	Tongue dry, brown coated
6.	Allium sativum	Sensation of hair on tongue
7.	Ammonium carbonicum	Vesicles on tongue, sour metallic taste
8.	Anacardium orientale	Tongue feels swollen, impending speech and motion
9.	Antimonium crudum	Tongue coated thick white as if white washed
10.	Antimonium tartaricum	Coated, pasty thick white with red edges and dry especially in the center, brown coated
11.	Apis mellifica	Tongue fiery red, swollen, sore with vesicles, feels scalded
12.	Argentum nitricum	Prominent papillae at the tip of the tongue, red, painful, tastes copper like ink
13.	Arnica montana	Tongue dirty brown, dark in the center, cyanosis, taste as from bad eggs
14.	Arsenicum album	Dry, clean and red stitching and burning pain in tongue, ulcerated with blue colour, metallic taste
15.	Arsenicum metallicum	White coated shows imprints of teeth
16.	Arum triphyllum	Red, sore tongue
17.	Aurum muriaticum	Burning stitches and induration
18.	Baryta carbonica	Paralysis of tongue, smarting, burning pain in tip of tongue
19.	Belladonna	Red on edges, strawberry tongue, swollen and painful
20.	Berberis vulgaris	Feels scalded, vesicles on tongue
21.	Bismuthum	Tongue white, swollen, black, gangrenous looking wedges on dorsum and sides of tongue
22.	Bryonia alba	Dryness, coated yellowish, dark brown, bitter taste in mouth
23.	Calcarea carbonica	Sour taste, dryness of tongue at night, burning pain at the tip of the tongue
24.	Calcarea flourica	Cracked appearance of the tongue with or without pain, induration of tongue
25.	Calcarea sulphurica	Tongue flabby resembling a layer of dried clay, sour, soapy, acrid taste, yellowish coating at base
26.	Cantharis annuum	Covered with vesicles, deeply furred, edges red
27.	Capsicum	Burning in tip of tongue
28.	Carbo vegetabilis	Tongue coated white or yellow, brown covered with apathae

No.	REMEDY	CHARACTERISTIC SYMPTOMS
29.	Myrica	Tongue furred with bad taste
30.	Causticum hahnemanni	Paralysis of tongue with indistinct speech
31.	Chamomilla	Tongue yellow, taste bitter
32.	Chelidonium majus	Tongue yellow with imprints of teeth, large and flabby, taste bitter, pasty
33.	Chionanthus	Broad with thick yellow layer
34.	Cinchona officinalis	Tongue coated thick, dirty tip, burns, bitter taste
35.	Colocynthis	Tongue rough as from sand, feels scalded
36.	Conium maculatum	Soreness about root of tongue
37.	Condurango	Cancer of tongue, ulcerated
38.	Cuprum mettalicum	Constant protrusion and retraction of tongue, paralysis of tongue
39.	Eupatorium	Yellow coated tongue, bitter taste
40.	Gelsemium sempervirens	Tongue numb, thick coated, yellowish, trembling, paralysed
41.	Graphites	Burning blisters on tongue
42.	Helleborus niger	Tongue red and dry
43.	Heloderma	Tongue cold, tender and dry
44.	Hydrastis canadensis	Peppery taste, tongue white, swollen, large, flabby, slimy shows imprints of teeth as if scalded, ulceration fissures towards the edges
45.	Hyoscyamus niger	Tongue dry, red, cracked, stiff and immovable, protruded with difficult speech
46.	Hypericum perforatum	Tongue coated white at the base, tip clean
47.	Ipecacuanha	Clean tongue
48.	Kalium bichromicum	Tongue mapped, red, shining, smooth and dry with dysentery, broad, flat, thickly coated, feeling of hair on tongue
49.	Kalium carbonicum	White tongue with backache, weakness, prostration
50.	Kalium muriaticum	White or grey coating at base of tongue, dry or slimy
51.	Kalium nitricum	Tongue red with burning pimples, burning at night
52.	Kalium phosphoricum	Tongue coated brownish like mustard
53.	Kalium sulphuricum	Tongue coated yellow and slimy
54.	Lac caninum	Tongue coated white with bright red edges, stiffness of tongue
55.	Lachesis mutus	Tongue swollen, burns, trembles, paralysed, yellowish red, bites easily, red, dry, cracked at tip, trembling
56.	Lathyrus	Burning pain at the tip of the tongue with tingling numbness as if scalded
57.	Lycopodium clavatum	Tongue dry, black, cracked and swollen, oscillates to and fro, blisters on tongue

No.	REMEDY	CHARACTERISTIC SYMPTOMS
58.	Medorrhinum	Tongue coated brown and thick blistered, canker sore, coppery taste
59.	Mercurius	Difficult speech on account of trembling tongue, furrow in upper surface of tongue, lengthwise. Tongue thick, heavy, moist coating, yellow, flabby, teeth indented, feels as if burnt with ulcers, with much salivation
60.	Mercurius dulcis	Tongue black
61.	Mercurius iodatus flavus	Coated thickly yellow at the base, tip and edges may be red and have imprints of teeth
62.	Morphinum	Tongue dry, brown, violet in middle
63.	Muriaticum acidum	Tongue pale, swollen, dry, leathery, paralyzed, deep ulcers on tongue, hard lumps in tongue
64.	Myrica	Tongue furred with bad taste
65.	Natrum chloratum	Sore irritable spots along sides of tongue swollen large flabby indented
66.	Natrum muriaticum	White coating on the tongue with ulcers on side, numbness tingling of tongue, vesicles and burning as if there was hair on it, mapped tongue
67.	Natrum phosphoricum	Blisters on tip of tongue with stinging in the evening, thin, moist coating on tongue
68.	Nux moschata	Tongue dry, adheres to the roof of the mouth but no desire for water, saliva like cotton, tongue numb, paralysed
69.	Nux vomica	First half of tongue clean, posteriorly covered with deep white yellow coating, cracked edges
70.	Opium	Tongue black, paralyzed
71	Ostrya virginica	Tongue yellow coated at the root
72.	Paris quadrifolia	Tongue dry, white, without thirst
73.	Phosphoricum acidum	Tongue swollen, dry with viscid, frothy mucus at night, bites tongue involuntarily
74.	Phosphorus	Tongue dry, smooth, red or white, thinly coated
75.	Physostigma venenosum	Tongue feels sore on tip with eye complaints, blisters on tongue, mapped, indented, fissured with yellow patch, down the center
76.	Phytolacca decandra	Tongue red tipped, feels rough and scalded, blisters on tongue, mapped, indented
77.	Plumbum mettalicum	Tongue tremulous, red on margin cannot put it out, seems paralyzed
78.	Podophyllum peltatum	Tongue broad, large, moist, burning sensation of tongue
79.	Ptelea trifoliata	Tongue coated white or yellow, feels rough, swollen, papillae red and prominent, coating may be brownish yellow
80.	Pulsatilla nigricans	Yellow, white tongue, feels rough, covered with tenacious mucus, biting, broad
81.	Pyrogenium	Tongue red and dry, clean, cracked smooth as if varnished
82.	Radium bromatum	Prickling sensation at the end of the tongue
83.	Ranunculus sceleratus	Tongue mapped, burning and rawness of tongue
84.	Rhamnus californica	Tongue with clean pink, central patch
85.	Rhus toxicodendron	Tongue red and cracked, coated except red triangular space at the tip, dry and red at edges

No.	REMEDY	CHARACTERISTIC SYMPTOMS
86.	Rhus venenata	Red at tip, fissured in the middle, vesicles on under side
87.	Salicylicum acidum	Tongue purplish, leaden coloured
88.	Sanicula aqua	Tongue large, flabby, burning, must protrude to keep cool, ringworm on tongue
89.	Sarsaparilla officinalis	Tongue white, apthae metallic taste
90.	Secale cornutum	Tongue dry, cracked, blood like ink exudes, thick, viscid, yellowish, cold, livid, tingling on the tip of the tongue which is stiff, swollen, paralyzed
91.	Sempervivum tectorum	Cancer of tongue, has ulcers, bleeds easily especially at night, much of tongue whitish
92.	Sepia officinalis	Tongue white, taste salty, putrid. Tongue foul, but clean during menses
93.	Silicea terra	Sensation of hair on tongue
94.	Spigelia anthelmia	Tongue fissured, painful
95.	Spongia tosta	Tongue dry and brown, full of vesicles
96.	Sulphur	Tongue white with red tip and borders
97.	Syphilinum	Tongue coated, teeth indented, deep longitudinal cracks
98.	Taraxacum officinale	Mapped tongue covered with a white film, feels raw, comes off in patches leaving red sensitive spots
99.	Terebinthinae oleum	Tongue dry, red, sore, shining burning in tip with prominent papillae
100.	Thuja occidentalis	Tip of tongue very painful, white blisters on side, close to root, painful, sore
101.	Veratrum album	Tongue pale, cold, cool sensation as from pepper mint, dry in center
102.	X-ray	Tongue dry, rough, sore, ulcerated, cancer of tongue

HOMOEOPATHIC DREAMS

No.	REMEDY	DREAMS
1.	Abrotanum	Frightful dreams and trembling, dreams of dogs
2.	Aconitum napellus	Anxious dreams with anxiety in chest, clairvoyance
3.	Agaricus muscarius	Dreams as if he was walking up and down the room
4.	Allium cepa	Dreams of being near water
5.	Alumina	Dreams of talking, laughing, of ghosts, of thieves, marriage, death
6.	Ammonium muriaticum	Lascivious dream, falling into water
7.	Anacardium orientale	Vivid dreams, recurred to him during day time, dreams of fire
8.	Antimonium crudum	Dreams of quarreling, dream of festival
9.	Apis mellifica	Dreams of journey, of flying
10.	Argentum nitricum	Dreams of departed friend, of ghost
11.	Arnica montana	Dreams of black dog, muddy water, robber
12.	Arsenicum album	Dreams of biting
13.	Baptisa tinctoria	Dreams of swimming in river
14.	Belladonna	Dreams about murder, of fire, swimming
15.	Borax veneta	Lascivious dreams, dreams of coition
16.	Bovista lycoperdon	Dreams of being bitten by a snake
17.	Calcarea arsenicosa	Dreams of people, forgotten
18.	Calcarea phosphorica	Dreams of travelling, cutting women into pieces
19.	Cannabis sativa	Dreams that room was turning round with her
20.	Cantharis vesicatoria	Dreams of forest
21.	Carbo animalis	Dreams of scientific subjects
22.	Cimicifuga	Dreams of limbs broken
23.	Cinnabaris	Dreams of spider as large as an ox
24.	Cyclamen europaeum	Dreams of money, dreams of gold
25.	Drosera rotundifolia	Dreams of being maltreated, of thirst, drinking
26.	Fluoricum acidum	Dreams of own death
27.	Glonoinum	Fearful dreams, weeping with fear
28.	Graphitis	Dreams of cat, fire
29.	Gratiola officinalis	Dreams of freezing

No.	REMEDY	DREAMS
30.	Hepar sulphuricum	Dreams of health, expectorating blood, pus
31.	Ignatia amara	Dreams of same subject throughout night, miscarriage
32.	Iodum	Dreams of eating, walking in mud
34.	Kalium carbonicum	Dreams of family
35.	Kalium phosphoricum	Dreams of being naked in public
36.	Kreosotum	Dreams of crying, urinating
37.	Lac caninum	Dreams of large snake in her bed
38.	Lachesis mutus	Dreams of death, funeral, snake
39.	Lilium tigrinum	Dreams of labour
40.	Lycopodium clavatum	Dreams of fight, frightful dreams
41.	Medorrhinum	Dreams of ghost, dead people
42.	Mezereum	Dreams of warts
43.	Natrum carbonicum	Dreams of being stabbed with a knife
44.	Natrum muriaticum	Dreams of murder, crime, poisoned
45.	Nux vomica	Dreams of accident, coffee, wine
46.	Oxalicum acidum	Dreams of water.
47.	Petroleum	Dreams of somebody lying along his side
48.	Pulsatilla nigricans	Dreams of fright, cat, ghosts
49.	Rhus toxicodendron	Dreams of exertion, fire
50.	Sarsaparilla officinalis	Feels as if in a dream all time
51.	Sepia officinale	Dreams are anxious, of rape, snake
52.	Silicea terra	Dreams of earthquakes
53.	Thuja occidentalis	Dreams of accident, death, falling from high places, misfortune
54.	Ustilago maydis	Dreams are amorous, anxious, frightful, unpleasant
55.	Valeriana officinalis	Dreams of confusion, nightmare
56.	Vinca minor	Dreams amorous
57.	Veratrum viride	Dreams frightful, vivid, of water
58.	Veratrum album	Dreams of jumping, misfortune, quarrel, robber, forgetful
59.	Zincum metallicum	Dreams of anger, anxious, continued
60.	Zingiber officinale	Dreams anxious, of health

MIASMATIC EVOLUTION

No.	PSORA	SYCOSIS	TUBERCULAR	SYPHILITIC
1.	**FUNCTIONAL CHANGES** Prepared from pus of psoric lesion	**STRUCTURAL CHANGES** Prepared from gonorrhoeal virus	**RECURRENCE** Collection from tubercular abscess	**DESTRUCTIVE CHANGES** Prepared from syphillitic virus
2.	**Mind:** Irritability, anger, fear of dark, fear of being alone, hurried, worried, self importance, disappointment in love. Suppressed anger	**Mind:** Irritability < contradiction, sluggish, stubborn, obstinate, slow, egoistic. Suppressed desire	**Mind:** Active, social, hardworking, fear of death, cosmopolitan, intelligent, artistic, friendly, hopeful about life, forgetful, hyperactive, schizophrenia, perverted sexual disorder	**Mind:** Idiotic, foolish, suspicious fear of death, accident, poverty, jealous, theft, robbery, revengefulness, antisocial, destructive, criminality
3.	**Skin:** Redness, irritability, contact dermatitis, dandruff, hair fall, eczema, acne scabies, vesicle, itching, suppressed skin diseases, cutaneous eruptions	**Skin:** Warts, moles, tumour, carbuncles, patchy hair loss, acne vulgaris, contageous skin diseases, cauliflower eruptions	**Skin:** Alopecia areata, grey hair, psoriasis, recurrent acne with pus	**Skin:** Grey hair, baldness, malignant skin, non-healing ulcers
4.	**Discharges:** White, clear, watery, transparent, bland, odorless	**Discharges:** Yellowish, green, offensive, ropy, sour taste	**Discharges:** Dark yellowish, offensive, clear, transparent with blood stain	**Discharges:** Black, dark, offensive, foetid odour, acrid, excoriating the part, blood stain
5.	**Gastro-intestinal system:** Nausea, vomiting, heartburn, water brash, acidity, dyspepsia, colic, worm infestation, itching, soreness in anal region	**Gastro-intestinal system:** Bilious vomiting, distention, belching, gastritis, bleeding or blind piles, enlarged liver, tenderness, polyps, fibrous tumour	**Gastro-intestinal system:** Haematemesis, flatulence, bleeding piles, hepatitis, ulcerative colitis, irritable bowel syndrome.	**Gastro-intestinal system:** Cancer of stomach, rectum, bleeding piles, offensive discharges, cirrhosis of liver
6.	**Respiratory system:** Cough, coryza, sinusitis, inflammed tonsils, rhinitis, otitis media.	**Respiratory system:** Diphtheria, kissing tonsils, adenoids	**Respiratory system:** Recurrent tonsillitis, deafness, epistaxis, haemoptysis, pneumonia, asthma, tetanus, bronchitis, tuberculosis, pneumonia, chickenpox	**Respiratory system:** Caries of nasal septum, oozing of offensive breath, pleural effusion, chronic asthma, bronchitis
7.	**Cardiovascular system:** Angina pectoris	**Cardiovascular system:** Hypertension, endocarditis, cardiomegaly	**Cardiovascular system:** Endocarditis, heart attack, myocarditis	**Cardiovascular system:** Cardiac arrest, myocardial infarction

No.	PSORA	SYCOSIS	TUBERCULAR	SYPHILITIC
8.	**Central nervous system:** Headache, migraine, vertigo, blurred vision, diplopia	**Central nervous system:** Benign tumour of brain, meningioma, space occupying lesion of brain, cephalhaematoma.	**Central nervous system:** Meningitis, transient ischaemic attack, chronic headache	**Central nervous system:** Hemiplegia, parkinsonism, retinal detachment
9.	**Genito-urinary system:** Burning micturition, increased urination	**Genito-urinary system:** Retension of urine, anuria, renal stone, gonorrhoea, spasmodic dysmenorrhoea	**Genito-urinary system:** Haematuria, recurrent urination, diabetic neuropathy.	**Genito-urinary system:** Past history of AIDS, VDRL, diabetes, gangrene, impotency, libido
10.	**Musculo-skeletal system:** Pain, swelling, tenderness, bleeding.	**Musculo-skeletal system:** Swelling, arthritis, rheumatism, gout	**Musculo-skeletal system:** Osteoarthritis, osteoporosis, tuberculosis of bone, pott's spine	**Musculo-skeletal system:** Osteochondrosis, ankylosis, spondylitis
11.	**Drugs:** Sulphur, Psorinum	**Drugs:** Thuja, Medorrhinum	**Drugs:** Tuberculinum, Bacillinum	**Drugs:** Syphillinum

TRIOS OF REMEDIES

(1) Diptheria

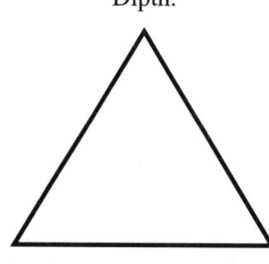

Dipth. / Phyt-b. / Merc.

(2) Sweat relieves

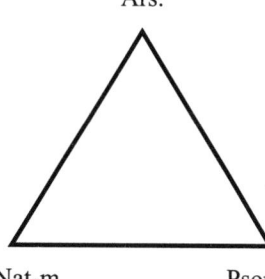

Ars. / Nat-m. / Psor.

(3) Sour smelling discharges

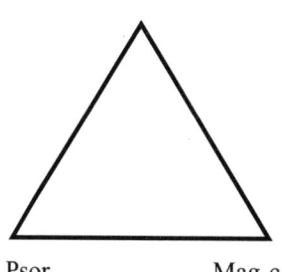

Rheum. / Psor. / Mag-c.

(4) Gonorrhoea

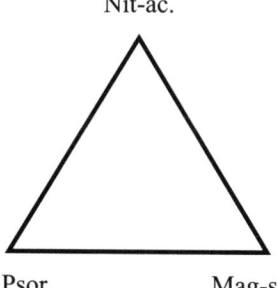

Nit-ac. / Psor. / Mag-s.

(5) Imprints of teeth

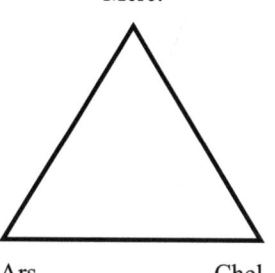

Merc. / Ars. / Chel.

(6) Acute inflammation

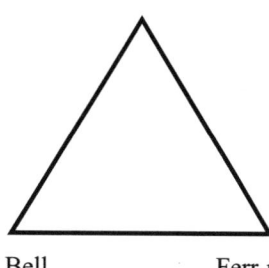

Acon. / Bell. / Ferr-p.

(7) Tinnitus

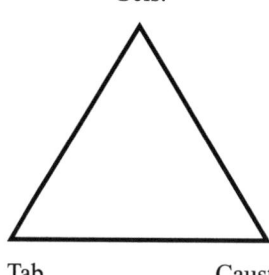

Gels. / Tab. / Caust.

(8) Alopecia

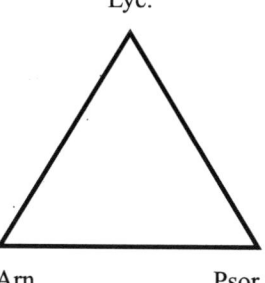

Lyc. / Arn. / Psor.

(9) Changeability of symptoms

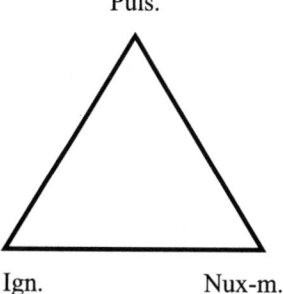

Puls. / Ign. / Nux-m.

(10) Warts

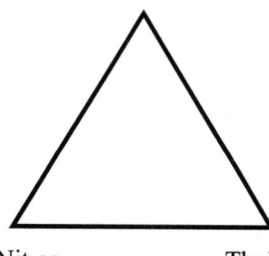

Caust. / Nit-ac. / Thuj.

(11) Colic

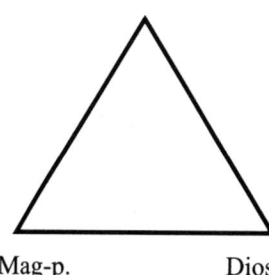

Coloc. / Mag-p. / Dios.

(12) Deafness

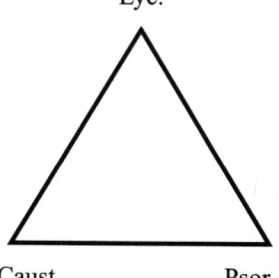

Lyc. / Caust. / Psor.

Trios of remedies

(13) Hysteria
Valer.
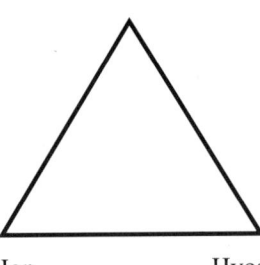
Ign.   Hyos.

(14) Vertigo
Rhus-t.
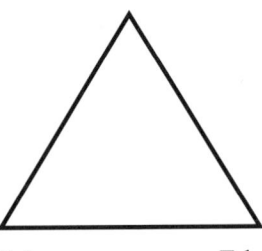
Gels.   Tab.

(15) Indifference
Sep.
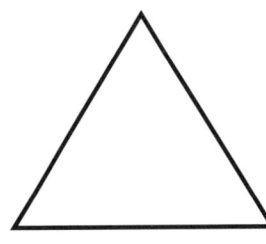
Fl-ac.   Ph-ac.

(16) Cancer of breast
Con.
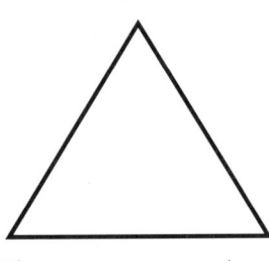
Phyt.   Aster.

(17) Sand in urine
Lyc.
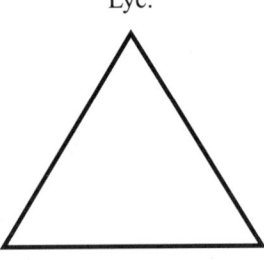
Borx.   Sars.

(18) Heart tonic
Dig.
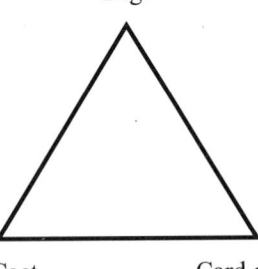
Cact.   Card-m.

(19) Bad effect of vaccination
Thuj.
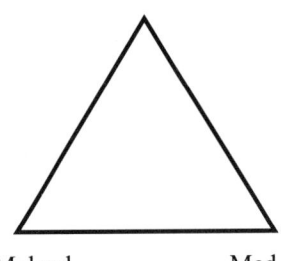
Maland.   Med.

(20) Abortion
Sabin.
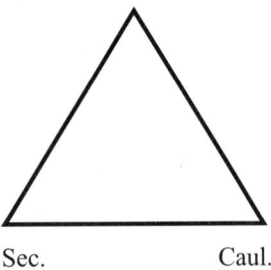
Sec.   Caul.

(21) Tobacco ailments from
Tab.
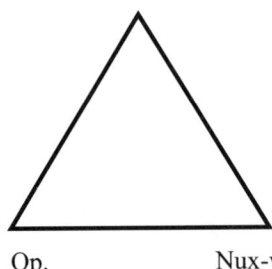
Op.   Nux-v.

(22) Mania
Hyos.
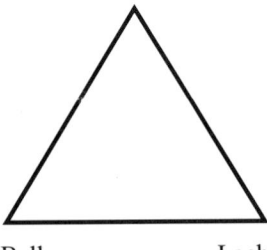
Bell.   Lach.

(23) Cholera
Carb-v.
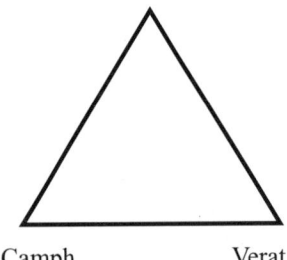
Camph.   Verat.

(24) Convulsion
Cupr.
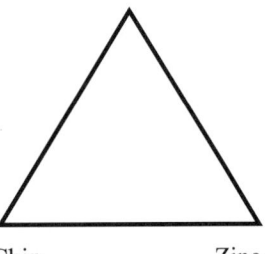
Chin.   Zinc.

(25) Renal colic
Berb.
Canth.   Tab.

(26) Paralysis
Gels.
Agar.   Caust.

(27) Constipation
Calc.
Alum.   Lyc.

(28) Injury
Arn.
Hyper.   Led.

(29) Periodical
Eup-per.
Chin.   Nat-m.

(30) Thirstless
Ip.
Puls.   Gels.

(31) Pain
Coff.
Bell.   Acon.

(32) Restlessness
Ars.
Acon.   Rhus-t.

(33) Constitutional trio
Calc.
Sulph.   Lyc.

(34) Loss of vital fluid
Carbo-v.
Caust.   Chin.

(35) Yellow coated tongue
Kali-bi.
Nat-m.   Chel.

(36) Epistaxis
Bry.
Ant-c.   Thuj.

Trios of remedies

(37) Emaciation
Nat-m.
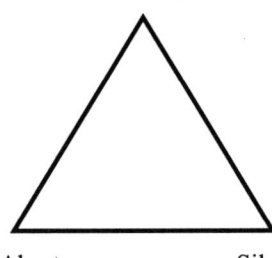
Abrot.   Sil.

(38) Corn
Thuj.
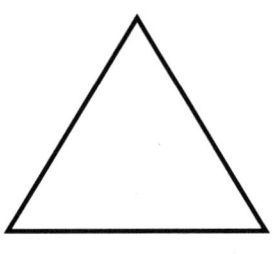
Ant-c.   Nit-ac.

(39) Liver remedy
Nat-s.
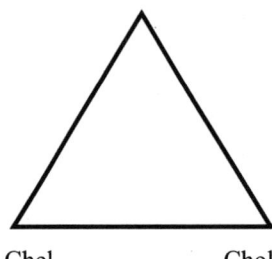
Chel.   Chol.

(40) Haemorrhoids
Aesc.
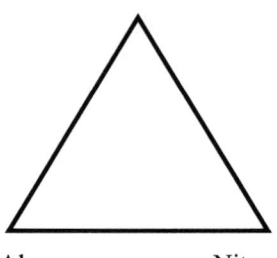
Aloe.   Nit-ac.

(41) Insomnia
Op.
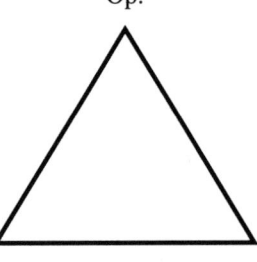
Nux-v.   Coff.

(42) Bad effects of vaccination
Thuj.
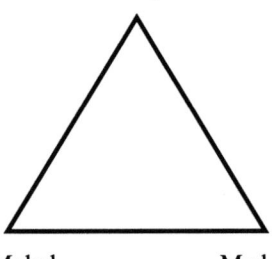
Malad.   Med.

(43) Burns
Canth.
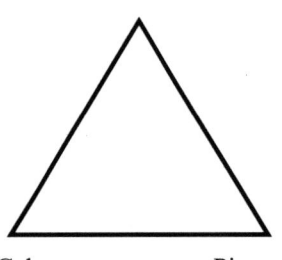
Calen.   Pic-ac.

(44) Psoriasis
Nat-m.
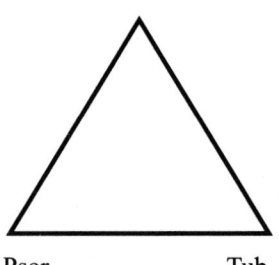
Psor.   Tub.

(45) Thinking of complaints <
Ox-ac.
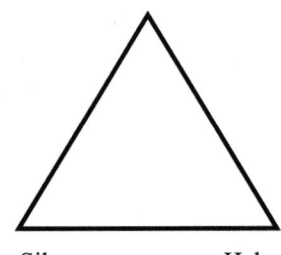
Sil.   Helon.

(46) Better by thinking
Phos.
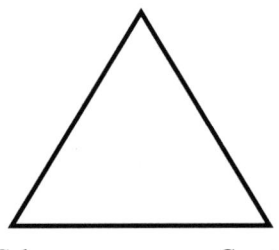
Calc-p.   Caust.

(47) Haemorrhage
Chin.
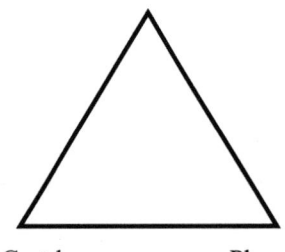
Crot-h.   Phos.

(48) Hernia
Lyc.
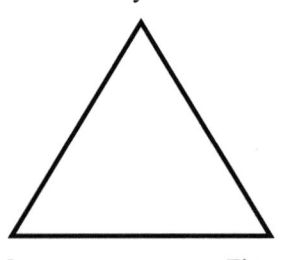
Nux-v.   Zinc.

(49) Stye
Puls.
Apis Kali-c.

(50) Whooping cough
Dros.
Cupr. Spong.

(51) Flatulence
Carb-v.
Lyc. Chin.

(52) Loss of memory
Kali-br.
Cann-i. Syph

(53) Leucorrhoea
Alum.
Con. Kreos.

(54) Oversensitivity
Bell.
Cham. Op.

(55) Hard goitre
Brom.
Iod. Thyr.

(56) Fistula-in-ano
Berb-v.
Calc. Sil.

(57) Gout
Ben-ac.
Nit-ac. Colch.

(58) Headache
Bell.
Nat-m. Psor.

(59) Post operative
Arn.
Calen. Rhus-t.

(60) Shock
Acon.
Carb-v. Pic-ac.

Trios of remedies

(61) Anxiety
Acon.
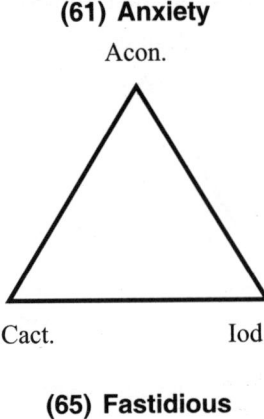
Cact.　　　　Iod.

(62) Confusion
Cann-i.
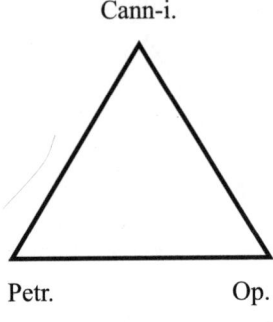
Petr.　　　　Op.

(63) Delirium
Ars.
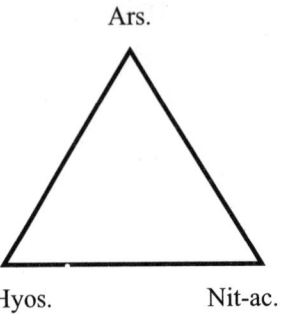
Hyos.　　　　Nit-ac.

(64) Delusion
Bell.
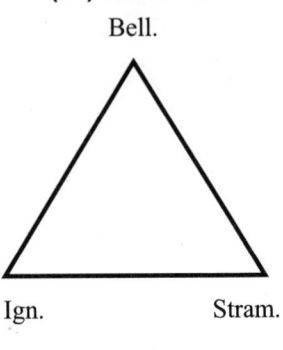
Ign.　　　　Stram.

(65) Fastidious
Ars.
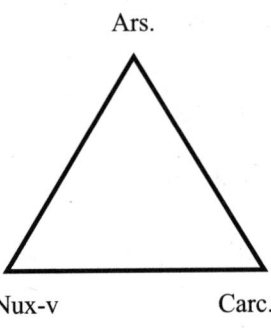
Nux-v　　　　Carc.

(66) Fear
Arg-n.
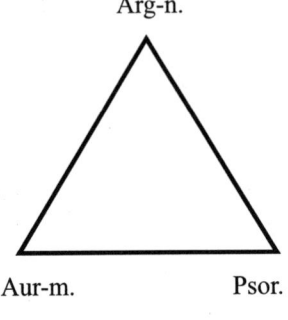
Aur-m.　　　　Psor.

(67) Forgetful
Bar-c.
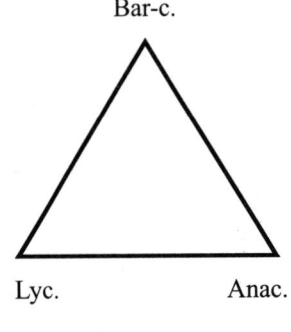
Lyc.　　　　Anac.

(68) Grief
Caust.
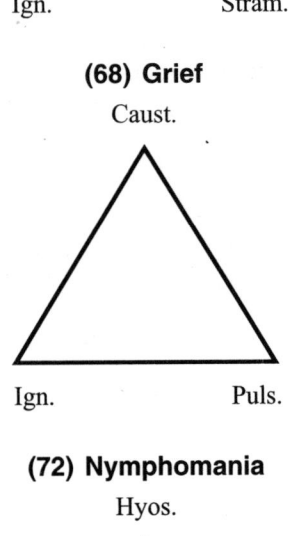
Ign.　　　　Puls.

(69) Homesickness
Caps.
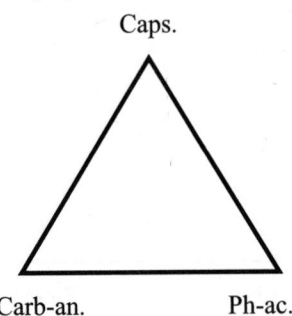
Carb-an.　　　　Ph-ac.

(70) Ozaena
Asaf.
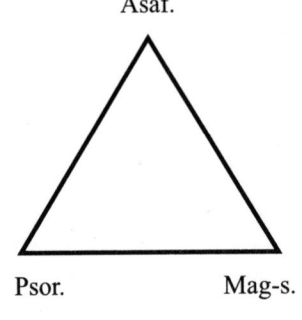
Psor.　　　　Mag-s.

(71) Loquacity
Hyos.
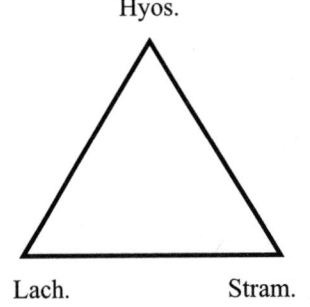
Lach.　　　　Stram.

(72) Nymphomania
Hyos.

Lach.　　　　Plat.

Complete Homoeopathic Materia Medica at a Glance

(73) Quarrelsome
- Aur.
- Ign.
- Tarent.

(74) Somnambulism
- Acon.
- Nat-m.
- Op.

(75) Suicidal disposition
- Aur.
- Nat-s.
- Arg-n.

(76) Superstitious
- Zinc.
- Lach.
- Con.

(77) Wickedness
- Cocc.
- Lach.
- Tarent.

(78) Cerebral haemorrhage
- Bell.
- Colch.
- Lach.

(79) Wen
- Graph.
- Kali-c.
- Sil.

(80) Cataract
- Calc-fl.
- Mag-c.
- Sil.

(81) Ptosis
- Caust.
- Con.
- Rhus-t.

(82) Glaucoma
- Spig.
- Phos.
- Sulph.

(83) Conjunctivitis
- Acon.
- Bell.
- Euph.

(84) Photophobia
- Arg-n.
- Graph.
- Nat-m.

Trios of remedies

(85) Pterigium
- Lach.
- Arg-n.
- Psor.

(86) Stammering
- Bell.
- Nux-v.
- Stram.

(87) Hypermetropia
- Calc.
- Sil.
- Arg-n.

(88) Myopia
- Phos.
- Puls.
- Phys.

(89) Coryza
- Bar-c.
- Carb-an.
- Phys.

(90) Mumps
- Puls.
- Brom.
- Bar-c.

(91) Toothache
- Cham.
- Plant.
- Merc.

(92) Aphthae
- Bapt.
- Merc-c.
- Sulph-ac.

(93) Tongue paralysis
- Caust.
- Gels.
- Op.

(94) Ranula
- Ambr.
- Nit-ac.
- Calc-s.

(95) Ascites
- Apis
- Ars.
- Apoc.

(96) Aversion to food
- Ars.
- Colch.
- Lil-t.

(97) Asthma

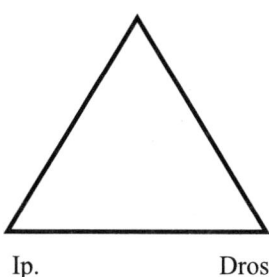

Ars. / Ip. / Dros.

(98) Asphyxia neonatorum

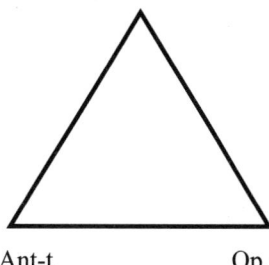

Arn. / Ant-t. / Op.

(99) Uterine fibroid

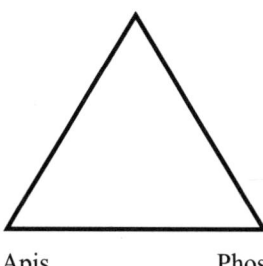

Calc-f. / Apis / Phos.

(100) Sterility

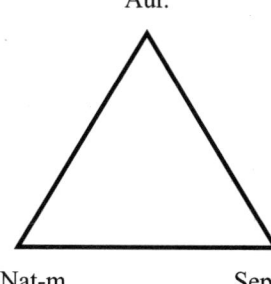

Aur. / Nat-m. / Sep.

(101) Retained placenta

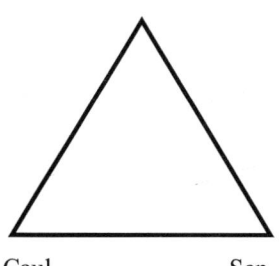

Canth. / Caul. / Sep.

(102) Masturbation

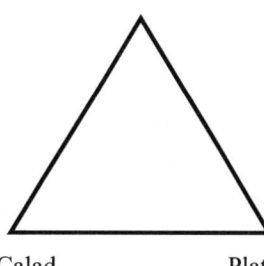

Bufo / Calad. / Plat.

(103) Lochia

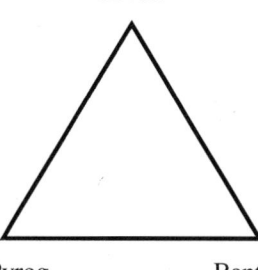

Kreos. / Pyrog. / Bapt.

(104) Varicocele

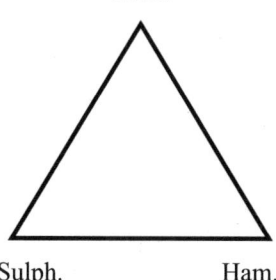

Lach. / Sulph. / Ham.

(105) Cancer of ovaries

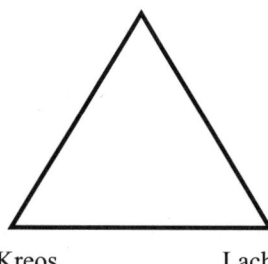

Con. / Kreos. / Lach.

(106) Sciatica

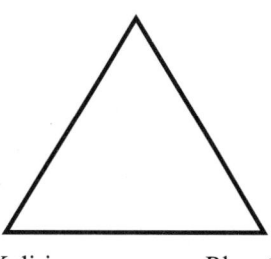

Bry. / Kali-i. / Rhus-t..

(107) Clubbing

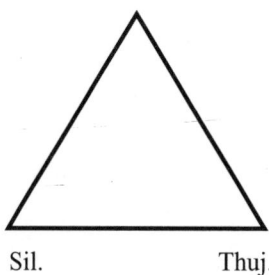

Graph. / Sil. / Thuj.

(108) Murmur

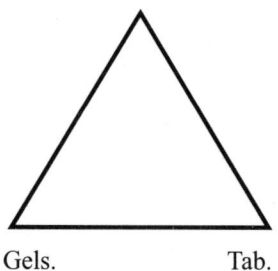

Rhus-t. / Gels. / Tab.

Trios of remedies

(109) Haemoptysis
- Sep.
- Fl-ac.
- Ph-ac.

(110) Gangrene
- Con.
- Phyt.
- Aster.

(111) Cyanosis
- Lach.
- Laur.
- Dig.

(112) Emphysema
- Hep.
- Ant-t.
- Lach.

(113) Measles
- Spong.
- Dros.
- Puls.

(114) Goose flesh
- Hell.
- Ign.
- Nux-v.

(115) Erysipelas
- Apis
- Bell.
- Euph.

(116) Carbuncle
- Sil.
- Tarent.
- Lach.

(117) Jaundice
- Chel.
- Nat-s.
- Sep.

(118) Dozing
- Berb.
- Canth.
- Tab.

(119) Cerebro-spinal fever
- Gels.
- Agar.
- Caust.

(120) Comatose
- Arg-n.
- Nux-v.
- Verat.

(121) Wound
Led.
Staph.   Op.

(122) Vomiting
Ars.
Puls.   Ip.

(123) Sycotic
Arg-n.
Thuj.   Kali-s.

(124) Syphilis
Aurum met
Kali-i.   Syph.

(125) Sun aggravation
Glon.
Nat-m.   Puls.

(126) Scurvy
Carb-v.
Merc.   Mur-ac.

(127) Parkinsonism
Merc.
Caust.   Nat-m.

(128) Plethora
Hyos.
Nat-m.   Sep.

(129) A/F nursing children
Borx.
Calc.   Puls.

(130) Moonlight aggravation
Graph.
Sil.   Thuj.

(131) Likes to be magnetised
Cupr.
Phos.   Calc.

(132) Leukaemia
Nat-ar.
Kali-p.   Thuj.

Trios of remedies

(133) Iron tonic abuse

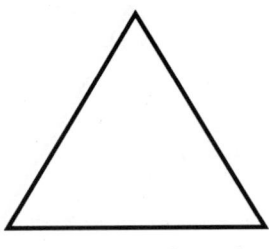

- Puls.
- Sulph.
- Zinc.

(134) Foggy weather

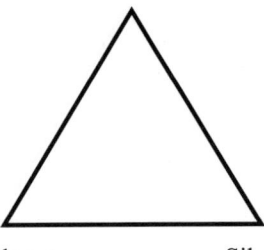

- Hyper.
- Rhus-t.
- Sil.

(135) Travel sickness

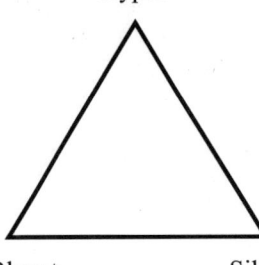

- Hyper.
- Rhus-t.
- Sil.

(136) Collapse

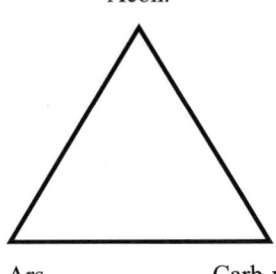

- Acon.
- Ars.
- Carb-v.

(137) Sprain

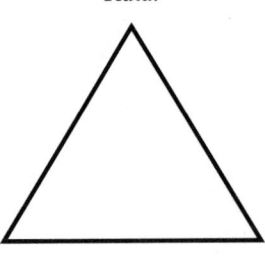

- Ruta.
- Bry.
- Arn.

(138) Stroke

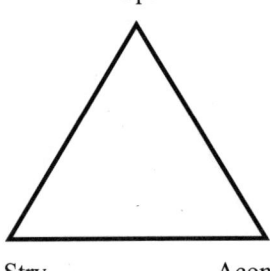

- Op.
- Stry.
- Acon.

(139) Fainting

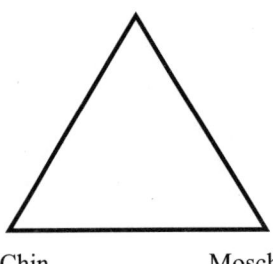

- Acet-ac.
- Chin.
- Mosch.

(140) Insect bite

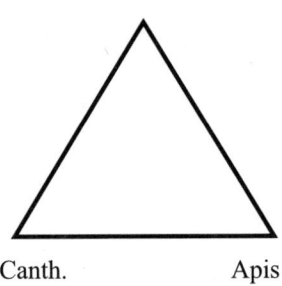

- Led.
- Canth.
- Apis

(141) Fever

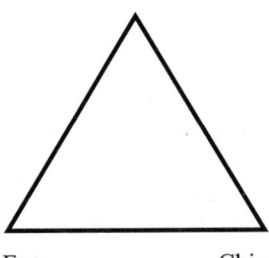

- Bell.
- Ferr.
- Chin.

(142) Dysmenorrhoea

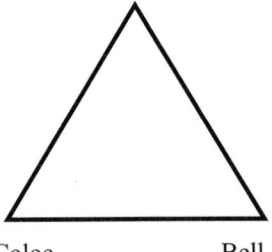

- Mag-p.
- Coloc.
- Bell.

(143) Gall stone

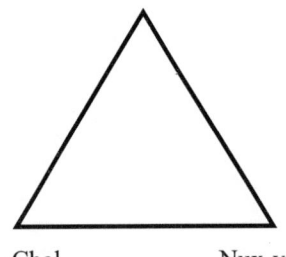

- Dios.
- Chol.
- Nux-v.

(144) Plague

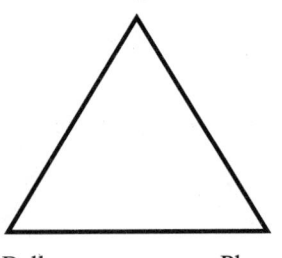

- Sulph.
- Bell.
- Phos.

(145) First aid
Arn.
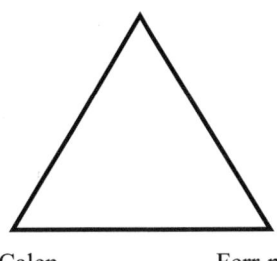
Calen. Ferr-p.

(146) Appendicitis
Bell.
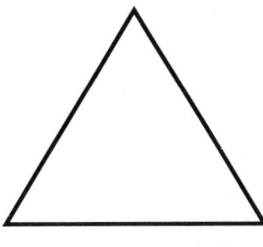
Bry. Psor.

(147) Small pox
Anti-c.
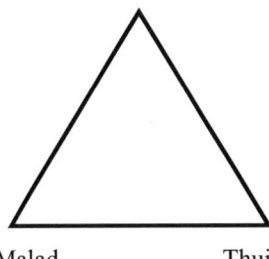
Malad. Thuj.

(148) Polio
Bar-c.
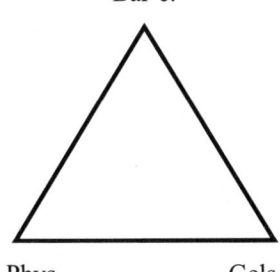
Phys. Gels.

(149) Gray hair
Psor.
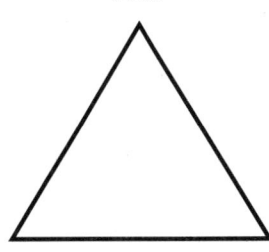
Thyr. Lyc.

(150) Leucoderma
Med.
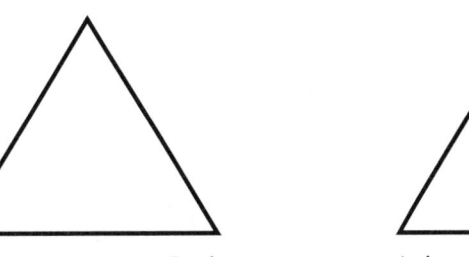
Tub. Lach.

(151) Herpes zoster
Sulph.
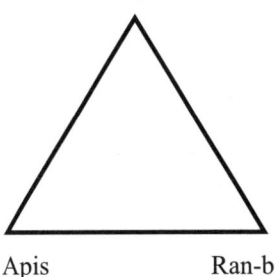
Apis Ran-b.

(152) Dandruff
Ars.
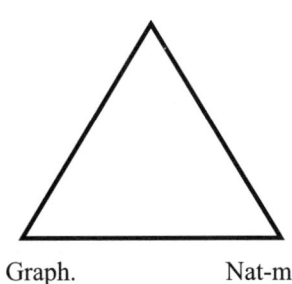
Graph. Nat-m.

(153) Urticaria
Acon.
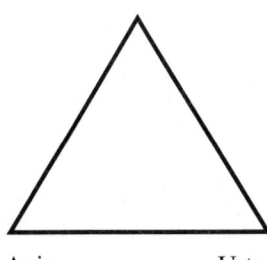
Apis Urt-u.

(154) Leprosy
Graph.

Hydrc. Sulph.

(155) Eczema
Ant-c.
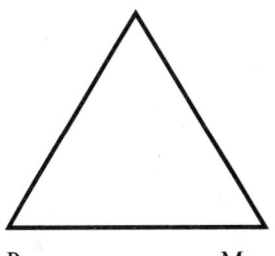
Psor. Mez.

(156) Acne rosacea
Kali-bi.
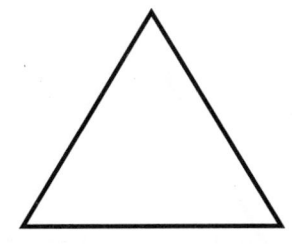
Berb-a. Ant-c.

Trios of remedies

(157) Chilblains
Abrot.
Borx.   Petr.

(158) Boil
Hep.
Sil.   Bell.

(159) Ringworm
Sulph.
Hep.   Tell.

(160) Halitosis
Bapt.
Borx.   Merc.

(161) Gingivitis
Merc.
Calc-fl.   Nat-m.

(162) Pyorrhoea
Kreos.
Sil.   Staph.

(163) Adenoids
Calc-fl.
Tub.   Bac.

(164) Strabismus
Gels.
Bell.   Hyos.

(165) Nasal polypus
Lem-m.
Kali-bi.   Thuj.

(166) Blepharitis
Psor.
Graph.   Hep.

(167) Diabetes
Uran-n.
Syzyg.   Lac-ac.

(168) Anorexia
Abrot.
Iod.   Lyc.

(169) Heart burn
Arn.
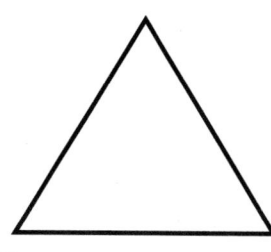
Hyper.　　　　Led.

(170) Gastroenteritis
Carb-v.
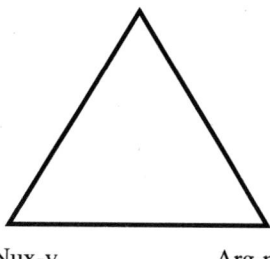
Nux-v.　　　　Arg-n.

(171) Worm infestation
Cina
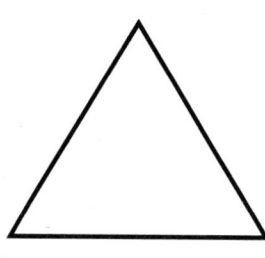
Stann.　　　　Teucr.

(172) Hiccough
Hyos.
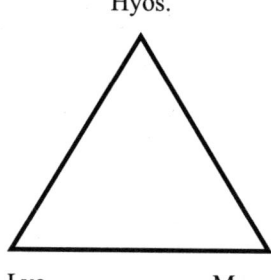
Lyc.　　　　Mag-c.

(173) Yawning
Ign.

(174) Epilepsy
Bufo

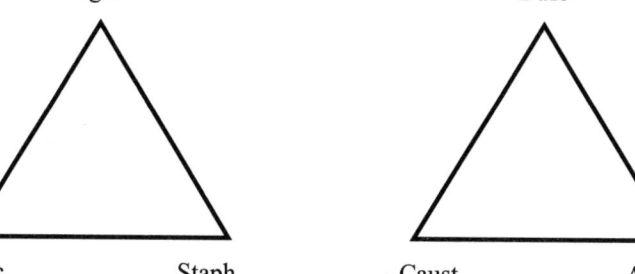

Lyc.　　　　Staph.　　　　Caust.　　　　Agar.

(175) Prostatitis
Thuj.

Ars.　　　　Sel.

(176) Urethral stricture
Canth.
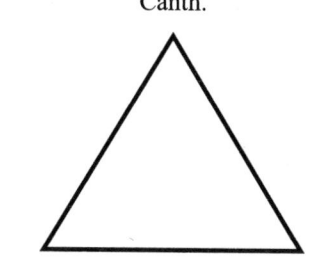
Merc.　　　　Cann-i.

(177) Ulcerative colitis
Carc.

Lil-t.　　　　Chloram.

(178) Urethral carcinoma
Carc.
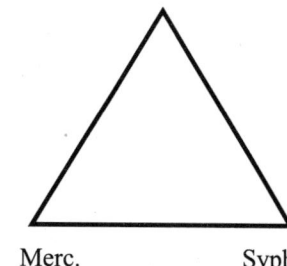
Merc.　　　　Syph.

(179) Azoospermia
Lyc.
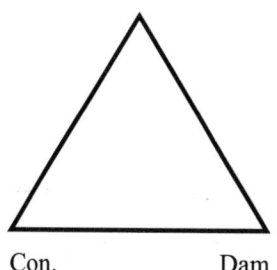
Con.　　　　Dam.

(180) Orchitis
Brom.
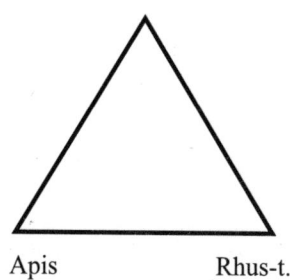
Apis　　　　Rhus-t.

Trios of remedies

(181) Impotency
- Lyc.
- Calc.
- Calad.

(182) Phimosis
- Apis.
- Bell.
- Canth.

(183) Rickets
- Sil.
- Calc-p.
- Calc.

(184) Backache
- Aesc.
- Kali-c.
- Merc.

(185) Shameless
- Bufo
- Anac.
- Op.

(186) Spiritless
- Cann-i.
- Cham.
- Bar-c.

(187) Writing mistake
- Bov.
- Fl-ac.
- Nux-v.

(188) Hydrocephalus
- Calc-p.
- Hyos.
- Sil.

(189) Thrombosis
- Lach.
- Sec.
- Both.

(190) Weils disease
- Phos.
- Coloc.
- Bell.

(191) Pyelitis
- Ter.
- Cupr-ar.
- Merc-c.

(192) Gumboil
- Bell.
- Merc.
- Phos.

Complete Homoeopathic Materia Medica at a Glance

(193) Sea sickness
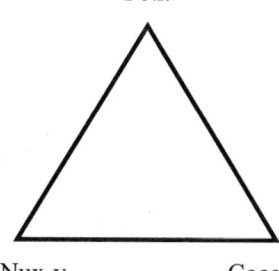
Petr.
Nux-v.   Cocc.

(194) Mushroom poisoning
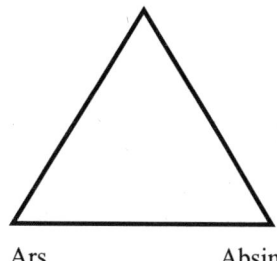
Nux-v.
Ars.   Absin.

(195) Swollen gland
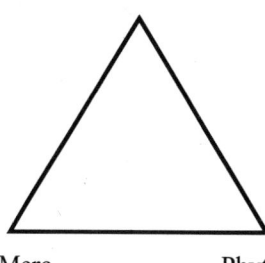
Bell.
Merc.   Phyt.

(196) Ganglion
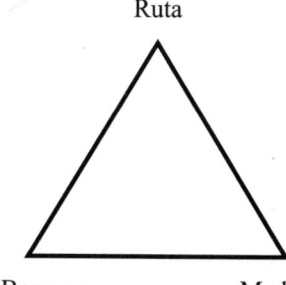
Ruta
Benz-ac.   Med.

(197) Milk leg
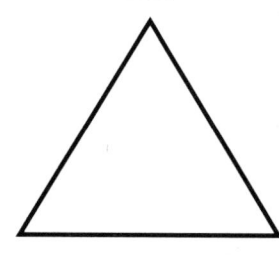
Puls.
Rhus-t.   Ham.

(198) Keloid
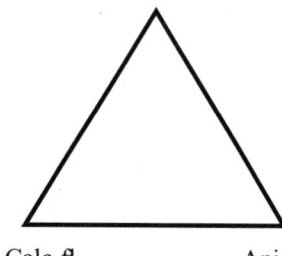
Fl-ac.
Calc-fl.   Apis

(199) Schizophrenia
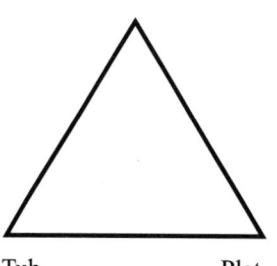
Nat-m.
Tub.   Plat.

Trios of remedies

BIBLIOGRAPHY

1. Hahnemann, S 2010, *Materia Medica Pura*, B. Jain Publishers, New Delhi.
2. Hering, C 1997, *Guiding symptoms of our Materia Medica*, 1st edn, B. Jain Publishers, New Delhi.
3. Kent, J T 1999, *Lectures on Homeopathic Materia Medica*, B. Jain Publishers, New Delhi, India.
4. Boericke, W 2004, *Pocket Manual of Homoeopathic Materia & Repertory*, 1st edn, B. Jain Publishers, New Delhi.
5. Tyler, M L 2010, *Homoeopathic Drug Pictures*, B.Jain Publishers, New Delhi.
6. Clarke, J H 2001, *Condensed Homoeopathic Materia Medica*, 1st edn, B. Jain Publishers, New Delhi.
7. Allen, H C 1999, *Allen's Keynotes*, 9th edn, B. Jain Publishers, New Delhi.
8. Farrington, E A 2004, *Clinical Materia Medica*, 1st edn, B. Jain Publishers, New Delhi.
9. Kent, J T, *Repertory of the Homeopathic Materia Medica*, B. Jain Publishers, New Delhi
10. Nash, E.B, *Leaders in Homoeopathic Therapeutics*, B. Jain Publishers, New Delhi
11. Von Douglas M. Borland, *Children's Types*, Narayana Verlag Publishers, Germany.